THE OXFORD HAN

PHILOSOPHY AND NEUROSCIENCE

THE OXFORD HANDBOOK OF

PHILOSOPHY AND NEUROSCIENCE

Edited by
JOHN BICKLE

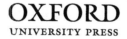

OXFORD
UNIVERSITY PRESS

OXFORD

UNIVERSITY PRESS

Oxford University Press is a department of the University of Oxford.
It furthers the University's objective of excellence in research, scholarship,
and education by publishing worldwide.

Oxford   New York
Auckland   Cape Town   Dar es Salaam   Hong Kong   Karachi
Kuala Lumpur   Madrid   Melbourne   Mexico City   Nairobi
New Delhi   Shanghai   Taipei   Toronto

With offices in
Argentina   Austria   Brazil   Chile   Czech Republic   France   Greece
Guatemala   Hungary   Italy   Japan   Poland   Portugal   Singapore
South Korea   Switzerland   Thailand   Turkey   Ukraine   Vietnam

Oxford is a registered trade mark of Oxford University Press
in the UK and certain other countries.

Published in the United States of America by
Oxford University Press
198 Madison Avenue, New York, NY 10016

© Oxford University Press 2009

First issued as an Oxford University Press paperback, 2013.

Library of Congress Cataloging-in-Publication Data
The Oxford handbook of philosophy and neuroscience /
edited by John Bickle.
p.   cm.
Includes bibliographical references.
ISBN 978-0-19-530478-7 (hardcover); 978-0-19-996550-2 (paperback)
1. Neurosciences—Philosophy.   I. Bickle, John.
II. Title: Handbook of philosophy and neuroscience.
[DNLM: 1. Neurosciences.   2. Philosophy. WL 100 O98 2009]
QP356.O94 2009
612.8—dc22   2008028323

Printed in the United States of America
on acid-free paper

Contents

Part VI: Neurophilosophy and Psychiatry

Part VII: Neurophilosophy

CONTRIBUTORS

KENNETH AIZAWA is Charles T. Beaird Professor of Philosophy at Centenary College of Louisiana. He is the author of *The Systematicity Arguments* and coauthor, with Frederick Adams, of *The Bounds of Cognition*. He works primarily in the philosophy of psychology.

COLIN ALLEN is Professor of History and Philosophy of Science and Professor of Cognitive Science at Indiana University, Bloomington, where he is also Adjunct Professor of Philosophy and a member of IU's Center for the Integrative Study of Animal Behavior. He has written extensively on philosophical issues in animal cognition and other issues at the intersection of philosophy of biology and philosophy of mind. He is engaged in several projects in Digital Philosophy, including directing the Indiana Philosophy Ontology project, and is serving as associate editor of the *Stanford Encyclopedia of Philosophy*.

WILLIAM BECHTEL is Professor in the Department of Philosophy and the interdisciplinary programs in Cognitive Science and Science Studies at the University of California, San Diego. His research focuses on the nature of mechanistic explanations and strategies for developing such explanations in the life sciences, including cell and molecular biology, neuroscience, and cognitive science. His recent books include *Connectionism and the Mind: Parallel Processing, Dynamics, and Evolution in Networks* (with Adele Abrahamsen, 2002), *Discovering Cell Mechanisms: The Creation of Modern Cell Biology* (2006), and *Mental Mechanisms: Philosophical Perspectives on Cognitive Neuroscience* (2007). He is also editor of the interdisciplinary journal *Philosophical Psychology*.

JOHN BICKLE is Professor and Head of the Department of Philosophy and Religion, Adjunct Professor in the Department of Psychology, and Fellow of the Institute for Imaging and Analytical Technologies (I²AT) at Mississippi State University. His research interests include philosophy of neuroscience, scientific reductionism, and cellular and molecular mechanisms of cognition and consciousness. He is the author of three books *(Psychoneural Reduction: The New Wave*, MIT Press, 1998; *Philosophy and Neuroscience: A Ruthlessly Reductive Account*, Springer, 2003; and *Understanding Scientific Reasoning*, 5th Ed., co-authors Ronald Giere and Robert Mauldin, Thomson, 2005), and more than 70 articles in philosophy and neuroscience journals, book chapters, and encyclopedias.

ANTHONY CHEMERO is Associate Professor in the Scientific and Philosophical Studies of Mind Program and the Psychology Department at Franklin and Marshall College. He is a cognitive scientist and philosopher of science whose work focuses on perception–action, dynamical systems modeling, and complex systems. His first book, *Radical Embodied Cognitive Science*, is soon to be published.

CHRISTOPHER CHERNIAK is a member of the Philosophy Department and its Committee for Philosophy and the Sciences at the University of Maryland. His research falls mainly in theory of knowledge and in computational neuroscience. His chapter in this volume is based on computational neuroanatomy that stemmed from his epistemology book, *Minimal Rationality*. His articles have appeared in, among other journals, *Journal of Philosophy*, *Physical Review*, and *Proceedings of the National Academy of Sciences (USA)*.

MAZVIITA CHIRIMUUTA is assistant professor in History and Philosophy of Science at the University of Pittsburgh and adjunct at the Pittsburgh Center for the Neural Basis of Cognition. Her research examines the relationship between neuroscience and the philosophy of mind and perception, with a particular interest in colour vision. As well has her work on the philosophy of perception, she has published articles on psychophysics and computational modelling of vision. She is currently writing a monograph on the philosophy of colour.

PATRICIA SMITH CHURCHLAND is Professor of Philosophy at the University of California, San Diego, and an adjunct Professor at the Salk Institute. Her research focuses on the interface between neuroscience and philosophy. She explores the impact of scientific developments on our understanding of consciousness, the self, free will, decision making, ethics, learning, and religion. She is author of the groundbreaking book *Neurophilosophy* (1986), coauthor with T. J. Sejnowski of *The Computational Brain* (1992), and coauthor with Paul Churchland of *On the Contrary* (1998). She has been president of the American Philosophical Association (Pacific Division) and the Society for Philosophy and Psychology, and she won a MacArthur Fellowship in 1991.

CARL F. CRAVER is Associate Professor in the Philosophy-Neuroscience-Psychology Program and the Department of Philosophy at Washington University in St. Louis. His research interests include the philosophy of neuroscience, scientific explanation, reduction and the unity of science, the history of electrophysiology, and the cognitive neuroscience of memory. He is the author of *Explaining the Brain: Mechanisms and the Mosaic Unity of Science* (Oxford University Press) and several articles in journals in history, philosophy, and neuroscience.

CHRIS ELIASMITH is Canada Research Chair and Director of the Centre for Theoretical Neuroscience at the University of Waterloo. He is jointly appointed to the departments of Philosophy and Systems Design Engineering. His research interests include large-scale, biologically realistic neural modeling, mental and neural representation, and neural dynamics. He is coauthor of the book *Neural Engineering*, which presents three principles for addressing such issues. He has published across a wide array of disciplines, with articles in journals including the *Journal of Philosophy, Synthese, Cognitive Science, Neural Computation, Journal of Neuroscience*, and *Cerebral Cortex*.

OWEN FLANAGAN is author most recently of *The Really Hard Problem: Meaning in a Material World* (2007). He is James B. Duke Professor of Philosophy at Duke University, where he also holds appointments as Professor of Neurobiology and Professor of Psychology and Neuroscience.

SHAUN GALLAGHER is Professor and Chair of Philosophy and Cognitive Science at the University of Central Florida and Professor of Philosophy and Cognitive Science at the University of Hertfordshire. He is the author of four books, including *How the Body Shapes the Mind* (Oxford University Press, 2005) and, with Dan Zahavi, *The Phenomenological Mind* (2008). He is currently editing the *Oxford Handbook of the Self*, and was recent coeditor of *Does Consciousness Cause Behavior?* (2006).

CARL GILLETT is Associate Professor of Philosophy at Northern Illinois University. His research interests cover foundational issues in the philosophy of psychology and neuroscience, the philosophy of science and metaphysics. He is a pioneer in the new research area of the metaphysics of science and is the author of numerous articles in journals such as *Nous*, the *Journal of Philosophy* and *Analysis*, among others. Presently, he is finishing a monograph on reduction and emergence in the sciences

IAN GOLD holds a Canada Research Chair in the departments of Philosophy and Psychiatry, and is Director of the Cognitive Science Program at McGill University in Montreal. His research, both empirical and theoretical, addresses the nature of delusions in psychiatric and neurological illness. He is also interested in questions concerning reductionism in neuroscience and psychiatry. He is the author of research articles and encyclopedia entries in the philosophy of perception and the philosophy of neuroscience, as well as a number of articles on delusion.

JAMES W. GRAU received his doctorate in psychology from the University of Pennsylvania in 1985. He was recruited to Texas A&M in 1987 and is currently Professor in both Psychology and Neuroscience. His research has been funded (since 1986) by NSF, NIDA, NIMH, NICHD, and NINDS. He was among the first to receive a University Faculty Fellow Award at Texas A&M and currently holds the Mary Tucker Currie Professorship in Liberal Arts.

RICK GRUSH is Professor of Philosophy at the University of California, San Diego. His research interests center on understanding the neural mechanisms underlying certain mental phenomena, including the representation of spatial and temporal aspects of experience, and the nature of demonstrative thought. He has published work on the philosophical, psychological, neurophysiological, and historical aspects of these issues.

VALERIE GRAY HARDCASTLE is Dean of the McMicken College of Arts and Sciences at the University of Cincinnati and Professor of Philosophy and Psychology. Her research interests include philosophical aspects of cognitive science, neurophilosophy, consciousness studies, and philosophy of science. Currently Editor-in-Chief of the *Journal of Consciousness Studies*, she has also published six books, most recently *Constructing the Self*, and numerous articles and chapters.

CHARLES HEYSER is Associate Professor at Franklin and Marshall College in the Department of Psychology. His research interests include behavioral neuroscience and psychopharmacology. He is the author of more than 50 articles and book chapters.

WILLIAM HIRSTEIN is Professor and Chair of the Philosophy Department at Elmhurst College, in Elmhurst, Illinois. He received his doctorate from the University of California, Davis, in 1994. He is the author of several books, including *On the Churchlands* (2004) and *Brain Fiction: Self-Deception and the Riddle of Confabulation* (2005). His other interests include autism, sociopathy, brain laterality, and the misidentification syndromes.

JUDY ILLES is Professor of Neurology and Canada Research Chair in Neuroethics at the University of British Columbia (UBC). She directs the National Core for Neuroethics at UBC and a research team devoted to ethical, legal, social and policy challenges specifically at the intersection of the neurosciences and biomedical ethics. These include advances in functional neuroimaging in basic and clinical research, commercialization of cognitive neuroscience, clinical findings detected incidentally in research, regenerative medicine, and stakeholder engagement on a global scale. She has written numerous books, edited volumes and more than 60 journal articles. Her book *The Oxford Handbook of Neuroethics* (J. Illes and B.J. Sahakian, Eds.) was published by Oxford University Press in 2011, and *Addiction Neuroethics* (A. Carter, W. Hall and J. Illes, Eds.) was published in 2012.

BRIAN L. KEELEY is Professor of Philosophy at Pitzer College in Claremont, California. He teaches in a variety of programs, including Philosophy, Neuroscience, Cognitive Science, and Science, Technology, and Society. In addition to publishing work on the strange epistemology of conspiracy theories and the nature of sensory modalities, he is the editor of *Paul Churchland*, a volume in the Cambridge University Press *Contemporary Philosophy in Focus* series of books.

ANTHONY LANDRETH is a postdoctoral researcher in neurobiology at UCLA. His research interests include the philosophy of science, moral psychology, mechanisms of motivation, and mechanisms of learning and memory. His experimental research is focused on genes for remote memory and the correction of learning deficits associated with neurofibromatosis.

PETER MACHAMER is Professor in the Department of History and Philosophy of Science at the University of Pittsburgh. He is also a member of the Center for the Neural Basis of Cognition, a joint Pitt-Carnegie Mellon University program. He is consciously interested in learning and memory.

PETE MANDIK is Professor of Philosophy at William Paterson University. He works on the neural basis for conscious experience. He has published over 30 articles on this and other topics, including mental representation, enactive and embodied cognition, and artificial life. He is author of *Key Terms in Philosophy of Mind* and *This is Philosophy of Mind: An Introduction*. He is coauthor of *Cognitive Science: An Introduction to the Mind and Brain* and coeditor of *Philosophy and the Neurosciences: A Reader*. He was a junior member and co-director of the McDonnell Project for Philosophy and the Neurosciences. He writes *Brain Hammer*, his intermittently neurophilosophical blog.

MARY W. MEAGHER received her Ph.D. from the University of North Carolina at Chapel Hill in 1989 in experimental and biological psychology with a minor in neurobiology. She trained postdoctorally in clinical psychology at Texas A&M University in 1993 and interned at the Audie L. Murphy Memorial VA Hospital in San Antonio, Texas, during 1993–1994. She is currently Professor of Clinical Psychology and Behavioral Neuroscience in the Department of Psychology, Faculty of Neuroscience, and the School of Rural Public Health at Texas A&M University.

JENNIFER MUNDALE is Associate Professor of Philosophy and Cognitive Sciences at the University of Central Florida. Her research interests include the philosophy of psychology, philosophy of psychiatry, and philosophy of neuroscience.

ERIC RACINE is Associate Research Professor and Director of the Neuroethics Research Unit at the Institut de recherches cliniques de Montréal (IRCM). He also holds other academic appointments at the University of Montreal and McGill University. He is the author of several papers and book chapters examining ethical issues in the application of neuroscience in research and patient care, including the monograph *Pragmatic Neuroethics* published at MIT Press (2010).

SARAH K. ROBINS is Assistant Professor of Philosophy at the University of Texas, El Paso. She has published in both philosophy and psychology, working on issues in memory and language acquisition. She was also co-organizer of the Future

Directions in Biology Series, a graduate student workshop in the philosophy of biology.

ALEX ROSENBERG is the R. Taylor Cole Professor of Philosophy at Duke University. He has held fellowships from the National Science Foundation, the American Council of Learned Societies, and the John Simon Guggenheim Foundation. In 1993, he received the Lakatos Award in the philosophy of science. In 2006–2007 he held a fellowship at the National Humanities Center. He was also the Phi Beta Kappa–Romanell Lecturer for 2006–2007. Rosenberg is the author of 11 books, including (most recently) *Darwinian Reductionism, or How to Stop Worrying and Love Molecular Biology* and *The Philosophy of Biology: A Contemporary Introduction* (coauthored with Daniel McShea). He has also written approximately 180 papers in the philosophy of biology and the philosophy of cognitive, behavioral, and social science.

ADINA L. ROSKIES is Assistant Professor of Philosophy at Dartmouth College. She has doctorates in both philosophy and in the neurosciences, and her primary research interests are in philosophy of neuroscience, philosophy of mind, and neuroethics. She has published extensively in both philosophy and neuroscience, in journals such as *Journal of Philosophy*, *Philosophy of Science*, *Trends in Cognitive Sciences*, *Science*, and *Journal of Neuroscience*. She is a project fellow in the MacArthur Project in Law and Neuroscience. When not thinking about the brain, she can often be found ascending or descending a mountain.

ALCINO J. SILVA pioneered the field of molecular and cellular cognition (MCC), and his laboratory had a key role in the development and expansion of MCC into an influential field with its own international society (MCCS; he was the society's founding president) and more than 300 laboratories worldwide. He is currently Professor of Neurobiology, Psychiatry, and Biobehavioral Sciences and Psychology at the University of California, Los Angeles. His laboratory is studying the biology of learning and memory. His research group is also unraveling mechanisms and developing treatments for learning and memory disorders. Recently, his studies in mice have led to clinical trials for the first targeted treatment for learning disabilities. He is also interested in the science of research, specifically in developing and testing hypothesis about the principles underlying scientific discovery.

C. MATTHEW STEWART is Resident Physician at the Johns Hopkins University in the Department of Otolaryngology, Head, and Neck Surgery. His primary research interest is in the interaction between the vestibular and visual systems, with an emphasis on assessing how specific types of visual motion processing centers compensate for dysfunctions in the balance apparatus of the inner ear. In addition, he has become involved in philosophy of neuroscience, with a focus on hypothesis and theory construction; data collection, interpretation, and validation; stimulus-response analysis; open- versus closed-loop biological system modeling; and brain imaging. He is the author of many articles and book chapters, in journals ranging from *Philosophy of Science* to *Journal of Neurophysiology.*

KENNETH SUFKA is Professor of Psychology and Pharmacology and Research Professor in the Research Institute of Pharmaceutical Sciences at the University of Mississippi in Oxford. His research interests include animal modeling of neuropsychiatric disorders, development of novel analgesic screening paradigms in chronic pain models, and philosophy of mind. He is the author of several book chapters and over 50 research articles in journals ranging from *Pain* to *Psychopharmacology* to *Philosophical Psychology.*

CHARLES WALLIS is Full Professor in the Department of Philosophy and the director of the Cognitive Science Group at the California State University, Long Beach. His research focuses on epistemology, philosophy of cognitive science, and the logic and philosophy of science. He has published and presented papers in computer science, philosophy, psychology, and science. His publications in Philosophy include journals such as *Philosophy of Science and Synthese.*

MORGAN WELDON is a senior psychology major with minors in classics and English in the Sally McDonnell Barksdale Honors College at the University of Mississippi. Upon graduation, she plans to enroll in a Ph.D. program in social psychology and conduct studies on achievement behavior.

WAYNE WRIGHT is Associate Professor and Department Chair in the Department of Philosophy at California State University, Long Beach. His research primarily focuses on foundational issues for the scientific studies of vision and color. His publications have appeared in journals such as *Erkenntnis, Philosophical Psychology, Philosophical Studies,* and *Review of Philosophy and Psychology.*

THE OXFORD HANDBOOK OF

PHILOSOPHY AND NEUROSCIENCE

INTRODUCTION

JOHN BICKLE

RESEARCH into the brain and nervous system has increased dramatically over the past four decades. Formed in 1970 with around 500 members, the Society for Neuroscience—the premier professional organization for scientists studying the nervous system at all levels—now boasts more than 35,000 members worldwide. Its annual week-long meeting now offers more than 14,000 scientific presentations, with attendance routinely over 30,000. In the popular media, one rarely picks up or clicks on the science section of a major newspaper or Web site and fails to find a report about a recent neuroscientific discovery. With so much professional scientific and popular interest, it is no wonder that some contemporary philosophers stay tuned. Bringing recent neuroscientific detail into philosophical discussion has opened new inquiries and breathed new life into old disputes. Increasingly one finds "philosophy of neuroscience" and "neurophilosophy" in listings ranging from course titles to individual statements of research specialization.

It seems reasonable to date the explicit start of the philosophy and neuroscience movement to 1986 and the publication of Patricia Churchland's *Neurophilosophy*. Of course, philosophers had been talking to neuroscientists professionally for many years before, but Churchland's book codified certain fundamentals. It set the stage for the issues that came to dominate the movement for the next two decades. These included focusing on theories (in psychology and the neurosciences) and intertheoretic relationships; militating against functionalism and the autonomy of psychology; and popularizing emerging trends in the cognitive neurosciences (neural networks, functional neuroimaging, and the neural correlates of consciousness come quickly to mind). At first, *neurophilosophy* served as a useful catch-all term for these inquiries. But soon philosophers began distinguishing the philosophy of neuroscience, which referred to philosophical reflections on neuroscience's emerging foundational questions. This research quickly took its place among other philosophies of specific sciences. These fields came to dominate English-speaking philosophy of science in the last decades of the twentieth century, as grand philosophical inquiries into science in general lost appeal. Neurophilosophy in turn came to stand more specifically for the application of neuroscientific discoveries to traditionally philosophical concerns.

"Philosophy *and* neuroscience" comfortably accommodates both endeavors and more. The more includes ongoing transdisciplinary interactions between philosophers and neuroscientists, where disciplinary boundaries get even blurrier. These inquiries are among the most exciting in all of recent philosophy, and it is time they received a broader professional hearing—hence this volume. There are chapters here that fall within philosophy of neuroscience typically conceived. There are also neurophilosophical chapters. But there are also chapters in which it is difficult to tell where the philosophy starts and the neuroscience ends, where the philosopher stops talking and the neuroscientist starts, and vice versa—even in single-authored chapters!

The "Philosophy and Neuroscience" title is also intended to bring in an extended audience—professional neuroscientists—and not just for the sake of greater sales. It is time for neuroscientists to see what recent interactions with philosophers have produced for some of their colleagues. The hope here is that the volume will not only inform but inspire. In the preface to *Neurophilosophy*, Churchland asserted that "it is now evident that where one discipline [neuroscience] ends and the other [philosophy] begins no longer matters, for it is in the nature of the case that the boundaries are ill-defined" (1986, ix–x). Back then, that slogan only had resonance with philosophers (and mostly only with wide-eyed Quineans). Gradually, however, it is becoming more than just a philosopher's rallying cry (or plea). The neuroscientists really are starting to pay attention.

So a principal goal of this volume is to give voice to some properly informed philosophers who are beginning to contribute directly to neuroscience. Most have not just waded into neuroscience's shallows but dived right into its practices alongside neuroscientists. This goal informed my choice of contributors, all of whom were invited. Many chapters are from younger scholars who, like me, cut their academic teeth within the first two decades of neurophilosophy. A number of these contributors have recently published or are now writing their first books. The time is thus ripe to showcase the work of these philosophers, providing them with wide latitude on the topics of their entries, in a book series as widely read and influential as the *Oxford Handbooks*.

I only imposed only two conditions on contributors. First, each chapter had to make direct appeal to data and evidence from some recognized field of current neuroscience. A wide net was cast. Appeals in these chapters range from functional neuroimaging, neuropsychological assessment, and computational neuroscience on down through behavioral and systems neuroscience, to functional microneuroanatomy, neurophysiology, and even molecular neuroscience. Second, I asked each contributor to consider collaborating with a neuroscientist. Coauthorship was not a requirement, and indeed many chapters are single-authored. (Despite their scientific interests, many philosophers still like to write alone.) But it is also clear, based on the amount and depth of neuroscientific coverage, that no author in this volume learned his or her neuroscience in a vacuum (or a vat).

Because philosophy and neuroscience is a field that continues to define itself, I did not ask contributors to focus on any particular topics, but instead to cover whatever they thought was most interesting. (Another goal of this volume is to characterize and classify the central issues in this field, according to its principal practitioners.) As I expected, most chapters congealed around a familiar set of issues, but in quite novel ways. In the remainder of this brief introduction, I'll list these basic themes and locate the various chapters within them.

Explanation, Reduction, and Methodology in Neuroscientific Practice

An interest in neuroscientific detail has long been correlated with evaluating mind–brain reductionism. A discussion of intertheoretic reduction, for example, occupied one of only four chapters in Churchland's *Neurophilosophy* that focused directly on philosophical concerns. Yet the traditional accounts of reduction from the philosophy of science have not borne up well in detailed applications to psychology-to-neuroscience cases. What relationships might replace these? All four chapters in this initial part address this question by focusing on detailed cases from actual neuroscientific practice. William Bechtel examines the long-term potentiation (LTP)–memory link, a favorite example of ruthless reductionists, and finds evidence in it instead for mechanistic reduction. He traces the mid-twentieth-century history of neuroscience, detailing the split between the ruthless reductionists who went on to become the Society for Neuroscience crowd, and the mechanistic reductionists who went on to develop behavioral, systems, and cognitive neuroscience as we know them today. Sarah Robins and Carl Craver examine recent work on circadian rhythms. They argue that causal-mechanistic explanations are central to this research, with multilevel mechanisms being the key explanatory posits. Their chapter is one of the more detailed applications in the literature of the "new mechanical" philosophy of science to a neuroscientific case study. Anthony Chemero and Charles Heyser examine the use of the object recognition memory paradigm in rodents, a laboratory favorite of reductionistic neuroscientists searching for cellular and molecular mechanisms of cognition. Their literature review of recent publications employing this procedure, and their own experiences with it as practicing behavioral neuroscientists, however, suggest that not only is mind–*brain* reductionism false, but its implicit adoption leads to methodologically flawed science. Alcino Silva and John Bickle advocate a new scientific field, the Science of Research, whose goal is to develop and test verifiable hypotheses about scientific practice. Focusing on cases from the young field of molecular and cellular cognition, they argue for two initial science of research hypotheses: the convergent four hypothesis about jointly sufficient conditions for establishing causal connections between phenomena in science, and the nature of actual reductionism within the practices of this reductionistic neuroscientific field.

Learning and Memory

The next section seeks to draw philosophical lessons from recent work in one of neuroscience's hottest fields: learning and memory. Of course, cases from this field are also prominent in chapters in the previous section; here, the philosophical lessons go beyond reduction, explanation, and methodology. Colin Allen, Jim Grau, and Mary Meagher discuss Grau, Meagher, and colleagues' behavioral neuroscientific research into the spinal cord–based learning capacities of spinally transected rats. These phenomena include numerous types of associative learning that fueled the cognitivist revolution in animal experimental psychology during the second half of the last century. This research, they argue, demonstrates that the boundaries of cognition lie beyond the brain itself. Alex Rosenberg details one current neurogenomic model of both implicit and explicit memory, and draws some negative implications for key aspects of computationalism in the philosophy of mind and psychology. However, his upshot is not entirely negative. Drawing on some comparisons between neurogenomics and developmental biology more generally, he argues that computationalism's emphasis on syntactic programs seems on its way toward neurobiological vindication. Peter Machamer employs citation indexes as a measure of particular papers' influence, and based on the highest cited papers, he argues that behaviorist methodologies remain prominent within current neuroscience. The specific nature of these methodologies creates a novel challenge for generalizing the experimental results to a full account of human learning and memory, one quite different from the standard challenges that defined the twentieth-century cognitivist revolution against behaviorism.

Sensation and Perception

Another area of great research interest and productivity in recent neuroscience has been sensation and perception. These results likewise generate interesting philosophical concerns. Valerie Hardcastle and Matthew Stewart remind us of long-standing philosophical speculation about cerebroscopes, devices that can read the brains of oneself and others, and ponder whether the modern technique of functional magnetic resonance imaging (fMRI) realize those philosophical speculations.

They turn specifically to attempts to image the brain in pain and point out serious methodological problems with this research. Nevertheless, they also point out that more than four years ago the Institute for Biodiagnostics of the National Research Council of Canada had already suggested that fMRI is potentially a cerebroscope for pain.

The other three chapters in this part speak to recently popular enactivist accounts of perception. Mazviita Chirimuuta and Ian Gold argue that some recent results from visual neuroscience cast doubt on the standard notion of a visual neuron's receptive field, at least in the sense that won David Hubel and Torsten Wiesel half of the 1981 Nobel Prize for Physiology or Medicine, and has since informed the hierarchical model of visual processing in the mammalian brain. They present numerous attempts to patch up the classical notion to account for these data, ranging from conservative extensions to radical replacements. One potential replacement they find intriguing, if not yet very well confirmed by experimental data, brings in resources from enactivist theories of perception. The response properties of visual neurons may reflect the complex interactions between perceiver and environment. Critical responses to enactivist theories dominate the final two chapters. Brian Keeley asks how enactivists propose to differentiate the senses and finds their account wanting in various empirical respects. The details of a pheromone-detecting vomeronasal sense seems in tension with what enactivist Alva Noë has said about it, as do the details of various visual prosthetic devices. Keeley argues that we're left with a crucial role for neurobiological research in differentiating the senses, a role he traces back to Aristotle and through the history of late-nineteenth-century neurobiology (specifically to Müller's law of specific nerve energies). Charles Wallis and Wayne Wright give enactivism a comprehensive cognitive-neuroscientific shakedown, and find it sorely lacking. They argue that not only have enactivists misdescribed the few neuroscientific details they've appealed to in defending their views, but that no evidence exists (yet) for the neural realization of the sensorimotor contingencies that ground enactivist theory.

NEUROCOMPUTATION AND NEUROANATOMY

Neural networks have been central to philosophy and neuroscience since Rumelhart and McClelland put together the two-volume *Parallel Distributed Processing* manifesto in 1986. Yet many philosopher fans of neural networks didn't keep up with developments in actual computational neuroscience. The authors in this section are strong exceptions to this common neglect. Rick Grush describes the computational details of his emulator framework and his previous applications of it to representations of egocentric (behavioral) space. He also applies it to behavioral time, including to some paradoxes of time consciousness made famous to philosophers by Daniel Dennett. He also discusses some novel neurophysiological work that suggests mechanisms of the emulator framework in mammalian cortex. Chris Eliasmith summarizes the basic principles of his neural engineering framework and its detailed application to modeling neural phenomena at various levels. He articulates lessons for philosophical topics ranging from levels in neuroscience and the relations between them, theory construction in the behavioral sciences, and the possibility and nature of a semantics for the resulting account of mental representations. Christopher Cherniak explains his group's work on brain wiring circuitries, providing an answer to the seeming paradox that nature hits on close-to-optimal wiring designs in brains, despite the limits of available space and the number of components. How does nature accomplish this? Cherniak draws inspiration from the anthropic principle of contemporary cosmology, generating an answer that potentially narrows the "hardware-independence" thesis of classic computational psychology.

NEUROSCIENCE OF MOTIVATION, DECISION MAKING, AND NEUROETHICS

Neuroethics is one area of philosophy and neuroscience that has made a significant mark on the broader philosophical community. It connects up with recent developments in social and affective neuroscience and has started to spawn related disciplines like neurolaw. But behavior and decision making in ethical situations are paradigmatically motivated, and so neuroethics might learn something from the latest work on the neuroscience of motivation. Anthony Landreth presents an account of this work, beginning with a well-known philosophical analysis. He grounds components of that analysis in a computational model drawn from reinforcement learning theory, and then suggests how components of the model might be realized by phasic and tonic activity in dopaminergic neurons in the midbrain and orbitofrontal cortex. Patricia Smith Churchland addresses the classic challenge to all naturalized ethical projects, the maxim of "no derivation of an ought from an is." She argues that ethical decision making isn't derivational but case-based. Thus, no logical prohibitions block strong nondeductive inferences of this sort to ought conclusions. She also grounds case-based ethical reasoning within both neuroevolutionary and neural network accounts. Adina Roskies surveys the comparisons and contrasts between neuroethics and more well-known genethics, arguing that the special causal proximity of brain to behavior generates unique ethical concerns. She documents four areas of recent neuroethical inquiry and some tantalizing ethical issues that have been raised in each. Eric Racine and Judy Illes consider possibilities for neural enhancement based on recent advances in brain–machine interfaces. They classify a variety of different kinds of ethical considerations that these developments raise. Then they argue that only an emergentist account of mind–brain relations, as opposed to strong reductionist and dualist accounts, can make sense of this full variety of ethical concerns.

Neurophilosophy and Psychiatry

Psychiatry over the past few decades has grown increasingly brain-based, and some philosophers have followed this trend. William Hirstein describes and classifies a variety of bizarre delusions of persons and their limbs, many replete with confabulatory symptoms. These patients make seemingly confident claims for which epistemologically strong counterevidence is readily available and often presented directly to them. Hirstein surveys the neural basis of these symptoms and suggests lessons for philosophical concerns such as rationality, our knowledge of the external world, and agency. Jennifer Mundale and Shaun Gallagher adjudicate a debate about delusional experience. Are delusional experiences immediate and noninferential, or rather the result of mistaken cognitive interpretations of relatively intact basic experiences? Based on both neural and phenomenological considerations, they defend the first option. Yet they also seek to integrate the concerns that have spawned top-down cognitive-processing accounts. Kenneth Sufka, Morgan Weldon, and Colin Allen provide a novel approach to the old question of whether nonhuman animals experience emotions similar to those of humans. The traditional approach is to seek structural homologies across species. Instead, they draw on research in which animals are used to model various features of neuropsychiatric disorders whose core symptoms involve changes in emotional processing. Their investigations produce a set of criteria implicit in this research to validate animal models in terms of shared etiologies, symptomatologies, pathophysiologies, and responses to treatments.

Neurophilosophy

The final section addresses some concerns squarely within neurophilosophy—the application of neuroscience results to reformulate and address traditional philosophical problems. Ken Aizawa and Carl Gillett insist that despite a recent flurry of philosophical challenges to the multiple realization argument about mental and physical kinds, neuroscientists readily accept a massive multiple realization hypothesis about human psychology. They defend this assertion with numerous detailed examples from recent neuroscience and locate it within a developed metaphysics of the realization relation. Their hypothesis need not trouble advocates of the importance of neuroscience for psychology, because this dependence is a consequence of their view (as opposed to the autonomy of psychology championed by some proponents of multiple realization). Owen Flanagan considers some grand claims about finding the neural seat of happiness based on behavioral and functional neuroimaging experiments on Buddhist priests. According to Flanagan, these claims, made by the neuroscientists doing the research and reported widely in the popular media, fail to acknowledge obvious limits on the experimental designs and results. They also fail to distinguish a variety of distinct types of happiness. Far more cautionary interpretations are warranted now, though the potential for future breakthroughs exists. Pete Mandik further develops his views on the neurobiological basis of subjectivity. Subjectivity is taken by many philosophers to be the defining feature of conscious experience, and some of these philosophers argue that no amount of neuroscientific data will ever illuminate it. Mandik provides both philosophical and neuroscientific evidence for an eliminativist conclusion (of sorts) about subjectivity. He argues that evidence exists for denying that we perceptually and introspectively experience properties that may be known in no other way.

The future of philosophy and neuroscience is difficult to foresee. Which (if any) of the topics making up this volume will generate future breakthroughs and interest? As neuroscience continues to develop, will it leave the use for philosophical reflection behind, or at least restrict it to professional philosophers? What new and revolutionary discoveries are waiting just over neuroscience's horizon, and will any of these spark new philosophical insights? None of us has a crystal ball, but we can hope that this volume, which purports to report the current state-of-the-art in this field, will keep some people pushing the traditional boundaries in the humanities, social sciences, and natural sciences.

REFERENCES

Churchland, P.S. (1986). *Neurophilosophy*. Cambridge, Mass.: MIT Press.
Rumelhart, D.E., McClelland, J.L., and the PDP Research Group. (1986). *Parallel Distributed Processing*, vols. 1 and 2. Cambridge, Mass.: MIT Press.

PART I

EXPLANATION, REDUCTION, AND METHODOLOGY IN NEUROSCIENTIFIC PRACTICE

CHAPTER 1

MOLECULES, SYSTEMS, AND BEHAVIOR: ANOTHER VIEW OF MEMORY CONSOLIDATION

WILLIAM BECHTEL

FROM its genesis in the 1960s, the focus of inquiry in neuroscience has been on the cellular and molecular processes underlying neural activity. In this pursuit, neuroscience has been enormously successful. Like any successful scientific inquiry, initial successes have raised new questions that inspire ongoing research. Although there is still much that is not known about the molecular processes in brains, a great deal of very important knowledge has been secured, especially in the past 50 years. It has also attracted the attention of a number of philosophers, some of whom have viewed it as evidence for a ruthlessly reductionistic program that will eventually explain how mental processes are performed in the brain in purely molecular terms. As neuroscience developed, however, there emerged a smaller group of researchers who focused on systems, behavioral, and cognitive neuroscience. These investigators also made impressive advances in the past 50 years, and they have been the focus of an even larger group of philosophers, who have appealed to systems-level understanding of the brain as providing the appropriate point of connection to the information processing accounts advanced in psychology.

Both the philosophers who appeal to cellular and molecular neuroscience and those who focus on systems and behavioral neuroscience are, from the point of view of mental activity, reductionists. But their construal of reduction differs, and it is those differences that are the focus of this chapter. John Bickle (1998, 2003, 2006) has been the primary champion of reduction of mental function to cellular and molecular processes, and he identifies his approach as *ruthless reduction*. The alternative approach, which appeals first to systems neuroscience to understand mental phenomena, I characterize as *mechanistic reduction*. Both approaches, as I show here, recognize that much is to be learned by understanding the cellular and molecular processes in the brain. Where they differ is in their conception of what is required to explain mental phenomena. The mechanistic approach emphasizes the need to identify all (or at least the major) operating parts of the mechanism responsible for the phenomenon of interest and to understand the way they are organized and how their operations are orchestrated to realize the phenomenon. For most mental phenomena, these working parts are characterized in terms of brain regions or cell populations, and their integration into networks constitutes the mechanisms responsible for the phenomena. The cellular and molecular processes targeted by the ruthless reductionist are typically not operating parts of these mechanisms, but are parts of their operating parts (or of the operating parts of the operating parts, etc.). They are themselves mechanisms at a lower level of organization. Understanding them is extremely important for the project of understanding the mechanisms responsible for the cognitive behavior; however, it is important to maintain a focus on the level at which they enter the explanatory account.

Focusing not on the appropriate philosophical analysis but on neuroscience itself, the contention of this chapter is that systems, behavioral, and cognitive neuroscience have a critical explanatory role to play. Whereas in the ruthless reductionist account, their role is primarily heuristic and preparatory for the ultimate account in terms of cellular and molecular processes, the mechanistic reductionist holds that there are real causal processes at different levels of organization, and appropriate research techniques are required to identify these causal processes and relate them in a mechanistic account. These tools are different from those developed in cellular and molecular neuroscience and require different skills for their application and interpretation of results. Such differences in research techniques and the explanations that researchers are seeking are often the basis for divisions into disciplines in science. In the last section of the chapter I explore the implications of this for the neurosciences, showing how the Society for Neuroscience is predominately focused on the cellular and molecular processes and investigations of systems and behavioral processes are often on the fringe of neuroscience proper and frequently pursued more directly in parts of psychology and increasingly in distinct fields that have adopted the names *behavioral neuroscience* and *cognitive neuroscience*.

1. Memory Consolidation: From Behavior to Molecular Processes

To make the discussion of contrasting accounts of reduction concrete, I focus on a particular mental phenomenon: memory consolidation. This is the phenomenon that for a period of time after an episode in which a new memory is encoded, the memory remains labile and is relatively easily disrupted. Some time later, after the processes referred to as consolidation are completed, the encoding acquires the robust and enduring characteristics of long-term memories. The phenomenon was already reported by Quintillian in the first century A.D. (Dudai and Eisenberg, 2004),[1] but it did not become the object of experimental investigation until the end of the nineteenth century with the research of Georg Elias Müller and Alfons Pilzecker in Göttingen (1900; see Lechner, Squire, and Byrne, 1999, for detailed analysis), who named the phenomenon *consolidation*. Only a decade earlier Hermann Ebbinghaus (1885) had pioneered a technique for studying the time course of memory in which he trained himself on lists of nonsense words and measured forgetting in terms of the number of retraining trials required before he could recite the list without error. Müller and Pilzecker adapted Ebbinghaus's procedures by testing subjects other than themselves and using syllable pairs, one of which would serve as the cue for the recall of the other. Their subjects reported a strong tendency for syllable pairs to come to mind between training trials despite efforts to suppress them. Müller and Pilzecker invoked the term *perseveration* for this phenomenon and appealed to it to explain a pattern of error they had observed—when subjects made incorrect responses, they often responded with other items that had been on the studied list, which may have become associated with the cue on subsequent rehearsals. This effect diminished with longer intervals between study and test. More significant, Müller and Pilzecker proposed that perseveration served the function of helping establish representations of the syllables in memory and strengthen the connections between them, for which they used the term *consolidate*:

> The experience of everyday life shows that perseverative tendencies of different parts of a train of thought can be weakened considerably by turning one's attention with energy to a different matter....One can question, however, whether the effect of such an intense mental occupation...immediately following reading of a list, simply reduces the frequency with which syllables of this list spontaneously regain conscious awareness. One might deem that the perseverative tendencies of syllables of a previously read list might also serve to consolidate the associations between these syllables...and that accordingly, weakening of the perseverative tendencies of syllables from a previously read list, due to other intense mental occupations, might have the additional effect of obstructing the associations between these syllables. (Müller and Pilzecker, 1900, p. 68; translated in Lechner et al., 1999, p. 79)

In additional experiments, they established that imposing another strenuous mental activity immediately after a learning and test episode would diminish later recall, but not if it was delayed even a few minutes.

William McDougall (1901) and William Burnham (1903) applied the results of Müller and Pilzecker to explain what Burnham referred to as *retroactive amnesia*, the loss of memory for the period immediately preceding shock or injury. Nearly 50 years later, Carl Duncan (1949) developed a procedure to create such amnesia experimentally using electroconvulsive shock in rats. As Lechner and colleagues note, explanations of retrograde inhibition in terms of inhibition of consolidation were generally superseded in psychological studies of memory by accounts in which subsequently encountered items were taken to interfere with the memory. Consolidation continued to figure in more biologically oriented studies of memory such as those inspired by Donald Hebb's (1949) account of gradual increases in cortical connections between neurons that spike together. Hebb's idea fostered an interest in a possible role for protein synthesis in establishing memories. Agranoff, Davis, and Brink (1966), for example, demonstrated that puromycin, a protein synthesis inhibitor, administered either just before or immediately after a training sequence in shock avoidance in goldfish had no effect on learning during a training session but eliminated all learning as measured 4 days later. This provided support for the hypothesis that protein synthesis is responsible for longer term memory formation but not short-term or working memory.

The path of research just described reflects a progression from behavioral-level studies relating shock or injury to amnesia to the identification of a molecular agent that brings about the same effect. Before following this path further, however, let me note what became the classic behavioral-level study of memory processes. In 1953, William Scoville performed a bilateral medial temporal lobe resection on a 27-year-old patient, H.M., who had experienced epileptic seizures since he was 10, presumably as a result of an accident in which he was knocked down by a bicycle. The surgery was successful in reducing the seizures, but it resulted in anterograde amnesia as well as temporally graded retrograde amnesia (i.e., memory loss is greater for more recently acquired memories than for ones acquired longer ago) of events for several years prior to the surgery (Scoville and Milner, 1957). The combination of graded retrospective amnesia with severe anterograde amnesia had been noted many decades earlier by Théodule-Armand Ribot (1882) and is expressed in Ribot's law ("progressive destruction advances progressively from the unstable to the stable") and provided strong support for the idea that a process of consolidation was required to stabilize memories.

What the case of H.M. made clear was that the medial temporal lobe, especially the hippocampus, plays an important role in the consolidation process. Research with this subject also helped differentiate types of long-term memory. Although H.M. has no memories for either episodes in his life (episodic memory) since the accident or for information presented to him since then (semantic memory), he has been able to acquire new skills (albeit denying that he has ever performed the skill prior to the test occurrence). This is taken to show that the hippocampus plays a critical role in encoding of episodic and semantic memories, but not in what is usually called *procedural* or *implicit* memory (Squire and Knowlton, 1995).

At approximately the same time that H.M. led researchers to focus on the hippocampus as involved in encoding of long-term explicit memories, a different line of research resulted in identifying in the hippocampus the process of long-term potentiation (LTP), the persisting enhancement in the response of a postsynaptic cell to a input from a presynaptic cell when the postsynaptic cell has readily spiked after inputs from the presynaptic cell. Although it is often reported that Tim

Bliss and Terje Lømo initiated research on LTP in 1973 in the wake of the memory deficits found in H.M. "to see whether the synapses between neurons in the hippocampus had the capability of storing information" (Squire and Kandel, 2000, p. 110), Carl Craver (2003) has shown that this line of research had a different origin. Already in the 1950s and 1960s, investigators, who were frustrated that electrical responses from cells in hippocampal preparations soon diminished, found that responsiveness could be revived by supplying a brief tetanus. From this grew numerous reports of increased potentiation of cell response in various areas of the hippocampus after tetanus. Moreover, during this period there was no direct linkage between the hippocampus and memory (if there had been, Scoville would probably not have been willing to remove it in H.M.). Rather, as Craver describes, the hippocampus was associated with a host of mental phenomena, such as olfaction, emotion, and autonomic regulation, sleep and respiration, sexual behavior, and so on. One of the major reasons to study the hippocampus was that it was thought to be involved in epileptic seizures, and the application of a tetanus to hippocampal cells was conceived as comparable to the repeated electrical stimulations thought to facilitate seizures. Another factor that Craver argues was particularly influential on Lømo's study of the hippocampus was that it was an anatomically well-characterized structure that was thought to provide a simpler model of cortical networks. It was thus well suited for studying synaptic mechanisms. In particular, it was possible to study monosynaptic pathways and focus directly on processes occurring at a given synapse.

Though the hippocampus was not viewed at the time as having a specific role in memory, researchers such as Per Andersen, Lømo's dissertation director, were very much interested in understanding learning, viewed as a process of neural plasticity. In an abstract for a conference of the Scandinavian Physiological Society, Lømo (1966, p. 128) reported an increase in "synaptic plasticity" that "may last for hours." Lømo was later joined by Bliss, and together they produced evidence for long-enduring LTP (Bliss and Lømo, 1973), although as Craver notes, there was great variability in the phenomena they elicited, and significant efforts in subsequent years were required to identify the conditions that regularly produced the phenomenon. One major aspect of this process was developing tissue-slice preparations in which the relevant circuits could be isolated, electrodes inserted to stimulate the presynaptic cell and to record from the postsynaptic cell, and investigated with a variety of probes, especially chemical ones.

Although they began their research for other reasons, in their 1973 paper, Bliss and Lømo proposed that the cellular phenomenon of LTP was a process involved in learning and memory. Demonstrating and regularizing the phenomenon of LTP was only the first step, though, in developing a cellular and molecular account of learning and memory. The next step involved discovering the mechanism through which LTP occurred. Bliss and Lømo themselves took a stand on what became one of the central issues concerning LTP—whether it involved changes in the excitability of the postsynaptic cell, changes in the presynaptic cell, or changes in synaptic efficacy. They adopted the latter view.

Discovering the mechanism required more than determining the locus of the phenomenon; it also required identifying the parts and operations of the mechanism and their organization. The major operations in a mechanism were discovered over the ensuing years and involve a number of molecules. In brief, when glutamate, the neurotransmitter that activates neurons exhibiting LTP, binds to N-methyl-D-aspartate (NMDA) receptors, they undergo a shape change that exposes pores in the membrane. These pores remain blocked unless the postsynaptic cell generates an action potential, in which case Ca^{++} ions flow into the cell and initiate a chemical cascade the alters the response properties of α-amino-3-hydroxy-5-methyl-4-isoxazole proprionic acid (AMPA) receptors, which also binds glutamate but in addition regulate the flow of Na^+ and K^+ ions that determine the voltage across the membrane of the postsynaptic cell. Beyond this immediate change in the postsynaptic cell, there is also a longer-term change that results in the synthesis of new proteins that alter such things as the dendritic spines on which receptors are lodged and the response properties of the AMPA receptors. The process of protein synthesis requires activation of DNA in the neuron's nucleus and the engagement of the protein synthesis machinery in the cytoplasm. Communication with the nucleus is realized by protein kinase A (PKA) that is released by the binding of cyclic adenosine monophosphate (cAMP) with cAMP-dependent PKA molecules. In the nucleus, PKA serves to phosphorylate cAMP response element binding protein (CREB), which in turn activates genes that initiate the synthesis of two proteins. One of these creates a positive feedback loop by destroying the regulatory subunits that bind with PKA to suppress its activity, and the other facilitates an increase in the number of active receptors in postsynaptic dendrites, thereby producing a structural change that alters the response of the postsynaptic cell to neurotransmitters.

This knowledge of the chemical processes involved in LTP has enabled researchers to begin to identify the particular genes involved in the overall activity. Thus, Silva and Bickle (chapter 4) describe gene knockout experiments in which mutant mice are created wherein activators of CREB are nonfunctional although the mice are otherwise normal. They showed that the mice that acquire normal associations between cues and shocks in the immediate setting (freezing when presented with the cue) that are evidenced in behavior when they are tested 1 hour later, fail to demonstrate learning when tested 24 hours later. Similar results were demonstrated in social recognition tasks and provide powerful evidence for the role of CREB in these behaviors.

2. RUTHLESS REDUCTIONISM

The path of research described in the previous section exhibits a progression from behavioral-level characterization of memory consolidation to identification of important components in the process at progressively lower levels. For the ruthless reductionist, this represents the form of explanatory advance that marks important progress in science. Bickle (2006) characterizes the project of the ruthless reductionist with the aphorism "intervene cellularly/molecularly and track behaviorally" which he then explicates:

- intervene *causally* at the level of cellular activity or molecular pathways within specific neurons (e.g., via genetically engineered mutant animals, as in the case study described in the previous section);
- then track the effects of these interventions under controlled experimental conditions using behavioral protocols well accepted within experimental psychology. (p. 425)

The strong claim in Bickle's account of reduction is the appeal to intervening *molecularly*. He articulates the standard for success in terms of finding cellular or molecular components on which intervention affects the phenomenon of interest: "One only claims a successful *explanation*, a successful *search for a cellular or molecular mechanism*, or a successful *reduction*, of a psychological kind when one successfully intervenes at the lower level and then measures a statistically significant behavioral difference" (2006, p. 425).

Bickle contrasts his ruthless reduction approach to that of philosophers who have appealed to cognitive neuroscience as the appropriate locus in neuroscience for explaining cognitive functions. He focuses the difference on the question of whether one can drop multiple levels down in explaining cognitive function:

> Many philosophers will still wonder how current neuroscience proposes to step across so many "levels" in a single bound. Between the behavioral and the molecular-biological levels lie (at least) the cellular, the neuroanatomical, the circuit (neuron networks), the regional, the systems (including the motor system, to generate measurable behavior), and perhaps even the information-bearing and -processing. Must not reductive "bridges" be laid between all these intermediaries before we can claim "mind-to-molecular pathway reductions"? And is not *cognitive neuroscience*—the branch of the discipline that at least some philosophers can claim familiarity with—having enough trouble "bridging" the higher levels to warrant reasonable worries about whether neuroscience will ever pull off the entire reduction? (2006, p. 412)

Appealing to examples such as the research already described on memory consolidation, Bickle embraces the project of molecular neuroscientists to "bridge the behavioral to the molecular pathway levels *directly*" (2006, p. 414).

3. MECHANISMS AND MECHANISTIC REDUCTION

A rather different account of reduction, one that takes very seriously the role of intervening levels that the ruthless reductionist disparages, results from focusing on what constitutes explanation in neuroscience. Whereas many philosophers of science, following the lead of the logical positivists in the early twentieth century, have emphasized the role of laws and viewed scientific explanation as involving logical deductions of the phenomena to be explained from these laws, neuroscientists (and more generally biologists and psychologists), tend to appeal to mechanisms for explanation. Thus, to explain a phenomenon such as memory consolidation, they seek to describe the mechanism responsible for producing it. Recently, a number of philosophers have sought to explicate the notion of mechanism to which these scientists have appealed and the way scientists develop and test models of mechanisms (Bechtel and Richardson, 1993; Glennan, 1996, 2002; Machamer, Darden, and Craver, 2000.) My preferred characterization is that a mechanism is "a structure performing a function in virtue of its components parts, component operations, and their organization" (Bechtel and Abrahamsen, 2005; Bechtel, 2006). In this account, I differentiate parts and operations (Machamer et al. similarly differentiate entities and activities) insofar as parts are structurally characterized, whereas operations are functionally identified as doing something (typically, altering themselves or something else in the process). Different research techniques are employed in decomposing a mechanism structurally into its component parts than are used to decompose it functionally into its component operations. Staining, for example, provides a means to identify neuron membranes, but electrodes are required to detect the electrical potential across the membrane. Ultimately, however, the parts of interests are those that perform the operations (which, following Craver, I refer to as *working parts*), and accordingly, it is important to link operations with parts (which I refer to as *localization*).

Insofar as a mechanistic explanation requires decomposing the mechanism into its working parts, and these are, in a well-delineated sense, at a lower level than the mechanism as a whole, mechanistic explanation is reductionistic. But critically, the working parts into which the mechanism is decomposed are just one level lower than the mechanism as a whole. These are the parts that are organized and whose operations are orchestrated so as to realize the phenomenon in question. In many cases the working parts of a mechanism will themselves be mechanisms consisting of their own working parts. Accordingly, the process of mechanistic explanation can often be iterated, and researchers may end up dealing with multiple levels of organization. It is important to attend to what phenomenon is being explained at each level of decomposition. The second round of decomposition is concerned with explaining how the working parts are constituted and organized so as to perform their operations.

From the mechanistic perspective, there is an important difference between intervening on a part, and intervening on a part of a part. To understand the mechanism responsible for the phenomenon of interest researchers must identify the various working parts of that mechanism and determine how they are organized to realize the phenomenon of interest. The working parts within these working parts are not themselves working parts of the first mechanism because they do not *directly* contribute to the phenomenon for which the first mechanism is responsible. They do so only as they are organized into the working parts of that mechanism.

This does not negate the importance of the parts of the parts and understanding what operations these subparts perform, but to make clear what the explanatory target is when focusing on these subparts—explaining how the parts of the larger mechanism perform their operations and not directly explaining the phenomenon realized in the larger mechanism. The whole organized part plays a causal role in the top-level mechanism, not each of the subparts taken individually. They contribute to the whole mechanism only insofar as they enable the part to perform its operation.

One strategy for developing and testing accounts of mechanisms shares much with Bickle's characterization of ruthless reductionistic research. Both use the strategy of intervening causally within the responsible mechanism and detecting the effects of intervention in the behavior of the whole system. The difference lies in the ruthless reductionist's emphasis on intervening *cellularly/molecularly*; the mechanistic perspective in contrast focuses on intervening on whatever components perform the operations that figure in the functioning of the mechanism. One version of this strategy for the mechanist involves removing or disabling a component to determine how the mechanism operates without it, thereby potentially gaining insight into what the component contributes to the normal functioning of the mechanism. The other involves stimulating a component to determine how the hyperoperation of the component affects the overall mechanism. (Yet another major strategy for the mechanist is to record, e.g., through single cell recording or functional neuroimaging, changes internal to the mechanism as it functions under various conditions. For discussion, see Bechtel, in press.)

Having identified differences between ruthless reduction and mechanistic reduction, I turn to the import that difference has to the practice of neuroscience. There is no doubt that the research Bickle cites as exemplary of ruthless reduction has provided important information about processes at work at some level of decomposition within the mechanism of memory consolidation. Moreover, information secured at such lower levels often places serious constraints on the accounts at higher levels. For example, if we learn that the subcomponents of a mechanism do not permit the component of the mechanism to perform the operation assigned to it by a higher-level decomposition, then the higher-level decomposition must be revised. But there is a major risk inherent in the strategy of ruthless reduction. Insofar as it focuses exclusively on a subcomponent (or a subsubcomponent) and relates it directly to behavior, it risks ignoring the other components of the mechanism and the organization that enables the components to work together to produce the phenomenon of interest. What is gained by paying attention to each level of organization identified in the course of decomposition is an understanding of the variety of roles that must be performed in producing the overall phenomenon.

Craver (2007) insists that a necessary condition on a good mechanistic explanation is that it accounts for the productive continuity between what he calls the start-up and termination conditions on the operation of a mechanism. Accounts that leave gaps in the characterization of the processes he counts only as sketches of mechanisms. Although I would argue that complete productive continuity is more than is needed in practice for good explanations (as well as resist the imposition of linearity that results from specifying start-up and termination conditions), the idea of productive continuity helps focus our attention on the need not just to identify a single component but to identify many of the parts and operations so that it is possible to conceptualize how the operations couple together to realize the phenomenon. Often such understanding is realized in mechanistic research by simulating the operation of the whole mechanism, either mentally or using physical or computational models. Only by including the major operations in the account can a researcher simulate the overall production of the phenomenon.

The shortcoming of the ruthless reductionist's approach is that it focuses on only one or a few subcomponents within the mechanism and fails to consider how those subcomponents are related to others in the realization of the phenomenon in question. The process of new protein synthesis activated by CREB is, it appears, an important operation in the process of memory consolidation (it may even be the crux point). But it is not the whole process. Other components, both within the hippocampus and elsewhere in the brain, also play a role in memory consolidation. One serious shortcoming of ignoring these other factors is the propensity to ascribe too much to the factors that are considered. (The legacy of focusing on genes as responsible for traits, ignoring the variety of factors involved in the regulation and expression of genes, illustrates the risks involved. Researchers often claim success in explaining biological traits as soon as they identify a responsible gene, failing to recognize that often many factors, including other genes as well as environmental processes, are required to generate the trait.)

4. From Molecular Processes Back to Systems

While great progress was being made in articulating the mechanisms of LTP, other advances were also being made with respect to the mechanisms involved in memory consolidation. Some of this research has been local to the hippocampus itself, although focusing not on the molecular processes within cells but on the neuroarchitecture of the hippocampus, which is distinctive and idiosyncratic. The hippocampal formation is organized as a loop involving a number of different regions. As shown in the schematic representation in figure 1.1, information from neocortical association areas in temporal, parietal, and frontal cortex enters the hippocampal formation via the parahippocampal gyrus and the perirhinal cortex. From these areas it is projected to the entorhinal cortex (EC), from which it is processed through a loop, ending up again in the EC, from which it is sent back out to the neocortical areas. The critical processing loop from the EC proceeds either directly on a pathway to the CA3 fields or via a route through the dentate gyrus (DG), which is unusual for

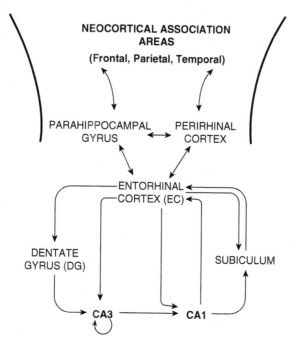

Figure 1.1. Schematic diagram of the hippocampal system. Information from widespread areas of neocortex converge on the parahippocampal region (parahippocampal gyrus, per-irhinal cortex, and entorhinal cortex, EC) to be funneled into the processing loops of the hippocampal formation. The tightest loop runs from EC into the core areas of the hip-pocampus (CA1 and CA3) and back; the loop through the dentate gyrus (DG) and the recurrent connections in CA3 are also important; the subiculum, which is not part of the hippocampus proper, provides an alternative return to EC. Not shown are a number of subcortical inputs and details of pathways and their synapses.

having quite a small number of neurons active in response to a given input. CA3's pyramidal cells are highly interconnected via recurrent connections (indicated by a small looping arrow); these cells also send activations forward to the pyramidal cells in CA1 via the small CA2 area (not shown). From CA1, activations are passed back to the EC directly or via an indirect pathway through the subiculum.

The distinctive architecture of the hippocampus has intrigued theorists as to its functional significance. The overall loop structure suggests that this may figure in the hippocampus's contribution to the ability, lost in H.M., to encode information over a several-year period until a more permanent engram is laid down outside the hippocampus and as playing a role in laying down that engram. As Edmund Rolls (1995; Rolls and Treves, 1998) conceptualized the activity of the hippocampus, it needed to be able to differentiate new events the organism encounters so it can develop new memories for them but not for mere variations on previous events. With these demands in mind, he developed a model with the same structure as the actual hippocampus of a rat but with fewer units for each structure. Thus, he employed 1,000 units each in his model of DG and CA3, whereas in the rat there are approximately 10^6 granule cells in the DG and 300,000 in CA3. To capture the sparseness of the coding found in the DG–CA3 pathway, he allowed each artificial DG units to activate only four CA3 units. The interconnections between CA3 cells were modeled by recurrent connections through which CA3 cells provided input to themselves and other cells. In the pathway from CA3 to CA1, each CA3 unit sent a projection to 60 of the 1,000 CA1 units, and in the pathway from CA1 to EC, each CA1 unit sent a projection to 200 of the 600 EC units.

Rolls employed his network to store 100 random patterns that were presented just once each as inputs to EC; storage was accomplished by adjusting weights between various units of the network by means of Hebbian learning. The architectural differences just noted affected how each part of the network functioned. Thus, after training, competitive learning in the pathways from EC to DG and from EC and CA3 to CA1 determined the activation patterns in DG and CA1; the pathways from EC to CA3 and from CA1 to EC functioned as pattern associators, whereas the very sparse connections from DG to CA3 served to differentiate patterns. After getting initial activation directly from EC and from EC via DG, CA3 ran 15 cycles on its recurrent connections to function as an autoassociative network. Activation then passed from CA3 to CA1 and from there back to EC, completing the processing loop.

Rolls measured the success of the model by its ability, when just part of each pattern was presented as input to the EC units, to regenerate the whole pattern on the same units (now as an output pattern). When the partial pattern was similar enough to the complete pattern—a correlation of just 0.40 was sufficient—the network could regenerate the complete pattern perfectly. In addition to obtaining this impressive overall result, Rolls was able to pin down some crucial design decisions. He already expected from the mathematical analysis and from the example of the rat hippocampus that varying the number of connections and sparseness would provide both separation and completion capacities. He also expected the recurrent connections in CA3 to be important and demonstrated that turning them off eliminated CA3's ability to complete patterns (the pathways beyond it could partially but not completely compensate).

The functions that Rolls tries to account for at the level of the hippocampus itself are very different than those the ruthless reductionist localizes within individual neurons but are ones still critical to memory consolidation. The Hebbian learning that Rolls assumes in his model requires a mechanism such as the enhanced protein synthesis initiated by CREB, but the overall model captures features of memory consolidation not explained at the molecular level involving, as it does, communication between populations of neurons.[2]

Memory consolidation is not limited to activity within the hippocampus. McGaugh (2000), for example, examined the contribution of the amygdala to memory consolidation, concluding that it plays an important role in allowing emotional arousal to modulate memory strength. This is shown, for example, by the fact that β-adrenergic receptor agonists infused into the basolateral nucleus of the amygdala enhance memory, whereas antagonists block the effects of systematically applied dexamethasone, which usually enhances memory. Inactivating the amygdala with lidocane infusions before retention tests does not impair enhanced memory, so

McGaugh concludes that it is not the locus of the memory: "It is clear from these findings that memory consolidation involves interactions among neural systems, as well as cellular changes within specific systems, and that amygdala is critical for modulating consolidation in other brain regions" (2000, p. 249).

The fact that patients such as H.M. retain memories acquired several years before damage to their hippocampus indicates that the ultimate result of consolidation involves encoding of information in parts of the brain other than the hippocampus. Lashley's (1950) failure to identify areas in neocortex that would eradicate particular memories when lesioned led many to turn away from seeking memory encodings (engrams) in neocortex. The reemergence of neural network modeling in psychology in the 1980s suggested an explanation for the failure to find engrams—in neural network models, information is often encoded in a very distributed fashion in which there is no single locus for the engram (accordingly, Rumelhart and McClelland, 1986, referred to such modeling as parallel distributed processing). These neural network models also employed a means of training such distributed representations through procedures involving gradual error reduction (Rumelhart, Hinton, and Williams, 1986a, 1986b). One consequence of such distributed representations is that they are subject to catastrophic interference as the learning of new information alters the connections that maintained the previously learned information (McCloskey and Cohen, 1989; Ratcliff, 1990). This was initially construed as a shortcoming of these models, but McClelland, McNaughton, and O'Reilly (1995) turned it to an advantage by suggesting that it explains why consolidation must be a drawn-out process. They proposed that by having the hippocampus serve to reinstate patterns repeatedly over time, it was possible for the connections in neocortex to develop so as to acquire new information without losing information acquired previously. They developed a computational model to simulate the gradual training of the neocortex via the hippocampus and showed that when this training procedure was interrupted, their simulated cortical networks exhibited retrograde amnesia much like that found in human and animal research.

The proposed interaction of hippocampus and cortical areas in consolidating memories is not just a theoretical model. Research on sleeping rats by Jones Leonard, McNaughton, and Barnes (1987) showed that induction of hippocampal LTP is blocked during non-REM sleep and Bramham and Srebo (1989) demonstrated that it did not impair maintenance of previously induced LTP. This led Wilson and McNaughton (1994) to explore activity in the hippocampus during non-REM sleep. Using multielectrode recording from CA1 cells, they established that cells that fired synchronously during a maze-learning training episode also produced correlated firing during non-REM sleep.[3] Hoffman and McNaughton (2002) have gone on to show that during periods of quiet wakefulness following a sequential reaching task cells in the posterior parietal, motor, and somatosensory cortices (but not in the prefrontal cortex) that produced correlated or sequential firing during the task continued to exhibit correlated or sequential firing. The authors are cautious in claiming that this reactivation of coordinated firing patterns is part of memory consolidation and how it relates to the synchronized activity in the hippocampus, but clearly anticipate a connection:

At present, the mechanisms leading to the observed widespread memory trace reactivation remain unknown, and the necessity of coherent memory trace reactivation for memory consolidation remains to be demonstrated. Nevertheless, the observation that memory trace reactivation is temporally ordered and concurrent across large areas of the primate neocortex is a critical prerequisite for this process to function as a mechanism for memory consolidation. (2007, p. 2073)

Further evidence of a need to focus on the whole mechanism involved in consolidation, not just local operations, is found in the recently renewed interest in what is called *reconsolidation*. Memory consolidation has often been construed as a one-time event, occurring in a period of approximately 24 hours (often much shorter) immediately after learning. Already in 1968, two studies suggested that after a memory is recollected, it must be reconsolidated or it will be lost. Schneider and Sherman (1968) were addressing the question of whether electroconvulsive shock produced amnesia when applied immediately after a single trial (in which rats were given a foot shock for stepping off a platform) was due to the connection with the learning or the arousal created by the foot shock. They investigated this by applying the electroshock after a second foot shock applied 30 seconds later (while the rats remained on the shock grids). This still produced amnesia, but the rats seemed to recover what they learned previously when tested a day later. The researchers then tried a 6-hour interval between the first and second foot shocks (the second accompanied by electroconvulsive shock) and found that it produced amnesia for the learning that was associated with the first foot shock, which was contingent on stepping off the platform. Moreover, the rats did not exhibit recovery when tested later. Misanin, Miller, and Lewis (1968) also demonstrated loss of memory when they applied electroconvulsive shock to rats immediately after presentation of a conditioned stimulus for which the rats had learned a response 24 hours earlier.

These results initiated a period of investigation into amnesia produced after exposure to cues that might re-elicit the initial learning using not just electroconvulsive shock but also hypothermia and inhibition of protein synthesis to block memory consolidation. These studies seemed to indicate that the amnesia was dependent on reactivating the memory traces and that reactivated memories were once again vulnerable and required consolidation (Lewis, Bregman, and Mahan, 1972). Other studies indicated that when memories were re-elicited, it was also possible to enhance the memory by applying electrical stimulation to the mesencephalic reticular formation (MRF), which also served to enhance memory when applied during learning episodes (DeVietti, Conger, and Kirkpatrick, 1977).

This line of research was largely eclipsed as the prevailing interest in the 1980s and 1990s focused on the molecular mechanisms of LTP emphasized by ruthless reductionists but were rekindled in part as a result of a review article by Susan Sara (2000). She encountered the phenomenon of memory reconsolidation herself in the course of a study on the effects of a NMDA receptor antagonist on rats performing a well-learned maze task. The antagonist had no effect on the immediate trials, but when rats were tested again 24 hours later, they exhibited amnesia. In the period since Sara's review, the phenomenon has again become the subject of multiple investigations. Many of the new studies applied protein synthesis inhibitors, such as anisomycin, to a range of species ranging from invertebrates to humans. When administered along with a retrieval task, usually a day after training involving punishment or aversive stimuli, the protein inhibitor caused behavior no longer to be guided by the memory of the recalled item. Nader, Schafe, and LeDoux (2000), for example, trained rats to associate a tone with a foot shock and respond by immediate freezing. Microinfusion of anisomycin into the lateral and basal nuclei of the amygdala could block either consolidation if applied immediately after training, or reconsolidation if applied immediately after retrieval, whether the retrieval was 1 or 14 days after conditioning. The investigators proposed the reconsolidation was required even for memories that had previously been well consolidated.

Some have viewed reconsolidation as employing the same mechanism as is responsible for consolidation to begin with, but substantial differences have also been observed in the two processes. For example, neither the central amygdala nucleus, required for acquisition of conditioned taste aversion, nor the basolateral amygdala, required for extinction, is required for reconsolidation (Bahar, Dorfman, and Dudai, 2004). Likewise, the hippocampus is required for consolidation, but not reconsolidation of passive avoidance in the rat (Taubenfeld, Milekic, Monti, and Alberini, 2001). At present findings such as these are suggestive of differences between the mechanisms involved in consolidation and reconsolidation, but a full understanding of the parts and operations in either mechanism are still to be worked out.[4]

Findings such as those discussed in this section, many of which resulted from studies taking off from the research on protein synthesis in memory consolidation, point to the limitations of the ruthless reductionist approach of focusing solely on the molecular constituents and processes of protein synthesis in postsynaptic cells, even when tested in behaving systems. What these findings point to is that there are many additional working parts in the mechanisms responsible for memory consolidation. The molecular cascade that Bickle emphasizes may play a role—indeed, an important role—in the overall process. But that role is situated within one of the constituent working parts of a much larger mechanism. Mechanistic reduction emphasizes the need to focus on identifying all the major components of the mechanism, determining their operations, and understanding how they are organized in the realization of memory consolidation. Ruthless reduction only identifies lower level constituents of one component part of the mechanism.

5. Disciplinary Settings

Whereas the term *neuroscience* is often applied retrospectively to research on the brain that began to be pursued in earnest in the nineteenth century, its origins are in the 1960s with a research program that focused on the physics and chemistry of the brain, especially its biophysics. The primary endeavor for which the term *neuroscience* was employed indeed reflects the project of ruthless reductionism, a narrowing of focus to the molecular processes within individual neurons. In this section, I begin by describing the disciplinary setting in which neuroscience itself developed, and then show how this project represented a radically narrowing of the research pursuits of inquiries into the structure and function of the brain that had preceded it. These broader aspirations are maintained in fields that append adjectives such as *systems, behavioral,* and *cognitive* to the core term *neuroscience.* One must look to the fields named using these adjectives for the realization of the older investigations in neuroanatomy and neurophysiology and the promise of understanding how cognition is realized in the brain.

The primary inspiration for the development of the interdisciplinary field of neuroscience came from advances in biochemistry, biophysics, and molecular biology in the middle decades of the twentieth century. The principal instigator for bringing these disciplines together was Francis Schmitt, who created what he called the Neurosciences Research Program (NRP) in 1962. Schmitt's own background was in biophysics, where he had contributed to deciphering the action potential in the giant squid axon as well as applying techniques such as electron microscopy to identifying structural components of neurons and muscle fibers. After moving to MIT in 1941 to head the Department of Biology and Biological Engineering, Schmitt established a large laboratory devoted to biophysical studies of collagen, muscle fibers, and neurons. Earlier in his career he had worked with Joseph Erlanger and Herbert Gasser at Washington University in St. Louis; they had pioneered techniques for recording from individual neurons and discovered that different neurons conducted impulses at different speeds (see Erlanger and Gasser, 1937, for an overview of their investigations). At MIT, Schmitt attempted to understand the processes within neurons that gave rise to action potentials. While working at the Marine Biological Station in Viña del Mar, Chile, he encountered the large squid, *Dosidicus gigas,* with a giant axon ranging up to 4 mm diameter. He studied both the constitution of its axoplasm and the mechanism of the action potential, studies that he continued at MIT using the smaller squid, *Loligo pealii,* found off New England (Schmitt, 1959).

In 1955, Schmitt became highly involved with creating scientific institutions to support biophysics, and with financial support from the Biophysical and Biophysical Chemistry Study Section of the National Institutes of Health (NIH), he organized a 4-week-long summer program in 1958 called the Intensive Study Program in Biophysics at the University of Colorado, Boulder. This brought together 200 biologists, chemists, physicists, psychologists, and engineers and culminated in the publication of *Biophysical Science: A Study Program* (Oncley, Schmitt, Williams, Rosenberg, and Bolt, 1959) that helped delineate the scope and chart the research agenda for the new enterprise. Schmitt's own interest in nerve transmission led him to focus on the question of how chemical processes could operate sufficiently rapidly to support information retrieval. He was inspired by a meeting with Manfred Eigen to begin considering ways in which elementary-charge carriers might be transported within neurofilaments and organized a symposium on the topic at MIT in the spring of 1960 and another the following spring on macromolecules and memory function (Schmitt, 1962). From the experience with these two symposia, Schmitt began to formulate plans for an interdisciplinary institute focused on what he called *mental biophysics* or *biophysics of the mind*, which would

> Investigate the "wet and dry" biophysics of central nervous system function, i.e., to study the physical basis of long-term memory, learning, and other components of conscious, cognitive behavior, by effective utilization of the biophysical and biochemical sciences, from the physical chemistry of neuronal and glial constituents (wet biophysics) through bioelectric studies (moist biophysics) to studies of fast transfer of elementary charged particles, organized microfields, stochastic models, and applications of computer science (dry biophysics).[5]

Schmitt identified nine basic disciplines comprising mental biophysics: solid-state physics, quantum chemistry, chemical physics, biochemistry, ultrastructure (electron microscopy and x-ray diffraction), molecular electronics, computer science, biomathematics, and literature research. Conspicuously absent from this list are neuroanatomy (above the ultrastructure level) and neurophysiology. Despite the inclusion of the word *mental* and the major developments that had transpired in psychology and linguistics in the previous decade (the advent of information processing models in psychology and transformational grammars in linguistics), these disciplines were also absent.

By September 1961, Schmitt was referring to his project as the Mens Project, reflecting a growing interest in the traditional phenomena associated with mind. The range of disciplines expanded, but mostly in the direction of including disciplines such as neurophysiology, neuroanatomy, and neurology (psychology, though, made it into the list of 25 fields that might be included in the project). When Schmitt convened an organizational meeting of 11 researchers in early 1962, most were from physics, biophysics, biochemistry, and molecular biology, plus one neurologist. The closest to psychology or neurophysiology was Heinrich Klüver, who was identified as representing biological psychology. Klüver is perhaps best known for his work with Paul Bucy that focused attention of the range of deficits following removal of the temporal lobe in monkeys. Klüver was led to this research as a result of his interest in determining whether removing the temporal lobe would block the hallucinations induced by mescaline. Although the lesion had no affect on the organism's response to mescaline, it did impair the monkey's ability to identify objects by sight alone. Klüver and Bucy (1938) characterized this condition as *psychic blindness* or *visual agnosia*. Although these results played an important role in understanding temporal lobe function and provided the foundation for later research by Karl Pribram and Mortimer Mishkin, they hardly represented the mainstream of work in psychology, which by the 1960s was increasingly influenced by researchers emphasizing information processing accounts (Miller, Galanter, and Pribram, 1960).

On the basis of this meeting, Schmitt made a proposal to the NIH and another to NASA to fund the Neurosciences Research Program (NRP). It is pretty clear that while the phenomena the NRP sought to consider were ones traditionally associated with psychology, the approaches it promoted were to be drawn from biophysics and other closely allied sciences. Figure 1.2, from the 1963 program report to the NIH, conveys the way the project was conceived. The first 27 associates are situated within a triangle in which physics, chemistry, and biology form the points and the edges are labeled physical chemistry, biophysics, and biochemistry.

One of the main functions of the NRP was to host meetings that would foster exchange. Some of these were limited to associates; Schmitt described the first meeting of the associates: it "lasted for five days, and we were tutoring each other day and night." In addition, the NRP sponsored several 3-day work sessions a year, in which senior scientists in the chosen fields would educate others about his or her field. The chairperson for each of these sessions was charged with writing a synthetic overview of the field and the discussions at the meeting, which was then published in *Neurosciences Research Program Bulletin* (MIT Press also published an annual anthology of material from the bulletin under the title *Neurosciences Research Symposium Summaries*). The work sessions for the first year give a flavor of the endeavors of the NRP:

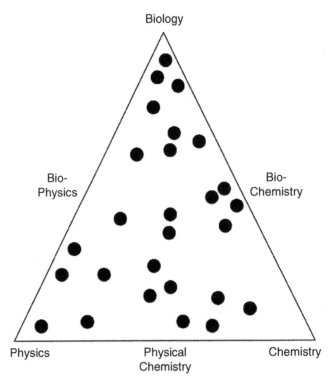

Figure 1.2. The distribution of base fields of associates of the Neurosciences Research Program, redrawn from a 1963 progress report to the National Institutes of Health. Disciplines represented: chemistry, 1; biochemistry, 2; neurochemistry, 1; physical chemistry, 5; chemical physics, 1; mathematics, 1; physics, 2; biophysics, 3; molecular biology, 2; electrophysiology, 1; neurobiology, 1; neuroanatomy, 2; psychology, 2; psychiatry, 1; clinical medicine, 1.

Report Title	Chair
Cell Membranes	A.L. Lehninger
Information Storage and Processing in Biomolecular Systems	M. Eigen and L.C.M. DeMaeyer
From Brain Structure and Functions to Memory	W.J.H. Nauta
Glial Cells	R. Galambos

The NRP became a spur behind the creation of the Society for Neuroscience in 1970, which has grown in 35 years from 500 members to more than 37,500. Although the society includes researchers who work at the systems and behavioral levels, the predominant emphasis remains on cellular and molecular neuroscience; as Bickle has pointed out, it reflects the approach of the ruthless reductionist. Nonetheless, the term *neuroscience* (or sometimes *neurobiology*) is often taken to have a much broader scope, one that is more reflective of traditions of investigating the brain that were largely set aside by the founders of the Society of Neuroscience. After briefly noting highlights of this history, I focus on the recent continuation of this history in systems, behavior, and cognitive neuroscience.

The study of the structure and function of the brain has a long history, but the nineteenth century proved particularly important in development of neuroanatomy and neurophysiology at both the neuronal and whole brain levels as well as the development of neuropathology. The last part of the century witnessed a controversy over whether neurons were discrete cells separated by a gap between them or whether there was continuity between cells either in their axons or dendrites. This was resolved with the introduction of a silver nitrate stain by Golgi and its use by Cajal to demonstrate the individuality of neurons, a conclusion notorious rejected by Golgi (Mundale, 2001). The electrical properties of neurons were demonstrated earlier in the century by Emil du Bois-Reymond (1848–84) and his student, Julius Bernstein, who at the beginning of the twentieth century advanced a proposal to explain electrical conduction in nerves as a result of the influx of potassium ions (Bernstein, 1912). One direction this research led was into the study of the mechanisms underlying the action potentials and LTP. Another was in the direction of recording from individual neurons and attempting to relate action potentials in neurons to external stimuli. This technique complemented approaches in the nineteenth century to studying brain regions either by analyzing deficits when areas were damaged or lesioned or by microstimulating neurons to determine the effects of their activity (Ferrier, 1876). By the early twentieth century, these techniques had revealed that many brain areas were laid out in topographical maps. Damage to selected regions revealed that different parts of the visual field are mapped onto different parts of the striate cortex (Holmes, 1918), whereas stimulation of areas near the central sulcus revealed the organization of somatosensory and motor cortex (Penfield and Boldrey, 1937).

As important as lesion and stimulation studies were, the ability to record from individual neurons while manipulating sensory inputs provided the greatest advances in understanding the large-scale organization of the brain. Following Stephen Kuffler's (1952) discovery of retinal cells that responded to the contrast between the stimulation in the center of their receptive fields and that in the surround, Hubel and Wiesel (1962, 1968) initiated their studies of cells in the lateral geniculate nucleus and Brodmann area 17 (subsequently known as V1), in the latter of which they found cells that responded to bars of light. They also identified other areas with topographical maps of the visual field (which came to be known as V2 and V3) and other researchers, especially Semir Zeki (1973, 1974), identified still other maps in areas that responded selectively to the color or motion of the stimulus. By the 1990s, 32 brain areas had been identified as principally involved in visual processing, taking up over a third of the cortex in the macaque monkey (Felleman and van Essen, 1991; for a historical review of this research, see Bechtel, 2008). Similar mapping of brain regions has been done for other sensory and motor areas and even in frontal cortex, where there is less ability to correlate activity with sensory stimuli or motor responses (Carmichael and Price, 1996). These efforts at identifying brain regions responsive to differing types of information, and increasingly on identifying the connectivity patterns linking them, constitutes the project of systems neuroscience. Although pursued by investigators who align themselves with neuroscience, systems neuroscience is recognized even by them as at the periphery of neuroscience. Thus, van Essen and Gallant, in introducing their work on the organization and functioning of different visual areas in *Neuron*, a leading neuroscience journal, comment:

> These explorations involve mainly physiological and behavioral techniques that are quite different from the cellular and molecular techniques most familiar to this journal's readership. Nonetheless, we hope that a review of recent progress in understanding visual cortex will interest a broad spectrum of neuroscientists who share the ultimate objective of attaining a continuum of explanations of brain function, from the most molecular to the most cognitive levels. (van Essen and Gallant, 1994, p. 1)

Historically, the term *behavioral neuroscience* reflects a development out of a tradition in psychology referred to as *physiological psychology*. Because physiological processes involved in behavior could often be studied most directly in nonhuman animals, physiological psychology was often linked with comparative psychology; in 1940 the *Journal of Comparative Psychology* was renamed the *Journal of Comparative and Physiological Psychology* and became the flagship journal for psychological studies that emphasized the biological basis of behavior. By the 1980s, comparative and physiological psychology went separate ways, and the publication split into two journals, one of which was named *Behavioral Neuroscience*. In an editorial announcing the split, Richard Thompson, who had been the editor of the combined journal and the first editor of *Behavioral Neuroscience*, commented on the scope of the field of behavioral neuroscience:

> Traditionally, physiological psychology emphasized certain approaches and techniques, particularly lesions, electrical stimulation, and electrophysiological

recording. Study of the biological bases of behavior is now much broader and includes genetic factors, hormonal influences, neurotransmitter and chemical factors, neuroanatomical substrates, effects of drugs, developmental processes, and environmental factors, in addition to more traditional approaches. All these variables act ultimately through the nervous system…The contemporary meaning of the term "behavioral neuroscience" is almost as broad as "behavior" itself. Behavioral neuroscience is the field concerned with the biological substrates of behavior. Judging by its current rate of development, behavioral neuroscience could well become a dominant field of science in the future. (Thompson, 1983, p. 3)

Cognitive neuroscience is the most recent of these three specialized domains of neuroscience, developing in the late 1980s. Part of the thrust for its creation stemmed from a perceived gulf between brain researchers and psychologists, which some researchers sought to overcome. In this spirit, brain researcher Joseph E. LeDoux and psychologist William Hirst edited a book, *Mind and Brain: Dialogues in Cognitive Neuroscience* (1986), which drew together neuroscientists and psychologists to review the state of the art in their own discipline and respond to the corresponding reviews of the other on four topics: perception, attention, memory, and emotion. These reviews reveal both the emergence of a desire of some practitioners in each area to be able to draw on the resources of the other, but also the large differences between the investigations pursued. As just one example of the differences, while most cognitive psychologists conducted their studies on adult humans, most neuroscience research was conducted on other species, where ethical constraints did not prevent insertion of electrodes into brains or making experimental lesions.

The term *cognitive neuroscience* was introduced somewhat earlier when Michael Gazzaniga established the Cognitive Neuroscience Institute with $500,000 provided by the Alfred P. Sloan Foundation. The grant was awarded to Gazzaniga and George Miller to attempt to draw inferences about cognitive function in normal individuals from deficits that followed brain injury. It was the only grant with a neural component in the 10-year, $17.4 million initiative the Sloan Foundation began in 1977 to support cognitive science, itself a fledging interdisciplinary endeavor involving principally psychology, linguistics, and artificial intelligence.[6] In 1986, the James S. McDonnell Foundation announced an initiative "to develop some specific programs to support research linking the biological with the behavioral sciences," and a month later Gazzaniga submitted a proposal to fund cognitive neuroscience. The foundation put together a panel to explore how to proceed (in addition to Miller and Gazzaniga, the panel included Marcus Raichle, Michael Posner, Terry Sejnowski, Gordon Shepherd, Emilio Bizzi, and Steven Hillyard; only Shepherd reflected the cellular and molecular focus typical in neuroscience). Concluding that there were "too many open questions, theoretical tangles and potential misunderstandings separating the two critical specialties—neuroscience and psychology—to proceed immediately," the panel elected first to constitute study groups. By 1988, the foundation was ready to fund a summer institute in cognitive neuroscience, and in 1989 it began a 10-year collaboration with the Pew Charitable Trusts to fund centers and individual research in cognitive neuroscience. In 1989, Gazzaniga established the

Journal of Cognitive Neuroscience and in 1994 cofounded the Cognitive Neuroscience Society, providing institutional identity to the new initiative. It is noteworthy that in contrast to the Society for Neuroscience, with over 37,500 members, the Cognitive Neuroscience Society currently has approximately 2,000 members.

Earlier, I noted a growing interest in brain researchers and psychologists in integrating their results, but what most advanced the endeavor of cognitive neuroscience was the development of a new research technique that permitted linking cognitive operations to brain regions. This involved, on the one hand, noninvasive means of measuring brain activity (actually, blood flow, which is assumed to be linked to brain activity) through either positron emission tomography (PET) or magnetic resonance imaging (MRI) and, on the other hand, ways of relating brain activity to operations in cognitive tasks. The most influential of the strategies for relating brain activity to cognitive tasks was provided by Michael Posner, a cognitive psychologist hired to satisfy a stipulation in a very large grant from the McDonnell Foundation to Washington University in St. Louis for the study of higher brain function, where Marcus Raichle was developing PET to study blood flow in the brain. Posner adapted a technique first introduced by nineteenth-century Dutch psychologist Cornelius Donders for using the difference in time required to perform two cognitive tasks differing in that one required an additional operation to determine the time required for that operation. Posner proposed measuring not increased time but increased blood flow between two tasks differing in one operation. In a pioneering study, Petersen, Fox, Posner, Mintun, and Raichle (1988) subtracted blood flow measured when subjects read nouns aloud from that measured when they generated a verb related to the noun and spoke that verb. The regions of increased blood flow—left dorsolateral prefrontal cortex, anterior cingulate, and right inferior lateral cerebellum—were taken to be involved in semantic processing.

In many ways, cognitive neuroscience can be viewed as the human counterpart of systems and behavioral neuroscience, and all three are counterpoised to cellular and molecular neuroscience. Their focus is not on individual neurons and the molecular processes within them, but on the interactions of multiple brain regions. Sometimes it appears that the main interest in these endeavors is to determine where in the brain cognitive activities occur, but in fact in most research the goal is to identify the various parts of the brain that are active in a given task, what each is contributing, and how these areas are organized so as to coordinate their operations in the performance of an overall task. In other words, they are engaged in identifying the mechanisms responsible for such tasks as identifying an object, detecting and responding to motion, processing language, encoding or retrieving memories, and so on. Researchers pursuing such research are fully aware that the brain regions they study are comprised of neurons and that processes such as the generation of action potentials and the altering of communication at synapses are crucial to the behavior of the brain regions. For systems and cognitive neuroscientists, however, those activities are at a lower level of organization; operations at that lower level can explain how the components they study perform their operations, but not how those operations together perform the overall cognitive task, which is their objective.

6. CONCLUSIONS

The two positions I have discussed in this chapter, ruthless reduction and mechanistic reduction, are both reductionist in that they recognize the importance of seeking knowledge of brain processes at different levels of organization to understand cognitive function. They are united in standing opposed to the attempts to divorce psychology and cognitive science from being constrained by our rapidly growing knowledge of brain processes. The principled arguments some philosophers have offered for psychology and cognitive science developing explanations ignoring the brain sciences are, on both views, a prescription for disaster.

The two accounts also agree that information about molecular and cellular processes, such as information about the molecular cascade involved in LTP and the genetic processes involved in synthesizing new proteins, is also of potentially great relevance to understanding memory consolidation. Bickle quote approvingly the following passage from Kandel, Schwartz, and Jessell's (2000, pp. 3–4) textbook, the leading textbook in neuroscience:

> This book…describes how neural science is attempting to link molecules to mind—how proteins responsible for the activities of individual nerve cells are related to the complexities of neural processes. Today it is possible to link the molecular dynamics of individual nerve cells to representations of perceptual and motor acts in the brain and to relate these internal mechanisms to observable behavior.

The language of linkages employed by Kandel and colleagues in this passage is instructive. Both ruthless reduction and mechanistic reduction accommodate linkages. Where they part company is on Bickle's gloss of this passage: "These 'links' are nothing less than *reductions* of psychological concepts and kinds to molecular-biological mechanisms and pathways." The molecular processes in cells to which Bickle proposes to reduce psychological concepts such as memory consolidation are, on the mechanistic reductionists account, processes within operating components of the relevant mechanism. They do not, on their own, explain the phenomenon of memory consolidation. Such an explanation requires identifying the full range of brain areas involved in memory consolidation and the operations each performs. The processes to which the ruthless reductionist appeals only figure in the subsequent attempts to explain these operating parts.

Although I have argued that Bickle is wrong in defending the ruthless reductionist approach to explanation, he has, as I have indicated, correctly captured the ethos in mainstream neuroscience, as represented by the Society for Neuroscience. Since its inception in the 1960s, the society has represented an attempt to explain mental phenomena at the cell and molecular level. As a result, systems neuroscience has only found a home at the fringe of neuroscience, and behavioral and cognitive neuroscience is pursued in enterprises outside the scope of neuroscience as characterized by the Society for Neuroscience. Researchers are increasingly looking to these projects for the explanation of phenomena such as memory consolidation.

The cellular and molecular accounts are parts of a subordinate (but certainly not unimportant) explanation of how the parts of the mechanism operate.

NOTES

1. Dudai (2004, p. 52) quotes Quintillian as reporting the "curious fact...that the interval of a single night will greatly increase the strength of the memory," and as raising the possibility that "the power of recollection...undergoes a process of ripening and maturing during the time which intervenes."

2. In terms of its differentiation and categorization capacities Rolls's network exhibits some of the same capacities as a neural network developed by Lynch and Granger (1989) to model olfaction that was based on the anatomy of the olfactory bulb, piriform cortex, and the EC and used a learning rule motivated by research on LTP. Bickle (1995) appeals to this model in support of his claim that there have already been successful reductions of psychological theories to purely neuroscientific theories. Without addressing the claim that the reducing theory is *purely* neuroscientific, I note that the reduction does not simply involve cellular and molecular analysis (as his more recent ruthless reductionism advocates) but an explanation in terms of a network (mechanism) involving multiple interacting components.

3. While these researchers were investigating non-REM sleep, others such as Elizabeth Hennevin (see Hennevin, Hars, Maho, and Bloch, 1995) focused on REM sleep and established an increase in it following learning and amnesia when animals or humans are deprived of REM sleep after learning. György Buzsáki (1998) proposes that both REM and non-REM sleep are critical for memory formation: During REM sleep, updated information is provided to CA3 from neocortical areas and bursting activity critical for synaptic plasticity and long-term memory consolidation is realized during non-REM sleep.

4. Bickle (2005) has himself appealed to the details of research on memory reconsolidation in responding to criticisms of ruthless reduction advanced by Looren de Jong and Schouten (2005) and has emphasized the role investigations at the cellular and molecular levels have played in recent research on memory reconsolidation. I agree that the interventions are often molecular in nature but maintain that the challenge in understanding memory reconsolidation, as in understanding memory consolidation itself, is to understand the full mechanism involved, not just the individual molecular components.

5. From a 1962 grant proposal quoted by Swazey (1975, p. 532).

6. Although the roots of the collaboration between these fields go back at least to a September 1956 symposium on information theory held at MIT in which Chomsky presented his work on transformation grammars, Newell and Simon introduced the first AI program, Logic Theorist, and George Miller identified informational limitations on cognitive processes involving the magic number 7, the term *cognitive science* itself first appears in two books published in 1975 (Bobrow and Collins, 1975; Norman and Rumelhart, 1975). The Sloan initiative was a major factor in developing cognitive science, fostering the creation of interdisciplinary programs at many institutions. One of these institutions, University of California, San Diego, used part of its grant to sponsor a conference, the La Jolla Conference on Cognitive Science, in 1979, which became the founding conference of the Cognitive Science Society. Two years earlier, a new journal,

Cognitive Science, was founded and subsequently was published by the Cognitive Science Society (for an account of the history of cognitive science, see Bechtel, Abrahamsen, and Graham, 1998).

REFERENCES

Agranoff, B. W., Davis, R. E., and Brink, J. J. (1966). Chemical studies on memory fixation in goldfish. *Brain Research* 1: 303–309.

Bahar, A., Dorfman, N., and Dudai, Y. (2004). Amygdalar circuits required for either consolidation or extinction of taste aversion memory are not required for reconsolidation. *European Journal of Neuroscience* 19: 1115–1118.

Bechtel, W. (2006). *Discovering Cell Mechanisms: The Creation of Modern Cell Biology.* Cambridge: Cambridge University Press.

Bechtel, W. (2008). *Mental Mechanisms: Philosophical Perspectives on Cognitive Neuroscience.* London: Routledge.

Bechtel, W. (in press). The epistemology of evidence in cognitive neuroscience. In R. Skipper, C. Allen, R. A. Ankeny, C. F. Craver, L. Darden, G. Mikkelson, et al. (Eds.), *Philosophy and the Life Sciences: A Reader.* Cambridge, Mass.: MIT Press.

Bechtel, W., and Abrahamsen, A. (2005). Explanation: A mechanist alternative. *Studies in History and Philosophy of Biological and Biomedical Sciences* 36: 421–441.

Bechtel, W., Abrahamsen, A., and Graham, G. (1998). The life of cognitive science. In W. Bechtel and G. Graham (Eds.), *A Companion to Cognitive Science.* Oxford: Basil Blackwell, 1–104.

Bechtel, W., and Richardson, R. C. (1993). *Discovering Complexity: Decomposition and Localization as Strategies in Scientific Research.* Princeton, N.J.: Princeton University Press.

Bernstein, J. (1912). *Elektrobiologie. Die Lehre von den elektrischen Vorgängen im Organismus auf moderner Grundlage dargestellt.* Braunschweig: Vieweg & Sohn.

Bickle, J. (1995). Psychoneural reduction of the genuinely cognitive: Some accomplished facts. *Philosophical Psychology* 8: 265–285.

Bickle, J. (1998). *Psychoneural Reduction: The New Wave.* Cambridge, Mass.: MIT Press.

Bickle, J. (2003). *Philosophy and Neuroscience: A Ruthlessly Reductive Account.* Dordrecht: Kluwer.

Bickle, J. (2005). Molecular neuroscience to my rescue (again): Reply to Looren de Jong & Schouten. *Philosophical Psychology* 18: 487–494.

Bickle, J. (2006). Reducing mind to molecular pathways: Explicating the reductionism implicit in current cellular and molecular neuroscience. *Synthese* 151: 411–434.

Bliss, T. V. P., and Lømo, T. (1973). Long-lasting potentiation of synaptic transmission in the dentate area of the unanaesthetized rabbit following stimulation of the perforant path. *Journal of Physiology* 232: 331–356.

Bobrow, D. G., and Collins, A. F. (1975). *Representation and Understanding: Studies in Cognitive Science.* New York: Academic Press.

Bramham, C. R., and Srebo, B. (1989). Synaptic plasticity in the hippocampus is modulated by behavioral state. *Brain Research* 493: 74–86.

Burnham, W. H. (1903). Retroactive amnesia: Illustrative cases and a tentative explanation. *American Journal of Psychology* 14: 382–396.

Buzsáki, G. (1998). Memory consolidation during sleep: A neurophysiological perspective. *Journal of Sleep Research* 7: 17–23.

Carmichael, S. T., and Price, J. L. (1996). Connectional networks within the orbital and medial prefrontal cortex of macaque monkeys. *Journal of Comparative Neurology* 371: 179–207.

Craver, C. (2003). The making of a memory mechanism. *Journal of the History of Biology* 36: 153–195.

Craver, C. (2007). *Explaining the Brain: What a Science of the Mind-Brain Could Be.* New York: Oxford University Press.

DeVietti, T. L., Conger, G. L., and Kirkpatrick, B. R. (1977). Comparison of the enhancement gradients of retention obtained with stimulation of the mesencephalic reticular formation after training or memory reactivation. *Physiology and Behavior* 19: 549–554.

Du Bois-Reymond, E. (1848–1884). *Untersuchungen über thierische Elektricität.* Berlin: Reimer.

Dudai, Y. (2004). The neurobiology of consolidations, or, how stable is the engram? *Annual Review of Psychology* 55: 51–86.

Dudai, Y., and Eisenberg, M. (2004). Rites of passage of the engram: Reconsolidation and the lingering consolidation hypothesis. *Neuron* 44: 93–100.

Duncan, C. P. (1949). The retroactive effect of electroshock on learning. *Journal of Comparative and Physiological Psychology* 42: 32–44.

Ebbinghaus, H. (1885). *Über das Gedächtnis: Untersuchungen zur experimentellen Psychologie.* Leipzig: Duncker & Humblot.

Erlanger, J., and Gasser, H. S. (1937). *Electrical Signs of Nervous Activity.* Philadelphia: University of Pennsylvania Press.

Felleman, D. J., and van Essen, D. C. (1991). Distributed hierarchical processing in the primate cerebral cortex. *Cerebral Cortex* 1: 1–47.

Ferrier, D. (1876). *The Functions of the Brain.* London: Smith, Elder.

Glennan, S. (1996). Mechanisms and the nature of causation. *Erkenntnis* 44: 50–71.

Glennan, S. (2002). Rethinking mechanistic explanation. *Philosophy of Science* 69: S342–S353.

Hebb, D. O. (1949). *The Organization of Behavior.* New York: Wiley.

Hennevin, E., Hars, B., Maho, C., and Bloch, V. (1995). Processing of learned information in paradoxical sleep: Relevance for memory. *Behavioural Brain Research* 69: 125–135.

Hoffman, K. L., and McNaughton, B. L. (2002). Coordinated reactivation of distributed memory traces in primate neocortex. *Science* 297: 2070–2073.

Holmes, G. M. (1918). Disturbances of visual orientation. *British Journal of Ophthalmology* 2: 449–468.

Hubel, D. H., and Wiesel, T. N. (1962). Receptive fields, binocular interaction and functional architecture in the cat's visual cortex. *Journal of Physiology* 160: 106–154.

Hubel, D. H., and Wiesel, T. N. (1968). Receptive fields and functional architecture of monkey striate cortex. *Journal of Physiology* 195: 215–243.

Jones Leonard, B., McNaughton, B. L., and Barnes, C. A. (1987). Suppression of hippocampal synaptic activity during slow-wave sleep. *Brain Research* 425: 174–177.

Kandel, E. R., Schwartz, J. H., and Jessell, T. M. (2000). *Principles of Neural Science*, 4th ed. New York: McGraw-Hill.

Klüver, H., and Bucy, P. (1938). An analysis of certain effects of bilateral temporal lobectomy in the rhesus monkey, with special reference to "psychic blindness." *Journal of Psychology* 5: 33–54.

Kuffler, S. W. (1952). Neurons in the retina: Organization, inhibition and excitatory problems. *Cold Spring Harbor Symposia on Quantitative Biology* 17: 281–292.

Lashley, K. S. (1950). In search of the engram. *Symposia of the Society for Experimental Biology, IV. Physiological Mechanisms in Animal Behaviour*: 454–482.

Lechner, H. A., Squire, L. R., and Byrne, J. H. (1999). 100 years of consolidation—remembering Müller and Pilzecker. *Learning and Memory* 6: 77–87.

LeDoux, J. E., and Hirst, W. (Eds.). (1986). *Mind and Brain: Dialogues in Cognitive Neuroscience*. Cambridge: Cambridge University Press.

Lewis, D. J., Bregman, N. J., and Mahan, J. (1972). Cue-dependent amnesia in rats. *Journal of Comparative and Physiological Psychology* 81: 243–247.

Lømo, T. (1966). Frequency potentiation of excitatory synaptic activity in the dentate area of the hippocampal formation. *Acta Physiologica Scandinavica* 68: 128.

Looren de Jong, H., and Schouten, M. (2005). Ruthless reductionism: A review essay of John Bickle's *Philosophy and Neuroscience: A Ruthlessly Reductive Account. Philosophical Psychology* 18: 473–486.

Lynch, G., and Granger, R. (1989). Simulation and analysis of a simple cortical network. *Psychology of Learning and Motivation* 23: 205–241.

Machamer, P., Darden, L., and Craver, C. (2000). Thinking about mechanisms. *Philosophy of Science* 67: 1–25.

McClelland, J. L., McNaughton, B., and O'Reilly, R. C. (1995). Why there are complementary learning systems in the hippocampus and neocortex: Insights from the successes and failures of connectionist models of learning and memory. *Psychological Review* 102: 419–457.

McCloskey, M., and Cohen, N. J. (1989). Catastrophic interference in connectionist networks: The sequential learning problem. In G. H. Bower (ed.), *The Psychology of Learning and Motivation*, vol. 24. New York: Academic Press, 69–105.

McDougall, W. (1901). Experimentelle Beitraege zur Lehre vom Gedaechtnis: Von G.E. Mueller und A. Pilzecker. *Mind* 10: 388–394.

McGaugh, J. L. (2000). Memory—a century of consolidation. *Science* 287: 248–251.

Miller, G. A., Galanter, E., and Pribram, K. (1960). *Plans and the Structure of Behavior*. New York: Holt.

Misanin, J. R., Miller, R. R., and Lewis, D. J. (1968). Retrograde amnesia produced by electroconvulsive shock after reactivation of consolidated memory trace. *Science* 160: 554–555.

Müller, G. E., and Pilzecker, A. (1900). Experimentelle Beiträge zur Lehre vom Gedächtnis. *Zeitschrift für Psychologie und Physiologie der Sinnesorgane. Ergänzungsband* 1: 1–300.

Mundale, J. (2001). Neuroanatomical foundations of cognition: Connecting the neuronal level with the study of higher brain areas. In W. Bechtel, P. Mandik, J. Mundale, and R. S. Stufflebeam (Eds.), *Philosophy and the Neurosciences*. Oxford: Blackwell.

Nader, K., Schafe, G. E., and LeDoux, J. E. (2000). Fear memories require protein synthesis in the amygdala for reconsolidation after retrieval. *Nature* 406: 722–726.

Norman, D. A., and Rumelhart, D. E. (1975). *Explorations in Cognition*. San Francisco: Freeman.

Oncley, J., Schmitt, F. O., Williams, R. C., Rosenberg, M. D., and Bolt, R. H. (Eds.). (1959). *Biophysical Science: A Study Program*. New York: Wiley.

Penfield, W., and Boldrey, E. (1937). Somatic motor and sensory representation in the cerebral cortex of man as studied by electrical stimulation. *Brain* 60: 389–443.

Petersen, S. E., Fox, P. T., Posner, M. I., Mintun, M., and Raichle, M. E. (1988). Positron emission tomographic studies of the cortical anatomy of single-word processing. *Nature* 331: 585–588.

Ratcliff, R. (1990). Connectionist models of recognition memory: Constraints imposed by learning and forgetting functions. *Psychological Review* 97: 285–308.

Ribot, T.-A. (1882). *Diseases of Memory: An Essay in the Positive Psychology* (W. H. Smith, Trans.). New York: Appleton-Century-Crofts.

Rolls, E. T. (1995). A model of the operation of the hippocampus and entorhinal cortex in memory. *International Journal of Neural Systems* 6 (supplement): 51–70.

Rolls, E. T., and Treves, A. (1998). *Neural Networks and Brain Function*. Oxford: Oxford University Press.

Rumelhart, D. E., Hinton, G. E., and Williams, R. J. (1986a). Learning internal representations by error propagation. In D. E. Rumelhart and J. L. McClelland (Eds.), *Parallel Distributed Processing: Explorations in the Microstructure of Cognition*. Vol. 1. *Foundations*. Cambridge, Mass.: MIT Press.

Rumelhart, D. E., Hinton, G. E., and Williams, R. J. (1986b). Learning representations by back-propagating errors. *Nature* 323: 533–536.

Rumelhart, D. E., and McClelland, J. L. (Eds.). (1986). *Parallel Distributed Processing: Explorations in the Microstructure of Cognition. Vol. 1. Foundations*. Cambridge, Mass.: MIT Press.

Sara, S. J. (2000). Retrieval and reconsolidation: Toward a neurobiology of remembering. *Learning and Memory* 7: 73–84.

Schmitt, F. O. (1959). Molecular organization of the nerve fiber. *Reviews of Modern Physics* 31: 455–465.

Schmitt, F. O., ed. (1962). *Macromolecular Specificity and Biological Memory*. Cambridge, Mass.: MIT Press.

Schneider, A. M., and Sherman, W. (1968). Amnesia: A function of the temporal relation of foot-shock to electroconvulsive shock. *Science* 159: 219–221.

Scoville, W. B., and Milner, B. (1957). Loss of recent memory after bilateral hippocampal lesions. *Journal of Neurology, Neurosurgery, and Psychiatry* 20: 11–21.

Squire, L. R., and Kandel, E. (2000). *Memory*. New York: Scientific American Library.

Squire, L. R., and Knowlton, B. J. (1995). Memory, hippocampus, and brain systems. In M. S. Gazzaniga (ed.), *The Cognitive Neurosciences*. Cambridge, Mass.: MIT Press, 825–837.

Swazey, J. P. (1975). Forging a neuroscience community: A brief history of the neurosciences research program. In F. G. Worden, J. P. Swazey, and G. Adelman (Eds.), *The Neurosciences: Paths of Discovery*. Cambridge, Mass.: MIT Press, 529–546.

Taubenfeld, S. M., Milekic, M. H., Monti, B., and Alberini, C. M. (2001). The consolidation of new but not reactivated memory requires hippocampal C/EBP_β. *Nature Reviews Neuroscience* 4: 813–818.

Thompson, R. F. (1983). Editorial. *Behavioral Neuroscience* 97: 3.

van Essen, D. C., and Gallant, J. L. (1994). Neural mechanisms of form and motion processing in the primate visual system. *Neuron* 13: 1–10.

Wilson, M. A., and McNaughton, B. L. (1994). Reactivation of hippocampal ensemble memories during sleep. *Science* 265: 676–679.

Zeki, S. M. (1973). Colour coding of the rhesus monkey prestriate cortex. *Brain Research* 53: 422–427.

Zeki, S. M. (1974). Functional organization of a visual area in the posterior bank of the superior temporal sulcus of the rhesus monkey. *Journal of Physiology* 236: 549–573.

CHAPTER 2

BIOLOGICAL CLOCKS: EXPLAINING WITH MODELS OF MECHANISMS

SARAH K. ROBINS AND CARL F. CRAVER

1. INTRODUCTION

What is required of an adequate explanation in neuroscience? Debates frequently arise among neuroscientists (and philosophers interested in neuroscience) about whether a proposed explanation for a given phenomenon is, in fact, the correct explanation. Does long-term potentiation explain the blocking effect in classical conditioning? Do size differences in hypothalamic nuclei or in the base pair sequence in particular genes explain sexual preferences? Do 40 Hz oscillations in the cortex explain feature binding in phenomenal consciousness? Although the answers to these questions depend in part on specific details about these diverse phenomena, they also depend on widely accepted (though largely implicit) standards for determining when explanations succeed and when they fail. Many of those implicit standards, we argue, can be captured by the claim that explanations in neuroscience describe multilevel mechanisms. In this essay, we summarize some key features of mechanistic explanation, say what it means for mechanistic explanations to span multiple levels, and show what is required to bridge levels of explanation.

We illustrate our view of mechanistic explanation by considering the mechanism of circadian rhythms. Circadian rhythms are periodic fluctuations in behavior, cognition, and physiological processes that are synchronized with the light–dark cycle of the environment. These rhythms have a period of about one 24-hour day. These fluctuations are controlled in part by an endogenous timekeeping mechanism (a biological "clock") that works via periodic changes in gene expression. Although many of the fine details of this example remain to be decided, enough is known about the cellular and molecular mechanisms regulating circadian rhythms to illustrate what is required of an adequate mechanistic explanation (for a helpful review, see Herzog and Schwartz, 2002). In fact, biological clocks stand out as a paradigm case of successful mechanistic explanation in neuroscience.

This case exemplifies our thinking about mechanisms, but it does not by itself justify the normative claim that neuroscientists ought to describe mechanisms in their explanations. The example shows merely that our view of mechanisms comports well with exemplars of successful explanation in neuroscience. The view thus honors and justifies the implicit and explicit standards that have been shaped through the reflective scrutiny of generations of neuroscientists, but that alone does not show that the scientists have developed the correct standards. Although we shall not argue for it here, we believe that a sufficient defense of these norms can be provided on instrumental grounds: Models that describe mechanisms are more useful for the purposes of manipulation and control than are scientific models that do not describe mechanisms. This distinguishes mechanistic explanations from purely descriptive models and simulations. In what follows, we provide an account of mechanistic explanation and some common failures of mechanistic explanation. We discuss the sense in which mechanistic explanations typically span multiple levels and we provide an account of what it means to integrate such levels.[1]

2. MECHANISMS

Neuroscientists rarely write about explanation in the abstract; instead, they write about mechanisms. Sometimes they use other terms—they describe *cascades, pathways, systems,* and *substrates.* We use the term *mechanism* for all of these. The word should not be understood as implying adherence to any strict metaphysical system. Clearly neural mechanisms are not generally understood as machines that work only through motion, attraction and repulsion, or the transmission of conserved quantities. Nor are they generally understood as Heroic simple machines, or machines that work according to the principles of Newtonian mechanics, or strictly deterministic systems in which laws of nature allow only one output for any input. The term *mechanism* as it is used in contemporary neuroscience has been liberated from these etymological strictures, allowing for a broader understanding of mechanistic organization as befits biological systems. One might worry, in fact, that the term has lost any determinate content that it once had and persists only as an honorific. We acknowledge that the notion of mechanism in contemporary neuroscience is far more liberal than its historical antecedents, but we disagree that the term has thereby been stripped of its meaning.

The central thrust of any causal-mechanical view of explanation is that to explain a phenomenon is to show how it is situated within the causal structure of the world (Salmon, 1984). Etiological explanations situate an item within the causal structure of the world by describing its antecedent causes and the mechanisms by which the *explanandum* phenomenon (the phenomenon to be explained) was produced. Constitutive mechanistic explanations, on the other hand, situate an item with respect to the causal structure internal to the phenomenon to be explained. They describe underlying mechanisms, such as the biochemical mechanism of protein synthesis and the ionic mechanisms of the action potential. In his classic defense of a causal-mechanical approach to explanation, Salmon focused almost exclusively on etiological explanations. Constitutive mechanistic explanation, in contrast, has been the focus of much recent work in the philosophy of science (see, e.g., Bechtel, 2005; Bechtel and Richardson, 1993; Craver, 2007; Darden, 2006; Machamer, Darden, and Craver, 2000).

Although there are minor disagreements among proponents of mechanistic explanation, they all agree with the schematic statement that constitutive mechanistic explanations describe entities and activities organized such that they exhibit the explanandum phenomenon. Mechanistic explanations explain by showing how the explanandum phenomenon, Ψ, is made up of the organization of component entities, X, and their activities, ϕ, as displayed in figure 2.1. The explanandum phenomenon is some behavior, property, or process of a mechanism as a whole. The *explanans* (the explanation of the phenomenon) includes the entities, activities, and organizational features that exhaustively make up the mechanism. Constitutive explanations are thus inherently interlevel; they explain the behavior of the whole in terms of the organized behaviors of its parts. In the remainder of this section, we discuss each of these components of mechanistic explanation (the explanandum phenomenon, entities, activities, and organization), lay out some criteria for

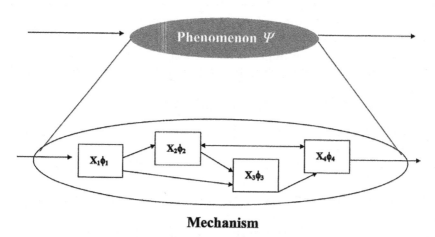

Mechanism

Figure 2.1 Schematic of a mechanism.

complete and successful mechanistic explanation, and describe some ways that mechanistic explanations can fail.

2.1. The Explanandum Phenomenon

All mechanistic explanations are framed by reference to the phenomenon that one is trying to explain. There are no mechanisms simpliciter, only mechanisms *of* a given phenomenon, such as the mechanism *of* protein synthesis or the mechanism *of* the action potential. The choice of the phenomenon and the depth with which the phenomenon is characterized determine what will and will not count as an adequate description of the mechanism that explains it.

In our example, the phenomenon to be explained is the circadian rhythm. These rhythms are widely conserved across the animal and plant kingdoms. Bread mold, crickets, sea hares, and fungi have circadian rhythms, as do hamsters and humans. The few organisms that do not display such cycles (or that have erratic cycles) live in aperiodic environments, such as caves (Poulson and White, 1969). Yet circadian rhythms are not controlled by environmental stimuli alone. Many plants and animals maintain circadian cycles for several generations after being transferred to aperiodic environments (Aschoff, 1960). The persistence of circadian rhythms in the absence of environmental stimuli has led to the general acceptance of the idea that the rhythms are regulated by an internal time keeper or clock.

In humans, the most obvious aspect of the circadian rhythm is the sleep–wake cycle. Under standard conditions, humans alternate between 16 hours of wakefulness and 8 hours of sleep. These cycles of sleep and wakefulness are accompanied by physiological changes, such as fluctuations in blood pressure, body temperature, brain metabolism, gastric motility, heart rate, respiration, and the concentrations of myriad circulating hormones. These cycles are also correlated with periodicities in behavior and cognition, including appetite, athletic performance, locomotion, mood, motivation, saccadic velocity, and sex drive (Van Dongen, Kerkhof, and Dinges, 2004). With some idealization, we can identify four aspects of the circadian rhythm phenomenon that must be accounted for by any adequate and complete explanation. These include the intrinsic timing of the clock; the entrainment (setting) of the clock to its environment; the effects of the clock on behavior, cognition, and physiology; and the patterns of disease and malfunction to which the system is susceptible.

The primary phenomenon to be explained is the timing mechanism of the clock itself. In the absence of environmental cues, humans enter a "free run" state, one full cycle of which is completed in roughly 24.3–24.7 hours.[2] Colin Pittendrigh (1954) is recognized as the first to document that the circadian rhythm persists in the absence of environmental cues. He exposed *Drosophila* larvae to different temperature and light conditions and measured the effect of these factors on their hatching cycle. *Drosophila* metamorphosis, from embryonic development through eclosion (hatching) from the pupal casing, takes 6 days. Pittendrigh's experiments demonstrated that larvae hatch on a consistent (although slightly shorter) schedule regardless of changes in temperature and light. When restored to normal environmental conditions, the larvae were able to readjust (lengthen) their cycles. This finding helped establish that rhythmic processes, at least in *Drosophila*, are endogenously regulated. Similar results were obtained for human subjects living in caves. They maintained regular sleep–wake cycles persisting in a free-run state repeating every 24.3–24.7 hours. Sleep and wake times thus gradually shifted forward (see figure 2.2a, b), cycling through the entire 24-hour solar day (Kleitman, 1963; Siffre, 1964).

The existence of a free-run rhythm in the absence of any relevant environmental input is taken as conclusive evidence that circadian rhythms are endogenously determined (Aschoff, 1981). Whether there is a particular clock mechanism within

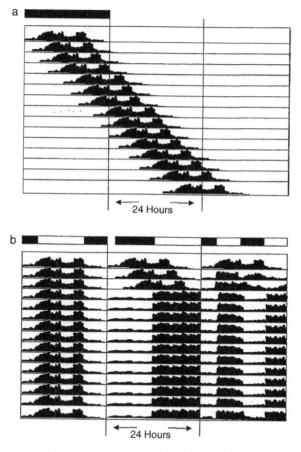

Figure 2.2 (a) A model actogram, or activity record, for an organism in freerunning rhythm. In many mammals this cycle is slightly longer than a 24-hour day, and so gradually decouples from environmental time. Horizontal lines represent one 24-hour day. Vertical lines are 24 hours apart. Activity is measured by the amount of spiking above each horizontal line, in terms of heart rate, body temperature, or specified motor activity (e.g., wrist movement in humans, wheel-running in rodents). (b) Actograms of entrainments to three environmental light schedules, as indicated by the bars above the actogram.

the organism that performs this function is a further question. As we will explain, the clock in humans (and many other mammals) is believed to be housed in the suprachiasmatic nucleus (SCN) of the hypothalamus (Moore and Eichler, 1972; Stephan and Zucker, 1972). Localized brain lesions to the SCN cause both the free-run and entrained rhythms to vanish (Klein and Moore, 1979; Moore and Klein, 1974; Rusak and Zucker, 1979). Any adequate explanation of the circadian rhythm must reveal the time-keeping mechanism of this clock and show why the rhythm has the free-run pattern it does.

An adequate explanation must also describe how the clock is entrained to the local time by environmental cues, or *zeitgebers* (Aschoff, 1960; Pittendrigh, Bruce, and Kaus, 1958).[3] Zeitgebers cause the free-run rhythm of the clock to undergo a phase shift, setting the clock's environmental cues. Light is the most familiar zeitgeber. The sensitivity of the human circadian clock to environmental lighting conditions allows international travelers to adjust to local time. It also allows shift workers to adjust (if only incompletely) to around-the-clock working conditions. Light is not the only zeitgeber: Exercise, humidity, smell, temperature, and food availability are all known to entrain the clock in some species (Pittendrigh, 1981). In humans and many other animals, of course, light is the dominant zeitgeber. Photoreceptors receive light information and pass it on to a subset of specific ganglion cells that project to the SCN (Moore, Speh, and Card, 1995). The pathway on which light travels from the photoreceptors to the SCN is known as the retinohypothalamic tract (Hendrickson, Wagoner, and Cowan, 1972; Moore and Lenn, 1972). A complete explanation of the circadian rhythm must explain how light changes the physicochemical responses of photoreceptors, how this "information" is encoded, how it is transmitted and preserved along the retinohypothalamic tract, and how that neural signal changes the behavior of the clock in the SCN in such a way as to produce a phase shift.

Third, an adequate explanation of the circadian rhythm must explain how the clock, entrained or not, exerts its influence on the diverse behavioral, cognitive, and physiological systems that participate in the rhythm.[4] The correlation among these diverse phenomena is thought to be explained by a common cause (the activities of the clock), and one goal is to elucidate the mechanism by which the clock is connected to each of these. Given the diversity of factors participating in this rhythm, it is unsurprising that circulating hormones have figured prominently in candidate mechanisms. The most studied such mechanism involves the regulation of melatonin release in the pineal gland (Wurtman, Axelrod, and Kelly, 1968). Increases in the concentration of circulating melatonin are known to make an organism drowsy, whereas decreasing circulating melatonin concentrations are known to produce extended wakefulness (McNamara, 2004). The neurons in the SCN project to the sub-paraventricular nucleus (PVN) (Watts, Swanson, and Sanchez-Watts, 1987) of the hypothalamus, a region known to play an essential role in the rhythmic release of melatonin from the pineal gland. Lesions to the PVN disrupt cyclic melatonin release from the pineal, as well as induce disturbances in the release of other hormones from the pituitary (Hastings and Herbert, 1986). In mammals, the release of melatonin is a function of the clock itself, because organisms can persist in regular melatonin release even when removed from all exogenous light cues (Axelrod, Wurtman, and Snyder, 1965). The clock plays an essential role in regulating daily rhythms in melatonin release, which participate in sleep–wake regulation (Illernová, 1991; McNamara, 2004). However, there are likely other direct and indirect pathways through which the clock regulates behavior, cognition, and physiological processes. For now, we leave this aspect of the mechanism behind. Nonetheless, any complete understanding of the circadian rhythm would necessarily have to detail the mechanism by which the clock maintains the tight correlation among these diverse features.

Finally, any adequate explanation should show how the phenomenon can break down in conditions of damage or disease. Blind people who lack retinal photoreceptors or have damaged optic nerves typically exhibit free-run circadian rhythms (Sack, Lewy, and Hoban, 1987). Damage to the retinohypothalamic tract can also cause the organism to become unresponsive to external photic cues and enter a persistent free-run rhythm. There are clinical cases of persistent circadian rhythm disturbance, in which the person never adapts to changes in the light–dark cycle. Some people suffer from delayed sleep phase syndrome, in which they chronically stay up until the early morning and sleep until the late morning or early afternoon. Some, especially the elderly, suffer from advanced sleep syndrome, in which patients fall asleep and wake up very early (Van Dongen et al., 2004). Any adequate explanation of circadian rhythms should explain the regularly observed ways the phenomenon can fail or falter and should also make sense of the effective strategies for preventing or ameliorating these forms of breakdown.

The fundamental normative constraint on a mechanistic explanation is that it should account for all and only the aspects of the phenomenon to be explained. If a model fails to explain all aspects of the phenomenon, or if it makes predictions that do not accord with aspects of the phenomenon as it is observed in the wild, then it is not an adequate description of a mechanism. For example, a model that can predict changes in the entrained cycle but does not predict the free-run rhythm produced in the absence of zeitgebers leaves out a crucial component of the explanation. Likewise, a model that explains the free-run and entrained rhythms of the mechanism only under standard or nonpathological conditions, and either makes no predictions or makes false predictions about the behavior of the system under such conditions, is not an adequate explanation. A mechanism includes all and only the entities, activities, and organizational features relevant to all aspects of the phenomenon to be explained (such as the four features of the circadian rhythm already described). Anything less is in some sense incomplete. Anything more adds nothing to the explanation.

Some will object that this requirement demands too much of explanations. Surely scientists (including those who work on the mechanisms of circadian rhythms) are often satisfied with less than complete explanations. Certainly it is possible to reach a level of explanatory detail beyond which further elucidation of the minute details of the mechanism would only cloud human understanding. We do not intend to deny either of these claims. Our project is to express what is required of a complete mechanistic explanation, not to give an account of when a given explanatory text is complete or detailed enough for the purposes at hand. Complete mechanistic models account for all aspects of the phenomenon and include all of the explanatorily relevant details of the mechanism. Most areas of science, perhaps all of them, traffic in partial models. This fact deserves further exploration, but it is not our focus here.

2.2. Component Entities

In mechanistic explanations, the behavioral profile of a mechanism as a whole (the phenomenon) is explained in terms of components of the mechanism organized and acting together. Mechanistic explanations are in this respect unlike procedural descriptions, such as the description of making a cake (Cummins, 1983). The cook breaks the egg, adds the flour, stirs the batter, and so on. This procedural description unfolds entirely at the level of the cook. He or she is the agent of all the component procedures. Mechanistic explanations, in contrast, describe interactions among the parts: the force of bowl on shell, the gaseous output of yeast, and the whir of components in the blender's clutch. Mechanistic explanations are also unlike interpretive explanations, in which the goal is merely to describe some program that could generate a certain class of outputs from a certain class of inputs. The components in mechanisms are not "as if" posits or functional descriptions abstracted from the details. Mechanisms are concrete, embodied in the details of a biological system, its working parts, and their actual spatial and temporal relations to one another. The circadian clock is not an abstract entity. It is not described equally well as a grandfather clock, a digital wristwatch, and an egg timer. Any number of mechanisms might possibly implement circadian rhythmicity in a given species: It might, for instance, be made up of metabolic processes, ionic processes, or genetic regulatory processes (Dunlap, 1999). The correct explanation for time keeping in that species specifies which is correct and describes how it works.

In humans and most mammals, the time-keeping mechanism is located in the SCN (Moore and Eichler, 1972). This mechanism can be characterized schematically as an oscillator, that is, as a system that exhibits regular periodic alternations between a positive loop, which moves a system variable toward an equilibrium state, and a negative loop, which makes the system deviate from that equilibrium state (Dunlap, 1999). In the SCN, these positive and negative loops involve mutually interacting cycles of gene regulation and protein production in the SCN's component cells (Van Gelder and Herzog, 2003). The positive loop activates gene expression; the negative loop suppresses it. Each loop inhibits the other, and each loop feeds back to turn itself off. The two loops are differentially responsive to environmental light: The positive loop is active in the morning, and the negative loop is active in the evening, accounting for the sleep–wake cycles. Genes and proteins are the featured entities in this oscillatory mechanism. An adequate explanatory model of the circadian rhythm in a given species will identify the component genes and the proteins that they produce.

The genetics of the circadian rhythm were first investigated in the fruit fly, *Drosophila melanogaster* (Konopka and Benzer, 1971). Researchers identified the first circadian gene, *period* (*per*, of which there are three known subtypes, *mper1*, *mper2*, and *mper3*)[5] in *Drosophila* through the creation of mutants (Reddy et al., 1984). This discovery was followed by *frequency* (*frq*) in the fungus *Neurospora* (McClung, Fox, and Dunlap, 1989) and *timeless* (*tim*) again in the *Drosophila* (Myers, Wager-Smith, Wesley, Young, and Sehgal, 1995). These genes are crucial for maintaining an organism's free-run rhythm. Organisms with mutations to one or more of these genes have radically altered circadian rhythms, and their deficits appear to be localized to rhythmic behaviors, indicating that these are indeed clock genes. In mammals, at least four clock genes are involved: *per*, *cryptochrome* (*cry*, sometimes called *clock*), *bmal1*, *tim* (*rev* in some species).[6] When these genes are expressed, they produce proteins that regulate the expression of other genes, moving the cell toward and away from the equilibrium state. A complete explanation of the circadian clock includes all of the relevant brain regions, neurons, molecules, and ions.

2.3. Activities

Mechanistic explanations also include the various activities of and interactions among the mechanism's parts. *Activities* are the causal components of mechanisms; they are what the entities do. Terms such as *cause* and *produce* are schema terms that are shown to have content when they are fleshed out in terms of the activities for which they stand.

Expression, repression, transcription, and translation figure prominently in genetic mechanisms. Consider some of the activities involved in the entrainment of the mammalian clock to light. The negative loop can be described as beginning when photic information (in the form of patterns of neural firing that are correlated with the presence of light) is transmitted to the SCN from the retina via the release of glutamate, a neurotransmitter. The glutamate causes *per* genes (such as *mper1* and *mper2*) to initiate transcription, expressing PER proteins. These proteins are phosphorylated by casein kinase (CKI_E) in the cytoplasm, binding with the CRY protein to form dimers (molecules comprised of protein subunits). These dimers then move into the nucleus, binding to the CLK:BMAL1 dimers. In the absence of the CRY dimers, the CLK:BMAL1 dimers bind to promoter sites on *cry*, *per*, and *rev* activating transcription of these genes. The binding of CRY dimers with CLK:BMAL1 dimers prohibits this, thereby suppressing gene transcription. This forms the negative loop of the SCN's oscillation. *Per* transcription yields suppression of further *per* transcription via feedback. The expression of PER ultimately down-regulates the expression of the *per* gene.

While the negative loop is active, the nucleus of the cell contains a maximal number of REV proteins, which inhibit activation of the positive loop (through repression of *bmal1* activation). As the concentration of REV drops, *bmal1* begins to express BMAL1. As BMAL1 proteins amass, they bond with CLK (forming CLK:BMAL1 dimers) to activate the transcription *per, cry,* and *rev*. This binding is made possible because the CRY and REV proteins, which are prominent during the peak of the negative loop, are at low levels as the positive loop begins. At this point, the negative loop begins to feed back on itself. The longer *bmal1* has been active, the more REV proteins begin to accumulate. These proteins bind to promoter sites on the *bmal1* genes (specifically retinoic acid receptor–related orphan receptor response element, RORE, promoter sites), which suppress further transcription in the gene. This decreases the level of BMAL1 proteins, allowing for the negative loop to reactivate. The two loops are thus interrelated, but they provoke different responses in the organism, creating the morning and evening loops that synchronize behavior to the light–dark cycle of the environment (for a video depiction of this process, see Van Gelder and Herzog, 2003).

Clearly, there are many different kinds of activity in this mechanism, all of which are familiar in biochemistry and genetics. In some cases (as our occasional use of filler terms in the foregoing description indicates), scientists do not know which activities explain the correlation between variables. They know that two variables of the system are correlated with one another, and, importantly, that one of the variables is sensitive to (that is, can be manipulated on the basis of) changes in another variable. For example, neuroscientists knew that light played a role in circadian rhythmicity long before they developed an understanding of how it influenced the genetic mechanisms of the clock. Neuroscientists can know that a protein influences gene expression even if they are at the time quite unsure as to the precise activities by which the protein affects the genetic regulatory mechanisms. Deeper explanations are often achieved by delving further into the detailed levels of mechanisms.

Several norms of explanation follow from the claim that mechanisms are partly constituted by activities and interactions. First, earlier events explain later events and not vice versa. If explanations cite causes, and causes precede their effects, then the factors cited in the explanans should precede the item in the explanandum.[7] When testing potential zeitgebers, researchers look for environmental factors that occur prior to a change in rhythmic behavior. As discussed, light is the most obvious and well-studied environmental influence on circadian rhythms, but there are many other factors that influence an organism's endogenous cycle. Exercise is one, although its effects are somewhat different across species (Mistlberger and Skene, 2004). To evaluate exercise's potential as a zeitgeber, studies have been designed where exercise is scheduled at a particular time in the organism's daily cycle, and subsequent phase shifts in other parts of the organism's routine are monitored (reviewed in Mistlberger and Skene, 2005). When evaluating nonphotic entrainment in humans and other organisms, the key first step is to establish the correct temporal relationship. Events that occur after phase shifts in the organism's free-run rhythm are not candidate explanations. Establishing precise temporal relationships is difficult in the case of circadian rhythms. An event that occurs long after a phase shift might be part of the explanation if it is so much later as to be part of a new cycle. But this merely reiterates the point under discussion: To establish a later event as relevant is to establish it as being part of a *new* cycle, and thus to establish that it precedes its effect.

Although it is important to locate temporally prior elements as potential causes, there is a second norm that moderates the first: Mere temporal sequences are not explanatory. Simply locating an event as occurring prior to the explanandum event does not thereby secure a causal relationship. The rooster crows before dawn, but the crowing does not explain the sunrise. Some sequences are explanatory, and some are not. In many (but not all) cases, explanatory sequences are underwritten by a mechanism. In the case of entrainment, there is a pathway through which the environmental factor sends information to the cells of the SCN, allowing for a phase shift in their free-run rhythms (Johnson, Elliott, and Foster, 2003). The pathways through which exercise and other nonphotic zeitgebers entrain the circadian clock are not fully understood at present. Exercise may have direct influence on circadian rhythmicity via an unknown pathway, as well as indirect influence on known pathways. For example, exercise is known to change pupil size, which may alter the amount of photic information that reaches the SCN via the retinohypothalamic tract (Ishigaki, Miyao, and Ishihara, 1991). Establishing the mechanistic details that ground the temporal relationship between an environmental cue and the biological clock is one way to illustrate the difference between a mere temporal sequence and a causal relation, but as we will see, it is not the only way.

Third, the apparent platitude that mechanisms are partly constituted by causal relations helps express the norm that mere correlations are not explanatory. The rooster's crow is correlated with the sunrise, the apparent motion of the stars, and fluctuations in the body temperature of cows. The correct explanation does not include such irrelevant correlates. In the early twentieth century, French scientist Henri Piéron proposed that the sleep–wake cycle was fundamentally a physiological response to self-inflicted toxicity. Piéron hypothesized that a particular toxin was active during the day and disappeared at night, accounting for the change in wakefulness across the 24-hour day. To test this view, Piéron performed experiments with dogs. He deprived a group of dogs of sleep for several days. Cerebrospinal fluid (CSF) from these dogs was then injected into another group of fully rested dogs, who promptly fell asleep for several hours. This led Piéron (1913) to conclude that there was indeed a chemical basis to circadian rhythmicity. However, further research cast doubts on the significance of Piéron's results. Schnedorf and Ivy (1939) were able to show that injecting CSF into an organism causes hypothermia, which then causes him or her to sleep (Kandel and Schwartz, 1981, p. 480). Thus, the original correlation between chemicals in CSF and sleep–wake cycles was shown not to be explanatory because the relation could be explained by the causal influence of a third factor, in this case, the experimental intervention itself. Causally irrelevant factors, those that fail to make a difference to the explanandum phenomenon, are not explanatory. The difference between the two is revealed, as this case illustrates, through the logic of controlled experiments, which we discuss next.

The idea that mechanistic explanations include activities and interactions should not be understood to preclude probabilistic explanations. In some cases, probabilistic explanations can be eliminated in favor of deterministic activities and causal relations, but we see no good reason to stipulate that this must always be the case. At any rate, explanations in neuroscience frequently, perhaps typically, must deal at best with probabilistic phenomena. The overall pattern of electrophysiological activity in the SCN is explained (at least in part) by appeal to stochastic interactions between the individual cells that compose it. These cells are tightly packed together so that they share extracellular ionic environments. It is thought that this proximity increases the probability of the cells firing synchronously.

The precise mechanism of this synchronization is unknown. However, it is known that no one cell, or set of cells, dictates the firing rate of any other (Prosser, 2000). Rather, it appears the close proximity of neurons increases the probability that they will undergo similar effects in response to changes in the extracellular fluid. The extracellular conditions that cause one SCN neuron to fire are likely to have an influence on surrounding neurons as well. The firing of one SCN neuron thus increases the probability that surrounding neurons will fire. When these firings become synchronized, the neurons in a given area fall into phase with one another, allowing the SCN to emit a single rhythm that is the amalgamation of many individual rhythms. We discuss the details of this process in section 3. Here we emphasize the fact that detailing the mechanistic interactions between individual neurons allows for an understanding of these stochastic relations.

One can fulfill all of these constraints on mechanistic explanation by demanding that the activities included in neural mechanisms sustain relationships of manipulability. Let X and Y be two variables whose values represent potential inputs to and outputs from one activity. For example, X could be the variable representing whether a gene is expressed, and Y could represent the concentration of a given protein in the nucleus. One should require that it be possible to change the value of the effect variable by changing the value of the cause variable. Somewhat more rigorously, variable X is causally relevant to variable Y if and only if one can possibly change the value of Y through an intervention,[8] I, that changes the value of X. The difference between activities and pseudo-activities (those that do and do not fulfill the norms of explanation already sketched) can thus be diagnosed with tests of manipulability: Activities and interactions sustain manipulability relations. To rule out possible confounds, one must require, in addition, that X changes Y only via the influence of intervening on X. In particular, one must rule out the possibilities that I changes Y directly, that I changes a causal intermediate between X and Y, or that I is correlated with some other cause of Y (for many of the details required to make this suggestion fully explicit, see Woodward, 2003; as applied to neuroscience, see Craver, 2007, chap. 3). This view has the virtue of keeping the notion of activity close to the epistemic criteria by which causal claims are evaluated. The restrictions on allowable interventions are precisely those placed on good experiments for testing causal claims. Legitimate activities in mechanistic explanation include all those that pass this test.

This manipulationist view of causal relevance has the virtue of satisfying the foregoing assumptions about activities in neuroscience. First, one cannot typically change causes by intervening to change effects. As discussed, exercise has been shown to cause a phase shift in the free-run rhythm of the biological clock in many different organisms (Mistlberger and Skene, 2005). Altering an organism's exercise routine does bring about changes in the subsequent stages of the organism's cycle, but the reverse does not hold. Intervening to induce a phase shift in the organism's clock does not alter the earlier exercise (although it will alter when the animal exercises in the future). Temporal sequences are explanatory only when it is possible to wiggle one stage of the mechanism by wiggling another. Exercise meets the manipulability criterion because changes in exercise alter preestablished rhythms. Variations in exercise intensity and duration further modulate the circadian response, suggesting an intricate relation of manipulability between these two variables (Buxton, Lee, L'Hermite-Baleriaux, Turek, and Van Cauter, 2003). The entraining activities of exercise thus robustly satisfy the manipulability criterion.

Third, correlations are explanatory only when one can change one correlate by intervening to change the other. Piéron's (1913) hypothesized relation between toxins in CSF and the sleep–wake cycle was shown to be a mere correlation because manipulations of the former were only relevant when accompanied by the onset of hypothermia in the organism (via pressure in the spinal column from the injection). Piéron's experiment violates the requirement that the intervention on X should not change Y directly. His manipulation itself caused the change in the outcome variable, giving misleading vindication to his hypothesized chemical mechanism. Failure to establish a more precise relation of manipulability between chemicals and rhythmicity prohibited Piéron's hypothesis from featuring in a complete explanation of biological clocks. Of course, it is no simple matter to identify possible confounds and to devise experiments that avoid them. Real causal relationships are revealed in appropriately controlled experiments.

Fourth, one cannot intervene into causally irrelevant factors to produce a change in the effect. As shown through Pittendrigh's (1954) classic experiments, changing the temperature at which *Drosophila* larvae are incubated does not alter their hatching schedule. The organism's rhythm is resistant to temperature change. The failure of temperature to satisfy this manipulability relation means that within a normal environmental range, temperature plays no entraining role in explanations of circadian rhythmicity in *Drosophila*.

Finally, low-probability effects can be explained when it is possible to change the probability of the effect by manipulating the cause. Varying the proximity of SCN cells should change the extent to which their oscillations are in phase. Through such manipulations, the mechanism by which single oscillations synchronize to create a central oscillator can be understood.

These norms of explanation are exhibited by the case of circadian rhythms and, indeed, by all other explanations in neuroscience with which we are familiar. These norms are taught through examples in contemporary neuroscience classes, they are used to design experiments, and they are implicitly invoked in the assessment of grant proposals and research reports. Mechanistic explanations satisfy these core norms on adequate explanations. Explanations that satisfy these constraints are, by definition, potentially useful for the purposes of manipulation and control. If one demands that explanations serve this end, one should demand that explanations describe mechanisms.

2.4. Organization

An adequate mechanistic explanation also shows how the entities and activities in a mechanism are organized spatially, temporally, and actively such that they exhibit the phenomenon to be explained. Spatial organization includes the locations, sizes, shapes, and orientations of component entities. Temporal organization includes the order, rate, and duration of the steps. Active organization includes the diverse inter-actions of the components in the mechanism. We consider these forms of organiza-tion in turn.

Location and connection are crucial aspects of spatial organization. The mam-malian biological clock is housed in the SCN, directly above the optic chiasm. Given the wide amount of converging evidence on the nature and function of the SCN, the clock is one of the strongest cases for functional localization in the entire brain (Herzog and Schwartz, 2002). The SCN has two subdivisions: The ventrolat-eral SCN receives information from the retinohypothalamic tract directly, and the dorsomedial SCN section receives input from the thalamus (Van den Pol, 1991). Environmental light information reaches the SCN via the retinohypothalamic tract (Hendrickson et al., 1972; Moore and Lenn, 1972). This is how the circadian clock receives (at least some of) its information regarding environmental time, which it then uses to synchronize the organism's internal clock with the surrounding envi-ronment.[9] Most synaptic connections from SCN cells are intrinsic and there are no direct connections between the SCN and motor pathways. From this, one can infer that the clock's regulation of behavior is largely indirect. To trace the location and points of contact between components of the mechanism is to reveal the spatially continuous structure that sustains the productive relations between stages of the mechanism.

Often, the connections between stages depend crucially on the structures of the entities in the mechanism and on those structured entities being oriented with respect to one another in particular ways. By detailing spatial constraints, anato-mists, protein chemists, and other scientists concerned with regular and persistent structures contribute to the study of neural mechanisms. Learning about the loca-tion of and connections between a mechanism's components often allows one to trace productive relationships through the mechanism. For example, the proximity of the SCN to the pineal gland, and the known anatomical connections between these two structures, helped establish the relation between circadian rhythmicity and melatonin release (Ralph and Lynch, 1970). Likewise, discovery of the retino-hypothalamic tract established the predominant route by which light entrains the oscillations of the SCN (Moore and Eichler, 1972).

Size, shape, and orientation are also important aspects of a mechanism. The parvocellular neurons that comprise the SCN are some of the smallest in the entire brain. In the rat, the average SCN cell has an area of $84\,\mu m^2$. Furthermore, these cells are densely packed: There are approximately 16,000 in the paired SCN of a rat (Van den Pol, 1980). The neurons of the SCN are organized into chains, with an average of only 15 to 20 nm of extracellular space between them. The chains run parallel to one another in a rostrocaudal direction (Van den Pol, 1991). These chains are held together by a neural cell adhesion molecule that is necessary for synchronizing the oscillations of individual neurons (Alvarez, 2004; Prosser, Rutishauser, Ungers, Fedorkova, and Glass, 2003). Thus, this tightly packed spatial organization of cells in the SCN is thought to be essential to its function as the organism's central oscillator.[10] The proximity of neurons increases the probability that these chains of cells will fire together. Changes in the ion concentration in the extracellular fluid around an SCN neuron are likely to influence several other neurons that share this extracellular fluid. Thus, changes in the membrane potential of one neuron are likely to be related with changes of the membrane potential in several surrounding neurons. Once a neuron's cell membrane is sufficiently depolarized (typically $-60\,mV$), an action potential begins. Thus, the shared extracellular space makes it probable that many cells in a row will experience sufficient depolarization and initiate action potentials simultaneously. This synchronized firing allows for synchronized oscillations. The convergence of multiple cellular oscillators to create a central oscillator is thought to make the circadian rhythm both precise and robust (Enright, 1980). As this example shows, learning about the shape and orientation of components in a mechanism further restricts the space of possible mechanisms for a given phenomenon.

Temporal constraints are also often crucial for a mechanism to work. The stages of mechanisms have a productive order from beginning to end, with earlier stages giving rise to later stages. The stages of mechanisms also have characteristic rates and durations that can be crucial to their operation. Because the biological clock is a time-keeping mechanism, issues of order, rate, duration, and frequency are of particular importance to keeping the clock in synchrony with its environment. Furthermore, the biological clock is a cyclical mechanism: Earlier stages give rise to later stages, which in turn reactivate the earlier stages in a continual feedback loop. These oscillations in individual SCN neurons synchronize to establish the precision of the organism's rhythm.

There are thus (at least) two levels of temporal organization in the mammalian biological clock. First, there are the temporal interactions involved in the positive and negative feedback loops of each individual SCN neuron. Second, there is the generation of one circadian time from the compilation of these individual oscillations. Understanding each of these levels of temporal organization is critical to a complete explanation of the mammalian clock mechanism. At the lower level, the negative and positive loops interchange, running for approximately 12 hours each and reaching their peaks at opposing times of day. The precise periods of expression for each of the involved clock genes are discovered through observations of mutants in aperiodic environments.[11]

At a higher level of organization, the SCN generates oscillations that are the average of these individual feedback loops. This averaging yields an incredibly precise mechanism. In the absence of environmental cues, there is less than 2 percent deviation in daily activity onset in rodents (Daan and Oklejewicz, 2003). However, there is a great deal of variability in the oscillation rates of individual neurons. Studies have revealed period deviations of up to 1.1 hours between SCN neurons measured in vitro. When the SCN explants are measured as a whole, there is less than 0.1 hour of variation (Herzog, Aton, Numano, Sakaki, and Tei, 2004). The mechanism for this averaging is not currently known. Discovering that mechanism, however, will involve calibrating temporal constraints across at least these two levels of organization.

These spatial and temporal aspects of the organization of mechanisms trace the productive relationships among the component stages—the relationship of giving rise to, driving, making, allowing, inhibiting, and preventing its successor. In this sense, mechanisms exhibit productive continuity from setup to termination. The discovery of mechanisms is often driven by the goal of eliminating gaps in the explanation of a mechanism's productive continuity.

2.5. Filler Terms and Mechanism Sketches

Models that describe mechanisms lie somewhere on the continuum between a mechanism sketch and an ideally complete description of the mechanism. By filling in the organizational features and satisfying the above constrains, one makes progress in turning sketches into ideally complete descriptions.

A *mechanism sketch* is an incomplete model of a mechanism. It characterizes some parts, activities, and features of the mechanism's organization, but it has gaps. Sometimes gaps are marked in visual diagrams by black boxes or question marks. More problematically, sometimes they are masked by *filler terms*. Words such as *activate, cause, encode, inhibit, produce, process,* and *represent* are often used to indicate a kind of activity in a mechanism without providing any detail about how that activity is carried out. Black boxes, question marks, and acknowledged filler terms are innocuous when they stand as placeholders for future work or when it is possible to replace the filler term with some stock-in-trade property, entity, activity, or mechanism. In contrast, filler terms are barriers to progress when they veil failures of understanding.

Although much is presently understood about the mammalian biological clock, black boxes and filler terms remain. Earlier, the positive loop of SCN oscillation was described as beginning with the activation of *bmal1* transcription. *Activation* serves as a filler term here. The precise mechanism through which this clock gene is activated is presently unknown. By highlighting this as a gap in our present understanding of the clock mechanism (Van Gelder and Herzog, 2003), the limit on current understanding is recognized and the search for the cause of the activation continues. If the term activation is used to stand for "some process we know not what" and if the provisional status of that term is forgotten, then one has only an illusion of understanding.

At the other end of the continuum are *ideally complete descriptions of a mechanism*. Such models include all of the entities, properties, activities, and organizational features that are relevant to every aspect of the phenomenon to be explained. Few (if any) mechanistic models provide ideally complete descriptions of a mechanism. In fact, such descriptions would include so many potential factors that they would be unwieldy for the purposes of prediction and control and utterly unilluminating to human beings. As a consequence, models frequently drop details that are irrelevant in the conditions under which the model is to be used. Ideally complete mechanistic models are the causal-mechanical analog to Peter Railton's notion of an *ideal explanatory text* that includes all of the information relevant to the explanandum, even if no single human could possibly understand it in all its complexity. Further work remains to be done to adumbrate the diverse pragmatic factors that affect this selective process.

As with most mechanistic explanations, the explanation of circadian rhythmicity in humans and other organisms that is presently available is somewhere between a mechanism sketch and an ideally complete mechanistic explanation. One sign that an explanation is incomplete or inadequate is that it fails to account for the full range of phenomena associated with the behavior in question. Although the explanation of clock oscillation is largely complete, there are still questions about various parts of the mechanism. For example, the activator of *bmal1* transcription in the positive loop of the oscillator is currently unknown (Van Gelder and Herzog, 2003). The decrease in REV proteins is thought to be part of this process, but the mechanism through which these two activities interact has yet to be discovered. Additionally, there is currently no explanation of what makes a particular species diurnal and another nocturnal (Herzog and Schwartz, 2002). Species differ in whether light cues cause them to be active during light or dark periods. Whether this is a difference in the type of entrainment or in the clocks themselves remains an open question. Despite these present limitations in our understanding of circadian rhythmicity, there is a great deal that is understood about how these clock mechanisms work. This understanding will lead to answers to these questions, as well as the identification of other areas where further inquiry is needed.

2.6. From How-Possibly to How-Actually Models

One last normative requirement should be made explicit. In providing an explanation, one seeks to describe an actual, not merely possible, mechanism. The components described in the model should correspond to components in the mechanism. The discovery of a mechanism typically begins with a description of the phenomenon and a range of possible mechanisms that could account for it. Progress is made in the search for mechanisms by adding constraints to the space of possible mechanisms, excluding mechanisms that are inconsistent with these and directing attention toward those that fit with the known constraints.

Models vary considerably in their mechanistic plausibility. *How-possibly models* are purported explanations, but they are only loosely constrained conjectures about the mechanism that produces the explanandum phenomenon. They describe how a set of parts and activities might be organized such that they exhibit the explanandum phenomenon. One can have no idea if the conjectured parts exist and, if they do, whether they can engage in the activities attributed to them in the model. Some computer models are purely how-possibly models. For example, the entrainment of biological clocks to various light–dark cycles can be simulated by providing a computer program with the basic temporal properties of the mechanism (order, duration, rate). Such models can help generate hypotheses about how an organism would respond to various situations, particularly in cases where such situations are not practically or ethically possible (e.g., with humans). How-possibly models are often heuristically useful in constructing a space of possible mechanisms, but they are not adequate explanations. In saying this, we are saying not merely that the description must be true (or true enough) but that the model must correctly characterize the details of the mechanism. *How-actually models* describe real components, activities, and organizational features of the mechanism that in fact produces the phenomenon. They show how a mechanism works, not just how it might work. Models lacking such detail invariably fare worse than those containing such detail for purposes of manipulative control because greater knowledge of the underlying mechanism affords more possibilities for intervention.

Between how-possibly and ideal explanations lies a range of *how-plausibly* models that are more or less consistent with the known constraints on the components, their activities, and their organization. Again, how accurately a model must represent the details of the internal workings of a mechanism will depend on the purposes for which the model is being deployed. If one is trying to explain the phenomenon, however, it will not do merely to describe some mechanisms that could produce the phenomenon. One wants the model, in addition, to show how the phenomenon is in fact produced by the system in question.

Philosophers of the special sciences, such as Robert Cummins (1975, 1983), Daniel Dennett (1998), Bill Lycan (1989), and Herbert Simon (1969), emphasize that explanations often proceed by functional analysis, reverse engineering, homuncular explanation, and decomposition. One begins with a complex phenomenon and then shows how that phenomenon can be produced by teams of subsystems whose organized behavior accounts for the behavior of the system as a whole. The behavior of the subsystems can often be explained in turn by postulating the behavior of further subsubsystems, and so on. As a first-pass description of the nature of explanation in sciences such as cognitive neuroscience, physiology, and molecular biology, this is a helpful descriptive framework. However, these accounts have yet to be developed to the point that they can distinguish how-possibly from how-actually functional analysis, reverse engineering, and homuncular explanation. Cummins (1975, 1983) sometimes speaks as if any description of a sequence of steps between input and output will suffice to explain a phenomenon. In speaking this way, Cummins erases the distinction between how-possibly and how-actually. Other times, he insists that such descriptions must ultimately bottom out in descriptions of neurological mechanisms (Cummins, 2000). According to our view, constitutive explanations require descriptions of real mechanisms, not mere how-possibly posits.

2.7. Summary

The detail provided here offers only a sketch of the entities and activities of the circadian rhythm mechanism. But this sketch suffices to illustrate the primary features of mechanistic explanation. First, the biological clock is identified relative to the phenomenon of interest: the circadian rhythm. The clock contains entities and activities organized together such that they display this phenomenon. Entities are the parts of the mechanism. These parts include the SCN, the neurons that compose it, the neurotransmitters by which those neurons interact, the clock genes, and the proteins they produce. Entities have various properties in virtue of which they act and interact with one another. These interactions constitute the activities of the mechanism, such as the firing rates of the neurons of the SCN, the expression and repression of the clock genes, and the bindings and activations of the gene proteins. Activities are the causal elements of mechanistic explanation. Finally, a mechanistic explanation involves specification of how the entities and activities are organized— in terms of spatial, temporal, and active structure. Detailing the mechanism's organization allows one to understand how the entities and activities of the biological clock are united to exhibit the phenomenon of rhythmicity.

An adequate mechanistic explanation includes all and only the entities and activities relevant to the phenomenon to be explained. The explanation does not include fictional items (such as souls or entelechies) or mere as-if posits, no matter how useful they might be for the purposes of prediction or simulation. The components in mechanisms are real parts of the causal structure of the world. They have stable clusters of properties, can be detected with multiple causally independent techniques, and can be used for the purposes of intervention (by adding, deleting, or accelerating parts and activities). Explanations with entities and activities that satisfy these criteria are more useful for the purposes of manipulation and control than are explanations adverting to fictional or as-if posits.

3. Levels of Mechanisms

So far, we have focused most closely on describing aspects of the circadian clock mechanism at a given level. We have emphasized the molecular, gene-regulation elements among the cells of the SCN. But the mechanism of the circadian rhythm spans multiple levels of organization.[12] There are behaviors of organisms, activities of physiological systems, action potentials in neurons, and the molecular cascades of the clock genes. Although there is some question as to how many levels there are, one can identify roughly four levels of mechanisms in this explanation. At the top is the circadian rhythm phenomenon, both the periodicities in behavior and physiology, the entrainment of those rhythms in response to environmental cues, and various facts about how the system can break down. One level down, the mechanism for this phenomenon involves three subsystems: a biological clock, an entrainment mechanism, and a mechanism regulating the behavioral and physiological effects of the clock. Focusing on the first of these, the clock can be broken down into further levels of mechanisms. The SCN itself is an oscillator, the resonance of which sets the time of all other systems in the body (e.g., the olfactory bulb, Granados-Fuentes, Prolo, Abraham, and Herzog, 2004). The SCN oscillator is a conglomeration of the individual oscillators housed within each neuron of the SCN (for an intriguing discussion of levels of explanation in circadian clocks, see Dunlap, 1999). Explaining the genetic basis of the oscillations of each SCN neuron is an essential component in the explanation of periodic behavior, but such an explanation necessarily falls short of explaining the circadian system itself.

These phenomena exist at multiple levels in the mechanism. In levels of mechanisms, some component X's ϕ-ing is at a lower level than S's Ψ-ing when and only when X is part of S, ϕ is part of Ψ, and X and its ϕ-ing are components in the mechanism for S's Ψ-ing. The clock mechanism as a whole is at a higher level of mechanisms than the cells in the SCN, which in turn are at a higher level of mechanisms than the genetic regulatory mechanisms controlling protein synthesis in those cells. Levels of mechanisms should not be confused with levels of theory or levels of science because a single theory in neuroscience often describes multiple levels of mechanisms and because single fields of neuroscience (such as chronobiology, the study of biological rhythms) often do research that spans multiple levels of mechanisms. Nor should levels of mechanisms be confused with levels of size (which need not involve a part–whole relationship, as levels of mechanisms do by definition) or levels of causes (because levels of mechanisms, as a part–whole relation, cannot interact causally). Nor should levels of mechanisms be confused with levels of realization. In levels of realization, one compares two distinct properties of one and the same object: S's Ψ-ing might be said to be at a higher level of realization than S's ϕ-ing if S has Ψ in virtue of having ϕ (that is, there can be no difference in S's Ψ-ing without a difference in S's ϕ-ing). Thus, the clock being an organized set of activities among the entities in the clock mechanism realizes the property of maintaining the free-run rhythm. Levels of realization are not a part–whole relation but a necessitating relationship between two properties of one and the same thing.

The failure to distinguish levels of mechanisms from levels of realization has led some philosophers and scientists to worry that higher level phenomena in neuroscience and psychology are causally (and so explanatorily) superfluous. The argument (most forcefully stated by Kim, 1998, who draws a parallel distinction) is that all of the causal powers at higher levels are inherited from the causal powers at lower levels. If so, then it appears that higher level items have no causal powers over and above the lower level items, and one is thereby warranted in rejecting the idea that the higher level item has any causal powers over and above the lower level items. This argument does not apply to levels of mechanisms. Nobody should deny that parts organized together into a mechanism can do things that the parts individually cannot do. The positive and negative loops in the genetic regulatory mechanisms of the clock can keep time, but individual clock genes, such as *per* or *tim*, by themselves cannot. This should be uncontroversial (Kim says it is "obvious," and indeed it is). Metaphysical arguments for rejecting the importance of higher level causes and higher level explanations, though often repeated, simply do not apply to levels of mechanisms as we have defined them.[13]

Let us take the notion of levels of mechanisms as unproblematic and ask what it means to bridge levels in a hierarchy of mechanisms. In our view, bridging levels is a matter of showing that items at different levels are related as mechanism to component: by showing that X and its ϕ-ing are components in the mechanism for S's Ψ-ing.

Interlevel relations of this sort are tested with experimental strategies that are in many ways like those used to test for causal relationships within a mechanism (as discussed in section 2.4) except that they link phenomena, entities, and activities at different levels in a hierarchical mechanisms. Interlevel relationships are not causal relations—they involve a part–whole relation—but they nonetheless are evaluated with similar experimental stimuli. There are four possible genres of interlevel experiment. They differ from one another depending on whether the interventions are excitatory or inhibitory and on whether the structure of the experiment is bottom-up or top-down.

In bottom-up inhibitory experiments, one intervenes to inhibit or remove a part of the mechanism (or to suppress one of more of its activities) and then detects the consequences of that intervention on the behavior of a mechanism as a whole. Given the centrality of gene expression in the oscillatory loop, perhaps the best example of bottom-up inhibition is the use of knockout mice (mutant species lacking in one or more of the relevant clock genes). Deleting any of the three *period* genes (*mper1*, *mper2*, or *mper3*) causes the organism to experience a shorter circadian rhythm than wild types (Alvarez, 2004). As discussed earlier, *period* genes play a key role in both the positive and negative loops of mammalian oscillation. Activation of *per* genes marks the initiation of the negative loop. The CLK:BMAL1 protein dimers formed during the positive loop bind to promoter sites on *per*. Period mutants thus lack a key element of each loop, which results in the accelerated rate of cycling observed in these knockout mice. Each of the three *period* genes produces distinct changes when it is selectively removed. *Mper1* knockouts can maintain their periodicity in constant darkness, whereas *mper2* knockouts cannot. The precise role of *mper3* is currently unknown, although it is thought to have a role in regulating transcription of other clock genes by generating partial proteins (Alvarez, 2004).

In bottom-up excitatory experiments, one intervenes to excite or stimulate a part of a mechanism (or to engage one of its activities) and then detects the consequences of that intervention for the behavior of the mechanism as a whole. In vitro experiments have shown that electrical stimulation of the SCN can cause phase shifts in the clock's free-run rhythm (Rusak and Groos, 1982). Depending on where the stimulation was received in the cycle, the stimulation could move the clock forward or backward. If the stimulation was received during early (subjective) night, the rhythm phase-shifted backward; if the stimulation was received during late (subjective) night, the rhythm phase-shifted forward. The ability to stimulate the SCN even once it has been removed from the organism provides supplemental evidence that this nucleus does indeed house an endogenous clock mechanism.

In top-down excitatory experiments, one intervenes to excite or activate the behavior of the mechanism as a whole and then detects the effects of that intervention on the workings of the component parts. The experiments discussed earlier regarding the testing of exercise as a possible zeitgeber are examples of top-down experiments. One can intervene to change the behavior of the organism (in this case, wheel running in rats) and detect changes in the onset of the oscillations in the organism's clock. Increasing the intensity and duration of an organism's exercise routine can be used to measure subsequent phase shifts in the free-run rhythm of the organism's clock.

In top-down inhibitory experiments, one intervenes to inhibit or suppress the behavior of the mechanism as a whole and then detects the effects of that intervention on the workings of the component parts. An example of such an experiment is the common method of placing an organism into a permanently dark environment and detecting SCN activity, gene expression, or protein levels. One intervenes to remove a driving force for the mechanism as a whole and monitors how that intervention changes the behavior of the components.

These experiments suggest a sufficient condition for integrating levels of mechanism in neuroscience: X's ϕ-ing is integrated with (or is shown to be a component of) S's Ψ-ing when it is possible to manipulate S's Ψ-ing by manipulating X's ϕ-ing and when it is possible to manipulate X's ϕ-ing by manipulating S's Ψ-ing. This condition is not necessary, because there are experimental situations in which one would not be able to satisfy these conditions even though the component is in fact part of the mechanism. Nonetheless, this condition on interlevel integration articulates clear guidelines for assessing interlevel relations and establishing a relationship of componency between a part and a mechanism as a whole.

4. CONCLUSION

One may perhaps object that mechanistic explanation is far too simple to fully express the complexity of real explanations in neuroscience. The parts of neural mechanisms are so intimately and massively interconnected that one might think that they are no longer truly separable. Or perhaps one thinks that neuroscientific explanations require emergent properties that cannot be explained by decomposition into the parts, activities, and organizational features that constitute the mechanism. Although we have found no evidence for these claims in our efforts to characterize the mechanism of the circadian rhythm, we cannot, on the basis of a single case, exclude the possibility that they might be true of some neural mechanism. Our purpose has been to provide a view of mechanistic explanation by reference to which such claims can be made explicit and assessed.

One aspect of this example that warrants further exploration is the chimeric structure of this mechanistic explanation. Different aspects of the phenomenon have been investigated in different experimental organisms. The resulting structure is thus a hodgepodge of models derived from the study of organisms as distinct as flies, mice, and humans. Although the parts that comprise the clock mechanism vary widely from species to species, all biological clocks share formal properties (e.g., control of internal time through gene regulation). It is unclear to us that a single model from beginning to end can be given for any of these species. Nor is it likely that the chimera produced by combining these different components into a single system would be viable (let alone keep time). However, understanding the chimeric relation between the mechanisms of various experimental organisms broadens our understanding of rhythmicity as a whole and (presumably) aids inquiry into the mechanisms of other organisms that have yet to be investigated. This feature is not unique to the mechanistic explanation of the circadian rhythm but can be found throughout the biological sciences. Yet this aspect of mechanistic explanation must await fuller discussion in a separate publication.

NOTES

1. For a more complete defense and elaboration of this view of mechanisms, see Craver (2007).

2. In other organisms, the freerunning cycle can be anywhere from 16 to 32 hours. Bread mold, for example, can have a period of 19 hours in constant darkness, whereas rats can express a period of nearly 26 hours in constant light (Herzog, personal communication).

3. For a review of the views of Pittendrigh and Aschoff on entrainment, see Daan (2000).

4. It is possible that there is no central time keeper, or that there are many different time keepers that work independently. Given the evidence for a clock, and its regulation of all other time keepers, we leave these possibilities aside.

5. In this chapter, we follow the convention of referring to a gene itself by its abbreviation in italics and the protein expressed by the gene in all capital letters, for example, *per* and PER.

6. For an overview of the genes involved in various organisms, see Dunlap (1999).

7. This principle arguably has exceptions in certain domains of physics (see Price, 1996), but we know of no exceptions in neuroscience.

8. In stochastic cases, one should require that the intervention on X change the probability distribution over possible values of Y.

9. There is additional light information that reaches the SCN via indirect pathways through the intergeniculate leaflet of the lateral geniculate nucleus and the intergeniculate leaflet (Card and Moore, 1982; Pickard, 1985), as well as presumed further pathways through which additional zeitgebers reach and entrain the circadian clock.

10. There are many peripheral oscillators that exist in bodily tissues outside the brain. Although the rhythms in these peripheral systems are influenced by the SCN's oscillations, these tissue-specific oscillators are thought to exert local control on rhythmicity to meet the individualized needs of particular areas (Alvarez, 2004).

11. For a summary of regulation in mammalian clock genes, see Albrecht (2002). The activated display by Van Gelder and Herzog (2003) provides animation of this process where gene activity is synchronized with zeitgeber time.

12. For further defense of the view that mechanistic explanations of circadian rhythms span levels, see Bechtel and Abrahamsen (2008).

13. We leave aside the question of whether the problem holds for levels of realization, the argument's intended target.

REFERENCES

Albrecht, U. (2002). Invited review: Regulation of mammalian circadian clock genes. *Journal of Applied Physiology* 92: 1348–1355.

Alvarez, J. D. (2004). Genetic basis for circadian rhythms in mammals. In A. Sehgal (Ed.), *Molecular Biology of Circadian Rhythms*. Hoboken, N.J.: Wiley-Liss, 93–140.

Aschoff, J. (1960). Exogenous and endogenous components in circadian rhythms. *Cold Springs Harbor Symposium on Quantitative Biology* 25: 11–28.

Aschoff, J. (1981). Freerunning and entrained circadian rhythms. In J. Aschoff (Ed.), *The Handbook of Behavioral Neurobiology, vol. 4: Biological Rhythms*. New York: Plenum Press, 81–93.

Axelrod, J., Wurtman, R. J., and Snyder, S. H. (1965). Control of hydroxyindole O-methyltransferase activity in the rat pineal gland by environmental lighting. *Journal of Biological Chemistry* 240: 949–954.

Bechtel, W. (2005). *Discovering Cell Mechanisms: The Creation of Modern Cell Biology*. Cambridge: Cambridge University Press.

Bechtel, W., and Abrahamsen, A. (2008). From reduction back to higher levels. In B. C. Love, K. McRae, and V. M. (Eds.), *Proceedings of the 30th Annual Conference of the Cognitive Science Society*. Austin, Tex.: Cognitive Science Society, 559–564.

Bechtel, W., and Richardson, R. C. (1993). *Discovering Complexity: Decomposition and Localization as Strategies in Scientific Research*. Princeton, N.J.: Princeton University Press.

Buxton, O. M., Lee, C. W., L'Hermite-Baleriaux, M., Turek, F. W., and Van Cauter, E. (2003). Exercise elicits phase shifts and acute alterations of melatonin that vary with circadian phase. *American Journal of Regulatory, Integrative, and Comparative Physiology* 284: R714–R724.

Card, J. P., and Moore, R. Y. (1982). Ventral lateral geniculate nucleus efferents to the rat suprachiasmatic nucleus exhibit avian pancreatic polypeptide-like immunoreactivity. *Journal of Comparative Neurology* 206: 390–396.

Craver, C. F. (2007). *Explaining the Brain: Mechanisms and the Mosaic Unity of Neuroscience*. Oxford: Oxford University Press.

Cummins, R. (1975). Functional analysis. *Journal of Philosophy* 72: 741–764.

Cummins, R. (1983). *The Nature of Psychological Explanation*. Cambridge, Mass.: Bradford/MIT Press.

Cummins, R. (2000). How does it work? Vs. what are the laws? Two conceptions of psychological explanation. In F. Keil and R. Wilson (Eds.), *Explanation and Cognition*. Cambridge, Mass.: MIT Press, 117–145.

Daan, S. (2000). Colin Pittendrigh, Jurgen Aschoff, and the natural entrainment of circadian systems. *Journal of Biological Rhythms* 15: 195–207.

Daan, S., and Oklejewicz, M. (2003). The precision of circadian clocks: Assessment and analysis in Syrian hamsters. *Chronobiology International* 20: 209–221.

Darden, L. (2006). *Reasoning in Biological Discoveries*. Cambridge: Cambridge University Press.

Dennett, D. (1998). Cognitive science as reverse engineering: Several meanings of "top-down" and "bottom-up." In *Brainchildren: Essays on Designing Minds*. Cambridge, Mass.: MIT Press, 249–260.

Dunlap, J. C. (1999). Molecular bases for circadian clocks. *Cell* 96: 271–290.

Enright, J. T. (1980). Temporal precision in circadian systems: A reliable neuronal clock from unreliable components? *Science* 209: 1542–1545.

Granados-Fuentes, D., Prolo, L. M., Abraham, U., and Herzog, E. D. (2004). The suprachiasmatic nucleus entrains, but does not sustain, circadian rhythmicity in the olfactory bulb. *Journal of Neuroscience* 24: 615–619.

Hastings, M. H., and Herbert, J. (1986). Neurotoxic lesions of the paraventricular-spinal projection block the nocturnal rise in pineal melatonin synthesis in the Syrian hamster. *Neuroscience Letters* 69: 1–6.

Hendrickson, A. E., Wagoner, N., and Cowan, W. M. (1972). An autoradiographic and electron microscopic study of retino-hypothalamic connections. *Zellforschungen* 135: 1–26.

Herzog, E. D., Aton, S. J., Numano, R., Sakaki, Y., and Tei, H. (2004). Temporal precision in the mammalian circadian system: A reliable clock from less reliable neurons. *Journal of Biological Rhythms* 19: 35–46.

Herzog, E. D., and Schwartz, W. J. (2002). Invited review: A neural clockwork for encoding circadian time. *Journal of Applied Physiology* 92: 401–408.

Illernová, H. (1991). The suprachiasmatic nucleus and rhythmic pineal melatonin production. In D. C. Klein, R. Y. Moore, and S. M. Reppert (Eds.), *Suprachiasmatic Nucleus: The Mind's Clock*. Oxford: Oxford University Press, 197–216.

Ishigaki, H., Miyao, M., and Ishihara, S. (1991). Change of pupil size as a function of exercise. *Journal of Human Ergology* 20: 61–66.

Johnson, C. H., Elliott, J. A., and Foster, R. (2003). Entrainment of circadian programs. *Chronobiology International* 20: 741–774.

Kandel, E. R., and Schwartz, J. H. (1981). *Principles of Neural Science*. New York: Elsevier.

Kim, J. (1998). *Mind in a Physical World*. Cambridge, Mass.: MIT Press.

Klein, D. C., and Moore, R. Y. (1979). Pineal N-acetyltransferase and hydroxy-indole-O-methyl-transferase: Control by the retinohypothalamic tract and the suprachiasmatic nucleus. *Brain Research* 174: 245–262.

Kleitman, N. (1963). *Sleep and Wakefulness*, rev. ed. Chicago: University of Chicago Press.

Konopka, R. J., and Benzer, S. (1971). Clock mutants of *Drosophila melanogaster*. *Proceedings of the National Academy of Sciences USA* 68: 2112–2116.

Lycan, W. (1999). The continuity of levels of nature. In W. Lycan (Ed.), *Mind and Cognition: A Reader*, 2nd ed. Malden, Mass.: Blackwell.

Machamer, P. K., Darden, L., and Craver, C. F. (2000). Thinking about mechanisms. *Philosophy of Science* 57: 1–25.

McClung, C. R., Fox, B. A., and Dunlap, J. C. (1989). The *Neurospora* clock gene *frequency* shares a sequence element with the *Drosophila* clock gene *period*. *Nature* 33: 558–562.

McNamara, P. (2004). Hormonal rhythms. In A. Sehgal (Ed.), *Molecular Biology of Circadian Rhythms*. Hoboken, N.J.: Wiley-Liss, 231–253.

Mistlberger, R. E., and Skene, D. J. (2004). Social influences on mammalian circadian rhythms: Animal and human studies. *Biological Review* 79: 533–556.

Mistlberger, R. E., and Skene, D. J. (2005). Nonphotic entrainment in humans? *Journal of Biological Rhythms* 20: 339–352.

Moore, R. Y., and Eichler, V. B. (1972). Loss of circadian adrenal corticosterone rhythm following suprachiasmatic lesions in the rat. *Brain Research* 120: 167–172.

Moore, R. Y., and Klein, D. C. (1974). Visual pathways and the central neural control of a circadian rhythm in pineal serotonin N-acetyltransferase activity. *Brain Research* 71: 17–33.

Moore, R. Y., and Lenn, N. J. (1972). A retinohypothalamic projection in the rat. *Journal of Comparative Neurology* 146: 1–14.

Moore, R. Y., Speh, J. C., and Card, J. P. (1995). The retinohypothalamic tract originated from a distinct subset of retinal ganglion cells. *Journal of Comparative Neurology* 352: 351–366.

Myers, M. P., Wager-Smith, K., Wesley, C. S., Young, M. W., and Sehgal, A. (1995). Positional cloning and sequence analysis of the *Drosophila* clock gene *timeless*. *Science* 270: 805–808.

Pickard, G. E. (1985). Bifurcating axons of retinal ganglion cells terminate in the hypothalamic suprachiasmatic nucleus and the intergeniculate leaflet of the thalamus. *Neuroscience Letters* 55: 211–217.

Piéron, H. T. (1913). *Le probleme physiologique du Sommeil*. Paris: Masson.

Pittendrigh, C. S. (1954). On temperature independence in the clock system controlling emergence time in *Drosophila*. *Proceedings of the National Academy of Sciences USA* 40: 1018–1029.

Pittendrigh, C. S. (1981). Circadian systems: entrainment. In J. Aschoff (Ed.), *The Handbook of Behavioral Neurobiology, vol. 4: Biological Rhythms*. New York: Plenum Press, 95–124.

Pittendrigh, C. S., Bruce, V., and Kaus, P. (1958). On the significance of transients in daily rhythms. *Proceedings of the National Academy of Sciences USA* 44: 965–973.

Poulson, T. L., and White, W. B. (1969). The cave environment. *Science* 105: 971–981.

Price, H. (1996). *Time's Arrow and Archimedes' Point*. Oxford: Oxford University Press.

Prosser, R. A. (2000). Serotonergic actions and interactions on the SCN circadian pacemaker: In vitro investigations. *Biological Rhythms Research* 31: 315–339.

Prosser, R. A., Rutishauser, U., Ungers, G., Fedorkova, L., and Glass, J. D. (2003). Intrinsic role of polysialylated neural cell adhesion molecule in photic phase resetting of the mammalian circadian clock. *Journal of Neuroscience* 23: 652–658.

Ralph, C. L., and Lynch, H. J. (1970). A quantitative melatonin bioassay. *General Comparative Endocrinology* 15: 334–338.

Reddy, P., Zehring, W. A., Wheeler, D. A., Pirrotta, V., Hadfield, C., Hall, J. C., et al. (1984). Molecular analysis of the *period* locus in *Drosophila melanogaster* and identification of a transcript involved in biological rhythms. *Cell* 38: 701–710.

Rusak, B., and Groos, G. (1982). Suprachiasmatic stimulation phase shifts rodent circadian rhythms. *Science* 215: 1407–1409.

Rusak, B., and Zucker, I. (1979). Neural control of circadian rhythms. *Physiology Review* 59: 449–526.

Sack, R. L., Lewy A. J., and Hoban, T. M. (1987). Free-running melatonin rhythms in blind people: Phase shifts with melatonin and triazolam administration. In L. Rensing,

U. Van der Heiden, and M. C. Mackey (Eds.), *Temporal Disorder in Human Oscillatory Systems*. Heidelberg: Springer-Verlag, 219–224.

Salmon, W. (1984). *Scientific Explanation and the Causal Structure of the World*. Princeton, N.J.: Princeton University Press.

Schnedorf, J. G., and Ivy, C. (1939). An examination of the hypnotoxin theory of sleep. *American Journal of Physiology* 125: 491–505.

Siffre, M. (1964). *Beyond Time*. New York: McGraw-Hill.

Simon, H. (1969). *The Sciences of the Artificial*. Cambridge, Mass.: MIT Press.

Stephan, F. K., and Zucker, I. (1972). Circadian rhythms in drinking behavior and locomotor activity of rats are eliminated by hypothalamic lesions. *Proceedings of the National Academy of Sciences USA* 69: 1583–1586.

van den Pol, A. N. (1980). The hypothalamic suprachiasmatic nucleus of the rat: Intrinsic anatomy. *Journal of Comparative Neurology* 191: 661–702.

van den Pol, A. N. (1991). The suprachiasmatic nucleus: Morphological, and cytochemical substrates for cellular interaction. In D. C. Klein, R. Y. Moore, and S. M. Reppert (Eds.), *Suprachiasmatic Nucleus: The Mind's Clock*. Oxford: Oxford University Press, 17–50.

Van Dongen, H. P. A., Kerkhof, G. A., and Dinges, D. F. (2004). Human circadian rhythms. In A. Sehgal (Ed.), *Molecular Biology of Circadian Rhythms*. Hoboken, N.J.: Wiley-Liss, 255–269.

Van Gelder, R. N., and Herzog, E. D. (2003). Oscillatory mechanisms underlying the murine circadian clock. *Science, STKE* 209: tr7.

Watts, A. G., Swanson, L. W., and Sanchez-Watts, G. (1987). Efferent projections of the suprachiasmatic nucleus: Studies using anterograde transport of Phaseolus vulgaris leucoagglutinin in the rat. *Journal of Comparative Neurology* 258: 204–229.

Woodward, J. (2003). *Making Things Happen: A Theory of Causal Explanation*. Oxford: Oxford University Press.

Wurtman, R. J., Axelrod, J., and Kelly, D. E. (1968). *The Pineal*. New York: Academic Press.

CHAPTER 3

METHODOLOGY AND REDUCTION IN THE BEHAVIORAL NEUROSCIENCES: OBJECT EXPLORATION AS A CASE STUDY

ANTHONY CHEMERO AND CHARLES HEYSER

1. INTRODUCTION

Before Ian Hacking's *Representing and Intervening* (1983) philosophers of science focused almost exclusively on scientific theories. The lasting impact of Hacking's book is that scientific experimental practices have also been shown to be of philosophical interest. One point Hacking made, on which no one seems to have followed up, is that the goal of laboratory experiments is the production of *effects*, reliably statistically significant changes in some (dependent) variable that result from experimenter manipulation of some other (independent) variable. Effects, Hacking points out, often survive changes in the theories that explain them. We can see this in the behavioral and neural sciences: Methodologies that reliably produce effects are often reused hundreds, even thousands of times by researchers with widely divergent theoretical outlooks. Consider as examples the operant conditioning chamber, a.k.a. the Skinner box, and the Morris water maze. This chapter focuses on a similar, widely used methodological innovation: object exploration procedures for rodents. Since being introduced in its current form in a 1988 paper by Enna-ceur and Delacour, this methodology has been used in hundreds of experiments to explore how drugs and gene manipulations (among others) affect recognition memory in rodents. By looking carefully at the object exploration methodology and reporting a few of our own experiments with it, we show that although it does reliably produce statistically significant effects, it is not clear that these effects result from the manipulations (of genes, neurotransmitter systems) that the experiment-ers single out as the independent measure. This leads us to argue that, in general, the psychological and cognitive sciences are not plausibly reducible to neuroscience. We also argue that the assumption that the higher level behavioral sciences are reduc-ible to neuroscience leads neuroscientists to perform flawed experiments. There are, that is, two reasons not to believe in reductionism: It is probably not true, and believing it can make you a bad scientist. Or so we will argue.

We proceed as follows. In section 2, we provide a very brief description of reduction and reductionism. This will serve as necessary background for the claims we will make later in sections 5 and 6. In section 3, we describe the object explora-tion methodology as it is used in behavioral neuroscience, behavioral genetics, and psychopharmacology. As part of this description, we discuss the results of a review of the literature on object exploration, first described in Chemero and Heyser (2005). The literature review shows that researchers are surprisingly careless concerning the nature of the objects they select to be explored in their experiments. These neuro-scientist are careless, we think, because they are acting like reductionists. In section 4, we discuss three of a series of experiments that we and our collaborators have done using the object exploration methodology. These experiments show that the affordances of the to-be-explored objects affect the way rodents explore objects. In section 5, we argue for some methodological conclusions. Most important, we argue that neuroscientists, even those who focus their research on genes or neurotrans-mitter effects, must attend closely to the details of behavior. In section 6, we draw some philosophical conclusions regarding psychoneural reduction. In particular, we argue that because affordances, which are features of extended brain–body–environment systems, affect the way rodents explore objects, one cannot account for the behavior of these rodents by focusing solely on their brains. That is, rodent psychology cannot be reduced to rodent neuroscience. We believe this generalizes to other mammals.

2. REDUCTIONISM AND REDUCTION

To make the claims we eventually make, we need to say something about the nature of reduction and reductionism. Because the world does not suffer a lack of writing on this topic, and because it is discussed in every introductory course in philosophy of science or mind, we are brief. (For a more thorough, but still brief overview, see Silberstein, 2002.) The word *reductionism* as it is commonly used refers to an amalgam of two views, an ontological thesis and an epistemological thesis. The ontological thesis, commonly discussed in the philosophy of mind, is the claim that entities or processes of one kind are identical to, supervene on, or are exhaustively causally determined by entities or processes of some other kind. For the purposes of the debate in question here, the reduced entities or processes are psychological, and the reducing entities or processes are neurological. We'll call this thesis "ontological reductionism." Ontological reductionism is one possible position in the venerable mind–body problem. The epistemological thesis, commonly discussed by philosophers of science, is the claim that the laws, generalizations, and regularities of one science can be accounted for by the laws, generalizations, and regularities of some other science, along with bridge principles. For the current purposes, the question is whether laws, generalizations, and regularities of psychology will be accountable in terms of the laws, generalizations, and regularities of neuroscience, along with bridge principles. We'll call the epistemological version of reductionism "intertheoretic reduction." Although for the most part we will be concerned with intertheoretic reductionism, we believe that the truth or falsity of intertheoretic reduction is the main kind of evidence one could offer for the truth or falsity of ontological reductionism; perhaps it is the only kind of evidence.

The classic formulation of intertheoretic reduction is Nagel (1961). Although Nagel's formulation was inspired by now unpopular positivist principles and has been subject to many modifications in the intervening years, it still forms the basis for most discussions of intertheoretic reduction. In Nagel's view, and subsequent modifications (e.g., Hooker, 1981a, 1981b, 1981c; P.M. Churchland, 1985, 1989; P.S. Churchland, 1986), a comparatively specific reduced theory has its laws, generalizations, and regularities accounted for in a comparatively general reducing or base theory. There is a range of ways the base theory might account for the subject matter of the reducing theory (Churchland and Churchland, 1990). In the ideal case, the reduced theory is simply *subsumed* by the more general base theory: The reduced theory is still taken to be true, but a special case of the base theory. For example, Newton's three laws of motion can be used, along with a few auxiliary assumptions, to derive Kepler's laws of planetary motion. Kepler's laws are simply a special case of Newton's more general theory. At the other end of the spectrum, the base theory might *falsify* the reduced theory. The base theory, that is, might account for the facts and generalizations of the less general theory in a way that shows the latter to be false. For example, Lavoisier's theory of combustion as oxidation showed the prior view of combustion as the release of immaterial phlogiston to be false. Most cases of intertheoretic reduction discussed in the literature (Newtonian physics to Einsteinian physics; classical thermodynamics to statistical mechanics) fall somewhere between simple subsumption and outright falsification.

In the cognitive and neural sciences, Paul and Patricia Churchland famously expect that folk psychology will be replaced and shown to be wildly false by future research in cognitive neuroscience. The Churchlands believe that the relationship between scientific psychology and cognitive neuroscience will be something more like subsumption. Ontologically speaking, they are eliminative materialists about folk psychology and reductionists about scientific psychology. Bickle (2003) has argued that the subsumption of scientific psychology will be by molecular and genetic neuroscience, bypassing cognitive neuroscience entirely. Because of this bypass, Bickle calls himself a *ruthless reductionist* and argues, ontologically speaking, for "mind to molecule reductionism."

The final point we wish to make here concerns the relationship between reductionism about psychology and recent work often collected under the umbrella phrase "extended cognition" (Chemero, 2009; Clark, 1997; Gibson, 1979; Hutchins, 1995; McClamrock, 1995; Thompson, 2007; Turvey, Shaw, Reed, and Mace, 1981; Varela, Thompson, and Rosch, 1991; Warren, 1984; Wilson, 2004). According to extended cognition, the cognitive system extends beyond the skin of the cognizer and includes portions of the environment. Correspondingly, extended cognitive science is the study of the combined brain–body–environment system, typically modeled using nonlinearly coupled differential equations (Beer, 1995, 1999; Chemero and Silberstein, 2008; Kelso, 1995; Kelso and Engstrom, 2006; Kugler and Turvey, 1987; Oullier, de Guzman, Jantzen, Lagarde, and Kelso, 2005). Although it may be obvious, it is worth stressing that extended cognition is incompatible with reductionism of either type. Ontologically, if cognitive systems are extended and include aspects of the environment, they cannot be identical to or supervene on anything strictly neural; brains are only proper parts of cognitive systems. Epistemologically, if extended cognitive science is an important component of scientific psychology, then neuroscience cannot subsume or replace scientific psychology. Because extended cognitive science consists in laws, generalizations, and regularities concerning brain–body–environment systems, neuroscience is not appropriate as a base theory. Neither cognitive neuroscience, which describes the computational properties of brain areas, nor molecular neuroscience, which describes chemical and genetic effects on neurons and synapses, is more general than extended cognitive science. The remainder of this chapter constitutes an empirical argument that cognition is extended and, hence, that reductionism is false in general. We make this case by showing that for at least one experimental methodology widely used in the neurosciences, one can only succeed experimentally by taking cognitive systems to be extended. That is, taking cognitive systems to be extended and therefore not reducible is required for successful neuroscience. The experimental methodology in question is object exploration. We now turn to that.

3. THE OBJECT EXPLORATION METHODOLOGY IN THE NEUROSCIENCES

Object exploration is an increasingly popular experimental paradigm in behavioral neuroscience. This task is appealing because there is no explicit need for food or water restriction, and several behavioral endpoints can be obtained rapidly, including general activity, reactivity to novelty, and learning. In addition, the task is fairly rapid, taking only 1–3 days to complete, providing a model system for high-throughput behavioral analysis in many different species including (but not limited to) mice (Sik, van Nieuwehuyzen, Prickaerts, and Blokland, 2003), rats (Berlyne, 1950; Ennaceur and Delacour, 1988), hamsters (Thinus-Blanc, Durup, and Poucet, 1992), dogs (Callahan, Ikeda-Douglas, Head, Cotman, and Milgram, 2000), ravens (Stowe et al., 2006), horses (Visser et al., 2002), rainbow trout (Sneddon, Braithwaite, and Gentle, 2003), parrots (Mettke-Hofmann, Winkler, and Leislser, 2002), and monkeys (Kim, Chae, Lee, Yang, and Shin, 2005; Zola-Morgan, Babrowska, Moss, and Mahut, 1983). The cross-species comparative nature of this task may be one of its strongest features. In general, animals are exposed to various objects for a certain amount of time, and their behavioral responses to the presentation of these stimuli are recorded for the duration of the trial. These initial exposures can be used to assess the organism's reactivity to novelty. In subsequent trials, objects can either be moved to a new location (spatial rearrangement), or a familiar object can be replaced with a novel object (substitution). During these exposures, one can continue to examine the animal's reactivity to novel change and memory (i.e., recognition memory). The basic premise is (1) animals will explore novel objects, (2) repeated exposure to the objects will result in decreased exploration (habituation), and (3) a change in spatial orientation (rearrangement) or object (substitution) will result in dishabituation of the previously habituated exploratory behavior. The resulting dishabituation will be expressed as a preferential exploration of the novel feature (spatial or object) relative to familiar features in the environment (i.e., recognition memory). The reliability of this habituation/dishabituation effect and the inference it licenses concerning recognition memory makes object exploration an attractive research methodology, especially if one wants to determine how some drug, gene, or lesion impacts memory.

One of the first papers to use this paradigm was by Berlyne (1950) using adult male Wistar rats. A more recent paper by Ennaceur and Delacour (1988) brought this paradigm to the attention of those in the behavioral neurosciences. Since then, various forms of the object exploration task have been used to examine the effects of drug exposure (e.g., Heyser, Pelletier, and Ferris, 2004; O'Shea, McGregor, and Mallet, 2006), genetic manipulations (e.g., Bourtchouladze et al., 2003; Ventura, Pascucci, Catania, Musumeci, and Puglisi-Allegra, 2004), and neurobiology (e.g., Aggleton, Blindt, and Rawlins, 1999; Ainge et al., 2006; Bussey, Saksida, and Murray, 2003; Lee, Hunsaker, and Kesner, 2005; Lee et al., 2006; Norman and Eacott, 2004; Save, Poucet, Foreman, and Buhot, 1992). Studies into the neurobiology of object recognition using the substitution paradigm have concluded that the perirhinal cortex is critical for performance on this task. The results of these experiments have been used to challenge the traditional theories of the medial temporal lobe memory systems in which the hippocampus, perirhinal, entorhinal, and parahippocampal cortices are exclusively involved in consolidating declarative memories (see Buckley and Gaffan, 2006, for a review).

Despite the priority of the Berlyne paper (1950), the interest in object exploration in the behavioral neurosciences is due largely to the later publication by Ennaceur and Delacour (1988). By June 2007, that paper had been cited at least 322 times (according to ISI Web of Science). Surprisingly, for a publication that is a methodological touchstone, Ennaceur and Delacour (1988) say only this about the objects used in the experiments: "The objects to be discriminated were made of glass, plastic or metal and existed in duplicate. Their weight was such that they could not be displaced by rats" (p. 48). This description of the objects is repeated verbatim (or nearly verbatim) in many of the object exploration studies done by Ennaceur (and various colleagues), one or more of which is cited by every object exploration study we have encountered. This sparse description of the to-be-explored objects provides very little guidance to those who want to use this methodology. Furthermore, this appears to show a lack of interest in the actual stimulus as if their selection was without consequences and only the details of the behavior of the animals were important, when in fact, the nature of the objects used in these studies may be critical to the behavior observed (i.e., initial exploration, response to novelty, and recognition memory). Casual observation and common sense suggest that different sorts of nondisplaceable, glass, plastic, or metal objects will be explored differently. For example, put a 2-year-old human in a room with a nondisplaceable, black metal cube and a nondisplaceable, brightly painted, plastic bunny. Or, more to the point for current purposes, put her in a room with one red plastic cube that she can climb on (and jump off of) and a red plastic cube that she cannot climb on. In this latter case especially, the to-be-explored objects have different affordances, leading to potentially *qualitatively* and *quantitatively* different exploratory behaviors (Renner and Rosenzweig, 1986).

One way to put the concern is to say that it seems obvious that the *affordances* of the to-be-explored objects might affect how objects are explored in these experiments. Affordances (Gibson, 1979) are opportunities for action by animals in the environment. In particular, affordances for particular activities are present when the relations among an animal's abilities and environmental features are such that that activity is possible. As such, they are definable only in terms of extended animal–environment systems (Chemero, 2003, 2009; Chemero and Turvey, 2007; Turvey, 1992). Given this, it is not particularly surprising that Ennaceur and Delacour are unconcerned with the affordances of the objects in their studies. Like other researchers who use the object exploration task, they do research in neuroscience, behavioral genetics, and psychopharmacology; that is, they are exactly the types of neuroscientists who, as Bickle (2003) points out, tend to be (ruthless) reductionists.

A recent literature review (Chemero and Heyser, 2005) shows that this lack of interest in the nature of the objects is widespread in the literature on object exploration. We reviewed 116 papers that used the object exploration methodology to see (1) whether there was a mismatch among the to-be-explored objects with respect to the affordance "climbability," and (2) whether the to-be-explored objects were described sufficiently to determine if there was a mismatch. We defined the affordance *climbability* as follows: Any two objects that

(1) are sufficiently sturdy to support the full weight of the animal without deformation, and

(2) have a surface that is
   a. parallel to the ground,
   b. at a height less than the full length of the animal (tail excluded),
   c. at least as wide as the distance between the animal's left and right feet, and
   d. at least as long as the distance between the animal's front and back feet
      afford the same behavior, climbing-on. (Chemero and Heyser, 2005, p. 411)

A few quick notes about this definition. First, it is animal-relative. Things that are climbable for monkeys will often not be climbable for mice; things that are climbable for adult mice may not be climbable for juvenile mice. Second, it individuates behaviors somewhat loosely. Objects that are climbable for some kind of animal are lumped together, even though it might take different muscle motions for that animal to climb them. Thus, stairs, deck chairs, bar stools, and tables are all climbable by most adult humans, even though you must do very different things to get onto a stair step and a bar stool. Third, this definition is in terms of the body scale of animals (following Warren's classic 1984 work), but affordances are not necessarily body-scaled (Cesari, Formenti, and Olivato, 2003; Chemero, 2003, 2009). Here, body scale serves as an easily measured operationalization of climbing ability. Finally, affordances are defined here, and generally, in terms of extended animal–environment systems.

Using this understanding of the affordance climbability, we found that of the 116 papers reviewed,[1] only 64 described the objects in enough detail to determine whether the objects were climbable by the animals being studied. Fifty-two of the papers did not describe the to-be-explored objects sufficiently to make a determination; many of these simply repeated the Ennaceur and Delacour description of the objects as nonmovable and made of plastic, metal, or glass. Of the 64 that did describe the objects in detail, 32 used objects that differed with respect to climbability—some were climbable by the animals studied, some were not. The remaining 32 used objects that were equivalent with respect to climbability. If the climbability of the objects used in the studies does impact the way animals explore them, the results of all but these 32 studies are methodologically suspect. They are suspect because if the climbability of the objects matters to how they are explored, the conclusions drawn concerning the effects of the drug, gene, or neurotransmitter manipulations may be instead the result of differences in the affordances of the objects used in the study.

Let us put this in perspective. Of the papers we reviewed, half of those that described to-be-explored objects in any detail described objects that conflicted in their climbability. Assume that these conflicts are also present in the same proportion of studies that do not describe their objects in detail. This would indicate that about half of the studies using object exploration methodology to study the effects of drugs, genes, and neurotransmitters on memory may have significant confounds. Given this, it is very important to determine whether the affordances of to-be-explored objects affect the way animals explore them in object exploration experiments. In the next section, we describe a few of a series of experiments we have done on affordances and object exploration.

4. Some Experiments

In this section, we describe a few of the experiments we have done to determine the effect of altering affordances on object exploration in mice and rats. The overall effect is that the affordances of to-be-explored objects do impact the way mice and rats explore them.

4.1. Object Exploration: Alcohol Withdrawal

One of our first experiments using an object exploration procedure was to examine the effects of alcohol withdrawal on recognition memory in rats. For this study, we used adult male Wistar rats, randomly assigned to two groups (control and withdrawal). Ethanol was administered in a nutritionally complete liquid diet at a concentration of 8.7 percent (w/v). Ethanol-treated rats were given 24-hour access to the ethanol liquid diet for 3 weeks. Control rats were given a liquid diet that was equivalent in terms of calories but did not contain alcohol. Withdrawal was initiated in ethanol-treated rats by removing the liquid diet. All rats were tested for object exploration 8 hours after the withdrawal of the liquid diet. Previous research has shown that the severity of the withdrawal syndrome is correlated with the blood alcohol concentration and that an observable withdrawal syndrome that includes hyperirritability, tremors, rigidity, hypothermia, and hyperexcitability is present 8 hours after the removal of alcohol (Macey et al., 1996).

Rats were tested in a square wooden open field ($64 \times 64 \times 49$ cm) located in a dimly lit soundproof room. A video camera was mounted above the apparatus, and all behaviors were scored from the videotaped sessions. The rats were given four successive 6-minute trials, each separated by a 3-minute interval. The first of the four trials was a familiarization phase in which the rats were placed in the empty open field (containing no objects). During trials 2 and 3, three objects were placed in the open field: a paint can (12×11 cm), a clear glass water bottle (18×7.5 cm), and a green metal cylinder (17×8.5 cm). As in other object exploration experiments, all objects were weighted such that the rats could not move them. The objects were positioned in a triangular arrangement. Of the initial objects, only the paint can was climbable by the rats (according to the criteria already presented). For trial 4, the climbable paint can was removed and a novel object (a wooden box, $13 \times 9.5 \times 11$ cm) was substituted to assess recognition memory. Recognition memory would be inferred from the behavioral response of preferential exploration of the novel object (in the last trial) over the familiar objects. The basic premise of this task is

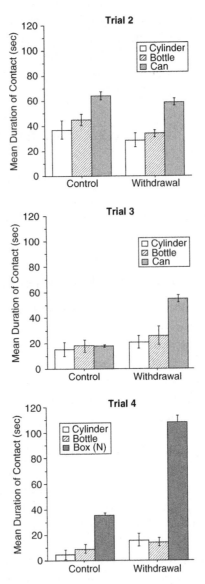

Figure 3.1. Mean (± SE) duration of contact (sec) for each object across the three trials in control animals and animals undergoing ethanol withdrawal. In trial 2, the rats explored the can significantly longer than the other two objects (P < 0.05). This trend continued in trial 3 for rats undergoing ethanol withdrawal. Both groups of rats showed preferential exploration for the novel object (the box) in trial 4. However, rats undergoing ethanol withdrawal explored the novel object significantly more than control animals (P < 0.05).

that repeated exposure to the same objects results in progressively less exploration (i.e., habituation), and by substituting a novel object for a familiar one, dishabituation should occur in the form of renewed exploration specific to the novel object. Several behaviors were recorded during trials 2–4, including line crosses, rears, grooming, the frequency and duration of contact with each object, and the latency to make first contact with each object within a given trial. The first three of these (line crosses, rears, grooming) are performance measures and relate to the testing of recognition memory only in the sense that the overall behavior of the animal is within expected ranges (i.e., are its action typical for the rat in this situation). For example, a reduction in line crosses following an experimental manipulation might lead to changes in object exploration. However, these alterations are likely to be unrelated to recognition memory. The other three (frequency and duration of contact with objects, and latency to first contact) are taken to be potential indicators of recognition memory.

Simply looking at the last trial (in which a novel object was substituted for a familiar object) it would appear that alcohol withdrawal improved recognition memory (see figure 3.1, bottom panel). Recognition memory would be manifest as preferential exploration of the novel object as compared to the familiar objects, an effect readily apparent in control rats. However, it is also clear that rats undergoing alcohol withdrawal spent significantly more time in contact with the novel object.

A more complete look at the data revealed that the animals (regardless of group assignment) spent significantly different amounts of time with the various objects at the start of the experiment (see figure 3.1, top panel). More specifically, both control and withdrawal rats spent significantly more time in contact with the climbable paint can as compared to the nonclimbable metal cylinder and the nonclimbable glass bottle. That is, these objects differed in their affordant properties; the rats preferentially explored the paint can (which they could touch, rear, and climb on) compared to the water bottle and metal cylinder, which could only be touched and reared on.

During the last trial, the paint can was removed and a novel object (the wooden box) was substituted in its place in the open field. The wooden box was also climbable by the rats. From our initial conclusion that alcohol withdrawal facilitates recognition memory, it is impossible to draw any conclusion with any certainty given that the rats spent more time with objects that afforded climbing. Our uncertainty stems from the fact that the resulting behavior may be due to novelty (e.g., reactivity to novelty or improved recognition memory) or simply due to the fact that they prefer exploring objects that can be climbed. To determine the effect of alcohol withdrawal on novel object exploration, we needed to control for climbability.

4.2. Object Exploration: Alcohol Withdrawal, Part II

We subsequently replicated the study with only one change—all objects were matched for their affordances for climbing, using a procedure identical to that already outlined. Control and alcohol withdrawal rats were tested using objects that could not be climbed; the only behavior possible was touching or rearing against the object. The objects were three identical clear glass water bottles (22.5 × 7.5 cm that tapered to a top 5 cm in diameter). For trial 4, one of the bottles was removed, and a novel object (a metal cylinder, 23 × 9 cm that tapered to a top 5 cm in diameter) was substituted to assess recognition memory. None of these objects are climbable by an adult male Wistar rat.

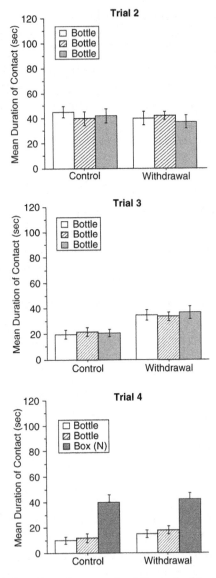

Figure 3.2. Mean (± SE) duration of contact (sec) for each object across the three trials in control animals and animals undergoing ethanol withdrawal. In trial 2, object exploration was equal across all objects. Rats undergoing ethanol withdrawal explored all objects significantly more than control animals (P < 0.05) during trial 3. Both groups of rats showed preferential exploration for the novel object (the box) in trial 4 (P < 0.05).

As can be seen in figure 3.2 (top panel), all animals showed equal levels of exploration across the objects. It is interesting to note that rats in the withdrawal group did spend more time exploring the objects (figure 3.2, middle panel). This could be related to changes in exploratory behavior or alterations in habituation in rats undergoing alcohol withdrawal. As can been seen in figure 3.2, there were no differences between the groups during the novelty substitution of trial 4. Given that animals from both groups exhibited preferential responding to the novel object, one could conclude that ethanol withdrawal does not appear to affect object recognition using the parameters of the present study. This conclusion is strengthened by the fact that the objects are matched for affordances, and as a result there are no apparent biases among the objects in terms of exploration. Therefore, the results of the initial study were in large part due to the fact that the animals were tested using objects that differed in their affordances.

4.3. Object Exploration: Not All Objects Are Created Equal

Given the results of the experiments examining alcohol withdrawal, we began a series of studies with rodents specifically to look at object selection and its impact on performance in the object exploration task. One experiment was conducted to characterize object exploration in adult male and female C57BL/6J mice under different object conditions. More specifically, the mice were tested either with objects that could be touched (TOUCH) and not climbed or with objects that could be touched and climbed (CLIMB). (These results were presented in Chemero and Heyser, 2005.)

Mice were tested in a large circular open field (120 cm in diameter) located in a dimly lit room. A video camera was mounted above the apparatus, and all behaviors were scored from the videotaped sessions. The mice were each given four successive 6-minute trials, each separated by a 3-minute interval. The first of the four trials was intended to be a familiarization phase in which the mice were placed in the empty open field (containing no objects). During trial 2, four different objects were placed in the open field. All objects were weighted such that the mice could not move them. The objects were positioned in a square arrangement equidistant from each other and from the outer wall of the open field. For mice in the TOUCH group, these objects consisted of a glass bottle (19 × 6.5 cm; tapered top), a metal rectangular can (7.5 × 4 × 13 cm), a set of plastic stacking squares (5.5. × 5.5 × 16 cm; tapered top), and a plastic toy barrel (19 × 6.5 cm; tapered top). These objects could not be climbed by the mice because they are too tall or too narrow or both (violating clause 2 of the definition of climbability in section 3). For mice in the CLIMB group, the objects were a plastic square (6 × 6 × 6 cm), a rectangular plastic bottle on its side (5 × 14 × 5 cm), a cardboard box (7.5 × 8 × 3 cm), and a plastic object with a hole in the center (6 × 12 × 6 cm). These objects were of a height that they could be climbed on. The same objects remained in the open field during trials 3 and 4. Several behaviors were recorded during trials 2–4, including line crosses, rears, grooming, the frequency and duration of contact with each object, and the latency to make first contact with each object within a given trial.

As can be seen in figure 3.3, mice in the CLIMB condition spent significantly more time in contact with the objects when compared with the contact scores in the TOUCH group. Thus, the type of object encountered had a significant impact on the duration of contact exhibited by the mice. In this case, climbable objects were explored for a longer period of time relative to those objects that could only be touched. In addition, in this experiment gender differences were only seen in the TOUCH group. Female mice explored TOUCH objects significantly less than male mice (see figure 3.3). No gender differences were observed in the CLIMB condition. So changing the affordances of the to-be-explored objects can cause a sex difference to appear or disappear. In addition, object type also affected the overall rate of habituation (as defined by a decrease in exploration across trials). More specifically, mice in the CLIMB condition exhibited the slowest rate of habituation as compared to mice in the TOUCH only condition (see figure 3.4). Although we do not show the individual object data for this experiment, it is important to note that within each condition (TOUCH or CLIMB) the objects were equally explored. These data

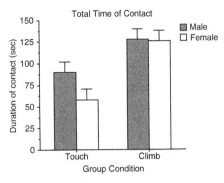

Figure 3.3. Mean (± SE) duration of contact (sec) for each object type in male and female mice. The mice explored the climbable objects significantly more than objects that could only be touched (P < 0.05). Female mice spent significantly less time in contact with objects that could only be touched than male mice (P < 0.05).

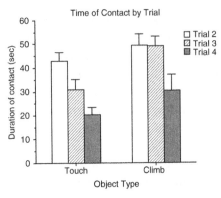

Figure 3.4. Mean (± SE) duration of contact (sec) for each object type across the three trials. The mice explored the climbable objects significantly more than objects that could only be touched (P < 0.05). A more rapid decrease in exploration was observed in the touch-only condition as compared with the climbable condition.

provide further evidence that exploratory behavior is significantly affected by the available affordances.

4.4. Object Exploration: Chronic Mild Stress, a Work in Progress

Recently we have begun to examine other factors that may impact exploratory behavior. Any activity-related behavior can be affected by the presentation of a stressor. For this study, we used adult male Wistar rats randomly assigned to two groups (control and stress). A chronic mild and variable stress procedure was used. In this procedure, mild unpredictable stressors are presented each day for a period of 3 weeks. The stressor used in the present study were crowding (six rats were placed in a large housing bin for 12 hours), cage tilt, strobe light (for 3 hours during the dark cycle), soiled bedding (500 ml water added to the cage bedding), a forced water swim (10 min), or nothing (there were days interspersed throughout the 3 weeks when no stressors were presented).

Rats were tested in a square wooden open field (64 × 64 × 49 cm) located in a dimly lit soundproof room. A video camera was mounted above the apparatus, and all behaviors were scored from the videotaped sessions. The rats were given four successive 6-minute trials, each separated by a 3-minute interval. The first of the four trials was intended to be a familiarization phase in which the rats were placed in the empty open field (containing no objects). During trials 2 and 3, two objects (22.5 × 7.5 cm that tapered to a top 5 cm in diameter) were placed in the open field. All objects were weighted such that the rats could not move them. The objects were equidistant from each other and from the sides of the open field. For trial 4, one glass bottle was removed and a novel object (a metal cylinder, 23 × 9 cm that tapered to a top 5 cm in diameter) was substituted to assess recognition memory. Several behaviors were recorded during trials 2–4, including line crosses, rears, grooming, the frequency and duration of contact with each object, and the latency to make first contact with each object within a given trial.

As can be seen in figure 3.5, object exploration significantly decreased across trials. In addition, rats exposed to chronic mild and variable stressor explored the objects significantly more than controls on both trials. There were no differences in the overall rate of habituation between the groups (see figure 3.5). Control and stressed rats exhibited preferential exploration of the novel object during trial 4. However, the preference for the novel object was significantly higher in control rats (71 percent of the exploration was directed toward the novel object) as compared to rats subjected to chronic mild and variable stressors (62 percent of the exploration was directed toward the novel object). Closer examination of the data revealed that both groups of rats explored the novel object the same amount (see figure 3.6). However, rats in the stress group continued to explore the familiar object significantly more than controls (see figure 3.6).

So what should one conclude from this study? Given the differences during the last trial (novelty substitution), one might conclude that stress had a disruptive effect on recognition memory—at least in the magnitude of that expression. However, this conclusion is less certain given that difference in exploration duration were evident during the early trials. Furthermore, stressor presentation typically results in a reduction of ongoing behavior. In fact, behavioral inhibition is one of the hallmark outcomes of this task for validation as animal models of depression (Willner, 2005). In the present study, contact with the objects was increased in rats in the stress group, which is opposite of what is predicted when one does not take

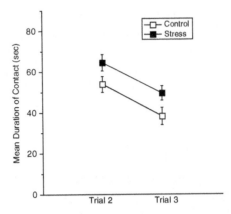

Figure 3.5. Mean (± SE) duration of contact (sec) across the two trials in stressed and control rats. The rats in the stress group explored the objects significantly more than those in the control group (P < 0.05). Both groups showed a significant decrease in exploration of the objects across the two trials (i.e., habituation).

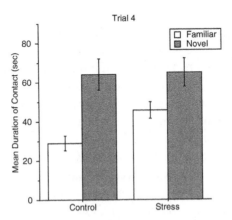

Figure 3.6. Mean (± SE) duration of contact (sec) during trial 4 for rats in the stress and control conditions. Both groups of rats showed preferential exploration for the novel object in trial 4 (P < 0.05). However, this preference was significantly greater in control rats (P < 0.05).

affordances into account. However, it is important to note that the objects selected for this study could not be climbed; in fact, they were very tall. It is tempting, therefore, to speculate that the animals may have been responding to the objects as walls. Stressors can also produce a wall-hugging behavior (thigmotaxis). If this is the case, then one would expect more contact with the objects. It is important to reiterate that this is speculative as further research needs to be conducted using objects that can be climbed over (i.e., that don't serve as walls or cover for the animals).

4.5. Object Exploration Summary

These four experiments, and many others we have performed, show unequivocally that the affordances of to-be-explored objects affect the behavior of animals in object exploration experiments. The alcohol withdrawal experiments (4.1 and 4.2) show that object choice can make apparent effects of alcohol withdrawal appear and disappear. The "not all objects are created equal" experiment (4.3) showed that object choice can produce novelty effects that in most object exploration experiments might be interpreted as improved recognition memory. Using climbable versus nonclimbable objects can also produce an artifactual gender effect. The results of experiment on chronic mild stress (4.4) are harder to interpret. One way to interpret those results is that stressed rats explored objects more than nonstressed animals, in violation of what is known about the depressive effects of stress on behavior. Looking at the relationship between the scale of the to-be-explored objects and the scale of the rats, it seems more likely that the stressed rats were using the objects as barriers, and engaging in expected thigmotaxis. Further experiments to sort this out are in progress.

That these effects result from the affordances of the to-be-explored objects is troubling. It indicates that in as many as half of the experiments using the object exploration methodology, the effects on recognition memory purportedly caused by drug, gene, or neurotransmitter manipulation may instead be caused by object choice.

5. Empirical and Methodological Conclusions

The object exploration methodology as it has been used recently in the neurosciences is a reliable generator of statistically significant effects. For this reason, it has been used hundreds of times in the past few years to study the effect of molecular and genetic neural manipulations on recognition memory. The four experiments described here suggest that in many cases the effects produced in these experiments may not be the result of the intentional neural manipulations that are identified as independent variables (i.e., gene, drug, or neurotransmitter manipulations); rather, these effects may be the result of the affordances of the objects selected for the animals being studied. That is, it is not always clear whether the small-scale neural manipulations the experimenter intends to investigate or inadvertent large-scale animal–environment system manipulations cause the observed effects. Furthermore, in many cases it is not clear that the observed effects are related to recognition memory. It is not clear, that is, whether animals recognize that things have changed, and therefore explore novel objects preferentially, or whether they simply prefer objects with particular affordances (climbing, thigmotaxis when stressed). We hasten to add that we believe these issues do not arise for experiments in which affordances of the to-be-explored objects for the animal are matched. That is, for the approximately 30 percent of published experiments that demonstrably do use objects with matched affordances, we believe that the effects are caused by the experimental manipulation and do provide evidence of effects on recognition memory. In the other 70 percent or so of studies, it is unclear what causes the effect.

This leads to the (perhaps obvious at this point) recommendation that experimenters need to take affordances into account when they design object exploration experiments. If one wants to study the effects of (say) alcohol withdrawal on recognition memory, one must explicitly and carefully control for the affordances of the to-be-explored objects for the species under study. We have looked at only one affordance of particular relevance for object exploration studies, climbability. To do these experiments correctly, however, all the affordances that might affect exploration need to be controlled for. This requires that the experiments be informed by a deep and detailed knowledge of the behavior of the animals being studied. Experimental animals cannot be treated as bags of chemicals or as containers for neural systems. Instead, they must be understood as endogenously active agents, engaging with their environments to satisfy their needs. To understand the way they engage with the environments they interact with in object exploration experiments, it is absolutely vital to understand the affordances of the to-be-explored objects for the animals. As noted, however, affordances are defined only in terms of extended animal–environment systems. Thus, to do object exploration experiments correctly, one must adopt an extended cognitive science approach, understanding the relevant object of scientific study as the brain–body–environment system. The experiments described herein point out that those who want to use object exploration to study the effect of micro-features (genes, neurotransmitters, drugs) of neural systems must do in terms of macro-scaled brain–body–environment systems. Ironically, these psychopharmacologists, behavioral geneticists, and other neuroscientists who focus on molecular-level neural systems must adopt extended cognition approach and design their experiments accordingly.[2]

A second consequence is less deep, but arguably more important. The methods sections of papers reporting object exploration must make it clear that the to-be-explored objects are matched for affordances. In approximately 45 percent of the papers we reviewed for Chemero and Heyser (2005) (see note 1), not enough was said about the objects used to determine whether they were matched for affordances.

This is a symptom of a more general problem, the trend in recent years toward shorter methods sections. In many cases, methods sections consist primarily of citations of other papers. The methods section is arguably the most important part of a scientific paper. It should be long enough to be very clear about what was done in the experiments; it should also not appear in small type after the main body of the publication, as happens in some of the highest profile scientific journals.

6. Philosophical Conclusions

The first scientific conclusion mentioned—that neuroscientists who use the object exploration methodology must adopt an extended cognition approach—is directly relevant to the philosophical debates over reductionism. As we discussed in section 2, the philosophical position of reductionism is actually two related positions: intertheoretic or epistemic reductionism and ontological reductionism. Reductionists typically believe both of these claims. None of these positions fare well, at least not as general truths, in light of the results discussed here.

Start with reductionism simpliciter, the mixed conviction that psychological phenomena are neural phenomena and that neuroscience will eventually be seen as the best explanation of psychological phenomena. As Bickle (2003) points out, neuroscientists themselves are typically reductionists in this sense, and molecular and genetic neuroscientists, like those who typically employ the object exploration methodology, are typically ruthless reductionists. Furthermore, we take it that Bickle's own ruthless reductionist position is this sort of hybrid reductionism. We believe that the problems with the object exploration methodology brought to light by our literature review and experiments occur precisely because the neuroscientists who employ the methodology are reductionists. Clearly, many of those who use the object exploration methodology are not concerned with the properties of the to-be-explored objects. Why else would they not bother to describe the objects? Why else would they use objects that are likely to invoke different sorts of behavior? We believe that the conviction that psychological phenomena just are molecular and genetic phenomena, and that studying molecular and genetic phenomena just is doing psychology, leads to this neglect of behaviorally relevant aspects of the environment and thereby to flawed experimental design. This amounts to a pragmatic argument against reductionism, ruthless or otherwise. If believing in reductionism leads neuroscientists to poor experimental methodology, neuroscientists should not believe in reductionism. Nor should philosophers of neuroscience encourage neuroscientists to believe in reductionism.

The results also imply that intertheoretic reduction fails. In intertheoretic reduction, one accounts for the laws, regularities, and generalizations of the reduced science using the laws, regularities, and generalizations of the reducing science, along with bridge principles. In the case at issue here, the reduced science is psychology or cognitive science and the reducing science is cognitive or molecular neuroscience. The experiments show that such a reduction is in general impossible. To do object exploration experiments correctly, one must adopt an extended cognition approach. That is, one must take the object of study for the cognitive sciences to be wide brain–body–environment systems. The laws, regularities, and generalizations of wide cognitive science cannot be accounted for using the resources of the neurosciences. The clearest reason to believe this to be the case is that the explanatory purview of the neurosciences is a proper spatial part of the explanatory purview of the cognitive sciences. We have shown that effectively investigating recognition memory requires extended cognitive science, a science of the coupled brain–body–environment system. Neuroscience is only a science of a portion of the coupled brain–body–environment system, and so cannot account for recognition memory. And recognition memory is only one of many phenomena that currently seem to require extended cognitive science.

We noted in section 2 that the best evidence for ontological reductionism, the conviction that psychological phenomena just are neural phenomena, is the truth of intertheoretic reductionism. We have a hard time imagining any other reason to believe in ontological reductionism. We have just argued that intertheoretic reductionism is false, which seems to pull the main support for ontological reductionism. Indeed, the same argument can be made, with bridge principles, against ontological reductionism. Ontological reductionism is the view that psychological phenomena are identical to or supervene on neural phenomena. The results described in sections 3 and 4 indicate that cognitive systems are extended brain–body–environment systems. Extended brain–body–environment systems neither are identical to nor supervene on neural systems. So ontological reductionism is false. Despite the translation, however, this argument really depends on the failure of intertheoretic reductionism. The main reason to believe that cognitive systems are extended is that certain aspects of them seem to demand extended cognitive science. Strictly speaking, though, the failure of intertheoretic reduction does not entail the failure of ontological reduction. One might set aside the failings of our feeble scientific theories and hold that the psychological and the neural are nonetheless identical. God or some other being much smarter than we are could account for all psychological phenomena in terms of neuroscience. It is hard to see any reason why one would believe this, other than some a priori principles concerning that essence of mental phenomena. Those who wish to invoke a priori principles concerning the essence of mental phenomena here are free to do so. But they should be unsurprised when cognitive and neural scientists, along with a growing number of philosophers, ignore them.

Given the results on object exploration we have argued that in general, reductionism fails pragmatically, epistemologically, and ontologically. The "in general" is very important. What we have shown is that neuroscientists should not believe that all psychological phenomena are reducible, that we will not be able to account for all of psychology's subject matter using the neurosciences, and that not all psychological phenomena are identical to or supervenient on neural phenomena.

What we've shown is that object exploration, and perhaps recognition memory, are extended cognitive phenomena, spanning brain, body, and environment. Given the current state of play in the cognitive sciences, many aspects of perception, development, motor control, and social coordination are also wide. (See works cited in the discussion.) There are also psychological phenomena that are plausibly reducible to neural phenomena—Bickle's favorite case, long-term memory consolidation and long-term potentiation, is a good candidate. It is open to the committed reductionist to try to argue that current extended cognitive science will be falsified by future neuroscience; in the future, coupled brain–body–environment explanations will be viewed the way that explanations that refer to phlogiston are today. A committed antireductionist could try a parallel argument and hold that current brain-internal explanations will be falsified by future extended cognitive science. Either argument would be, to put it mildly, steeply uphill. They would required making a convincing case that every one of today's convincing extended explanations will be falsified by more convincing future neural explanations (or vice versa), in advance of having any of those explanations. It's hard to imagine such an argument that does not rely on a priori principles concerning the essence of mental phenomena.

In contrast to the committed reductionist and antireductionist we imagined in the last paragraph, we believe we should embrace our current patchwork of explanatory styles in the cognitive and neural sciences. That is, we endorse explanatory pluralism (Chemero and Silberstein, 2008), according to which some psychological phenomena are best accounted for in terms of molecules and genes, some in terms of large-scale neural dynamics, and some in terms of extended brain–body–environment systems. To say this is to say that given the current state of play in the cognitive and neural sciences, there is no reason to believe that either reductionism or antireductionism about psychology is true across the board. Or to put the same point another way, there in no reason to believe that the psychological sciences will be unified. This implies, of course, that discussions of the essence of mental phenomena are simply beside the point.

NOTES

1. Since 2004 (when we wrote Chemero and Heyser, 2005), we have reviewed approximately 200 more publications in which object exploration experiments are described. Though we have not kept track formally, we believe that the proportions we report here generalize to the literature at large.

2. In comments on an earlier draft of this chapter, Bickle points out that neuroscientists need only take extended cognitive science into account for the purpose of designing experiments, but need not adopt extended cognitive science as a theoretical perspective. Although we acknowledge that there is something more to adopting a theoretical perspective than using it to design experiments, we believe that for the practicing experimentalist, there is no more important role for a theoretical perspective. Furthermore, when we say that neuroscientists must adopt the ecological approach, we are

not suggesting that they begin doing experiments on affordances or attending meetings of the International Society for Ecological Psychology. Rather, we mean that they ought to treat the insights of extended cognitive science the way they treat results from research on operant and classical conditioning, that is, as part of the knowledge base they need to understand and take to be true to do neuroscience correctly.

REFERENCES

Aggleton, J. P., Blindt, H. S., and Rawlins, J. N. P. (1989). Effects of amygdaloid and amygdaloid-hippocampal lesions on object recognition and spatial working memory in rats. *Behavioral Neuroscience* 103: 962–974.

Ainge, J. A., Heron-Maxwell, C., Theofilas, P., Wright, P., de Hoz, L., and Wood, E. R. (2006). The role of the hippocampus in object recognition in rats: Examination of the influence of task parameters and lesion size. *Behavioural Brain Research* 167: 183–195.

Beer, R. (1995). Computational and dynamical languages for autonomous agents. In R. F. Port and T. van Gelder (Eds.), *Mind as Motion*. Cambridge, Mass.: MIT Press, 121–147.

Beer, R. D. (1999). Dynamical approaches to cognitive science. *Trends in Cognitive Sciences* 4: 91–99.

Berlyne, D. E. (1950). Novelty and curiosity as determinants of exploratory behaviour. *British Journal of Psychology* 41: 68–80.

Bickle, J. (2003). *Philosophy and Neuroscience: A Ruthlessly Reductionist Account*. Boston: Kluwer.

Bourtchouladze, R., Lidge, R., Catapano, R., Stanley, J., Gossweiler, S., Romashko, D., et al. (2003). A mouse model of Rubinstein-Taybi syndrome: Defective long-term memory is ameliorated by inhibitors of phosphodiesterase 4. *Proceedings of the National Academy of Sciences USA* 100: 10518–10522.

Buckley, M. J., and Gaffan, D. (2006). Perirhinal cortical contributions to object perception. *Trends in Cognitive Sciences* 10: 100–107.

Bussey, T. J., Saksida, L. M., and Murray, E. A. (2003). Impairments in visual discrimination after perirhinal cortex lesions: Testing "declarative" vs. "perceptual-mnemonic" vies of perirhinal cortex function. *European Journal of Neuroscience* 17: 649–660.

Callahan, H., Ikeda-Douglas, C., Head, E., Cotman, C. W., and Milgram, N. W. (2000). Development of a protocol for studying object recognition memory in the dog. *Progress in Neuro-Psychopharmacology and Biological Psychiatry* 24: 693–707.

Cesari, P., Formenti, F., and Olivato, P. (2003). A common perceptual parameter for stair climbing in children, young, and old adults. *Human Movement Science* 22: 111–124.

Chemero, A. (2003). An outline of a theory of affordances. *Ecological Psychology* 15: 181–195.

Chemero, A. (2009). *Radical Embodied Cognitive Science*. Cambridge, Mass.: MIT Press.

Chemero, A., and Heyser, C. (2005). Object exploration and the problem with reductionism. *Synthese* 147: 403–423.

Chemero, A., and Silberstein, M. ((2008). After the philosophy of mind. *Philosophy of Science* 75: 1–28.

Chemero, A., and Turvey, M. (2007). Hypersets, complexity and the ecological approach to perception-action. *Biological Theory* 2: 23–36.

Churchland, P. M. (1985). Reduction, qualia, and the direct introspection of brain states. *Journal of Philosophy* 82: 8–28.

Churchland, P. M. (1989). *A Neurocomputational Perspective*. Cambridge, Mass.: MIT Press.

Churchland, P. M., and Churchland, P. S. (1990). Intertheoretic reduction: A neuroscientist's field guide. *Seminars in the Neurosciences* 4: 249–256.

Churchland, P. S. (1986). *Neurophilosophy*. Cambridge, Mass.: MIT Press.

Churchland, P. S. (2002). *Brain-Wise*. Cambridge, Mass.: MIT Press.

Clark, A. (1997). *Being There*. Cambridge, Mass.: MIT Press.

Ennaceur, A., and Delacour, J. (1988). A new one-trial test for neurobiological studies of memory in rats. 1: Behavioral data. *Behavioural Brain Research* 31: 47–59.

Hacking, I. (1983). *Representing and Intervening: Introductory Topics in the Philosophy of Natural Science*. Cambridge: Cambridge University Press.

Heyser, C. J., Pelletier, M., and Ferris, J. S. (2004). The effects of methylphenidate on novel object exploration in weanling and periadolescent rats. *Annals of the New York Academy of Sciences* 1021: 465–469.

Gibson, J. J. (1979). *The Ecological Approach to Visual Perception*. Boston: Houghton Mifflin.

Hooker, C. A. (1981a). Towards a general theory of reduction. Part I: Historical and scientific setting. *Dialogue* 20: 38–59.

Hooker, C. A. (1981b). Towards a general theory of reduction. Part II: Identity in reduction. *Dialogue* 20: 201–236.

Hooker, C. A. (1981c). Towards a general theory of reduction. Part III: Cross-categorial reduction. *Dialogue* 20: 496–529.

Hutchins, E. (1995). *Cognition in the Wild*. Cambridge, Mass.: MIT Press.

Kelso, J. (1995). *Dynamic Patterns*. Cambridge, Mass.: MIT Press.

Kelso, J. A. S., and Engstrom, D. (2006). *The Complementary Nature*. Cambridge, Mass.: MIT Press.

Kim, D. Chae, S., Lee, J., Yang, H., and Shin, H.-S. (2005). Variations in the behaviors to novel objects among five inbred strains of mice. *Genes, Brain and Behavior* 4: 302–306.

Kugler, P., and Turvey, M. (1987). *Information, Natural Law, and the Self-Assembly of Rhythmic Movement*. Hillsdale, N.J.: Erlbaum.

Lee, A. C. H., Buckley, M. J., Gaffan, D., Emery, T., Hodges, J. R., and Graham, K. S. (2006). Differentiating the roles of the hippocampus and perirhinal cortex in processes beyond long-term declarative memory: A double dissociation in dementia. *Journal of Neuroscience* 26: 5198–5203.

Lee, I., Hunsaker, M. R., and Kesner, R. P. (2005). The role of hippocampal subregions in detecting spatial novelty. *Behavioral Neuroscience* 119: 145–153.

Macey, D. J., Schulteis, G., Heinrichs, S. C., and Koob, G. F. (1996). Time-dependent quantifiable withdrawal from ethanol in the rat: Effect of method of dependence induction. *Alcohol* 13: 163–170.

McClamrock, R. (1995). *Existential Cognition*. Chicago: University of Chicago Press.

Mettke-Hofmann, C., Winkler, H., and Leislser, B. (2002). The significance of ecological factors for exploration and neophobia in parrots. *Ethology* 108: 249–272.

Nagel, E. (1961). *The Structure of Science*. New York: Harcourt, Brace, World.

Norman, G., and Eacott, M. J. (2004). Impaired object recognition with increasing levels of feature ambiguity in rats with perirhinal cortex lesions. *Behavioural Brain Research* 148: 79–81.

O'Shea, M., McGregor, I. S., and Mallet, P. E. (2006). Repeated cannabinoid exposure during perinatal, adolescent or early adult ages produces similar long-lasting deficits in object recognition and reduced social interaction in rats. *Journal of Psychopharmacology* 20: 611–621.

Oullier, O., de Guzman, G. C., Jantzen, K. J., Lagarde, J. F., and Kelso, J. A. S. (2005). Spontaneous interpersonal synchronization. In C. Peham, W. I. Schöllhorn, and W. Verwey (Eds.), *European Workshop on Movement Sciences: Mechanics-Physiology-Psychology*. Cologne: Sportverlag Strauss, 34–35.

Renner, M. J., and Rosenzweig, M. R. (1986). Object interactions in juvenile rats (*Rattus norvegicus*): Effects of differential experiential histories. *Journal of Comparative Psychology* 100: 229–236.

Save, E., Poucet, B., Foreman, N., and Buhot, M.-C. (1992). Object exploration and reactions to spatial and nonspatial changes in Hooded rats following damage to parietal cortex or hippocampal formation. *Behavioral Neurosciences* 106: 447–456.

Sik, A., van Nieuwehuyzen, P., Prickaerts, J., and Blokland, A. (2003). Performance of different mouse strains in an object exploration task. *Behavioural Brain Research* 147: 49–54.

Silberstein, M. (2002). Reduction, emergence and explanation. In P. Machamer and M. Silberstein (Eds.), *The Blackwell Guide to the Philosophy of Science*. New York: Blackwell.

Sneddon, L. U., Braithwaite, V. A., and Gentle, M. J. (2003). Novel object test: Examining nociception and fear in the rainbow trout. *Journal of Pain* 4: 431–440.

Stowe, M., Bugnyar, T., Loretto, M.-C., Schloegl, C., Range, F., and Kortschal, K. (2006). Novel object exploration in ravens (*Corvus corax*): Effects of social relationships. *Behavioural Processes* 73: 68–75.

Thinus-Blanc, C., Durup, M., and Poucet, B. (1992). The spatial parameters encoded by hamsters during exploration: A further study. *Behavioural Processes* 26: 43–57.

Thompson, E. (2007). *Mind in Life: Biology, Phenomenology, and the Sciences of Mind*. Cambridge, Mass.: Harvard University Press.

Turvey, M. T. (1992). Affordances and prospective control: An outline of the ontology. *Ecological Psychology* 4: 173–187.

Turvey, M. T., Shaw, R. E., Reed, E. D., and Mace, W. M. (1981). Ecological laws of perceiving and acting: In reply to Fodor and Pylyshyn. *Cognition* 9: 237–304.

Varela, F., Thompson, E., and Rosch, E. (1991). *The Embodied Mind*. Cambridge, Mass.: MIT Press.

Ventura, R., Pascucci, T., Catania, M. V., Musumeci, S. A., and Puglisi-Allegra, S. (2004). Object recognition impairment in Fmr1 knockout mice is reversed by amphetamine: involvement of dopamine in the medial prefrontal cortex. *Behavioural Pharmacology* 15: 433–442.

Visser, E. K., van Reenen, C. G., van der Werf, J. T. N., Schilder, M. B. H., Knaap, J. H., Barneveld, A., et al. (2002). Heart rate and heart rate variability during a novel object test and a handling test in young horses. *Physiology and Behavior* 76: 289–296.

Warren, W. H. (1984). Perceiving affordances: Visual guidance of stair climbing. *Journal of Experimental Psychology: Human Perception and Performance* 10: 683–703.

Willner, P. (2005). Chronic mild stress (CMS) revisited: Consistency and behavioural-neurobiological concordance in the effects of CMS. *Neuropsychobiology* 52: 90–110.

Wilson, R. (2004). *Boundaries of the Mind*. New York: Cambridge University Press.

Zola-Morgan, S., Babrowska, J., Moss, M., and Mahut, H. (1983). Enhanced preference for perceptual novelty in the monkey after section of the fornix but not after ablation of the hippocampus. *Neuropsychologia* 21: 433–454.

CHAPTER 4

THE SCIENCE OF RESEARCH AND THE SEARCH FOR MOLECULAR MECHANISMS OF COGNITIVE FUNCTIONS

ALCINO J. SILVA AND JOHN BICKLE

1. INTRODUCTION: TWO PUZZLES ABOUT RECENT SCIENCE

In this chapter, we propose a new general framework for understanding contemporary science. We begin by introducing two puzzles. The first is specific to the neurobiology of cognitive functions. Most of the scientific details we appeal to in this chapter are drawn from recent work in this field. The second is more general, pertaining to some recently noticed inefficiencies in institutionalized science across the board. We contend that both of these puzzles can only be addressed in a rigorous, scientific fashion within a framework for discovering and testing hypotheses about science. We introduce the *science of research* (SR) as just this sort of a framework, develop two initial SR hypotheses, articulate scientific evidence that supports them, and show how they solve both of our puzzles.

1.1. Our First Puzzle, Specific to the Neurobiology of Cognition

One need not travel far into current mainstream neuroscience to discover a thriving psychoneural reductionism. The principal textbooks suffice. For example, in the introduction to the fourth edition of their *Principles of Neural Science*, Eric Kandel, James Schwartz, and Thomas Jessell write:

> This book...describes how neural science is attempting to link molecules to mind—how proteins responsible for the activities of individual nerve cells are related to the complexities of neural processes. Today it is possible to link the molecular dynamics of individual nerve cells to representations of perceptual and motor acts in the brain and to relate these internal mechanisms to observable behavior. (2001, pp. 3–4)

These "links" are based directly on experiments tying observable measures of psychological and cognitive concepts to neurophysiological processes and, most recently, molecular-biological mechanisms and pathways.

Many philosophers and cognitive scientists are simply baffled by assertions of such links. Of course, philosophical arguments still abound against reducing psychology to any physical science. But even setting those arguments aside, there remains a multilevel picture of mind–brain relations ingrained into contemporary thought. Armed implicitly with this picture, many "higher level" investigators of mind will wonder how current mainstream neuroscience proposes to descend so many levels in single experimental bounds. According to this picture, between the behavioral measures routinely used to indicate particular cognitive functions and intraneuronal molecular pathways lie at least the following levels: information bearing and processing, neural systems (including the motor systems generating the measurable behaviors), neural regions, neural circuits (networks), intercellular signaling, cellular activity, and synapses. Various cognitive-scientific and neuroscientific fields address these different levels. So mustn't reductive bridges first be built between each of these intermediate levels before "mind-to-molecules" linkages can legitimately be claimed? Isn't cognitive neuroscience having enough trouble bridging just the behavior/information processing levels with neural systems and regions?

It is difficult to overestimate how ingrained this multiple intermediate levels picture of the mind–brain is. Even Patricia Churchland—hardly an enemy of reductionism—assumes it. In her book, *Neurophilosophy*, which systematically articulated the field we see developed and reflected in the chapters in this volume, she undertakes the project of linking the known neurophysiology and functional neuroanatomy of basic neuroscience with "higher neurofunctional kinds":

> Fine-grained detail has accumulated concerning such things as the molecular structure, location, synthesis, blocking agents, and enhancing agents of the

various neurochemicals, but there is still nothing remotely resembling a comprehensive theory of what they do or of how the known psychological effects result from tinkering with them.... Until we have higher-level concepts to describe what configurations of neurons are doing, *we have no means of bridging the gap* between molecular descriptions and molar [systems-level] descriptions. (Churchland, 1986, p. 82; emphasis added)

In the longest chapter of her book (1986), and in even more detail in her computational neuroscience primer coauthored with Terry Sejnowski (1992), Churchland seeks explicitly to provide the necessary neurofunctional kinds to affect the higher steps in the chain of reductions that will ultimately link mind to molecules—*in the only manner of linkage possible*, given the multiple intermediate levels picture.

Philosophers of neuroscience have followed Churchland's lead. Most have simply ignored developments in cellular and molecular neuroscience over the past three decades and instead focused exclusively on cognitive neuroscience. They seek psychoneural linkages among information processing models, neural systems, and neural networks. The experimental tools they are familiar with are mostly limited to functional neuroimaging, neuropsychological and neurological assessments, and neurocomputational modeling. Even Churchland retains her commitment to the multiple intermediate levels picture of the mind–brain and subsequently to the implausibility of direct mind-to–molecular pathways links. Nearly two decades after *Neurophilosophy* first appeared, in her recent book, *Brain-Wise*, she writes: "The idea of 'explanation in a single bound' does stretch credulity, and neuroscientists are not remotely tempted by it" (2003, p. 193).

Our first puzzle about recent science, the one specific to the neurobiology of cognition, can now be expressed succinctly. How do recent proponents of mind-to–molecular pathways linkages justify their claims? What kinds of experimental results do they take as evidence for such claims, and when do they claim to have enough (sufficient) evidence? Lurking just below the surface of this puzzle is the broader methodological question of how we discover and *test* answers to such questions.

1.2. Our Second Puzzle, Concerning Inefficiencies in Institutionalized Science

Over the past 100 years, science has grown at a vertiginous pace and has changed every aspect of the world around us. In the process, scientific discovery has also been transformed from an activity that attracted a few people into an industrial occupation in developed countries that employs a significant percentage of the population and uses a sizable fraction of national resources. Academic and private research efforts employ millions of people and attract hundreds of billions of dollars worldwide. The U.S. National Science Foundation (NSF) estimated that in 2004 the U.S. investment in research and development (R&D) was approximately $312.1 billion (compared to $152 billion in 1990), with approximately a third of that figure coming from federal sources. The U.S. R&D share of the gross domestic product (GDP) in 2004 was nearly 3 percent, compared to 1.4 percent in 1953. This growing commitment to R&D

is not unique to the United States. Most developed countries currently spend more than 2 percent of their GDP in R&D (Shackelford, 2006). This growing social and economic investment in science is paralleled by an increasing societal dependency on the products of science. These products range from communication and transportation means that have had an incalculable effect on intellectual and commercial interchanges, to the perennial technological advances that power the world's economic engines. Thus, science and its products have become deeply woven into the fabric of the world's cultures and economies (Tansey and Stembridge, 2005).

Despite this unprecedented growth of R&D budgets, there have been few concerted efforts to systematically study and analyze the scientific process. Scientists use objective methods to analyze their subject matter (within physics, chemistry, biology, and the rest of the sciences), but they have hardly ever used scientific methods to study how they do science. Instead, this type of analysis has been the domain of philosophers of science. However well intentioned and inspired these efforts have been, they have always lacked (and continue to lack) the objectivity, testing, and systematic character associated with scientific research. Yet the unprecedented expansion of science over the past century has recently been accompanied by a growing awareness among scientists of significant inefficiencies in science. Some of these inefficiencies were uncovered initially by analyses of the scientific literature (Cole and Cole, 1972), but new electronic scientific databases allow for far quicker data collection. For example, a query into the Institute for Scientific Information (ISI) Web of Knowledge (isiwebofknowledge.com) in August 2006 using the key word *cognition* yielded 26,262 articles. Surprisingly, 13,268 of these—more than half—had been cited in other publications only two times or fewer. A similar query at the same time using the key words *learning* and *memory* yielded 22,261 articles—7,492 of which had been cited two times or fewer. This suggests that a very large percentage of the published literature on cognition, and on one of its best-studied aspects, has had little to no impact.

This puzzle about troublesome inefficiencies is not unique to the science of cognition. All databases of scientific publications demonstrate that a significant percentage of published articles are either never cited or cited only a very small number of times (e.g., fewer than three times; Hamilton, 1990, 1991). Citation indexes are admittedly a crude measure of scientific contribution, but they are nevertheless revealing when we consider costs. In the biological sciences alone, this total number of rarely cited publications may amount to more than 7 million articles, that all together took at least 7 billion hours of research time (based on a conservative estimate of 1,000 research hours total, by all members of the research team, per published paper—including experimental design and controls, data gathering and analysis, and manuscript writing and revising). This is a staggering estimate of physical and economic resources. Even though these rarely cited efforts might have had some influence on institutionalized science (e.g., doctoral degrees generated, tenure award decisions), it is difficult to determine what of significance they added to the growth and development of knowledge in their disciplines.

Another aspect of this puzzle stems from clear evidence of dramatic differences between the productivity of individual scientists. Although social factors as well as variations in natural abilities such as intelligence, perseverance, creativity, and drive undoubtedly play a role in an individual's success, it is almost certain that training on principles of scientific discovery, implicit or explicit, also plays a role. Several informal studies of influential scientists have revealed a strong lineage effect, suggesting that training has an effect on future success (Kanigel, 1993; Zuckerman, 1967). How might we determine, in an objective, scientific fashion, whether Nobel laureate trees are due to social factors (i.e., influential mentors opening exclusive doors for their students, brilliance attracting brilliance), or whether they are due to objective principles and skills that dramatically increase the probability of discovery, still being passed on apprentice-style from mentor to students? The influence of the mentor–student relationship is difficult to ignore. Out of the 92 U.S. Nobel Prize winners in the sciences that received their prizes by 1972, 48 had worked in junior positions with other Nobel winners (Kanigel, 1993; Zuckerman, 1967). Is this just the result of "Mathew's effect"—those with a lineage of scientific prominence get an unfair share of exposure and credit in science (Merton, 1968)—or is it a consequence of a modus operandi that is implicitly or explicitly passed on from mentor to students and could be taught objectively and widespread across disciplines? This specific concern points glaringly to the broader methodological question already mentioned. How can we proceed to get a grip on these puzzles in a way that will lead to objective, testable hypotheses about their root causes? Opinions abound on these topics. But short of answers to these broader methodological questions, they are destined to remain only that—opinions.

We contend that a new framework for understanding science scientifically is required to responsibly address puzzles like the ones we've sketched in this section. The results from an analysis derived from such a framework could have an enormous effect on how we fund, teach, publish, and carry out science. They should be especially useful in young disciplines, such as the neurobiology of cognition, toward developing research methodologies and theoretical frameworks for incorporating experimental data.

2. THE DISCIPLINE OF SR

2.1. SR Characterized

We propose a new scientific discipline, SR—the science of research (with *research* construed very broadly, as will become apparent). This new discipline will investigate and test general principles of scientific practice. Its key project is a scientific analysis of how successful science works, with an explicit goal being that of improving the training and practices of scientists. At bottom, then, it is as much a practical as a theoretical discipline. It is related to numerous other studies of science, including its mother discipline, the philosophy of science. Aspects of the latter discipline have sought to provide an analysis of the history and intellectual frameworks that govern science, including the structure and dynamics of its products. Yet SR requires the systematic testing of hypotheses, beyond logical analysis and epistemological intuition, for their comportment with actual scientific practices. A useful analogy here is medical research, an ultimate goal of which is the understanding and systematic development of pragmatic practices that improve the efficiency of health care, disease treatment, and prevention. By contrast, the philosophy of science has traditionally been based on individual insights, opinions, and arguments whose validation does not depend on either systematic testing or the general acceptance of other practitioners (i.e., other philosophers). This has led, mistakenly in our view, to an overemphasis on the *results* of science—theories, explanations, large-scale historical transitions within broad disciplines—rather than the processes and practices by which these results are achieved.

2.2. The Emergence of New Scientific Disciplines

As a new scientific discipline, SR will proceed through the developmental stages that characterize the emergence of (most) new scientific disciplines. Here we feel that the historical research of Thomas Kuhn (1962) has much to offer. Kuhn was originally a historian of physics, so his historical hypotheses were tested against the actual histories of specific fields in that discipline. SR is not equivalent to history of science. Instead, it is concerned with the general principles governing current scientific practice, and so must answer principally to case studies of current research programs. But in this subsection we make a point about the development of new scientific disciplines, so this part of our project connects with Kuhn's historical analysis. We are especially interested in an aspect of Kuhn's historical account that is less well known than his accounts of anomalies, crisis science, and scientific revolutions. This is Kuhn's characterization of how the first stage of "normal science" in a given discipline emerges out of a "preparadigm" phase. Kuhn's discussion of this process occupies only one chapter in his classic (1962) book (chapter 2, "The Route to Normal Science"—and unfortunately, in that chapter Kuhn spends as much time discussing the impact of first-emergent paradigms as he does of the process of their emergence). According to Kuhn, each discipline, from physics to medicine to economics, begins with isolated efforts by individual practitioners and their lineage of apprentices. In this initial stage, core practices are not systematically tested and evaluated, but are instead guided by tradition and mostly implicit principles passed on individually from a mentor to his or her apprentices. Not only is there widespread disagreement among practitioners about the basic theoretical principles that lead to successful results, but also about good experimental practices, useful methodological assumptions, the ranking of problems in terms of their importance for furthering knowledge, and the ways that all of these are taught to future practitioners. Kuhn's two examples (described very briefly!) are the study of physical optics prior to Newton's *Optiks* (Kuhn, 1962, pp. 12–13) and the history of electrical research in the first half of the seventeenth century prior to Franklin's

Electricity (pp. 13–18). He insists, however, that the history in these two examples is typical, and he lists numerous other examples of preparadigm sciences.

What finally emerges from the chaos of preparadigm science is "normal science." The key to this step is the emergence of a paradigm. Kuhn's notion of paradigm quickly became a trendy term of art in pop philosophy of science. But in his more historically focused writings, Kuhn was somewhat clearer about a paradigm's basic components, even if his use of the term was highly ambiguous. As his brief descriptions of the physical optics and electricity cases show, the first-emergent paradigm in a discipline is far more than a shared commitment to a single theory. It also consists of principles of systematic data evaluation and formalization, and the sharing of those principles and ideas among recognized participants that comprise the discipline. As normal science emerges from preparadigm science with the general acceptance of a single paradigm, a concerted effort to extract, state, and defend general principles of scientific practice becomes a part of the discipline. Consequently, when a discipline acquires the standing of normal science, students no longer depend solely on the implicit or explicit knowledge of their particular mentors. There is a shared body of knowledge that introduces them to fundamental principles that are central to the practice of their discipline. Central components of the paradigm are communicated through a core set of shared laboratory experiences and problems that all students are expected to master. Students do not just memorize the generalizations and laws of the discipline's theories; they learn the central applications of these generalizations in the discipline's activities. Of course, medical students learn about general biological principles that guide medical practice, financial analysts use economic principles in evaluating investments, and budding chemists learn the laws of synthesizing new compounds. But all of this theoretical learning takes place in normal science against a background of shared *practical* training.

We contend that SR at present remains a preparadigm endeavor, suffering from the host of shortcomings that Kuhn's analysis revealed of preparadigm examples from science's history. The discipline needs a first-emergent paradigm to move forward.

Despite Kuhn's initial attempts to make his account of science's dynamics answer to the actual history of various disciplines, there remains an air of relativism about it. Why, in a given discipline, did *that* paradigm first take hold? He suggests, in his brief discussion of Franklin and electricity that the explanation of one particular phenomenon (the Leyden jar) "provided the most effective of the arguments that made his theory a paradigm," and that "to be accepted as a paradigm, a theory must seem better than its competitors" (1962, p. 17). Yet these vague remarks didn't stop Kuhn's followers, particularly in the sociology of science, from quickly attributing these outcomes to "subjective" factors—sociological forces impinging on the discipline at the time, psychological factors that influenced key practitioners, and the like. Even now, scientists still lack validated general principles of how to maximize the probability of discovery, improve the chances that their work will contribute further knowledge in their discipline, and impact the work of other scientists. We propose that these lacks are due to SR still being in a preparadigm stage. Shared general principles about scientific practice, verified by their successful application to actual case studies in specific disciplines, have not yet been agreed on. Training on the procedures of scientific discovery still mostly depends on implicit practices passed on from individual scientists to their students and collaborators. The lesson from Kuhn's historical account of preparadigm to normal science is that two events forecast this transition: an explicit effort to extract and test general principles that guide the practice of the discipline, and an attempt to disseminate these principles so that others can use and build on them. The focus shifts from individual practitioners and their untested ideas to large groups of practitioners and an evolving body of shared, tested principles that guide their activities. One goal of the remainder of this chapter is to provide a first step toward achieving this outcome for SR.

2.3. The Many "Sciences" of Science

Even now, scientists learn how to identify important problems, devise research strategies, spot unique scientific opportunities, make research choices, and determine when a problem is solved, mostly from years of experience and implicit examples and interactions with their mentors and colleagues. Although methods to determine the properties of celestial bodies, derive new chemical compounds, and analyze the functional organization of the brain, for example, are subject to constant development and shared analysis, the workings of the processes by which progress on these matters is made are not. Disciplines as diverse as dialectics, heuristics, theology, and epistemology have been referred to as the science of science by various authors throughout the ages. Nevertheless, none of these disciplines ever involved the systematic analysis of scientific practice using techniques of science itself, the derivation and testing of key principles of scientific activity against detailed evidence of actual scientific practice, or the explicit aim of improving the overall efficiency and productivity of scientific activity. Certainly none ever came close to acquiring the status of the first normal science of science in Kuhn's sense. Toward achieving these aims, we propose SR as first and foremost a pragmatic discipline whose key goal is to extract and test principles that guide scientific research and increase the efficiency of science—just as the tested laws of, say, chemistry, economics, and medicine increased the efficiency and efficacy of their respective disciplines. Ultimately SR's methods, practices, and results must be accepted and developed further by practicing scientists. Nothing less will constitute success.

2.4. SR and Scientific Creativity

It is important to stress that the derivation of general principles of scientific investigation is not meant to undermine the creativity of individual scientists. After all, the accepted and largely shared general principles of, for example, medicine, economics, and chemistry do not undermine the creativity of the best surgeons, investors, and chemists. In each of these fields, individual acts of creative scientific genius are easily found and acknowledged. Yet these instances seem recognized as such by practitioners in these fields because of shared commitments to practices, methods, and goals—including largely shared rankings of the important from the peripheral problems and what constitutes solutions for them. Genuine creativity seems only recognizable as such against a shared background of "the normal."

2.5. SR Is Not History, Sociology, Cognitive Neuroscience, or Heuristics of Science

SR stems from the need to make explicit what successful scientists do. It seeks to generate general hypothesis about the principles underlying their success, develop new informatic tools such as electronic databases and computer modeling to test these hypotheses, share emerging findings among scientists who can then develop them further, and ultimately use these findings to shape the education of young scientists. We've already noted that this investigative work is best done by practicing scientists, because their implicit grasp of their disciplines and accumulated practical insights will best guide initial attempts to make these principles explicit. In stating general SR principles, it will be necessary to have a sense of what pushes science forward. Emerging SR knowledge holds great promise for impacting the education and activities of scientists. Even a small increase in the efficiency of science could have an exponential effect on discovery and innovation. Did Galen imagine that his pioneering efforts toward making principles of medical practice explicit would one day lead to average life expectancies of nearly 80 years in medically advanced societies? Did Lavoisier ever imagine that the elemental chemistry he was explicating would feed, clothe, house, transport, cure, and entertain the world? SR seeks similar impacts on the practice of science itself.

Some social scientists will argue that SR already exists, in the disciplines of history and sociology of science. But SR is not the study of the history or sociology of science, nor of the cognitive processes underlying scientific activities. These neighboring disciplines can be of great interest to SR practitioners, but they do not represent the central goals of the discipline. The accumulation of heuristics about the practices of scientists, such as those described in George Polya's (1945) inspired work *How to Solve It* is also not the goal of SR. Although valuable and insightful, these heuristics are not scientifically derived principles that have been either tested or validated. SR is not concerned with accumulating or cataloging untested insights about science but on generating and testing hypothesis concerning the general principles that underlie successful scientific practice.

Tool development has been a central focus of historians and sociologists of science, and rightly so. Tool development is central to the genesis and growth of all scientific disciplines, and it will also be so for SR. For example, the influence and impact of the work of pioneers of memory research, such as Ebbinghaus (1885) and Pavlov (1927), can be traced back not only to their theoretical insights but equally to their developing new tests and apparatus to test their ideas and develop their concepts. Experimental tools often determine which ideas and hypothesis can be rigorously evaluated first, and therefore which aspects of the discipline's phenomenology are first investigated and then built on.

3. SR in Practice: The Convergent Four Hypothesis

3.1. Introduction

So far our discussion has been entirely abstract. To ground the practices and goals of SR, we next describe an initial SR hypothesis, the *convergent four*. This hypothesis specifies four criteria that we claim are jointly sufficient for fully establishing causal hypotheses in actual, current scientific practice. (An earlier statement of similar criteria can be found in Elgersma and Silva, 1999; see also Silva, 2007). We derive these criteria and the case for their joint sufficiency directly from paradigmatic case studies of published scientific results. We assume that one key goal of science is to explain natural phenomena by establishing networks of causal connections among them. Single causal connections do not sit alone but are located within a network of other connections. Ours are not the first proposed criteria for establishing causal hypotheses in science. Previous attempts, however, were mostly focused on specific problems, such as Koch's postulates (1884) for studying pathogens and infectious diseases. We discuss some historical precedents of the convergent four in section 4.

Before we present the convergent four hypothesis, however, it is crucial to distinguish between two different scientific activities: investigating causal hypotheses relating distinct phenomena as contrasted with articulating and documenting the phenomena and concepts involved in causal hypotheses. A useful metaphor here is the difference between specifying the connections in a network versus specifying the nodes that get connected. For example, in memory research the initial distinction between short-term and long-term memory, or the fragmentation of memory into distinct kinds or types (e.g., iconic, working, declarative, implicit), are not matters of offering and testing causal hypotheses between distinct phenomena, but rather of articulating and documenting phenomena and concepts—although, of course, once articulated and documented, these phenomena and concepts figured prominently in causal hypothesizing and testing (in establishing causal connections). *The convergent four hypothesis only speaks to the practices involved in establishing causal hypotheses, not to the practices of articulating and documenting concepts and phenomena* (except indirectly).

To illustrate an earlier statement of the convergent four hypothesis, one of us (Silva, 2007) previously described two concrete cases: the widely accepted connection between DNA and heredity, and the still controversial connection between synaptic plasticity and learning (Morris et al., 2003; Silva, 2003). In this chapter, we focus on a more specific case from recent molecular and cellular neuroscience: the established experimental connections between cyclic adenosine monophosphate response element binding protein (CREB) activity in individual neurons and *memory consolidation* in mammals. Our detailed presentation of this research will not only illustrate and test each component the convergent four hypothesis but will also show philosophers and cognitive scientists how molecular pathways in neurons have been bridged, directly and experimentally, with cognitive functions. (Recall that was our first puzzle in section 1). Toward the end of this section, we show how the convergent four hypothesis addresses the second, more general puzzle about institutionalized science's inefficiencies.

Over the next five subsections we introduce far more molecular-biological detail than philosophers and cognitive scientists typically encounter. These details matter, however, because without them the strength and extent of the actual experimental linkages now in place between molecular mechanisms and cognitive functions will simply be missed. However, we urge readers less familiar with current molecular biology to not lose sight of the forest for the trees. We present these scientific details both to address the first puzzle sketched in section 1 and illustrate the convergent four hypothesis.

3.2. Basic Biochemistry and Molecular Biology of CREB

Good descriptions of the basic biochemistry and molecular biology of CREB can be found in numerous textbooks. CREB is a member of the CREB/ATF (activating transcription factor) family of gene transcription proteins that control the transcription of messenger RNA (mRNA) complementary to a strand of DNA in a variety of genes and many types of biological tissue. Some isoforms of CREB are transcription activators, turning on gene transcription; others are transcription repressors, inhibiting transcription. Evidence suggests that interactions between activator and repressor CREB isoforms are involved in regulating CREB activity; for simplicity, we focus exclusively on CREB activators. CREB activators are themselves activated via phosphorylation (attachment of a phosphate group), with a critical phosphorylation site being the serine residue at position 133. One mechanism of CREB phosphorylation starts with the binding of the neurotransmitter dopamine to postsynaptic receptors. This binding primes adenylyl and adenylate cyclase molecules in the postsynaptic terminal to convert adenosine triphosphate (ATP) into cyclic adenosine monophosphate (cAMP). Increased cAMP molecules bind to the regulatory subunits of cAMP-dependent protein kinase (PKA) molecules. This binding frees PKA catalytic subunits that translocate to the neuron nucleus. There the catalytic PKA subunits phosphorylate CREB transcription activators. When phosphorylated, CREB molecules bind at cAMP response element (CRE) sites in promoter regions of various genes, recruit other transcription elements on the promoter, change the configuration of the DNA molecule in the gene's control region to bring them in contact with the RNA polymerase docked further down in the promoter region, and turn on mRNA transcription.

The gene targets of phosphorylated CREB are numerous and varied, but in neurons undergoing late-long-term potentiation (L-LTP) two types of targets are crucial. (LTP is a well-studied form of activity-dependent synaptic enhancement that, since its earliest systematic investigations more than three decades ago, has been suggested as a key mechanism for certain forms of learning and memory. L-LTP is the form persisting for many hours to days at individual potentiated synapses, and requiring new gene expression and protein synthesis.) The first type are genes for regulatory proteins, like ubiquitin carboxyl-terminal hydrolase (uch). The protein binds to a proteosome to destroy free regulatory subunits of PKA, providing a feedback mechanism for keeping catalytic subunits in protractedly active states. The second type of targets for phosphorylated CREB are immediate early genes for proteins that serve as transcription activators for structural proteins. These last proteins restructure active synapses, keeping them potentiated for hours to days.

What does all of this biochemistry and molecular biology have to do with cognition? Over the past decade, numerous experiments have linked the cAMP-PKA-CREB-gene targets pathway in individual neurons to *memory consolidation*—the conversion of labile, easily disrupted short-term memories into stable, long-term form. The experimental evidence linking the CREB pathway to memory consolidation can be grouped under four distinct yet converging lines. Each line is one component of the convergent four hypothesis. We explicate each of these components separately, using illustrations drawn from the experimental literature linking CREB activity and memory consolidation in mammals.

3.3. Observation

Observation refers to experiments designed to determine whether one natural phenomenon regularly follows another. Observation experiments do not intentionally alter the phenomena being investigated, and as far as there is any experimental interference, this is typically an unwanted consequence. Good observation experiments document strong correlations between occurrences of the phenomena hypothesized to be causally related. The temporal aspect of observation experiments relies on the standard assumption in mechanistic science that causes precede their effects. But good observation experiments show more than simply this. They carefully document the exact temporal dimensions of the two phenomena. This is especially important in studies of the causal mechanisms of cognitive functions. What gets related in such studies is the occurrence of the hypothesized cellular or molecular mechanism and the observed behaviors being employed as experimental measures for the cognitive phenomenon. Often, though not always, meeting the observation condition is the first experimental step toward establishing a cellular or molecular mechanism for a cognitive phenomenon. However, it is never the only step, at least not in current molecular and cellular cognition.

In section 3.1 we distinguished the investigation of causal hypotheses from the articulation of concepts that figure into causal hypotheses. Recall that we offer the convergent four as an SR hypothesis about only the former activity. This is especially important to keep in mind when considering the observation component. Observation experiments also play a key role in articulating and elaborating scientific concepts. However, the observation experiments discussed here are limited to those used to investigate causal hypotheses in science—the connections, not the nodes.

Numerous observational studies correlate CREB functioning within the cAMP-PKA-CREB-gene targets pathway with accepted measures of memory consolidation in mammals. A good recent example comes from Paul Colombo and his colleagues (Countryman, Orlowski, Brightwell, Oskowitz, and Colombo, 2005). They used a long-term version of the social transmission of food preferences (STFP) in rats. In the STFP task, a "demonstrator" animal is first fed food cued with a specific odor that is retained on the animal's breath. Demonstrators then interact with "observer" animals. Following a delay period after the social interactions (typically 1–30 minutes for short-term STFP, and 24–48 hours for long-term STFP), observer rats are offered a choice between the cued and uncued food. The percentage of cued food eaten by the observers during the test phase relative to the amount of uncued food eaten is taken as a measure of short-term or long-term STFP memories. (Experimenters control for prior preferences for cued and uncued foods in observer animals.)

Previous lesion studies had shown that an intact hippocampus is necessary in rats for long-term STFP. To correlate increased CREB activity with the memory consolidation aspect of long-term STFP, Countryman et al. (2005, experiment 2) used a standard immunocytochemical reactivity technique to count the number of neurons in ventral and dorsal hippocampus (as well as a control brain region that has nothing to do with STFP) that were positive for phosphorylated CREB (indicating recent CREB activity in those neurons). This nonintervening, measurement-correlational observation study "tested the extent to which acquisition and recall, when measured independently, induced CREB phosphorylation...and demonstrates that

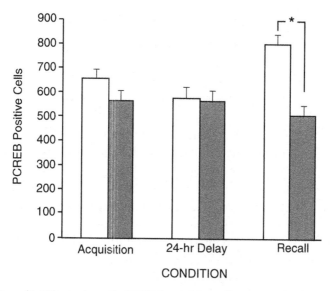

Figure 4.1 Mean (± SE) number of pCREB-ir positive cells per standard area measured in rat ventral hippocampus of STFP experimental (black bars) and social interaction control (gray bar) observers after acquisition, a 24-hour delay, or 48-hour recall of the social transmission of food preference. *$P < 0.05$. Reprinted with permission from Countryman et al. (2005), figure 9, p. 63.

learning-induced activity of the transcription factors is most robust in the ventral hippocampus" (Countryman et al., 2005, p. 65). The results correlated increased CREB activity in ventral hippocampus neurons with consolidation of the long-term STFP memories. Increases in CREB phosphorylation were not observed after a number of other control conditions (see figure 4.1).

3.4. Negative Alteration

Negative alteration refers to experiments in which the probability of one natural phenomenon is decreased and the effect on another (typically on its probability) is tested. Negative alteration experiments, as the name suggests, involve experimental interventions into proposed causal mechanisms and networks. When investigating the cellular and molecular mechanisms of cognitive functions, negative alteration experiments typically proceed by a controlled manipulation to decrease the hypothesized mechanism. A decrease in the behaviors used to indicate the cognitive function of interest is predicted. (The exception is when the mechanism is inhibitory, in which case the behavior is predicted to increase.) With the earlier advent of specific pharmacological techniques, and more recently the widespread use of genetically manipulated rodents, negative alteration experiments have been the experimental bread and butter of molecular neuroscience for more than two decades.

Thus, numerous negative alteration experiments have linked CREB activity in the cAMP-PKA-CREB-gene target pathway in individual neurons to memory consolidation in mammals. In CREB$^{\alpha\delta-}$ mutant mice, the gene for activator α and δ isoforms of CREB is interrupted with a method that deletes the gene in embryonic stem cells, which are then used to generate a line of mutant mice. (This is the negative alteration of CREB function.) These mutants have been used in memory consolidation experiments ranging from standard Pavlovian fear conditioning to contextual fear conditioning, the Morris water maze, STFP, place learning, and even social recognition memory. In all of these studies, the behavioral results are the same: CREB$^{\alpha\delta-}$ mutants display intact short-term memory compared to wild-type (nonmutated) littermate controls but deficient long-term memory. Recently, Satoshi Kida, Alcino Silva, and their colleagues developed a more sophisticated mutant mouse with an inducible-reversible repressor form of CREB that, when activated by tamoxifen (TAM), produces a temporally limited CREB-deficient mouse (the CREB^{IR} mutant). TAM injections activate the transgenic mutant CREB and this activated protein was shown to interfere with CREB-dependent transcription; at all other times, CREB activity is normal (Kida et al., 2002).

Kida et al. (2002) showed the usual pattern of behavioral results for decreased CREB functioning in CREB^{IR} mutants who had received TAM injections. They used both hippocampus-requiring and strictly amygdala-dependent memory tasks. The hippocampus-requiring task was contextual fear conditioning, in which animals are exposed to a new environment for 2 minutes and then shocked, and then placed back in the environment after a delay of 30 minutes to 1 hour for short-term test, and 24 hours for long-term test. The strictly amygdala-dependent task was classic Pavlovian fear conditioning, in which a neutral tone is paired with a shock, and the tone presented 30 minutes to 1 hour later for short-term test and 24 hours later for long-term test. On both tasks, the behavioral measure for memory is amount of time the animal spends freezing for 2 minutes after the conditioned stimulus is presented. Freezing is a characteristic rodent fear response in which the animal ceases all movement except breathing. CREB[IR] mice given the activator TAM showed normal memory for both tone and contextual conditioning 30 minutes but not 24 hours after training (see figure 4.2). Thus these induced CREB mutants displayed the usual memory consolidation deficit.

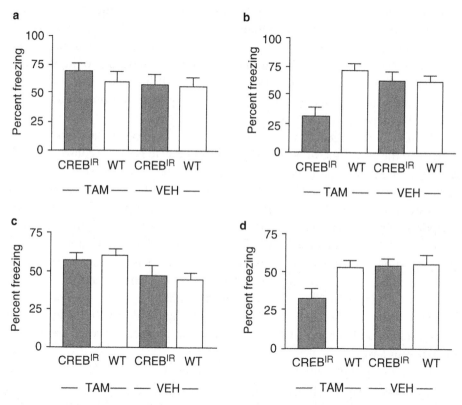

Figure 4.2 Activating the CREB repressor disrupted long-term (LTM) but not short-term (STM) conditioning for contextual and Pavlovian (tone) fear conditioning. (a) Activating CREB[IR] does not affect 2-hour memory (STM) for contextual fear conditioning (CREB[IR]/TAM, n = 9; WT/TAM, n = 6; CREB[IR]/VEH, n = 4; WT/VEH, n = 6). (b) Activating CREB[IR] disrupted 24-hour memory (LTM) for contextual fear conditioning (CREB[IR]/TAM, n = 14, WT/TAM, n = 5; CREB[IR]/VEH, n = 10; WT/VEH, n = 21). (c) Activating CREB[IR] does not affect 2-hour memory (STM) for tone fear conditioning (CREB[IR]/TAM, n = 9; WT/TAM, n = 11; CREB[IR]/VEH, n = 6; WT/VEH, n = 9); (d) Activating CREB[IR] disrupted 24-hour memory (LTM) for tone fear conditioning (CREB[IR]/TAM, n = 10; WT/TAM, n = 10; CREB[IR]/VEH, n = 10; WT/VEH, n = 11). Reprinted with permission from Kida et al. (2002), figure 2c–f.

3.5. Positive Alteration

Positive alteration refers to experiments wherein the probability of one natural phenomenon is increased and the effect on another (typically on its probability) is tested. Positive alterations, like negative alterations, involve experimental interventions into proposed causal mechanisms and networks. When investigating the cellular and molecular mechanisms of cognitive functions, positive alteration experiments typically proceed by a controlled manipulation to increase the hypothesized mechanism. An increase in the behavior used to indicate the cognitive function of interest is predicted. (The exception is when the mechanism is inhibitory, in which case the behavior is predicted to decrease.) So far, successful positive alteration experiments in molecular and cellular cognition have been difficult to achieve. One successful example involved increasing the number of N-methyl-D-aspartate receptor (NMDAR) 2B genes, which increased the amount of NMDAR 2B protein in the brain and the probability of synaptic plasticity (Silva, 2003). This protein is a subunit of NMDA receptors that, among other things, contribute to the activation of calmodulin kinase II (CaMKII) (Schulman, 2004). Behaviorally, mice that inherited the extra copies of the NMDAR 2B gene showed better learning of a type that is known to depend on those synapses (Tang et al., 1999).

More recently, Sheena Josselyn, Alcino Silva, and colleagues have linked CREB activity in the cAMP-PKA-CREB-gene target pathway to memory consolidation in a positive alteration experiment (Han et al., 2007). They microinjected replication-deficient herpes simplex virus (HSV) vectors fused with a gene expressing green fluorescent protein (GFP) and either the wild-type CREB gene for the α and δ transcription enhancer isoforms (*CREB^{WT}*) or a LacZ gene for a protein that has no effect on CREB function (as a control for any effects of viral transfection). The GFP gene insertion and subsequent protein synthesis makes infected neurons easy to image and count. Infected neurons synthesize a protein that distributes throughout their cytoplasms and literally glows green in microscopic images. The *CREB^{WT}* insertion is the positive alteration: It increases the amount of CREB α and δ proteins available and enhances CREB functioning in infected neurons over normal endogenous levels.

Using this positive alteration technique, Han et al. (2007) first manipulated CREB expression in a population of CREB^{αδ-} mice (the genetically mutated mice with greatly reduced levels of CREB transcription enhancers). These mutants displayed the characteristic memory consolidation deficit for Pavlovian auditory fear conditioning—intact short-term memory but greatly diminished long-term memory. They only froze about 20 percent of time after exposure to the conditioned tone during the testing phase 24 hours after tone-shock pairings. Wild-type littermate control mice, by contrast, froze about 60–70 percent of time. Han et al. (2007) microinjected HSV vectors containing genes for GFP and either CREB^{WT} or LacZ into the lateral nucleus of the amygdala (LA) of CREB^{αδ-} mutants or wild-type littermates prior to the training phase of auditory fear conditioning. Although the viral vector only infected around 18 percent of LA neurons in all groups, CREB^{WT} injections completely rescued long-term auditory fear conditioning in CREB$^{\alpha\delta-}$ mutants. CREB$^{\alpha\delta-}$ mutants receiving the LacZ control vector displayed the usual failure to consolidate long-term auditory fear conditioning memories. They froze only about 20 percent of time following exposure to the conditioned tone 24 hours after training. By contrast, wild-type mice microinjected with either CREB^{WT} or LacZ froze around 70 percent of time. Yet CREB$^{\alpha\delta-}$ mutants receiving microinjection of CREB^{WT} froze about 75 percent of time, statistically identical to wild-type performances (see figure 4.3). Han et al. (2007) controlled explicitly for the possibility that increasing CREB activity in LA neurons in CREB$^{\alpha\delta-}$ mutants simply increased freezing behavior. So increasing CREB function via a positive alteration using viral vector microinjections in less than 20 percent of LA neurons completely rescues the consolidation of long-term auditory fear conditioning in CREB-deficient mice.

In this experiment, the authors could not measure an enhancement in memory in WT mice driven by the CREB virus because the strong training conditions were designed to demonstrate that even after training that drives control mice to ceiling performances, CREB mutants still show clear memory deficits that can be rescued by the CREB virus. To see the effects of the CREB virus in wild-type mice, the authors used milder training conditions that allowed them to measure an enhancement in memory driven by the CREB virus. They used low-intensity shocks (0.4 mA as compared to 0.7 mA) during the training phase that elicit a less-than-maximal freezing response in the testing phase 24 hours later—typically about 40 percent of time as compared to 60–70 percent. Indeed, wild-type mice receiving the LA LacZ control vector froze about 40 percent of time following tone exposure 24 hours after training. Wild-type mice receiving the LA CREB^{WT} vector, however, froze about 75 percent of time, behaving as though they had been trained with maximally effective shocks. This difference is a statistically significant

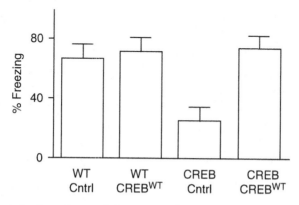

Figure 4.3 Microinjection of control (Cntrl; n = 8) or CREB^{WT} (n = 9) vector into the LA did not change the high levels of freezing in WT mice, whereas microinjection of CREB^{WT} (n = 9) but not control (n = 8) vector into CREB-deficient mice rescued this memory deficit [Genotype × Vector interaction F(1,30) = 6.64, P < 0.05]. Reprinted with permission from Han et al. (2007), figure 1D.

increase in tone-shock association due to increased CREB availability over normal endogenous levels.

Positive alteration experiments are unquestionably a key component in making compelling causal connections in science. In neuroscience, they often provide the missing piece of evidence for sufficient experimental justification of a hypothesized mechanism for a specific cognitive function. They provide key evidence in the search for cognitive enhancers with potential clinical applications. They provide the evidence that separates a genuine mechanism from frivolous counterexamples to the convergent four hypothesis, e.g., "altering the amount of O_2 in the animals' environment affects behavior on memory tasks. Is environmental O_2 therefore a mechanism of memory?" No, because positively altering—increasing—environmental O_2 beyond normal range does not increase memory behavior.

3.6. Integration

Integration refers to a general class of scientific activity that does not directly involve either manipulation or observation, but focuses instead on hypothesizing, ordering, and cross-referencing connections between phenomena. James Watson and Francis Crick's (1953a, 1953b) proposed connection between the biochemical properties of DNA and heredity is a monumental example from the previous century. It suggested a way that one phenomenon is part of a chain of causes that ultimately produces an effect: how the combinatorial possibilities of the bases (A, G, C, T) along a strand of DNA could be used to encode many different genes and in turn how the complementarity of the two strands of a DNA molecule could account for the propagation of genes between cell divisions, and thus ultimately the transmission of traits between generations. Sometimes one of the two phenomena being connected has never even been observed. A nice example was Hebb's (1949) proposal that learning is due to a hypothetical mechanism that modulates the communication between neurons. Even the rudiments of modifiable cell–cell communication (i.e., synaptic plasticity) took another two decades to establish (e.g., Bliss and Lømo, 1973). Hebbian-inspired ideas of how synaptic plasticity could be used to store information were an essential part of the body of work that connects synaptic plasticity with learning and memory (Silva, 2003). It is important to note that integration efforts do not always precede efforts in the other three components of the convergent four. Often, integration work accompanies developments propelled by observation, negative alteration, and positive alteration results.

The unifying effects of integration efforts result in the formation of numerous clusters of causal interconnections between related phenomena. Individual connections do not stand alone but in groups of other related connections that together form networks of available interconnected information. The experimental strength of one connection between two specific phenomena contributes to the strength of other connections in the cluster. The established connection between the postsynaptic cAMP-PKA-CREB-gene targets pathway and memory consolidation has recently been part of such an iterative integration process. pCREB is deactivated by dephosphorylation, the removal of the phosphate group from its P box. One molecular mechanism of this removal involves the activation of protein phosphatase 1 (PP1) within the neuron's nucleus. When activated, PP1 binds to pCREB proteins to remove the phosphate group, rendering CREB unable to transcribe mRNA. However, PP1 itself is inactivated via (phosphorylated) inhibitor 1 (I1). By integrating this chain of reasoning, if transgenic mice could be bred with an inducible inserted transgene for I1, then when that transgene is activated, those mice should have an abundance of I1 available for phosphorylation, and hence a reduction in the amount of activated PP1, and thus an increase in amount and duration of activated CREB. Given the CREB–memory consolidation link already established, there should be some memory tasks that these animals perform better when the I1 transgene is switched on: a novel positive alteration experiment.

Genoux et al. (2002) developed exactly such a transgenic mouse: the $I\text{-}1^*$ mutant. Expression of the $I1$ transgene was regulated by feeding the mice doxycycline (DOX). The transgene was under the control of a CaMKIIα promoter, so expression was limited primarily to hippocampus and cortex. Genoux et al. (2002) used a standard nonspatial hippocampus-dependent object recognition task as their behavioral measure of memory. Mice were first exposed to an object. The object was then removed from the environment for a specified delay period, and then the previously presented object was returned to the environment along with a novel object. A discrimination ratio was computed, based on the amount of time the mouse spent exploring the novel object as compared to the amount of time it spent exploring the previously presented object. (A 50 percent score indicates chance performance and no recognition of the previously presented object.)

Genoux et al. (2002) used three different training regimes. Equal amounts of training time (exposure to the first-presented object, 25 minutes) were used in all regimes, but in *massed training*, the entire 25 minutes occurred in a single training session. In *brief interval distributed training*, the 25 minutes were divided into five 5-minute training sessions, with 5-minute intertrial intervals (ITIs) between each session. In *longer interval distributed training*, the ITIs between the 5-minute training sessions were increased to 15 minutes. Mice were then tested for object recognition 5 minutes, 3 hours, and 24 hours after training. It has been known for more than a century that longer interval distributed training (within ITI limits) generates stronger memories than massed or brief interval distributed training. Genoux et al. (2002) obtained this familiar result with their control mice. Yet when they switched on the transgene in the $I\text{-}1^*$ mutants during brief interval distributed training, the animals' memory performances in the object recognition task exceeded that of brief interval distributed training controls at all testing periods and matched that of longer interval training controls. This positive alteration was reversible by turning off the $I1$ transgene (allowing DOX to be metabolized and not refeeding it). Control and DOX-treated animals (wild-types and $I\text{-}1^*$ mutants) spent the same percentages of training time exploring the object, indicating no motivational effect of the induced transgene (see figure 4.4).

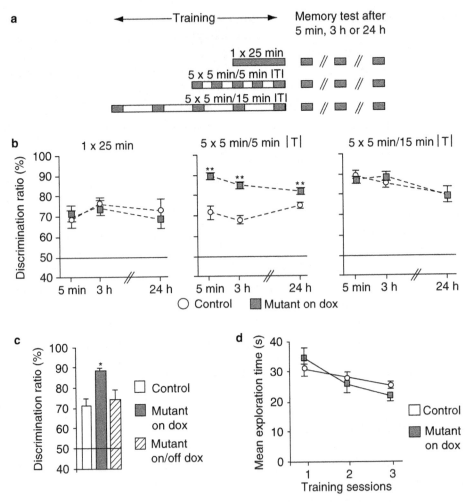

Figure 4.4 Distributed training improves performance in the object recognition task. (a) Scheme of training and testing protocols. ITI, intertrial interval. (b) Discrimination ratios in control mice 5 min ($F(1,23) = 10.296$, $P < 0.01$, for 5 min versus 15 min ITI), 3 hours ($F(1,9) = 22.976$, $P = 0.001$ for 5 min versus 15 min ITI), or 24 hours after training with either one of the protocols described in (a). Discrimination ratios in mutant mice 5 min ($F(1,13) = 16.565$, $P = 0.001$ for 1 × 25-min versus 5 × 5 min/5-min ITI), 3 hours ($F(1,13) = 5.217$, $P < 0.05$ for 1 × 25-min versus 5 × 5 mikn/5-min ITI), or 24 hours ($F(1,20) = 14.823$, $P = 0.01$ for 1 × 25-min versus 5 × 5 min/5-min ITI) after training. Lines at 50 indicate chance level. Dox, doxycycline. (c). Reversibility of the enhancement in performance. Mutant mice (n = 9) were treated with dox, trained with a set of objects for five 5-min sessions with 5-min ITIs and tested 5 min later (Mutant on dox). Dox was withdrawn and the animals were trained 2 weeks later with five 5-min sessions/5-min ITIs using a second set of objects, then tested 5 min later (Mutant on/off dox; $F(1,14) = 6.816$, $P < 0.05$ mutant on dox versus mutant on/off dox). Control mice n = 22. (d) Representative graph of total exploration during training in control (n = 22) and mutant (n = 7) mice. Decrease in total exploration per object across training sessions (1 to 3) indicates habituation to the objects. Control groups in these experiments were treated or not treated with dox. Results from these groups were similar and therefore were pooled. Reprinted with permission from Genoux et al. (2002), figure 1, p. 971.

Interestingly, PP1 is activated at high levels in hippocampus and cortical neurons during object recognition mass and brief interval distributed training. This increase is due to increased neuronal activity during these training regimes. (The usual mechanisms of PP1 activation are dependent on neuronal activity level.) Genoux et al. (2002) linked their positive alteration result directly to increased CREB activity in cortical neurons to a decrease in PP1 activation that normally occurs during brief interval distributed training (and not to some other mechanism of I1's action). They measured CREB-regulated expression of an inserted gene for β-galactosidase in neurons across cortex. This enzyme produces a blue color in its neuron substrates under standard microscopic conditions. CREB activity, as measured by β-galactosidase expression, was higher in cortical neurons (averaged across multiple cortical sections) when the I1 transgene was not switched on. When the transgene was activated, CREB function in mutants during brief interval training also increased to levels similar to those measured during longer interval distributed training in both *I-1* mutants with the transgene activated and controls (see figure 4.5). This collection of results from Genoux et al. (2002) nicely illustrates the iterative nature of integration practices we already stressed. Connections moved from the initially well-established cAMP-PKA-CREB-gene targets pathway to memory consolidation, to connections between other molecules that affect CREB activity (PP1, I1), and finally to new alteration experiments manipulating these additional molecules. The final experimental results of this integrative study suggested an answer at the level of molecular mechanism to a long-standing observation in experimental psychology, namely, increased learning during distributed versus massed training.

From the perspective of the convergent four hypothesis, scientific fields (like the study of learning and memory) consist of large networks of clusters of causal connections. Disciplines (like neuroscience) consist of interconnected groupings of these networks of clusters. One can imagine all scientific knowledge at a given

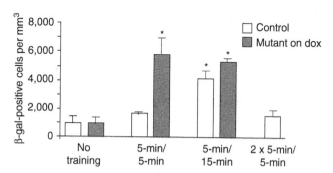

Figure 4.5 Enhanced CREB activity and phosphorylation. CREB transcriptional activity during training. Bar graphs are measurements of β-galactosidase positive cells per volume of cortex before training (no training, control, n = 4; mutant on dox, n = 3) and either after 5-min training followed by a 5-min delay (5-min/5-min, control, n = 3; mutant on dox, n = 3), 5-min training followed by a 15-min delay (5-min/15-min, control, n = 3; mutant on dox, n = 3), or two sessions of 5-min training followed by a 5-min delay (2 × 5-min/5-min, control, n = 3). Reprinted with permission from Genoux et al. (2002), figure 3a, p. 972.

time as a multidimensional information space populated by groupings of these networks of connection-clusters. Temporary disciplinary boundaries consist of areas where connections between groupings of these networks remain scarce. As science advances, this geography of connections fills in—and so does the taxonomy of the fields and disciplines. The goal of science is to fill this information space with additional networks of clusters that are optimally interconnected, both seamlessly and continuously. The general field of cognition has recently seen exactly this kind of integrative development, with the rise of *molecular and cellular cognition*. As Bozon et al. have stressed:

> A more profound, paradigmatic shift has been set in motion: no sooner was LTP discovered and a wealth of molecular information on its underlying mechanisms made available, then the beginnings of a new era in the cellular and molecular exploration of memory under both normal conditions and in disease states were framed. This has been driven by the increasing knowledge about LTP mechanisms, and also by the development of novel technologies specifically designed to exploit these molecular data. The net result has been a closer interaction between the fields of molecular, cellular, system and cognitive neuroscience that culminated in the past decade in the birth of the field of molecular and cellular cognition. (2003, p. 330)

We've discussed numerous examples of these interconnections in this section, limited to just a single molecular component of the cAMP-PKA-CREB-gene targets pathway and memory consolidation. Many similar specific connections have been formed, and are being formed as we write, and as does the CREB–memory consolidation link, many of these others also share the virtue of currently meeting all components of the convergent four.

In the distant future, disciplinary boundaries—areas of low densities of connections within science's overall information space—will only be due to fundamental ethical and physical limitations on experimentation. Hopefully, even as potential intervention techniques develop, humans will continue to find it unethical (and hence unacceptable) to carry out positive and negative alteration experiments to directly test links between the properties of molecular-biological, biochemical, and subatomic physical phenomena and the sociology of human populations. But that does not mean links will not exist between these phenomena. It means that the gaps between molecular biology/biochemistry/particle physics and sociology will only be filled by the collective strength of the myriad of interconnected clusters that reside between the information space that separates these disciplines and by extensive integration efforts that will require considerable amounts of computing power. There are many instances in science where technical and ethical problems limit the types of experiments that could be designed to test individual links in the networks of connections that define a scientific area or field. In these cases, the strength of each connection becomes very much dependent on the strength of the overall network. Thus, networks of knowledge can become stable and reliable even when individual connections do not fully fulfill the requirements of the convergent four hypothesis.

The convergent four hypothesis asserts that all four components are equally important for a sufficient evidential case for having established a causal connection scientifically between two phenomena. The synergy between these four different lines of evidence confers the total strength of evidence supporting any one proposed connection. In the case of CREB and particular forms of memory consolidation, this total evidence is strong. In the case of some other hypothesized molecular mechanisms for other cognitive phenomena, this total evidence may be weaker. Armed with the convergent four hypothesis, and its illustration by this single cluster of connections from recent molecular and cellular cognition studies, we extend our first SR hypothesis and answer the more general puzzle with which this chapter began.

3.7. Addressing the Puzzle about Institutionalized Science's Inefficiencies

Why do so many costly, time-consuming scientific publications, on topics of widespread interest, go unnoted within their disciplines? The convergent four hypothesis suggests an answer: *because those studies and results contribute to one of the convergent four conditions for which overwhelming experimental evidence already exists.* Those papers do not get cited across their specific disciplines because the specific component of the convergent four that they support is already strong enough for the phenomena they connect. They contain competent science—they were peer-reviewed and published, after all. But they provide the nth published observational study linking phenomenon A to phenomenon B, or the mth time that a specific negative alteration technique applied to A decreased the probability of B's occurrence. All the while, perhaps no positive alterations of A have been successful, or the integrative link between A and B still has significant gaps. This answer, based directly on the convergent four hypothesis, is objectively testable. We can survey the existing experimental literature linking A to B and group the most cited publications under the appropriate convergent four category. We can then assess the strength and variety of evidence for each category for linking A to B. We can then consider representative examples of undercited papers, arranged by date of publication, and see if they constitute simply more evidence for an already strong case for the category they fall under. Searchable electronic databases of scientific publications allow for easy collection of the relevant data.

Should our answer to this first question about science's inefficiencies bear out experimental testing, the impact on particular disciplines could be enormous. If editors and reviewers of the discipline's most prominent journals, grant and fellowship officials, review panels, and lab directors had an explicit, objective grasp of where specific hypotheses linking phenomena in their field stood with regard to the convergent four, both research resources and time could be directed to filling in the gaps. Inevitably, evidence sufficient for linking phenomena A and B leads to new hypotheses linking related phenomena. Our scientific case study in this section linking CREB activity to memory consolidation illustrated exactly this point. Evidence meeting the convergent four linked activity-dependent, stable synaptic plasticity (like LTP) to various forms of memory. This paradigmatic result was very much dependent on more specific hypotheses. For example, CREB activity in individual neurons is a key mechanistic component of the stability of synaptic changes, and the stability of these changes is central to the permanence of acquired information. A community of scientific researchers has been involved in the experimental work needed to establish the myriad of experimental threads that support the monumental finding that the changes in synaptic function are central to information storage in the brain. Major scientific cornerstones, such as the connection between synaptic plasticity and learning, are dependent on many mechanistic threads, each of which must fulfill all components of the convergent four. This not only adds to the weight of evidence supporting these key findings, it also provides mechanistic insights that elaborate on how one phenomena (i.e., synaptic plasticity) is connected with the other (learning, memory). Explicit statement and applications of the convergent four could hasten and streamline this process.

This potential impact applies to the education of individual scientists as well. Armed with the convergent four, a young scientist entering a new lab could survey its recent publications, group each under the appropriate convergent four category, and then develop and pursue research projects that fill in the gaps. Perhaps, for example, the lab has recently published a number of observational studies linking A to B and has filled in some experimental details about B that integrate the phenomena. If so, then the time is ripe in that lab for alteration experiments on A. One would hope that lab directors and heads would work with lab members and collaborators to develop such research strategies in light of the convergent four hypothesis (lab meetings are often concerned with less efficient topics). Our answer also suggests a way to test the influences of mentor–student interactions. Are Nobel lineage trees simply the result of biased sociological factors? Or are successful students of outstanding researchers often at least learning implicitly to pursue the gaps between phenomena as illuminated by the convergent four or other SR ideas that will undoubtedly emerge in the future? Do these students learn, perhaps by unconscious habituation, fundamental SR principles, such as looking for gaps according to the convergent four that their mentors' work has left open? The publication records of successful mentor–student relationships provide us with data to test this additional SR answer. If the data bear it out, research strategies based on the convergent four could become a part of basic scientific training, tailored to specific scientific disciplines. The potential here is quite exciting and nicely illustrates the pragmatic focus of SR.

3.8. One Limitation of the Convergent Four Hypothesis as Currently Articulated

The convergent four hypothesis does not pertain to several critical activities in science. One of these is the development of new tools for observing, altering, and manipulating natural phenomena. For example, in the neurobiology of learning and memory, new pharmacological tools like highly specific NMDA receptor antagonists and new genetic tools like mice with CaMKII mutations were central to initial efforts to connect synaptic plasticity to behavior (Silva, 2003). Tool development is an ideal topic for SR investigation. The results should lead to improved efficiency. Molecular and cellular cognition could serve as the subject for this SR investigation. It abounds with both new scientific tools and the direct application of tools developed in other disciplines (e.g., molecular biology, psychology, electrophysiology, etc.) to its experimental purposes.

3.9. The Sobering Reminder

Many scientists with whom we have discussed the convergent four hypothesis, especially molecular biologists, recognize it as an explicit statement of part of the implicit modus operandi of their discipline. This acknowledgment is promising. However, SR is itself a scientific discipline, so this hypothesis and its implications must be tested rigorously and objectively. We've already suggested ways that these tests can proceed. Tool development will figure prominently in such testing (see Silva, 2007, for an extended discussion). Our sobering reminder at the end of this section is that this work must be done before we accept the convergent four as an established SR result.

4. COMPARISONS AND CONTRASTS WITH PRIOR ATTEMPTS

In this section we survey briefly some prior attempts to characterize conditions on sufficient evidence for causal hypotheses in science. The first one we consider was developed specifically to test hypotheses about the causal agents of infectious diseases. The second was proposed as a model for testing causal hypotheses generally. We compare and contrast both with the Convergent Four.

4.1. Koch's Postulates

The *Koch (Henle) Postulates* (Henle, 1938; Koch, 1884) refer to criteria that must be fulfilled before a given pathogen could be taken as proved to cause a specific infectious disease (e.g., cholera, tuberculosis). The four requirements include (1) consistent isolation of the agent from disease cases, but not from normal subjects (although this second part was eventually abandoned by Koch when he found asymptomatic carriers of cholera); (2) propagation of the agent in culture; (3) reproduction of the disease by the isolated purified agent; and (4) reisolation of the agent from cases in (3). It is easy to see commonalities between Koch's postulates and two of the experimental categories described in the convergent four hypothesis. Koch's postulates (1), (2), and (4) are specific instantiations of the observation criterion. The hypothesized causal agent must be observed in association with the disease and must be seen to reproduce in appropriate media. Koch's postulate (3) is a specific implementation of positive alteration.

However, the convergent four hypothesis predicts that Koch's postulates will not be taken as sufficient to compel accepting a hypothesized causal connection between an agent and a specific disease. This prediction is verified by several attempts to revise Koch's postulates, proposed explicitly to address its experimental limitations (see, for example, Evans, 1976; Hill, 1965). The convergent four hypothesis asserts that in addition to Koch's postulates, it is critical to show that deleting the infectious agent from the subject (i.e., using antibiotics that eliminate the pathogen) cures the disease. This result would be a specific instance of negative alteration. The convergent four hypothesis also predicts that a credible explanation would have to be developed for how the pathogen causes the disease symptoms, based on detailed studies of the agent itself and the disease symptomatology. This result would be an instance of integration. Indeed, a recent revision of Koch's postulates proposes a number of changes that include specific instantiations of both the negative alteration and integration requirements of the convergent four hypothesis (Fredericks and Relman, 1996).

These limitations on Koch's postulates permit us to restress an important point about the application of the convergent four at particular developmental phases of individual scientific disciplines. The convergent four hypothesis provides an outline for the kinds of experiments and evidence required for an ideally compelling and efficient scientific test of a causal hypothesis. It is possible to make an acceptable case for a causal connection even in the absence of one (or more) of the four components. This absence in specific cases can be due to insurmountable ethical or technical limitations. In the case of Koch's original postulates, for example, negative alterations in the form we suggested didn't really exist as viable experimental tools at the time of their formulation, so it is not a great mystery as to why the importance of this strategy was missed. An acceptable case for a causal connection can rest on extensive amounts of evidence in the other three categories of the convergent four. A useful metaphor is the four legs of a chair. Even two- or three-legged chairs can stand and support some weight if the existing legs are sufficiently thick, strong, and properly placed. Influential causal connections in science are never isolated but always occur within networks of other related connections. This suggests that strengthening related connections can also serve to strengthen particular connections. Perhaps mathematical network theory analysis could be useful toward a formal analysis of this process (Newman, 2003).

4.2. Mill's Methods

In his classic logic book, *A System of Logic*, nineteenth-century British philosopher John Stuart Mill (1843) proposed several methods for discovering and confirming causal connections scientifically. Together, these have come to be called *Mill's methods*. Their statement and application was a monumental step forward in science's development. They were completely general, in the sense that they were intended to be applicable to all scientific disciplines. Mill stated them originally in terms of observations, but they are easily adapted to experimental interventions, as we will discuss them here.

Mill's first and simplest method is *agreement*: Look for a common factor that is present in all cases in which the effect occurs—for some respect in which all the different cases of the effect agree. When physicians confront numerous instances of a new symptomology, they begin looking for common factors among the cases: same food ingested, same virus in the bloodstream, and so on. Mill's second method is *difference*: Take away the hypothesized causal factor, hold every other potential causal factor constant across all cases, and see whether the effect still occurs. If the effect does not occur, this constitutes evidence that the removed factor is its cause. The method of difference, of course, is the rudiment of controlled experimentation. In both everyday reasoning and scientific practice, the methods of agreement and difference are often combined. This is Mill's *joint method of agreement and difference*, and it is important for establishing the necessity *and* sufficiency of a hypothesized cause. Agreement alone provides evidence that the hypothesized cause is sufficient for the effect. It shows that the effect can occur in the absence of any other factor, and hence that none of the other factors is necessary. But to tell whether the hypothesized factor is necessary, we must see whether the effect can occur in the absence of that factor—exactly what the method of difference investigates.

Mill's last two methods require the ability to quantify the effect. Suppose that a quantifiable effect occurs in the presence of several known causal factors a, b, c, and that it has already been established that c is responsible for one part of the effect and b is responsible for another part. Mill's method of *residues* asserts that the remainder of the effect (the "residue") must be caused by a. A classic logic textbook example is a person weighing a small, active dog. The person cradles the dog in his arms and steps on the scale, causing the scale to register 198.9 pounds. Prior to holding the dog, the man established his own weight at 171.4 pounds. Hence the dog's weight of 27.4 pounds constitutes the residue of the combined weighing effect. Finally, Mill's method of *concomitant variation* associates a quantitative change in the effect with quantitative changes in the hypothesized causal factor. If the hypothesized causal factor really is a causal factor, then we should see correlated quantitative changes in the occurrence of the effect when we make or observe quantitative changes (positive or negative) in the occurrence of the factor.

How do Mill's methods relate to the convergent four? We should not expect great differences. Mill's methods have been accepted principles of the inductive, experimental sciences for more than 150 years. In many ways, they constitute a detailed presentation of "the scientific method," as presented to students from grade school through postgraduate education. It would be remarkable if an SR study of actual current scientific practice revealed them to be grossly wrong. Mill's method of agreement is basically the observation component of the convergent four—one observes to find the common factor in various instances of the effect. Mill's method of difference is basically idealized negative alteration—one intervenes experimentally to eliminate the hypothesized causal factor, holding all other potential causal factors constant (to the extent possible), and simply measures whether the effect still occurs. Mill's joint method is the common combination of observation and negative alteration in experimental studies. Mill's method of concomitant variation is a crude, conflated statement of more sophisticated observation, negative, and positive alteration experiments—ones sensitive to the probabilistic nature of most causes. It fails to separate positive and negative interventions, however, and we saw ample reasons in section 3 to make this separation explicit. In molecular and cellular cognition studies, at least, negative alteration results are easier to achieve and must be interpreted with more caution. The convergent four thus makes explicit a separation that Mill's methods gloss over.

Mill's method of residues is best seen as an aspect of the practice of articulating scientific concepts, not testing causal hypotheses. It is a method for fragmenting a concept into its separate components. We drew this distinction between these two kinds of scientific endeavors early in section 3. The convergent four hypothesis thus has the further advantage over Mill's methods of keeping these two distinct scientific activities explicitly separated, as it pertains only to the testing of causal hypotheses. Finally, nothing in Mill's methods answers to the integration component. Similarly, there is no clear indication that *all* of Mill's methods must be fulfilled to provide a complete experimental justification for a causal hypothesis. Indeed, the usual reading of Mill's methods is that the satisfaction of any one of them, especially the joint method or the method of concomitant variation, is sufficient to establish a causal hypothesis. Thus in contrast to the convergent four, the standard interpretation of Mill's methods is logically too weak. The convergent four hypothesis predicts that there will be evidence judged sufficient for establishing a causal hypothesis according to Mill's methods, which *will not* be accepted as sufficient in actual scientific practice.

Perhaps the most reasonable upshot about these comparisons and contrasts is this: in the preparadigm stage of SR, still currently in place, Mill's methods constituted an important advance. They made explicit *some aspects* of the evidence deemed sufficient to establish causal hypotheses in actual scientific practice, were by and large accepted by many practitioners, and became a part of the education of young scientists. Unfortunately, they conflated practices that need to be kept distinct, ignored key components, and failed to notice that evidence from all these converging activities are required to make a completely sufficient case for a causal hypothesis. They were a useful first approximation to the convergent four. But in light of the deeper analysis of more detailed experimental case studies from more recent science (like the CREB–memory consolidation story we sketched), the next step toward "normal" SR is to replace Mill's methods with the convergent four in both their evaluative and educational uses.

5. A Second (Already Tested) SR Hypothesis

5.1. Reductionism in Actual Scientific Practice

Theories about the nature and scope of *reductionism* populate the philosophy of science literature. These theories have been especially influential in the philosophy of mind and cognitive science. Presently, two basic accounts of scientific reduction dominate philosophical discussion. How well do each of these accounts articulate reductionistic practices in actual science? (See Bickle, 2008, for extended discussion of the topic in this section.)

The first account, *intertheoretic reduction*, had its clearest and most influential statement in Ernest Nagel's (1961) book, *The Structure of Science*. According to Nagel, intertheoretic reduction is *logical deduction* of the laws or explanatory generalizations of the reduced theory from those of the reducing. Nagel was aware that in cases where the reduced theory contains terms that are not contained in the reducing, only trivial valid derivations of the former by the latter alone are possible. In such "heterogeneous" reductions, which Nagel acknowledged were typical in actual science, the premises of the derivation also required "rules of correspondence" that "bridge" all terms unique to the reduced theory with terms from the reducing. (For example, in the derivation of the ideal gas laws from the principles of statistical mechanics, a rule of correspondence relates "temperature" to "mean molecular kinetic energy of constituent gas molecules.")

Nagel also realized that actual scientific reductions often *correct* the reduced theory. To accommodate this, he added to the premises of the derivation counter-to-fact limiting assumptions and boundary conditions on the applicability of the reducing theory's laws. Thus, a corrective reduction would not imply the falsity of the reducing theory serving as premise of the derivation. Unfortunately, attempted applications of Nagel's basic model to increasingly well-described cases of reduction from science's history were failures. Ultimately, philosophers of science suggested fundamental revisions to his basic derivational account (see Hooker, 1981; Schaffner, 1967). Despite these challenges in the philosophy of science, however, Nagel's basic model was assumed to be the correct account of scientific reductionism by philosophers of mind well into the 1990s. It was assumed to provide the required relationship for the reduction of psychological to neurobiological theories by both proponents and opponents of psychoneural reduction.

In the mid-1990s, mostly due to influential work in the new discipline of consciousness studies, a new model of scientific reductionism gained philosophical prominence (Chalmers, 1996; Levine, 1993). Dubbed "functional reduction," this approach characterized scientific reduction as a two-stage process. The first stage involves "functionalizing" the concept targeted for reduction—characterizing it exhaustively in terms of its causes and effects. The second stage involves the normal experimental work in lower level sciences to discover which mechanisms in the actual world play the causal role ascribed to the target reduced concept. (Interestingly, this account was a key premise in one of the most influential arguments against the reducibility of the qualitative aspects of consciousness to brain events.)

Suppose we adopt the following SR approach toward characterizing real reductionism in real scientific practice (as Bickle has adopted in numerous recent studies, e.g., 2006a, 2006b). We find a clear example of a reductionistic field of scientific inquiry, dubbed so not only by its practitioners but also by scientists working in other related fields. Molecular and cellular cognition is an excellent candidate. Then, as unencumbered by epistemological and metaphysical assumptions as we can be, we investigate some paradigmatic examples of recent research from that field. Next we analyze the shared practices across these examples that differentiate this field from other, less reductionistic scientific fields investigating related phenomena. In cases drawn from molecular and cellular cognition, this will mean looking especially at experiments meeting the positive and negative alteration components of the convergent four. Such experiments, along with their implications for integration, constitute the special contribution that molecular and cellular cognition studies make to the science of cognition. The resulting analysis will be one of real reductionism in real scientific practice, as contrasted with artificial accounts of scientific reductionism that rest instead on philosophical assumptions about "what reduction has to be." In following this strategy, do we end up describing anything that resembles intertheoretic or functional reduction?

We contend that we do not (see Bickle, 2008, for more detailed arguments). Instead, we find that real reductionism in the actual practices of molecular and cellular cognition amounts to

> *Intervening causally* into increasingly lower levels of biological organization (i.e., cellular physiology, molecular pathways),

and then

> *Tracking* the effects of these interventions on the behavior of organisms using a variety of experimental procedures that are well accepted as measures of the cognitive phenomenon under investigation.

When the behavioral measures of the intervened organisms are statistically different than those of nonintervened controls, *in light of at least some aspects of an integration account that links the hypothesized cellular or molecular mechanism to the behaviors*, a reduction is claimed. Our best causal-mechanistic explanation for the behavioral data is then taken to reside at the lowest level into which we can intervene and for which an integrative account with the behaviors exists. Molecular and cellular cognitivists then speak of having found "a molecular biology of cognition" (Bailey, Bartsch, and Kandel, 1996), a "framework for a molecular understanding" of a specific cognitive function (Abel et al., 1997), or of its "molecular basis" (see www. molcellcog.org).

Unlike intertheoretic reduction, real reductionism in molecular and cellular cognition does not require an explicit, complete set of laws or explanatory generalizations that characterize the behaviors of reduced and reducing kinds in all contexts or circumstances. This is because reduction is not characterized as a logical relationship between collections of such laws or generalizations (theories). That is a good thing, because it is widely acknowledged that current scientific psychology does not offer such laws. For the record, neither does current molecular biology: Many specific details are known about the structure and dynamics of biological molecules, but that knowledge does not take the form of lawlike statements, even in molecular biology textbooks. Unlike "functional" reduction, real reductionism does not require the targeted reduced concepts to be characterized exhaustively in terms of their causes and effects. Instead, it requires cognitive concepts to be operationalized methodologically, in terms of specific behavioral measures for the purposes of controlled experiments. The methods of molecular and cellular cognition are also not even usefully approximated by the description of stage 1 of the functional reduction procedure. If you doubt this, we invite you to try to reconstruct an actual methods section of a typical molecular and cellular cognition publication in terms of the resources made available by functional reduction.

5.2. The Role of Higher Level Sciences

With SR still in early development, much can be learned by comparing and contrasting its initial results and hypotheses with recent work in the philosophy of cognitive science (see Bickle, 2008). For example, the SR result sketched in this section puts to rest a popular philosophical worry about reductionism. Some critics have charged that reductionism requires us to eschew or at least minimize the importance of higher level scientific investigations. But real reductionism, derived from the convergent four hypothesis, clearly does not require this. Notice that all four components *require* higher level scientific investigations. To establish the required observations, alterations, and integration between hypothesized molecular mechanisms and behaviors, we need precise knowledge about what the system does under controlled experimental conditions. This means having both precise data about the system's behaviors (as grist for our lower level mechanistic explanations) and good behavioral measures for the cognitive phenomenon at issue. These jobs require techniques from cognitive and experimental psychology. We need to know where to start inserting our cellular and molecular interventions. The "decomposition and localization" strategies of cognitive neuroscience are crucial for obtaining this (Bechtel and Richardson, 1993). We need to know what types of neuronal activity to intervene into: Action potential frequency? Action potential dynamics? Field potentials? Synaptic plasticity? Something else entirely? Neurocomputational modeling and computer simulations are important here. Each of these distinct neuronal activities is underlain by distinct molecular mechanisms and so requires different molecular-biological intervention techniques. Molecular and cellular cognition requires a lot of higher level cognitive science and neuroscience to achieve its potential reductions. Now it regularly draws on these sciences to get these details right. Molecular and cellular cognition is acknowledged to be a reductionistic brand of current neuroscience, perhaps even "ruthlessly" so. (That is why we drew paradigmatic cases from it to get an analysis of real reductionism in real scientific practice.) But that in no way precludes the use of higher level cognitive science by its practitioners. This common philosophical worry about reductionism is a red herring.

This point is worth dwelling on further, because more is at stake than just soothing philosophers' worries. Traditionally, the neuroscientific study of cognition has involved at least seven general disciplines: molecular neurobiology, neurophysiology, systems neuroscience, behavioral neuroscience, cognitive neuroscience, neuropsychology, and computational neuroscience/cognitive science. Each of these disciplines has its own experimental traditions and modus operandi that produce biases toward one or two components of the convergent four. For example, the typical functional neuroimaging study carried out in cognitive neuroscience is an observation experiment. Measured activation of brain region X regularly accompanies performance of behavior Y; therefore, activation of region X mediates behavior Y. Traditional neurophysiology also relies heavily on observation experiments. Many studies characterize synaptic, neuronal, and glial responses under different experimental conditions (see Bliss and Collingridge, 1993). Neurophysiology has also depended heavily on negative alteration experiments, using pharmacological and more recently molecular biological tools such as viral vectors and transgenic mice. The results are used to evaluate the causal connections between a given molecular process and a specific aspect of brain physiology (i.e., the role of NMDA receptors in LTP). Traditional behavioral neuroscience is also very much dependent on negative alteration experiments, where the function of a brain region is inferred from the behavior of experimental animals lacking that brain region due to surgical, electrical, or chemical lesions. In contrast, traditional computational neuroscience has focused on integration studies, using models to explore possible functional properties of molecular, physiological, or neuroanatomical mechanisms.

Recall that, according to the convergent four hypothesis, any finding that does not have convergent evidence from all four components still calls for further experimental work. Therefore, traditional behavioral neuroscientific lesion studies (negative alteration experiments) should be combined with observation, positive alteration, and integration studies. From the perspective of the convergent four hypothesis, it is clear why hypotheses about the function of a specific brain region supported by both cognitive neuroscientific observation experiments (functional imaging studies) and behavioral neuroscientific negative alteration experiments (lesion studies in experimental animals) invariably carry more weight among practicing scientists than those supported by only one of these approaches (Dade, Zatorre, and Jones-Gotman, 2002). And yes, this same point applies to successful positive and negative alteration experiments from molecular and cellular cognition. Without observation and integration experimental backing, such studies will rightfully have little long-term impact. For example, think of how little influence early studies by James V. McConnell (in which planaria ate the ground-up nervous tissue of conspecifics trained on a simple maze learning task and learned the task faster) had on the development of molecular and cellular cognition in its present form. Even positive alteration results get ignored in the long run if the integration component connecting hypothesized mechanism to measured behavior fails to be fulfilled.

The drive for integration in neuroscience has motivated researchers to venture into each other's traditional disciplines. Yet numerous SR questions remain. *How many* of the intermediate steps from intraneuronal molecular mechanism to behaviors need to be in place to justifiably connect up such phenomena? The convergent four is a good qualitative start toward answering these kinds of questions, but more detail will be needed to address quantitative SR questions. Are there a priori limitations on which phenomena can be connected directly? For example, most neuroscientists agree that it is unlikely that the physical properties of quarks will ever be experimentally connected to the behavior of societies. What reasons compel this view? Are properties of NMDA receptors and CaMKII as tightly connected experimentally to spatial learning as the properties of DNA are connected to heredity? If not, why not? What else needs to be added to currently available evidence and why? How do we know when there is enough evidence in each component to substantiate a connection between a brain phenomenon and a cognitive function? SR—systematic, testable, objective evidence-requiring attempts to answer these questions—will not only affect our perception of the state and reliability of our current knowledge. It will also improve the efficiency with which we explore this immense but tremendously exciting problem space. The convergent four hypothesis and the account of real reductionism in actual scientific practice are just the first baby steps along this path.

6. A Brief Concluding Remark on Searchable Publication Databases

Over the past 20 years a number of organizations have taken advantage of advances in computing and the ever decreasing price of data storage to develop comprehensive searchable electronic indices of scientific publications. MEDLINE and INSPEC are two well-known examples. By the end of 2005, MEDLINE had referenced more than 15 million articles in the biological sciences, from more than 4,600 journals, dating back to the 1950s. INSPEC listed nearly 10 million articles in physics, engineering and computer science, going back to 1898. These databases are not just being used as research tools. There have been significant efforts to use them to evaluate the success of individual scientists and the impact of their contributions. As we discussed in section 1, the ISI has developed a searchable database of citations. With this service it is straightforward to determine the number of citations associated with individual articles, scientists, and topics. Admittedly, these are crude measures of scientific contributions. Yet metrics such as these are now being used to estimate the influence of specific publications, individual scientists and even institutions (Cole, 2000; Hirsch, 2005). Like them or not, their use in such judgments is here to stay.

Within SR, we are proposing a different use for these extensive electronic records of science and its products. We're proposing to use them to chronicle the development and impact of concepts and ideas in science, to characterize the stages that define the evolution of influential ideas, and to extract and test explicitly stated hypotheses that govern these processes. In other words, we propose using them to begin the scientific study of science itself. Even people opposed to the use of these resources to evaluate scientific contributions should not fear their use for SR purposes. Hopefully the impact of their use in this way will have the same feedback dynamics we've stressed as one of SR's promises throughout this essay: building on and improving these crude beginnings.

ACKNOWLEDGMENT

Special thanks go to Marica Bernstein, whose comments on earlier versions of this chapter greatly improved its content and style.

REFERENCES

Abel, T., Nguyen, P. V., Barad, M., Deuel, T. A., Kandel, E. R., and Bourtchouladze, R. (1997). Genetic demonstration of a role for PKA in the late phase of LTP and in hippocampus-based long-term memory. *Cell* 88: 615–626.

Bailey, C. H., Bartsch, D., and Kandel, E. R. (1996). Towards a molecular definition of long-term memory storage. *Proceedings of the National Academy of Sciences USA* 93: 13445–13452.

Bechtel, W., and Richardson, R. C. (1992). *Discovering Complexity*. Princeton, N.J.: Princeton University Press.

Bickle, J. (2006a). Reducing mind to molecular pathways: Explicating the reductionism implicit in current mainstream neuroscience. *Synthese* 152: 411–434.

Bickle, J. (2006b). Ruthless reductionism in recent neuroscience. *IEEE Transactions on Systems, Man, and Cybernetics* 36: 134–140.

Bickle, J. (2008). Real reductionism in real neuroscience: Metascience, not philosophy of science (and certainly not metaphysics!). In J. Hohwy and J. Kallestrup (Eds.), *Being Reduced*. Oxford: Oxford University Press, 34–51.

Bliss, T. V., and Collingridge, G. L. (1993). A synaptic model of memory: Long-term potentiation in the hippocampus. *Nature* 361: 31–39.

Bliss, T. V., and Lømo, T. (1973). Long-lasting potentiation of synaptic transmission in the dentate area of the anaesthetized rabbit following stimulation of the perforant path. *Journal of Physiology (London)* 232: 331–356.

Bozon, B., Kelly, A., Josselyn, S. A., Silva, A. J., Davis, S., and Laroche, S. (2003). MAPK, CREB and *zif268* are all required for the consolidation of recognition memory. In T. V. Bliss, G. Collingridge, and R. Morris (Eds.), *Long-Term Potentiation: Enhancing Neuroscience for Thirty Years*. Oxford: Oxford University Press, 329–345.

Chalmers, D. (1996). *The Conscious Mind*. Oxford: Oxford University Press.

Churchland, P. S. (1986). *Neurophilosophy*. Cambridge, Mass.: MIT Press.

Churchland, P. S. (2003). *Brain-Wise*. Cambridge, Mass.: MIT Press.

Churchland, P. S., and Sejnowski, T. (1992). *The Computational Brain*. Cambridge, Mass.: MIT Press.

Cole, J. (2000). A short history of the use of citations as a measure of the impact of scientific and scholarly work. In B. Cronin and H. Atkins (Eds.), *The Web of Knowledge*. Medford, N.J.: Information Today, 281–300.

Cole, J., and Cole, S. (1972). The Ortega hypothesis. *Science* 178: 368–374.

Countryman, R. A., Orlowski, J. D., Brightwell, J. J., Oskowitz, A. Z., and Colombo, P. J. (2005). CREB phosphorylation and c-fos expression in the hippocampus of rats during acquisition and recall of a socially transmitted food preference. *Hippocampus* 15: 56–67.

Dade L. A., Zatorre, R. J., and Jones-Gotman, M. (2002). Olfactory learning: Convergent findings from lesion and brain imaging studies in humans. *Brain* 125: 86–101.

Ebbinghaus, H. (1885). *Über das Gedchtnis. Untersuchungen zur experimentellen Psychologie*. Leipzig: Duncker and Humbolt.

Elgersma, Y., and Silva, A. J. (1999). Molecular mechanisms of synaptic plasticity and memory. *Current Opinion in Neurobiology* 9: 209–213.

Evans, A. S. (1976). Causation and disease: The Henle-Koch postulates revisited. *Yale Journal of Biology and Medicine* 49: 175–195.

Fredericks, D. N., and Relman, D. A. (1996). Sequence-based identification of microbial pathogens: A reconsideration of Koch's postulates. *Clinical Microbiological Review* 9: 18–33.

Genoux, D., Haditsch, U., Knobloch, M., Michalon, A., Storm, D., and Mansuy, I. M. (2002). Protein phosphatase 1 is a molecular constraint on learning and memory. *Nature* 418: 970–975.

Hamilton, D. P. (1990). Publishing by—and for?—the numbers. *Science* 250: 1331–1332.

Hamilton, D. P. (1991). Research papers: Who's uncited now? *Science* 251: 25.

Han, J.-H., Kushner, S. A., Yiu, A. P., Cole, C. J., Matynia, A., Brown, R. A., et al. (2007). Neuronal competition and selection during memory formation. *Science* 316: 457–460.

Hebb, D. O. (1949). *The Organization of Behavior*. New York: John Wiley.

Henle, J. (1938). *On Miasmata and Contagie*. Baltimore: Johns Hopkins University Press.

Hill, A. B. (1965). The environment and disease: Association or causation? *Proceedings of the Royal Society of Medicine* 58: 295–300.

Hirsch, J. E. (2005). An index to quantify an individual's scientific research output. *Proceedings of the National Academy of Science USA* 102: 16569–16572.

Hooker, C. A. (1981). Toward a general theory of reduction. Part I: Historical and scientific setting. Part II: Identity in reduction. Part III: Cross-categorial reduction. *Dialogue* 20: 38–59, 201–236, 496–529.

Kandel, E. R., Schwartz, J., and Jessell, T. (2001). *Principles of Neural Science*, 4th ed. New York: McGraw-Hill.

Kanigel, R. (1993). *Apprentice to Genius: The Making of a Scientific Dynasty*. New York: Macmillan.

Kida, S., Josselyn, S. A., Pena de Ortiz, S., Kogan, J. H., Chevere, I., Masushige, S., et al. (2002). CREB required for the stability of new and reactivated fear memories. *Nature Neuroscience* 5: 348–355.

Koch, R. (1884). Die Aetiologie der Tuberkulose. *Mitt Kaiser Gesundheit* 2: 1–88.

Kuhn, T. S. (1962). *The Structure of Scientific Revolutions*. Chicago: University of Chicago Press.

Levine, J. (1993). On leaving out what it's like. In M. Davies and G. W. Humphreys (Eds.), *Consciousness: Psychological and Philosophical Essays*. London: Blackwell, 121–136.

Merton, R. K. (1968). The Matthew effect in science. *Science* 159: 56–63.

Mill, J. S. (1843). *A System of Logic, Ratiocinative and Inductive*. In J. M. Robson (Ed.), *The Collected Works of John Stuart Mill*, vols. 7–8. Toronto: University of Toronto Press, 1963.

Morris, R. G., Moser, E. I., Riedel, G., Martin, S. J., Sandin, J., Day, M., et al. (2003). Elements of a neurobiological theory of the hippocampus: The role of activity-dependent synaptic plasticity in memory. *Philosophical Transactions of the Royal Society of London, B: Biological Sciences* 358: 773–786.

Nagel, E. (1961). *The Structure of Science*. New York: Harcourt, Brace, and World.

Newman, M. E. J. (2003). The structure and function of complex networks. *SIAM Review* 45: 167–256.

Pavlov, I. P. (1927). *Conditioned Reflexes*. Oxford: Oxford University Press.

Polya, G. (1945). *How to Solve It: A New Aspect of Mathematical Method*. Princeton, N.J.: Princeton University Press.

Schaffner, K. F. (1967). Approaches to reduction. *Philosophy of Science* 34: 137–147.

Schulman, H. (2004). Activity-dependent regulation of calcium/calmodulin-dependent protein kinase II localization. *Journal of Neuroscience* 24: 8399–8403.

Shackelford, B. (2006). U.S. R&D continues to rebound in 2004. *InfoBrief Science Resources Statistic*. Washington, D.C.: National Science Foundation, Directorate for Social, Behavioral and Economic Sciences, 1–6.

Silva, A. J. (2003). Molecular and cellular cognitive studies of the role of synaptic plasticity in memory. *Journal of Neurobiology* 54: 224–237.

Silva, A. J. (2007). Understanding the strategies for the search for cognitive mechanisms. *Journal of Physiology (Paris)*.

Tang, Y. P., Shimizu, E., Dube, G. R., Rampon, C., Kerchner, G. A., Zhuo, M., et al. (1999). Genetic enhancement of learning and memory in mice. *Nature* 401: 63–69.

Tansey, M., and Stembridge, B. (2005). The challenge of sustaining the research and innovation process. *World Patent Information* 27: 212–226.

Watson, J. D., and Crick, F. H. (1953a). Genetical implications of the structure of deoxyribonucleic acid. *Nature* 171: 964–967.

Watson, J. D., and Crick, F. H. (1953b). Molecular structure of nucleic acids: A structure for deoxyribose nucleic acid. *Nature* 171: 737–738.

Zuckerman, H. (1967). Nobel laureates in science: Patterns of productivity, collaboration and authorship. *American Sociological Review* 32: 391–403.

PART II

LEARNING AND MEMORY

CHAPTER 5

THE LOWER BOUNDS OF COGNITION: WHAT DO SPINAL CORDS REVEAL?

COLIN ALLEN, JAMES W. GRAU, AND MARY W. MEAGHER

1. Introduction

Why should philosophers care about the spinal cord? After all, philosophers have mostly cared about neurons at all only insofar as they are relevant to the mind–body problem, and the assumption that the brain is where all the cognitively interesting action lives is practically built into the jargon of philosophy. Thus, the mind–body problem is often recast as the *mind–brain* problem, and generations of philosophers have cut their teeth on the mind–brain identity thesis. Similarly, the compound term *mind–brain* is frequently used by authors to signal their materialist bona fides, as in "We are interested in how consciousness arises in the mind–brain." This association of mind with brain is not just built into the discipline of philosophy, for neuroscience institutes from Johns Hopkins to Sydney to UC San Diego to Lausanne all have some permutation of *mind* and *brain* in their titles.

Ironically, the ubiquitous example used by philosophers to illustrate the mind-brain identity thesis is that pain is identical to C-fiber stimulation. Yet, as Puccetti (1977) pointed out long ago, this is hardly a good candidate for mind–brain identity given that C-fibers are located well outside the brain, existing as a subset of the sensory neurons that project to the spinal cord. Even more incongruously, many philosophers who haven't bothered to study their neuroanatomy have relocated C-fibers inside the brain in their expositions of the identity thesis, and this error has made it into at least one textbook that is still in print.

Complementary to this mind–brain association is the idea that the parts of the nervous system that lie outside the brain, including the spinal cord and the peripheral sensory and motor neurons, are mere conduits of sensory information and motor commands. As such, they constitute the trunk and branches of an extensive signal relay system that conveys sensory and proprioceptive information to the brain and relays its signals back to the muscles and organs. The implicit assumption for those who identify mind with brain is that there is no cognition outside the brain. Indeed, behavioral responses to sensory stimuli that do not involve brain mediation are often called "spinal reflexes," suggesting that they are fixed, automatic, and noncognitive in nature.

In this chapter, we review animal research that challenges this picture by showing the (rat) spinal cord to be a flexible and interesting learning system in its own right, and we discuss the consequences of these findings for philosophical understanding of the relationship between learning, cognition, and even consciousness. Although spinal plasticity has been hinted at for many years, the extent of its flexibility remains underappreciated. In a sense, it is hardly surprising that the nervous tissue in the spinal cord should have many of the same self-organizing and adaptive capacities as nervous tissue in the brain, but our view is that a full appreciation of the sophistication of the spinal cord raises some important questions about cognition. To answer our opening question, philosophers who master the details of these results will be in a much better position to discuss mind–body relationships.

It is currently fashionable in the philosophy of mind to discuss the "extended mind" hypothesis that the human mind literally extends outside the boundaries of the human organism into our interactions with "cognitive technologies," such as writing and the World Wide Web (Clark, 2003). Given such a radical environment, our discussion of whether cognition extends into the spinal cord may seem rather timid. We think that a good look at the actual science of spinal cord learning has more potential for helping philosophers understand the boundaries of cognition than any number of thought experiments about cognitive technologies. In the end, we do *not* argue that the spinal cord is either cognitive or conscious. We do argue, however, that the sophistication of spinal learning mechanisms in the rat, and presumably in all mammals and most other vertebrates, places certain long-held assumptions about the concepts of cognition, mind, and consciousness under the spotlight. (See Rockwell, 2005, for another biologically inspired but more radical approach to extended mind.)

An additional reason for philosophers to care about the spinal cord concerns questions about the relationship between behavioral evidence and cognitive attributions. At various stages of our careers, we have each advocated taking a cognitive approach to animal behavior. But data that Grau and Meagher have collected over the past two decades have challenged our thinking about these issues. In particular, these findings suggested that some of the data taken to demonstrate cognitive processing in nonhuman animals could also be obtained in the absence of a brain. Specifically, spinal systems appear to be sensitive to distraction, exhibit cue competition, and show a form of learned helplessness. Distraction and cue competition are typically connected with "attention," a central notion in cognitive science, whereas learned helplessness has been linked to a cognition of no control (Maier and Jackson, 1979; Maier and Seligman, 1976). We are not arguing that these phenomena as manifested in the spinal cord are identical to what's found in intact organisms when brains are fully engaged. We are saying, however, that apparent evidence of attentional phenomena must be treated carefully if a strong case for mental state attribution is to be made. A central issue here is just how similar a pattern of results has to be to demonstrate a level of functional equivalence that makes the use of cognitive terms anything more than a handy metaphor that helps scientists remember the overall pattern of the data.

We also believe that concepts of learning deserve more attention from theorists, including philosophers of the neural and behavioral sciences. Organisms may have multiple mechanisms for encoding relations between events in the environment and between those events and their own behaviors. A properly neuroscientific approach to those mechanisms will seek to characterize them at the "neurofunctional" level (Grau and Joynes, 2005a, 2005b) rather than, as was traditionally the case among psychologists, in terms of experimental methods. These issues are relevant to philosophers interested in issues of multiple realization of functional kinds. Aside from its philosophical interest, the research described here may have important implications for managing spinal cord injuries (Grau and Hook, 2006), as we'll explain further later.

2. ANTINOCICEPTION AND CONDITIONED ANTINOCICEPTION

The spinal cord has long been a focus of investigation of pain researchers. The Melzack-Wall gate theory (Melzack and Wall, 1965; Wall and Melzack, 1962) located a significant part of the regulatory control of vertebrate pain signals in the dorsal horn of the spinal cord, where peripheral A and C fibers relaying signals from nociceptors (neurons functionally specialized to sense noxious stimuli) converge with descending neurons from the brain. Traditionally, pain inhibitory effects due to learning, memory, and other cognitive processes were assumed to come top-down from the brain. Grau's initial research on spinal mechanisms of nociception was conducted within this conceptual framework.

The first unexpected result emerged from some studies on shock-induced antinociception (a form of stress-induced analgesia). It had been shown in several laboratories in the early 1980s that exposure to a mildly aversive shock can induce an inhibition in pain reactivity (Grau, 1987a). Pain reactivity was often measured using the tail-flick test, which assesses the latency at which a rat withdraws its tail from a radiant heat source. Tail flick is a reflexive response organized by neurons within the spinal cord (i.e., a spinal reflex). Because the response is spinally mediated, a tail withdrawal from noxious heat can be elicited after a mid- (thoracic) spinal cord transection. This transection completely eliminates all sensory–motor communication between neurons within the lower spinal cord and the brain, producing a form of paraplegia. Consequently, brain mechanisms remain unaware of stimuli presented below the transection. Because rats normally rely on their forelimbs to guide locomotor activity, a paraplegic rat has little trouble moving about its home cage, shows little evidence of pain or distress, and continues to eat and drink on its own.

In normal, intact, rats the tail flick reflex is modulated by brain systems through descending fibers that regulate the incoming pain signal. Grau (1987a) had worked to develop a model of when these descending inhibitory mechanisms are engaged, suggesting an account linked to Wagner's "Sometimes Opponent Processes" (SOP) model of automatic memory processing (Wagner, 1981). Grau had found that mildly painful electric shock could reduce reactivity to a subsequent noxious stimulus; for example, a few brief shocks to the tail would result in slower responses to a subsequent application of heat as measured by the tail-flick latency. This phenomenon of "antinociception" (reduction of nociception) seemed explainable in terms of brain-based short term memory of the initial painful event (the shock) causing modulation of subsequent nociception (from the heat stimulus). In casual terms, it was as if the memory of the aversive event maintained the pain inhibition, driving the descending circuits for 10 minutes or more.

2.1. Distractor-like Effects

Cognitive psychologists (beginning, e.g., with Atkinson and Shiffrin, 1968) have conceptualized short-term memory in humans as a kind of limited-capacity buffer where information is temporarily maintained but is subject to distraction by the intrusion of new information. Wagner (1981) showed that short-term memory in rats was also subject to distraction. Such a model predicts that if one could displace the memory of shock, the pain inhibition should disappear. Supporting this, Grau (1987a) showed that presenting a visual distractor (a flashing light) after a few brief shocks caused the shock-induced antinociception to rapidly decay. He then pushed the hypothesis a bit further, asking whether adding a better end could reduce the antinociception. (See Kahneman, Fredricksom, Schreiber, and Redelmeier, 1993, for a report of this phenomenon in humans.) The better end was generated using a weak shock that produced few signs of pain and little antinociception. If the memorial account is correct, a weak shock distractor should displace the memory of an earlier moderate shock and again cause the antinociception to decay more rapidly. Grau (1987b) confirmed that this occurred in intact animals. (See Grau, 2002, for a review of these and other experiments that appeared to confirm a role for short-term memory in antinociception in rats.)

Grau had assumed that the pain modulatory effects observed after moderate shock depended on brain systems, which influenced tail-flick latencies through descending fibers. Supporting this, moderate tail shock has no effect on tail-flick latencies when communication to the brain is cut by a thoracic transection (Meagher, Grau, and King, 1990). However, Meagher showed that when shock intensity is dramatically increased, it can generate antinociception in spinally transected rats (Meagher, Chen, Salinas, and Grau, 1993). Apparently, intense nociceptive input can directly engage mechanisms within the spinal cord that inhibit tail withdrawal from radiant heat. It was assumed, however, that this was a simple unconditioned response that had nothing to do with memory—at least not in the cognitive terms assumed by Grau (1987a). At this point, a difference of opinion arose between Grau and Meagher. Grau believed that when isolated from the brain, spinal mechanisms should not exhibit memory-like effects. Here, presenting a weak shock distractor should not cause the antinociception to decay more rapidly. If anything, increasing the duration of shock exposure should amplify the antinociception. In contrast, Meagher argued that spinal systems might exhibit simple forms of learning and memory-like phenomena similar to those observed in even simpler invertebrate organisms by Eric Kandel and colleagues (Carew, Hawkins, and Kandel, 1983; Dale, Schacher, and Kandel, 1988; Walters, Carew, and Kandel, 1981). If so, then the presentation of the weak shock could function as a distractor, displacing the memory of the more intense shock.

To begin to explore this issue, they performed an experiment modeled after the weak shock distractor study performed in intact rats. In this experiment, spinally transected rats received a brief intense shock followed by a weaker shock that produced little antinociception in transected subjects. Much to Grau's surprise, the weak shock distractor caused the antinociception to decay more rapidly, a pattern identical to that observed in intact rats (Grau, Salinas, Illich, and Meagher, 1990). Suspecting an artifact, Grau examined whether the temporal order of the stimuli mattered—a distractor should only have a disruptive effect when it is presented after the target event. When spinally transected rats received a weak shock before an intense shock, it had no effect; when the weak shock followed the intense shock, it caused the antinociception to decay more rapidly, as predicted by a memory-oriented account. Here, then, was a process that seemed formally equivalent to what had been found in the intact rats, albeit requiring higher levels of stimulation, but with no brain involvement at all.

2.2. Conditioning

Learning can also impact pain, and again, these effects were assumed to require a brain. Clearly, this is the case in many situations. For example, when an auditory or visual cue is paired with a moderately aversive shock, the cue acquires the capacity to elicit a conditioned antinociception on the tail-flick test (Fanselow, 1986). This effect reflects a form of Pavlovian conditioning, wherein the auditory or visual cue serves as the conditioned stimulus (CS) and the moderate shock acts as the unconditioned stimulus (US).

When a visual or auditory cue is employed, the brain must play a role. But what if a cutaneous cue was used instead? Under these conditions, perhaps lower level mechanisms within the spinal cord could support a simple form of conditioned antinociception. Grau and colleagues explored this possibility using mild shock to a rear leg as a CS and a strong shock to the tail as the US in spinally transected rats. The CS was applied either to the rats' left or right hind legs in one of two conditions: paired with a strong shock to the tail (CS+), or unpaired (CS−). During the conditioning phase, rats received either the CS+ or the CS− 30 times. One hour later, tail-flick latency was tested during reexposure to the CS. Shocks delivered to the same leg previously used for the CS+ produced longer tail flick latencies (i.e., an antinociceptive effect) than shocks to the CS− side, the same outcome observed in intact rats. Evidently, even the spinal cord is sensitive to CS–US relations (for a review of this literature see Patterson, 2001). Furthermore, as predicted by standard learning theory, the CS+/CS− difference extinguished across test trials. Conditioned antinociception appears not to require the involvement of the brain.

Latent Inhibition and Overshadowing

Given evidence that spinal neurons are sensitive to a CS–US relation, Paul Illich (Illich, Salinas, and Grau, 1994) explored whether this system could support some more complex Pavlovian phenomena, such as latent inhibition and overshadowing. Latent inhibition is the phenomenon whereby preexposure to a CS reduces its associability with the US. Intuitively, it is as if the organism has ceased attending to the CS because of the preexposure (habituation) and therefore fails to notice that the preexposed cue predicts the US. Overshadowing is observed when a compound CS, formed from two cues that differ in noticeability (salience), is paired with the US. Even though the less salient cue can support conditioning when it is presented alone, subjects typically fail to learn about it when it is presented in compound with a more salient cue.

To test for latent inhibition in the spinal cord, two groups of spinally transected rats were preexposed to the CS alone prior to conditioning. For one group (CS+ preexposed), the preexposed cue was subsequently paired with the tail shock US. For the other group (CS− preexposed), the preexposed cue was presented in an unpaired fashion with the US during conditioning. In both cases, stimulation to the left or right hind leg served as the CS (counterbalanced across groups). A third group (no preexposure) remained untreated during the preexposure phase. As expected, rats that received no stimulation during the preexposure phase exhibited longer tail-flick latencies during the CS+ (i.e., they predictably showed conditioned antinociception). Preexposure of the CS− had no effect (i.e., conditioned antinociception was observed when subjects were conditioned using stimulation to the opposite leg). But rats that experienced the CS+ alone prior to training exhibited little conditioned antinociception after the training regime was applied using the same side as the preexposure—that is, the stimulus preexposure produced latent inhibition.

To test for overshadowing, Illich and colleagues manipulated stimulus salience by having two different intensities of CS. One group of spinally transected rats was conditioned using the less intense CS (B) paired with the US, and, as expected, they showed conditioned antinociception in the form of longer tail-flick latencies compared with controls. Another group of spinally transected rats were given B in conjunction with the more intense CS (A). When these animals were subsequently tested with B alone, their tail-flick responses were not significantly different from controls. An additional control showed that the intense cue only disrupted learning about the less salient cue when the stimuli were presented in compound. These results suggested that spinal systems support overshadowing as well as latent inhibition.

The discovery of analogs to latent inhibition and overshadowing in the spinal cord was astonishing, for when brain mechanisms are involved, these phenomena are often accounted for in terms of attentional mechanisms. If one was dealing with an intact organism, one might be tempted to say that the rat's attention was directed away from the less salient cue and toward the more salient one when both are present, so that only the attended association with the US was learned.

We need to acknowledge that whatever mechanisms are operating in the spinal cord, they don't have all the functional capacities associated with Pavlovian conditioning in intact animals. Indeed, detailed analyses of the underlying mechanisms suggest that it may abide by simpler rules, and we assume that it is unable to support some complex phenomena. For instance, the capacity of the hippocampus to learn about temporal and spatial ordering greatly increases the range of relationships among stimuli beyond those that can be learned by the spinal cord alone. Likewise, in intact animals latent inhibition is sometimes characterized as involving a context-CS association (Wagner, 1981), but there is currently no evidence that spinal neurons can learn about contextual cues (although this has not been thoroughly investigated). The observed inhibition in the spinal cord is probably due to a simple nonassociative, single-stimulus habituation-like effect (the simplest version of latent inhibition). Despite these differences, Grau and Joynes (2005a, 2005b) have argued that results from the spinal cord suggest that it is important to keep a clear conceptual distinction between the learning phenomena associated with an experimental method, namely, Pavlovian conditioning, and the variety of neurofunctional mechanisms that can encode stimulus–stimulus relations in multiple ways. A similar point holds for instrumental (response–outcome) conditioning.

3. INSTRUMENTAL CONDITIONING

If the spinal cord exhibits Pavlovian conditioning, what about instrumental learning? In instrumental conditioning, delivery of a reinforcer (positive or negative) is made contingent on the organism's behavior, subsequently altering the probability of that behavior. Whereas in Pavlovian conditioning the key relation is between two stimulus events (the CS and US), in an instrumental paradigm learning depends on the relationship between a response (R) and an outcome (O). Most assume that this form of learning requires a brain, but here, too, recent data suggest otherwise.

To separate the role of the animal's own behavior in conditioning from the contribution of the reinforcing stimuli alone, it is necessary to use a yoked design, where one group of animals (the master group) is reinforced contingently on their own actions, and the yoked group receives the reinforcement on exactly the same schedule. The subsequent change in behavior in these two groups is compared to a third group of controls who receive no reinforcement at all. If outcome for the master group is significantly different from both the yoked and unreinforced groups, then it is reasonable to attribute the difference to the instrumental relationship between the animal's own behavior and the reinforcement.

Others (Buerger and Chopin, 1976) had previously explored whether spinal neurons are sensitive to response–outcome (R–O) relations, but this work had been dismissed on methodological grounds (Church and Lerner, 1976). Grau, Barstow and Joynes (1998) developed a set of procedures that overcame the limitations of past studies to provide evidence that spinal neurons are capable of a simple form of instrumental learning. In their paradigm, spinally transected rats are placed in an apparatus that allows both hind legs to hang free. Master rats are given a shock to one hind leg whenever that leg is in an extended position. Subjects in a second group are experimentally coupled (yoked) to the master subjects and receive shock at the same time as their master partner, independent of leg position. Master rats soon learn to keep the shocked leg lifted, effectively minimizing net shock exposure. This learning is not observed in the yoked subjects. To discount alternative interpretations of these results, Grau tested the subjects under common conditions with controllable leg shock. Previously trained rats (master) quickly reacquired the task, exhibiting positive transfer relative to a control group that had never been trained. Surprisingly, yoked subjects that previously received uncontrollable shock failed to learn, and this was true independent of whether they were tested on the same or opposite leg (for a recent review, see Grau et al., 2006).

Further work has shown that uncontrollable nociceptive stimulation has a lasting (>24 hours) inhibitory effect on spinal learning and impacts recovery after a spinal contusion injury. In the latter study, the spinal cord was bruised, rather than cut, using a device that emulates a human spinal injury. This produces a nearly complete paralysis that wanes over the course of a few weeks as subjects regain some hind limb function. Many spinal cord injuries in humans are accompanied by tissue damage that can provide a source of uncontrolled nociceptive input. Using an animal model, Grau et al. (2004) showed that uncontrollable nociceptive stimulation after injury impairs recovery. Importantly, nociceptive input has no adverse effect on recovery when it is controlled by the subject. These results imply that independent of philosophical debates, understanding how spinal cord neurons process signals could have important clinical implications. Indeed, the emergence of techniques to span a spinal injury with neural bridges has brought to the fore a potentially greater challenge—encouraging the new neurons to select the appropriate pattern of synaptic connectivity. Selecting appropriate connections is a process that will depend on a form of dynamic tuning that is shaped through the process of learning. Rewiring the spinal cord will depend on its capacity for learning.

In intact animals, it is well established that uncontrollable stimulation can induce a lasting impairment in learning and performance, a phenomenon known as learned helplessness. A key variable in this literature is the perception of control—subjects that receive the same amount of aversive stimulation, but can control its presentation, generally exhibit far fewer ill effects (Peterson, Maier, and Seligman, 1993). Moreover, a history of controllable stimulation can "immunize" subjects against the adverse effect of uncontrollable shock. Conversely, the presumed cognition of no control induced by uncontrollable shock can be reversed by exposing rats to controllable stimulation ("therapy"). Is the same true for spinal mechanisms? Eric Crown ran the analogous experiments in spinally transected rats and showed, as before, that uncontrollable shock disrupted subsequent learning (Crown and Grau, 2001). Subjects that had previously received controllable shock did not exhibit a learning deficit after uncontrollable shock. Conversely, coupling behavioral training with a pharmacological manipulation that fostered learning had a therapeutic effect that reversed the learning deficit. Once again, the overall pattern bears a remarkable similarity to the results obtained in studies of learned helplessness.

As with the Pavlovian conditioning, some caution is warranted. The learning capacities of the spinal cord are much more restricted than those of intact animals. In examining instrumental learning within the spinal cord, there are several criteria that must be met (adapted from Grau, Barstow, and Joynes, 1998):

A. *Minimum Criteria (Instrumental)*

1. Instituting a relationship between the response and an outcome produces a change in behavior (performance).
2. The effect is neurally mediated.
3. The modification outlasts (extends beyond) the environmental contingencies used to induce it.
4. The behavioral modification depends on the temporal relationship between the response and the outcome.

B. *Advanced Criteria (Operant)*

5. The nature of the behavioral change is not constrained (e.g., either an increase or decrease in the response can be established).
6. The nature of the reinforcer is (relatively) unconstrained (a variety of outcomes can be used to produce the behavioral effect).

The experiments performed by Grau and colleagues (Grau, Barstow, and Joynes, 1998; Grau, et al., 2006) have addressed the first four criteria, providing solid evidence that spinal neurons are sensitive to R–O relationships. At the same time, it's clear that many examples of operant behavior in intact animals exhibit a range of flexibility that seems well outside of what the spinal cord might accomplish. At the level of the cord, both the response options and available reinforcers are much more constrained (a failure to meet criteria 5 and 6). A third factor may involve the ease with which behavior can be inhibited by circuits in the brain. Intact rats can exhibit a range of behavior, can be trained with a variety of outcomes (though, here too, biological limits impose constraints), and can inhibit their actions—capacities that seem well outside the limits of spinal learning. Still, even though full operant conditioning appears to require mediation by circuits in the brain, Wolpaw and Lee (1989) showed that a spinal reflex could be modified by means of brain-dependent operant learning and that the behavioral change was preserved after spinal transection, locating the operant memory itself in the spinal cord.

4. PHILOSOPHICAL IMPLICATIONS

More than three and half centuries ago, Descartes argued that animals are automata: reflex-driven machines with no intellect or other cognitive capacities. A little more than two centuries later, T. H. Huxley traced the philosophical development of the idea that animals are automata, giving special attention to spinal cord reflexes (Huxley, 1874). Huxley reported a series of experiments on a frog, which showed that much of its reflexive behavior was preserved even when its spinal cord had been severed, or large portions of its brain removed. He argued that equivalence between the behavior of an intact frog and a frog with its brain removed implied that consciousness was superfluous to the explanation of either.

We have reviewed research showing that spinal neurons belonging to the nociceptive system are sensitive to both Pavlovian and instrumental relations, and they exhibit a number of phenomena that when studied in normal, intact organisms, including human beings, are frequently described in cognitive or attentional terms. These phenomena include a distractor effect, latent inhibition and overshadowing, and learned helplessness effects. Thus, like Huxley, we have suggested a kind of equivalence between spinal mechanisms and cerebral mechanisms. Rather conveniently for his thesis, Huxley ignored the fact that a brain-damaged frog is much less reactive to its environment than it was before (Crowley and Allen, 2008). We have indicated ways we think spinal mechanisms are much more restricted in their capacities than brain mechanisms. Nevertheless, it is clear that any view that treats learning and memory as brain-bound processes must confront these surprising findings about the adaptive capabilities of the rat spinal cord.

The exact mechanisms of spinal learning remain controversial, but the existence of spinal learning should no longer be. Grau et al. (2006) argue that the behavioral evidence for spinal learning was adequate even though some neuroscientists were reluctant to admit it before a role for NMDA (*N*-methyl-D-aspartic acid) receptors and LTP (long-term potentiation) in spinal neurons was demonstrated, thereby establishing a parallel to learning in the hippocampus. The attitudes of the skeptical neuroscientists, disbelieving of spinal learning until shown evidence for the engagement of specific molecular mechanisms, seems in line with Bickle's (2003) "ruthless reductionism" (exemplified by his view that memory consolidation has been reduced to the neuromolecular mechanisms of LTP). But much remains to be discovered about spinal learning, and the exact nature of the link between the behavioral results and mechanisms of synaptic plasticity is a long way from being established. It is also worth bearing in mind that newly emerging dynamical systems approaches to neural networks can provide models for associative learning without synaptic plasticity at all (Phattanasri, Chiel, and Beer, 2007). Whatever the outcome of this program of research into spinal cord learning, we do not believe it is necessary to take a strong stand on the question of whether all learning mechanisms will turn out to be constructed from the same molecular or neural components, although we would not be terribly surprised to find that the basic mechanisms are highly conserved by evolution (see also Bickle, 2003, chapter 3).

One foundational question raised by these findings, then, is "What is learning?" Is it a behavioral type or a neurological type? Traditionally, learning theorists (coming from the behaviorist tradition) have characterized it in terms of the procedures they use to study it, for example Pavlovian conditioning or instrumental conditioning—an approach which has the unfortunate consequence of making discovery of the underlying mechanisms seem relatively unimportant. An alternative perspective suggests that these apparently different forms of learning may instead reflect the deployment of similar neural mechanisms in the service of different adaptive functions. Thus, Pavlovian conditioning in the spinal cord seems tightly coupled to regulating nociception, a task where sensitivity to stimulus–stimulus relationships is important (Grau et al., 1990), whereas instrumental learning is functionally related to the central pattern generator involved in locomotor activities such as stepping (Edgerton, Roy, de Leon, Tillakaratne, and Hodgson, 1997) where the task is to adapt behavior to sensory feedback. These distributed learning systems may be organized in a lattice hierarchy that organizes and regulates behavior (Gallistel, 1980), with higher circuits being capable of associating more abstract relationships within the lattice. The project of mapping the details of the relationships among the distributed learning components will require attention to both their functional capacities and the neurobiological mechanisms, hence the neurofunctionalism advocated by Grau and Joynes (2005a, 2005b). From this perspective, although some aspects of learning and memory may be ruthlessly reduced to specific neuromolecular events in synapses, the degree of abstraction at which such reductions occur will not entirely suit the needs of behavioral scientists who want to understand how brain and spinal systems interact to produce adaptive behavior. Learning is neither solely a behavioral type nor solely a neural type.

Are spinal circuits beneath the lower bounds of cognition in this lattice? We don't know where to draw the line, or even whether it is worthwhile to try to do so. What we find interesting and challenging about these results is the recognition that neurons, wherever they are found, are capable of adaptively responding to relationships among their inputs. When those relationships are essentially uncorrelated, as in the yoked animals in the instrumental learning experiment already described, the effect on the neural mechanisms is to make future learning more difficult. Conversely, the master animals that had already been trained on one task were subsequently capable of learning a much more demanding task than the unyoked and untrained controls (Crown, Ferguson, Joynes, and Grau, 2002). Thus, the capacity to learn is itself a function of past experience, even in the spinal cord. Furthermore, under normal developmental conditions, spinal cord mechanisms are coupled to brain mechanisms with influence running in both directions. It seems likely that a full understanding of the cognitive and learning capacities of intact organisms will require significant attention to how these neural systems develop and interact.

At the high end of the spectrum, the discovery of spinal learning mechanisms also suggests a reassessment of philosophical arguments about the functional role of conscious experience in working memory for intact organisms (see Allen, 2004, for discussion). For example, it has often been suggested that the intrusion of conscious experience of pain into working memory serves as a signal that facilitates learning about how to behave when confronted with actual or possible tissue damage. But the finding that instrumental conditioning can take place without the involvement of the brain, and arguably therefore without consciousness, shows a need for more specificity about the exact role that brain-based systems associated with consciousness may play in learning about how to avoid noxious stimuli (Allen, Fuchs, Shriver, and Wilson, 2005). Bickle (2003, p. 163) lists learning and memory among the categories of behavior having "an obvious link with consciousness." Given the results we have described from the Grau laboratory, the obviousness of that link can no longer be simply assumed.

Acknowledgments

Funding for the experiments described within this chapter was provided by the National Institute of Neurological Disorders and Stroke Grant NS41548. C.A. is a grateful for input from the Biology Studies Reading Group in the Department of History and Philosophy of Science at Indiana University and for questions and comments received from an Indiana University cognitive lunch audience.

REFERENCES

Allen, C. (2004). Animal pain. *Noûs* 38: 617–643.

Allen, C., Fuchs, P. N., Shriver, A., and Wilson, H. (2005). Deciphering animal pain. In M. Aydede (Ed.), *Pain: New Essays on the Nature of Pain and the Methodology of Its Study*. Cambridge, Mass.: MIT Press, 352–366.

Atkinson, R. C., and Shiffrin, R. M. (1968). Human memory: A proposed system and its control processes. In K. W. Spence and J. T. Spence (Eds.), *The Psychology of Learning and Motivation: Advances in Research and Theory*, vol. 2. New York: Academic Press, 742–775.

Bickle, J. (2003). *Philosophy and Neuroscience, A Ruthlessly Reductive Account*. Boston: Kluwer.

Buerger, A. A., and Chopin, S. F. (1976). Instrumental avoidance conditioning in spinal vertebrates. *Advances in Psychobiology* 3: 437–461.

Carew, T. J., Hawkins, R. D., and Kandel, E. R. (1983). Differential classical conditioning of a defensive withdrawal reflex in *Aplysia californica*. *Science* 219: 397–400.

Church, R. M., and Lerner, N. D. (1976). Does the headless roach learn to avoid? *Physiological Psychology* 4: 439–442.

Clark, A. (2003). *Natural Born Cyborgs*. New York: Oxford University Press.

Crowley, S., and Allen, C. (2008). Animal behavior: *E Pluribus Unum?* In M. Ruse (Ed.), *The Oxford Handbook of the Philosophy of Biology*. New York: Oxford University Press, 327–348.

Crown, E. D., Ferguson, A. R., Joynes, R. L., and Grau, J. W. (2002). Instrumental learning within the spinal cord: II. Evidence for central mediation. *Physiology and Behavior* 77: 259–267.

Crown, E. D., and Grau, J. W. (2001). Preserving and restoring behavioral potential within the spinal cord using an instrumental training paradigm. *Journal of Neurophysiology* 86: 845–855.

Dale, N., Schacher, S., and Kandel, E. R. (1988). Long-term facilitation in *Aplysia* involves increase in transmitter release. *Science* 239: 282–285.

Edgerton, V. R., Roy, R. R., de Leon, R., Tillakaratne, N., and Hodgson, J. A. (1997). Does motor learning occur in the spinal cord? *Neuroscientist* 3: 287–294.

Fanselow, M. S. (1986). Conditioned fear-induced opiate analgesia: A competing motivational state theory of stress analgesia. *Annals of the New York Academy of Sciences* 467: 40–54.

Gallistel, C. R. (1980). *The Organization of Action: A New Synthesis*. Hillsdale, N.J.: Erlbaum.

Grau, J. W. (1987a). The central representation of an aversive event maintains the opioid and nonopioid forms of analgesia. *Behavioral Neuroscience* 101: 272–288.

Grau, J. W. (1987b). The variables which control the activation of analgesic systems: Evidence for a memory hypothesis and against the coulometric hypothesis. *Journal of Experimental Psychology: Animal Behavior Processes* 13: 215–225.

Grau, J. W. (2002). Learning and memory without a brain. In M. Bekoff, C. Allen, and G. M. Burghardt (Eds.), *The Cognitive Animal: Empirical and Theoretical Perspectives on Animal Cognition*. Cambridge, Mass.: MIT Press, 77–88.

Grau, J. W., Barstow, D. G., and Joynes, R. L. (1998). Instrumental learning within the spinal cord: I. Behavioral properties. *Behavioral Neuroscience* 112: 1366–1386.

Grau, J. W., Crown, E. D., Ferguson, A. R., Washburn, S. N., Hook, M. A., and Miranda, R. C. (2006). Instrumental learning within the spinal cord: Underlying mechanisms and implications for recovery after injury. *Behavioral and Cognitive Neuroscience Reviews* 5: 191–239.

Grau, J. W., and Hook, M. A. (2006). Spinal neurons exhibit a surprising capacity to learn and a hidden vulnerability when freed from the brain's control. *Current Neurology and Neuroscience Reports* 6: 77–80.

Grau, J. W., and Joynes, R. L. (2005a). A neural-functionalist approach to learning. *International Journal of Comparative Psychology* 18: 1–22.

Grau, J. W., and Joynes, R. L. (2005b). Neurofunctionalism revisited: Learning is more than you think it is. *International Journal of Comparative Psychology* 18: 46–59.

Grau, J. W., Salinas, J. A., Illich, P. A., and Meagher, M. W. (1990). Associative learning and memory for an antinociceptive response in the spinalized rat. *Behavioral Neuroscience* 104: 489–494.

Grau, J. W., Washburn, S. N., Hook, M. A., Ferguson, A. R., Crown, E. D., Garcia, G., et al. (2004). Uncontrollable nociceptive stimulation undermines recovery after spinal cord injury. *Journal of Neurotrauma* 21: 1795–1817.

Huxley, T. (1874). On the hypothesis that animals are automata, and its history. *Nature* 10: 362–366.

Illich, P. A., Salinas, J. A., and Grau, J. W. (1994). Latent inhibition, overshadowing, and blocking of a conditioned antinociception response in spinalized rats. *Behavioral and Neural Biology* 62: 140–150.

Kahneman, D., Fredricksom, B. L., Schreiber, C. A., and Redelmeier, D. A. (1993). When more pain is preferred to less: Adding a better end. *Psychological Science* 4: 401–405.

Maier, S. F., and Jackson, R. L. (1979). Learned helplessness: All of us were right (and wrong): Inescapable shock has multiple effects. In G. H. Bower (Ed.), *The Psychology of Learning and Motivation*. New York: Academic Press.

Maier, S. F., and Seligman, M. E. P. (1976). Learned helplessness: Theory and evidence. *Journal of Experimental Psychology: General* 105: 3–46.

Meagher, M. W., Chen, P. S., Salinas, J. A., and Grau, J. W. (1993). Activation of opioid and nonopioid hypoalgesic systems at the level of the brainstem and spinal cord: Does a coulometric relation predict the emergence or form of environmentally-induced hypoalgesia? *Behavioral Neuroscience* 107: 493–505.

Meagher, M. W., Grau, J. W., and King, R. A. (1990). The role of supraspinal systems in analgesia: The impact of spinalization and decerebration on the analgesia observed after very brief versus long shocks. *Behavioral Neuroscience* 104: 328–338.

Melzack, K., and Wall, P. D. (1965) Pain mechanisms: A new theory. *Science* 150: 971–979.

Patterson, M. M. (2001). Classical conditioning of spinal reflexes: The first seventy years. In J. E. Steinmetz, M. A. Gluck, and P. R. Solomon (Eds.), *Model Systems and the Neurobiology of Associative Learning: A Festschrift in Honor of Richard F. Thompson*. Mahwah, N.J.: Erlbaum, 1–22.

Peterson, C., Maier, S. F., and Seligman, M. E. P. (1993). *Learned Helplessness: A Theory for the Age of Personal Control*. New York: Oxford University Press.

Phattanasri, P., Chiel, H. J., and Beer, R. D. (2007). The dynamics of associative learning in evolved model circuits. *Adaptive Behavior* 15: 377–396.

Puccetti, R. (1977). The great C-fiber myth: A critical note. *Philosophy of Science* 44: 303–305.

Rockwell, W. T. (2005). *Neither Brain nor Ghost: A Nondualist Alternative to the Mind-Brain Identity Theory*. Cambridge, Mass.: MIT Press.

Wagner, A. R. (1981). SOP: A model of automatic memory processing in animal behavior. In N. E. Spear and R. R. Miller (Eds.), *Information Processing in Animals: Memory Mechanisms*. Hillsdale, N.J.: Erlbaum, 5–47.

Wall, P. D., and Melzack, R. (1962). On the nature of cutaneous sensory mechanisms. *Brain* 85: 331–356.

Walters, E. T., Carew, T. J., and Kandel, E. R. (1981). Associative learning in *Aplysia*: Evidence for conditioned fear in an invertebrate. *Science* 211: 504–506.

Wolpaw, J. R., and Lee, C. L. (1989). Memory traces in primate spinal cord produced by operant conditioning of H-reflex. *Journal of Neurophysiology* 61: 563–572.

CHAPTER 6

LESSONS FOR COGNITIVE SCIENCE FROM NEUROGENOMICS

ALEX ROSENBERG

ASSUME that cognitive science is the research program of computationalism, acting on a wager about how the mind works inspired largely by philosophical arguments. The wager is roughly that thinking shows powers of creativity, systematicity, and productivity that can only be explained as the purely syntactical processing of symbolic representations. Optimists about the wager hope that computational neuroscience will make good this hypothesis about thought that cognitive science advances to explain the powers of thought, by showing how the wet stuff substantiates, explains, systematizes, and improves these hypotheses. Pessimists about cognitive science will expect cognitive neuroscience to show why findings about the brain limit the prospects of the research program computationalism motivates. In this chapter I argue that it is not too early to begin to take sides on whether the optimists or the pessimists are going to turn out to be correct. I argue that what is already known in cognitive neuroscience, and has been known for a decade or so, is enough to significantly affect our expectations of the shape that cognitive science will take, and that shape will be significantly different from what computationalism leads us to expect.

In particular, I argue that work by some of the leading figures in the field, employing the resources of neurogenomics, has already provided strong grounds to be pessimistic about the representations to which a computational theory of mind is committed, but to be optimistic about the syntactic character of processes of think-ing and reasoning in the brain. Many philosophers will hold that the most pressing philosophical problem of computationalism is to explain how propositional repre-sentation in the brain is even possible, let alone actual, as much cognitive neurosci-ence presumes. There is no general agreement on how physical states can embody representations of distinct and different propositions as we individuate them and express their differences in speech and writing—that is, in media with "derived intentionality" (Searle, 1980). The failure to provide an adequate account of rep-resentation is, however, easily explained by findings in neuroscience, which I shall expound. These findings strongly suggest that brain states cannot represent distinct propositions as we apparently individuate them in spoken and written language but can come asymptotically close to doing so. If this is correct, propositional content is explained away as a natural and perhaps useful heuristic foisted on us in ordinary life by the closeness of the approximation to it that the brain attains. Whether this heuristic assumption is one that a cognitive science should also exploit is another matter on which pessimism may be in order. On the other hand, if the study of the brain reveals the same sorts of processes that molecular biology has uncovered else-where in development and operation of bodily processes, computationalism's com-mitment to discovering a syntax of thought may already be guaranteed. The only question that remains will be whether it will be much like a "language of thought" that some computationalists urge cognitive science to look for.

1. From Developmental Molecular Biology to Neurogenomics

The work by neuroscientists discussed here deals with neural mechanisms of mem-ory storage and memory recall that originated in the work of Eric Kandel and now includes a large number of other laboratories. It has accelerated over the past decade largely due to advances in genomics and proteonomics,[1] methods that enabled experimenters first to identify the genes whose products are differentially expressed in the various tissues of the body, then to switch them on and off or even selectively increase and decrease the levels of their expression, and eventually to assay for indi-vidual proteins, locate their concentrations in parts of cells, identify their structure, and quantify their enzymatic roles in chemical reactions.

To understand its significance requires a quick run-through of developments in molecular developmental biology. This discipline has now provided the details of embryological development across the phylogenetic spectrum from the *Drosophila* to mammals. What the details show is that across this spectrum, development is the result of switching on and off pretty much the same structural genes at different times by a diversity of regulatory genes, and differences among these regulatory genes result in the obvious differentiation on organismal body plans and behavioral capacities. This discovery reduces the surprise associated with the discovery that humans and mice have roughly the same number of genes, and only small multiples of the number of genes in much simpler systems such as fruit flies, the worm, *C. elegans*, and the sea slug *Aplysia*. Indeed, so far as development is concerned, one set of genes of central importance—the so-called *Hox* genes—differ across this spectrum largely in their copy numbers, so that increasing complexity of animals is the result of successive duplication and mutation of the same original set of regulatory genes. In the case of *Drosophila*, molecular biologists have been able to identify a literal program of development (one that can also be implemented on a desktop or laptop computer) involving some 30 genes and their gene products and by the repeated implementation of a structure of subprograms that builds the *Drosophila* embryo.[2] Biologists have been able to do this because advances in gene sequencing and computational biology have enabled them to locate both the structural genes and the regulatory ones that switch them on and off.

What these breakthroughs first provided for developmental biology, they soon began to provide for the understanding of the working of normal adult cells and groups of them. Having located genes on the chromosome, it became possible to precisely knock out these genes (and only them) in the germ line of an organism so the resulting deficits among offspring will enable the experimenter to identify the gene's somatic function. Subsequent breakthroughs—RNAi (*i* for interference) and double-stranded RNA—now enable experimenters to temporarily silence individual genes in cells of the body or simply reduce the number of protein products they express. Because everything that goes on in and at the surface of a cell is a matter of switching on and off genes and chemical reactions—catalytic or transformational—of their protein products, this technology will eventually enable the molecular biologist to learn all the details of cell physiology down to the level of the individual molecule.

This research has already had three sorts of results relevant to the present matter. First, as in development, it is now evident that many of the processes of cellular physiology are also well understood as the operation of structured digital programs instead of analog mass-action chemical reactions. Second, the diverse programs realized within and among cells are often structured iterations of subprograms to be found ubiquitously in many different processes in many different tissues of the body. These subprograms have come to be called *motifs*, owing to their repetition in diverse molecular processes; the search for these motifs and larger programs built out of these motifs have become a recognized research program under the label "systems biology" (Alon, 2006). Third, a class of genes has been identified as immediate early genes. These genes, already implicated in development, physiology, and learning, are, as the label implies, switched on and off in quick response to molecular stimuli. Among the immediate early genes already identified are ones with profound roles in behavior. The *fos-B* gene, for example, when knocked out seems to destroy normal nurturance behavior while leaving no other detectable deficits in mice (Brown, Ye, Bronson, Dikkes, and Greenberg, 1996; Gingrich and Hen,

2000). Similarly, knockouts for selective olfactory protein genes in male mice can by themselves inhibit males learning of appropriate courting behavior in these males (Swaney et al., 2006). The discovery of such genes made it clear how somatic cells, neurons especially, can respond in quantitatively and qualitatively profound ways to stimuli, rapidly expressing large quantities of catalytic molecules that quickly affect behavior.

2. More Than You Wanted to Know about Short-Term and Long-Term Implicit Memory

Kandel, Bailey, and Bartsch (1996) ask the question: "Can molecular biology provide novel insights into the mind?" Then the article turns technical, and few specific claims about human cognition are broached therein. But the publication had important and unnoticed consequences for the nature of human cognition.

Kandel, Bailey, and Bartsch begin by distinguishing "explicit" or what they call *declarative* memory, "the conscious recall of knowledge about people, places, and things" well developed in the vertebrate brain, from "implicit" nondeclarative nonconscious recall of motor skills, classical conditioning, and sensitization (1996, p. 13445). The seats of these two types of memories appear to be separated in the brain. Explicit memory is subserved by structures in the temporal lobe of the cerebrum (especially the hippocampus), whereas implicit learning involves learning processes in the sensory–motor pathways of organisms, including invertebrates like *Aplysia* that do not have anything like a cerebrum. Both explicit and implicit memory is characterized by distinct short-term and long-term capacities, and both of these are dependent on the number of training trials to which the neural circuits are exposed. Owing to advances in neurogenomics—the use of knockout and gene silencing techniques in the study of neurons—the macromolecular differences between short- and long-term implicit memory in *Aplysia*, *C. elegans*, and *Drosophila* are now relatively easy to study. They reveal unsurprisingly enough that the difference between short-term and long-term memory is a fairly obvious difference between establishing temporary covalent bonding relationships between molecules that degrade quickly and building more lasting anatomical structures.

Short-term implicit learning results from conditioning in which a chain of molecular signals and ambient catalytic molecules produce a short-lived modification in the concentration and the confirmation (secondary and tertiary structure or shape that changes binding and/or catalytic activity) of neurotransmitter molecules in preexisting synapses. Specifically, most neuroscientists hold, the conditioning begins when dopamine or (in invertebrates) serotonin molecules are released at the synapse between neurons in a pathway from a stimulated sensory neuron. The serotonin molecules bind receptor molecules at the sensory neuron, which in turn activate molecules of the enzyme adenylyl cyclase that catalyze the formation of cyclic AMP, and it in turn activates a kinase protein molecule PKA. This kinase catalyzes the release of another transmission molecule at the synapse between the sensory neuron and a motor neuron. The chain thus laid down will result in the same motor neuron firing again later when another weaker instance of the same stimulus (i.e., lower concentrations of the same molecules at every prior node), provided it occurs soon enough after the initial stimulation. The neural pathway has "remembered" how to respond to the stimulus. The sea slug *Aplysia* was important in Kandel's original research on the neurophysiology of learning because the relevant pathway for a given learned behavior is large enough to have been located and examined even before the tools of neurogenomics became available.

Long-term implicit memory appears to be mainly the result of the stimulation of somatic genes to orchestrate the production of *new* synapses connecting sensory and motor neurons. In long-term implicit memory, the initial steps are the same as in short-term learning: The repeated stimulus causes increases in and persistence of serotonin at the synapses of interneurons and sensory neurons, where receptor molecule's activation of the adenylyn cyclase repeatedly catalyzes the production of more cyclic AMP and thus activates PKA. But at this point something different from the short-term pathway's chain of events happens: Some of the larger number of PKA molecules (that result from repeated stimulation) diffuse to the sensory neuron's nucleus, where they activate a protein that binds to the DNA and switches on a number of genes whose molecular products form new synaptic connections between the sensory neurons and the motor neurons. Long-term implicit memory is realized by an anatomical change at the cellular level that involves a protein the binds to gene-promoter sequences. The cyclic AMP or cAMP response element binding protein of type 1 (CREB-1) and the cAMP response element, a gene that is a promoter or on switch for a suite of genes, are key players in this pathway. Each of the new synaptic connections work in the same way as the smaller number of connections laid down for short-term implicit memory, but their larger number means that the learned response will be manifested even if a significant number of the synaptic connections degrade, as happens over time. Thus, the new construction of additional synaptic connections provides for long-term implicit memory.

What is stored in implicit memory, long- or short-term? Kandel and neuroscientists in general describe what is stored in implicit memory as learned behavioral dispositions or capacities. This is what philosophers at least as far back as Ryle (1949, chap. 5) have called "knowledge how." It is nonpropositional, and there are no questions of its requirement to be "represented" in the neural structures that realize it. To the extent that a neural structure realizes knowledge of *how to respond*, for example, to aversive stimuli, an account of its "content" appears to be unproblematic. The content of the system of interneurons, sensory neurons, and motor neurons that intervene between painful stimuli and withdrawal of the body part painfully stimulated can be characterized variously in our language. For example, we may accord the pathway or some part of it the content "potential or actual tissue damage at bodily location A." But we do so without any temptation to attribute concepts such as "potential" or "tissue" or even "bodily location," still less some propositional attitude to a sea slug or a fruit fly. We accept that the experimenter's attribution of knowledge how to the simple pathway must take some propositional form, but we don't take the particular proposition chosen seriously as *the* content; we don't suppose that any experiment could narrow down the actual complete content to any particular unique proposition, nor is there any need to do so to fully understand the nature of implicit memory, short- or long-term. It would not be difficult for neuroscientists to narrow down the set of propositions that more completely characterize what is stored in implicit memory by varying stimuli or stimulating peripheral neurons that intervene between stimulus and the sensory–motor neurons. Such experiments enable the experimenter to identify more narrowly what features of the stimuli or peripheral neurons are detected (i.e., responded to) by the pathway.

3. How Are Explicit Memories Stored?

Explicit memories, recall, are those which Kandel, Bailey, and Bartsch (1996, p. 13445) identified as declarative: "the conscious recall," or better, storage "of knowledge about people, places and things" that is particularly well developed in the vertebrate brain. Storage of course is hardly even conscious, and it's clear that what Kandel and colleagues are interested in is information that *can be recalled* to consciousness, expressed propositionally, and presumed to be represented in the brain. (I have nothing more to say about consciousness hereafter.)

Explicit memory storage is localized to the temporal lobe, especially the hippocampus,[3] structures nonexistent in *Aplysia* and far from the sensory pathways in vertebrates that are homologous to the ones storing implicit memories—short- or long-term—in the sea slug. Studies of neural processing in these regions of the temporal lobe began with the determination that neural pathway there are subject to long-term potentiation (LTP), the process in which synapses become much more sensitive when they are repeatedly stimulated. In particular, repeated stimulation by the same concentrations of neurotransmitters of the neurons in the hippocampus results in much higher production of neurotransmitters that stimulate downstream neurons. This increased sensitivity can endure for long periods. LTP occurs in three different pathways in the hippocampus (mossy fiber, Schaffer collateral, and medial perforant) and goes through three different stages: short-term, early, and late LTP. There is of course a great deal of evidence that LTP in the hippocampus constitutes information storage in laboratory animals, especially mice.

Kandel, Bailey, and Bartsch's (1996) studies of the stages of LTP in these distinct pathways showed that the *same* molecular mechanisms, involving the same somatic genes that build new synaptic connections in the *Aplysia* implicit long-term sensory motor memory, are responsible for all the forms of LTP in all the hippocampal pathways that subserve explicit memory in vertebrates. They write:

> Similar to the presynaptic facilitation in *Aplysia*, both mossy fiber and Schaffer collateral LTP [two of the three types of LTP] have distinct temporal phases.... The early phase is produced by a single titanic stimulation [release of neurotransmitters], lasts 1–3 hours, and requires only covalent modification of preexisting proteins. By contrast, the late phase is induced by repeated titanic stimulations, and is dependent on new proteins and RNA synthesis. As is the case with long-term memory in *Aplysia*, on the cellular level there is a consolidation switch, and the requirement for [gene] transcription in LTP has a critical time window. In addition, the late transcription-dependent phase of LTP is blocked by inhibitors of PKA.... Recent studies by Nguyen and Kandel now indicate that these features of LTP also apply to a third major hippocampal pathway, the medial perforant pathway.... Thus, as in *Aplysia* presynaptic facilitation, cAMP-mediated transcription appears to be the common mechanism for the late form of LTP in all three pathways within the hippocampus. (1996, p. 13452)

Note the role of PKA and cAMP, which has been demonstrated to be the same in both implicit and explicit memory. Moreover, the presence of RNA synthesis implicates gene expression in the manufacture of new synapses. One thing missing from Kandel, Bailey, and Bartsch's (1996) account of the mechanism of LTP in the hippocampus was the identification of the same genes and their transcription factors—CREB-1, CREB-2 (or analogs—already known to be at work in implicit learning—as responsible for the RNA synthesis Kandel reports in explicit memory LTP. This would demonstrate that the same genes build the same new anatomical structures in explicit as in implicit memory. Kandel, Bailey, and Bartsch observed, "It will be of particular interest to investigate whether cAMP-dependent transcription factors...are also required for long term synaptic modification in mammals" (1996, p. 13452). Many studies subsequent to this article vindicated the expression of interest in this question. The answer appears to be a resounding *yes*.[4]

With understandable caution, Kandel, Bailey, and Bartsch concluded: "The apparent similarity of the molecular steps that underlie learning-related synaptic plasticity may reflect the fact that long-term memory for both implicit and explicit storage is associated with structural changes" (1996, p. 13452). Not just changes, but the very same structural changes—down to the same genes, transcription factors, and proteins, most of them identical at the molecular level.

What happened in the next 10 years or so turned this speculation about the identity of explicit and implicit memory storage into well-grounded theory. To understand the basic outlines of how Kandel's picture has been filled in, we need to introduce the NMDA receptors (so named because they can be stimulated by the drug N-methyl-D-aspartate, by contrast to other receptors, which cannot be so stimulated). These receptors are to be found elsewhere in the brain, including in the sensory–motor cortex, where implicit knowledge is stored.[5] When NMDA or the amino acid glutamine binds to these receptors, their shape changes and opens a channel into the neuron through which calcium ions flow, increasing the sensitivity of the neuron to subsequent electrical impulses. Work in one important region of the hippocampus, the CA1 region, has shown that when NMDA receptors are bound by a drug so that they cannot respond to the NMDA or glutamate molecules, LTP does not occur; when genes in the neurons produce below-normal quantities of NMDA, no LTP occurs; and when these genes produced above-normal quantities of NMDA, the neuron's susceptibility to LTP and animals' abilities to store explicit information is enhanced. This research further substantiates Kandel's hypothesis that long-term implicit and explicit memories are realized at the individual synaptic level by the same mechanisms of somatic gene regulated multiplication of anatomical structures.

Although there remains a substantial possibility that something entirely new in kind will be reported, several decades of work now strongly point to the conclusion that the molecular mechanisms of implicit and explicit memory, both short- and long-term, differ only in kind. Before drawing several of the obvious morals of this story for the nature of representation in the cerebrum, it is worth summarizing what is now known about the mechanism of information recall, to go along with what we know about information storage.[6]

4. HOW THE BRAIN RECALLS MEMORIES

Recall is a capacity associated only with explicit or declarative memory, of course, and if it is a matter of accessing representation laid down in explicit memory, it must take place in the hippocampus. Research on recall of stored information has focused on both the CA1 and the CA3 regions, which project on to the CA1 cells, on which the work reported in section 2 was focused. The strategy for studying how recall is effected unsurprisingly involves modulating the presence or the behavior of the NMDA receptor proteins on the surface of neurons. Tonegawa et al. (2002) were able to provide an account of the molecular mechanism of how stored information is recalled in response to environmental clues by knocking out genes that code for an important component of NMDA receptor proteins, NR1 (for NDMA receptor). The work also shows how information is degraded in the brain, and how degraded information can be recalled and used effectively.

Normal mice trained in a Morris water maze to recall the location of an underwater platform (on which they can rest) continue to do so without difficulty even when most of the environmental clues to the platform's location have been removed from the maze. Tonegawa et al. (2002) called this behavior "pattern completion." Mice in which the genes for NR1 have been knocked out showed normal behavior and normal protein distributions through development and maturation. But by week 18, the NR1 protein had disappeared from the CA3 region while remaining at normal levels elsewhere (including the CA1 region) in the brains of knockout mice. The cytoarchitecture of the mutant hippocampus was otherwise normal, and LTP elsewhere in the hippocampus (even LTP requiring NR1 in CA1) was unaffected by the gene deletion. Knockout and normal mice showed no difference in ability to acquire and retrieve explicit spatial memories of the location of the underwater platform in a Morris water maze with four cues on the surrounding walls. But when three of the four cues were removed and the animals retested, knockout mice were significantly worse at finding the platform. The experimenters excluded the hypothesis that the difference was due to memory loss by showing that the knockout mice did as well as controls when all four cues were restored. "In summary, under the full-cue conditions, both mutant and control mice exhibited robust memory recall, When three out of the four major extramaze cues were removed, control mice still exhibited the same level of recall, whereas the mutants' recall capacity was severely impaired" (Tonegawa et al., 2002, p. 215). What neural mechanisms underlie this deficit?

Recall what the research described in section 2 showed about explicit memory storage in the CA1 region of the hippocampus. Assuming that neural processing in this region stores memory, a comparison between cellular activity at the CA1 regions of normal and knockout mice subjected to the same water maze training regime and then tested with and without cues would show whether knocking out the NR1 gene impairs memory storage in CA1. The result of this experiment strongly suggests that mutant mice memory storage in CA1 is *unaffected* by the knockout. *Retrieval* is affected. Because the absence of NR1 proteins effects storage in CA3, Tonegawa advanced a two-stage theory of memory retrieval involving connections between the CA1 and CA3 neurons. Information, in this case spatial information about cues that indicate location of the underwater platform, is stored in neurons in both CA1 and CA3. A normal CA3 circuit stores full cue information and in the presence of full cue inputs stimulates the CA1 neurons to produce the hippocampal output that leads to rapid arrival at the platform. In mutant animals, the NR1 deficit impairs memory storage in the CA3 areas but has no effect on the CA1 storage, which in the presence of all four cues produces behavior indistinguishable from that of normal mice. Partial cue removal reduces the input stimulus to the CA3, but in normal mice these circuits are sufficiently strengthened by previous stimulation that they drive the full output pattern of the CA1 neurons. In mutant mice, the number of CA3 neurons providing input to CA1 neurons is significantly reduced and the corresponding CA1 neurons are not driven to produce the full output pattern of normal mice. Tonegawa and colleagues conclude that their "results reflect a primary deficit in NR dependent memory formation in CA3 that is then revealed as a deficit in recall under limited cue conditions" (2002, p. 218). Tonegawa and his collaborators were not reluctant to draw inferences from this research about CA3 cells in humans. They connect these results to the previously established neurochemical alternation in CA3 cells of some Alzheimer's patients.

The data from these experiments, along with the work of Kandel and others, led Tonegawa to propose a schematic probabilistic synaptic program for memory storage and recall realized by the CA1 and CA3 cells, along with the rest of the architecture of the region of the hippocampus (the entorhinal cortex, the dentate gyrus, the Schaffer and recurrent collateral neurons, mossy fiber neurons, and the perforant pathway) (2002, p. 217). The model suggests multiple memory locations of the same information; its probabilistic output mirrors the fact that memories are imperfect even in normal animals, and that the deficit produced by knocking out the gene coding for NR1 protein in CA3 cells reduces the probability of correct recall from a very high level to a much lower one. But the take-home lesson for our purposes is the distinctive recurrence of the same neurogenomic motifs across different parts of the brain, and different organisms, engaged in different memory-expressing behaviors.

5. Each Explicit Memory Is Just a Lot of Implicit Memories

It may not be safe to assume that human memory is realized in human brains by the same mechanism that realizes it in rat and mice brains, but there seems to be great deal of evidence in favor of it, and none against it. It seems equally reasonable to adopt as a working hypothesis that the differences between implicit and explicit or declarative memory is a matter of location and degree. The former is realized by the number and sensitivity of neuronal connections in the sensory motor areas of the vertebrate brain, and the latter is realized in the cerebrum and particularly the hippocampus. More significantly, the molecular biology of long-term implicit memory and explicit memory appears also to be substantially the same, indeed, identical except for the particular molecular configuration of the neurotransmitters and the nucleic acid sequence differences of the genes and RNAs that regulate changes in the microarchitecture of synaptic connections.

If the difference between the details of the neural connections that constitute long-term storage of implicit memory—storage of knowledge how—differs only by number of connections from long-term storage of explicit memory—knowledge that—then it is reasonable to consider whether long-term explicit memory storage differs only in degree from long-term implicit memory storage. In other words, it's worth considering whether propositional knowledge is nothing but a large number of synaptic connections, each one of which is a bit of associative learning, a neural circuit that realizes a conditional disposition to respond to stimuli in an environmentally appropriate way, a little bit of knowledge how.

Recall the point that the sensory–motor pathway produced by classical conditioning in the *Aplysia* constitutes the stored disposition to respond to noxious or positively rewarding stimuli in an environmentally appropriate manner. In these cases, it is natural to attribute content to the circuits owing to their functional role. Nevertheless, there is no temptation to attribute specific propositional content to such circuits, still less to identify a "language of thought" in which sentences expressing propositions about the presence of noxious or rewarding stimuli are written in the arrangements of neurotransmitters. The intentional attributions are instrumental, shorthand, heuristic. When, as we have seen, a large number of these circuits are "grown" owing to somatic gene expression involved in long-term memory, an organism like *Aplysia* persistently responds distinctively to stimuli. Under these conditions we may be tempted to accord the relevant circuits, when switched on, content *derived* from our own "original" intentionality, our representations to ourselves of the presence of aversive stimuli in the sea slug's immediate environment. But derived intentionality is not original intentionality, and it is no more problematic than the intentionality of the pixels or ink marks now reflecting light on to your retinas.

Move the same circuits to the hippocampus, multiply their numbers by several orders of magnitude, and the result is long-term explicit memory. Recall that Kandel called this explicit memory *declarative* and labeled it as conscious, meaning presumably that in humans the information stored can often be recalled at will, that when it is recalled it can be verbalized and be the subject of conscious awareness, events of successful recall at will, and verbalization in humans at least. Now, mere change of location cannot turn individual circuits that do not represent and lack intentionality into ones that do so and have it. Nor can it turn large packages of circuits that might have derived intentionality into ones with original intentionality. *Natura non facit saltum.* At least change in location and numbers cannot change structures that don't represent and are not intentional into ones that do and are, unless this change is merely a matter of degree, something no one should grant.

How do the circuits at CA1 or CA3 or the circuits that include synaptic connections from CA1 to CA3 and all the other subregions of the hippocampus, acquire the original intentionality that we believe reposes in the human brain? If the storage of information in the hippocampus is not a matter of original intentionality, then there seem to be only two options.

1. Representational states in the human (or primate or mammalian or vertebrate, take your pick) brain, the ones with true, real, original intentionality, are not to be found in exclusively in the hippocampus; other parts of the brain are necessary, and they are responsible for the original intentionality.

2. Some (much, all?) representations are fully located in the hippocampus, and there is no original intentionality to be found anywhere in these representational states; intentionality is an illusion foisted on us by the shear numbers of synaptic connections that produce such exquisitely fine-grained responses that mistakenly attributing specific propositional content is overwhelmingly natural to creatures like us, and heuristically invaluable.

Available neuroscience does not recommend the first alternative. As I have said, there are always surprises in science. Cross-phylogenic inference from experiments on rodent brains to ours is always to some degree fraught. Deficit, lesion, fMRI,

PET scan studies in humans tomorrow may show that memories accessible to consciousness are also stored elsewhere (note 3) or that their storage spans regions that include more than just the hippocampus. But for the moment, the betting must be against these alternatives.

Let's consider alternative 2 somewhat further. *Aplysia* is a wonderful model for understanding how the neuronal network realizes conditioning, but it is limited by the narrow repertoire of behavioral responses that *Aplysia* makes to a range of stimuli. This narrow range prevents us from attributing much discrimination of its environment to the sea slug. The more nuanced the differences in behavior as a function of the presence of different stimuli, or differing quantities of the same stimuli, the more content it is convenient to attribute to the neural networks intervening between stimuli and behavior. Though of course, in the case of sensory motor networks in these organisms, the attributions of content are merely heuristic (like those familiar from molecular biology's description of molecules as, e.g., "recognizing second messengers"). The number of different kinds of such synaptic pathways multiplies as the peripheral sensory neurology of organisms becomes more differentiated and the number of central neural synaptic connections that are possible increases. As this process proceeds in phylogeny, attributions of content will become increasingly specific. Once we get to *Drosophila* it will be natural to attribute information about self-location, local temperature, the direction and nature of nearby vegetation and food sources, the presence of fertile females or sexually aroused males, and so on. Of course, when we get to vertebrates, the attributions will become very fine-grained indeed. At this point, common sense and cognitive science will begin to attribute content not just heuristically but literally. However, once we recognize that what is going on neurophysiologically in these cases is just more of the same as what happens all the way down to *Aplysia*, we should want to resist such attributions and explain them as heuristic devices fostered by the wonderfully sophisticated behavioral responses that these trained neural pathways give rise to.

When we get to the human case, we are treating systems with hippocampuses composed of millions of cells. The rat CA1 area is estimated to contain upward of 355,000 pyramidal cells, each making synaptic contact with hundreds or thousands of interneuron cells. Though the difference between what transpires in the rat hippocampus and in the sea slug sensory motor system differs only by degree, it is a difference of at least five orders of magnitude. This is a difference in degree large enough to so finely narrow the range of propositions heuristically attributable as content to sets of synaptic connections in the hippocampus that literal ascription becomes overwhelmingly tempting.

In the human case, we may be able to add a further order of magnitude difference in degree from the rodent (even though the number and structure of the relevant somatic structural and regulatory genes seem to be similar). What this vast multiplication of synaptic structures does for the human is to asymptotically approach the literal content ascriptions common sense and cognitive science make. Our use of verbal and inscriptional sentential expressions to express our thoughts strongly suggests that we have particular propositions "in mind" that are expressed by the voice or the hand. Agreement and disagreement with others suggests a common acceptance of the same propositions. But of course experiences with ambiguity and differences in the meaning of sentences, expressed and inscribed, long ago taught all of us that each person may have a different proposition in mind when they assert or assent to the same sentence inscribed or vocalized in a natural language.

The approach to content inspired by the continuity of implicit and explicit memory storage takes us only a little way beyond this lesson. What it shows is that the set of circuits in the hippocampus or elsewhere in the brain that realize some information about the world are equally well described by more than one particular proposition from a set of only very slightly different ones, because the neural architecture does not in fact literally realize *any* propositional content at all. Rather, the circuitry is connected to a set of behavioral dispositions that will equally support any one of the members of this set of extremely similar propositions, and there are circumstances we can arrange that will enable us to further narrow down this set of equally well-supported propositions. But they won't narrow it down to a unique proposition that fully and completely expresses the representational content of the synaptic connections in question. For, like the much smaller number of otherwise similar synaptic connections in *Aplysia*, they are not capable of representing propositional content. They are not capable of original intentionality. Note that if the neural architecture cannot represent unique single propositions, it cannot represent precise (or fuzzy) sets of them either, because to begin with, if it did so, it would also have to represent the unique precise single (vague or nonvague) proposition that is constituted by the disjunction of the member of the set, an even harder task than literally representing one of the members of the set.

6. Farewell to Original Intentionality

But wait, if there is derived intentionality, as surely there is (just look at the words on this page), there must be original intentionality somewhere in the universe from which the derivation comes. Surely this original intentionality must be realized in the human hippocampus if it is instantiated anywhere. These rhetorical issues ride roughshod over several possibilities that need to be ruled out before we accept the indicative claims they really express.

Does an inscription having any derived content at all require that there be something else—a brain state—with some original intentional content or other on which the inscription's intentional content is dependent? Assume the answer is *yes*. By modus tollens, therefore, it follows from the denial of original intentionality in the brain that there is no real derived intentionality, that inscriptions, vocalizations, and other signs are not really *symbols*. This means of course that our attribution to them of the literal status of "symbol" is mistaken. But what if it turns out that treating them as symbols is a heuristic device we employ owing to the same considerations that lead us heuristically to ascribe intentional states to the synaptic circuits of the *Aplysia*?[7] Owing to the asymptotic approach of our neural circuitry to representing particular propositions, we mistake our heuristic attribution of derived intentionality for the literal attribution to signs of symbolizing—of representing specific propositions. Derived intentionality, if any, is dependent on original intentionality. Mutatis mutandis, the asymptotic approach of signs to derived intentionality is dependent on the asymptotic approach of neural architecture to original intentionality.

It is worth noticing how the present account of explicit memory as being on a continuum with implicit memory deals with one of the most persistent recent objections to a teleosemantic account of intentionality: the so-called disjunction problem (Fodor, 1991). This is the challenge to teleosemantic theories' attribution of representations to neural pathways that they cannot distinguish cases in which such pathways mistakenly realize a *false* propositions from cases in which they correctly realize a *disjunctive* proposition. An illustration will help. Suppose some neural pathway is said to realize "raven here now" owing to the environmental appropriateness of the behavior to which it leads in the circumstances in which it occurs. Now suppose that the same pathway is instantiated by a treepie (a black magpie, a bird of the same family as the raven, with much the same appearance). Any account of neural representation (for example, a teleosemantic account) must provide a principled distinction between the contents, "raven here now" and "raven or treepie here now." Tokening the former content is a natural mistake creatures can easily make. Tokening the latter is presumably rare, especially among nonlinguistic creatures. If a theory cannot distinguish between them, it does not have the resources to account for unique specific representational content, or so the argument goes.

The view that explicit memory is a huge number of implicit memories asymptotically approaching representation deals with this problem naturally and easily. To begin with, it holds that all representations are disjunctive, in the sense that there is no unique proposition realized by a set of synaptic connections; rather, there is always a disjunction of them each equally suited to a heuristic attribution of content. Do a synaptic network's connections make it natural to attribute "raven here now" or "raven or treepie here now?" That depends on a previous history of discriminations and failures to discriminate ravens and treepies. If there is no such history, the two propositions are on a par, along with indefinitely many other propositions, all of which it makes sense to attribute in the light of stimuli and subsequent behavior. The most complex neural architecture never represents a unique single proposition, because it never represents any propositions at all. Only rarely will it be the case that there is a unique nondisjunctive proposition that it is unavoidable heuristically to attribute.[8]

Fodor, who famously taxed teleosemantics with the disjunction problem, has advocated a theory of (original) intentional content that he claimed is not held hostage by the problem. It is his theory that intentional states are ones that are involved in relations of asymmetrical causal dependence. Consider a synaptic network, call it SN_1. Adapting Fodor's theory, the conditions SN_1 must meet for it to represents "raven here now" are roughly these:

1. There are occasions on which the presence of a treepie causes a synaptic network to produce raven-appropriate behavior. Call this synaptic network SN_2.
2. When SN_2 obtains, it does so because SN_1 is in place, but not vice versa.

While the theory of heuristic attribution advanced here does not actually involved literal attribution of original or any other intentionality, it explains perfectly well why a theory like Fodor's should look attractive. If a synaptic network SN_1 is trained up to produce long-term raven-appropriate behavior in the presence of ravens, this will be due to building a large number of new synaptic connections, as we have seen. Such connections will facilitate ocurrent behavior of the sort that leads from treepies to raven-present behavior that otherwise would not obtain. After all, under some conditions some treepies look very much like some ravens. But the reverse dependence does not obtain. Heuristically attributing "raven here now" to SN_1, as opposed to "black-colored bird or black-colored prey or black-colored moving object here now," requires that the behavior SN_1 produces be rather specific, specific enough to exclude "treepie here now" as a heuristically useful attribution. It is evident that on its initial occurrence, SN_2—the "raven here now" synaptic system caused by a treepie and resulting in raven-appropriate behavior—does not causally contribute to the initial appearance of, presence of, or long-term buildup of SN_1 synaptic connections. Whence the asymmetrical causal dependence Fodor thinks is the essence of original intentionality.[9]

7. Is Knowledge How Computable?

The claim that explicit declarative memory is just large quantities of implicit memory realizing behavioral dispositions but not inscribed with propositions, may be resisted, owing to an attachment to the computational theory of the mind—the thesis that cognition is at least often a process of syntactical manipulation of representational states with semantic content. To a first approximation, this theory holds that thinking is a mathematical or inferential process, familiar to logicians and computer scientists, in decidable procedures and algorithmic programs, that operates syntactically on symbols—inscriptions with semantic meaning—to produce further representations and ultimately behavior. Insofar as the view defended here is inhospitable to the literal attribution of representational content to synaptic networks, it may be viewed as hostile to a computational approach to cognition. But there are important aspects or components of computationalism to which this approach is quite amenable. It holds out the promise of actually providing a concrete program of research that will substantiate an important component, indeed, the most important component, of computationalism.

Begin by separating the computational theory of the mind into two well recognized components: (1) the claim that cognition is literally intentional, that brain states are symbols with (original or derived) intentionality; and (2) the claim that cognition is a form of reasoning that consists in the formal or purely syntactic manipulation of these brain states. The second of these claims is what neurogenomics holds the promise of vindicating.

It is of course obvious that synaptic connections and the somatic genes that construct and regulate them can realize the truth-functional connectives familiar in syntactical symbol processing. But that is only the tip of the computational iceberg, whose proportions are now becoming familiar in neurogenomics and proteonomics. To begin with, the computational character of development has become well understood in the early stages of the embryological development of many species (see Rosenberg, 2006, for examples), and it appears to embody many of the same subprograms across the phylogenetic spectrum from insects to humans. As mentioned, these subprograms are called motifs, and the term has become common in neurogenomics as well. The aims of systems biology are to uncover these motifs and, indeed, higher order motifs composed of repeated iterations of a small number of such motifs in much the way that structured programs in computer science are composed. The identification of computational programs realized by sets of structural and regulatory genes and their protein products is the major current focus of molecular biology. This is equally true in neurobiology as in developmental biology. Illustrations of this interest are easy to find. Once recent example is provided by the elucidation of sensory information processing in *C. elegans* (Chasalani et al., 2007). In the presence of certain food-related odors, this worm will move toward their sources, and in the absence of them engage in a characteristic random turning-and-moving behavior. Neurobiologists have now identified the molecular steps in the neuronal pathways from the worm's nose through the sensory motor neuron pathway. In particular, they have shown the existence of a circuit of switches, called AIB and AIY, that probabilistically start and stop turning behavior, subject to parallel but opposite regulation by a pair of initial peripheral neurons, AWC[on] and AWC[off].[10] One thing they have shown is how a sudden removal of stimulation in the olfactory neurons produces a sustained level of excitation in downstream neurons that start and keep the worm in its search-behavior mode, thereby accounting for "how 'working memory' of a transient stimulus is maintained" (Chasalani et al., 2007, p. 35). It is no surprise that the molecular signals realizing this program—glutamate molecules—are of the same general type as in implicit and explicit memory across the phylogenetic spectrum. More significantly, the olfactory pathway thus elucidated by Chalasani and colleagues is described by a commentator as:

> a circuit motif that seems to be used in several contexts in different organisms. In vertebrate vision, information flow through parallel channels of opposite signs is crucial for contrast sensitivity. The use of a similar functional motif in *C. elegans* olfaction emphasizes the efficiency of this circuit in processing sensory information, and supports the idea that systems of very different complexities

may nevertheless use shared strategies to perform similar tasks. In other words, much within man might still be worm.[11]

Examples can be multiplied and in effect have been in section 2. Thus, the process of memory recall elucidated there constitutes a computation program that, when operating normally, takes reduced cue data as input and uses stored memories to compute a probable location for the underwater platform in the water maze. When certain somatic genes are knocked out, the computation cannot be effected. The subprograms of this computation established by LTP are identical to those computed in the interneuron–sensory–motor pathway of *Aplysia*. It is early days in the search for the motifs that phylogenetic and genomic continuity lead one to expect across the metazoan sensory and neural equipment.

It seems safe to say that current research in neurogenomics is identifying the physical systems that realize data structures and the physical processes that employ them to compute outputs of various kinds, following a variety of nested, parallel, and independent programs, and that the programs are not just "curve-fitting overlays" but reflect what is really going on in the brain. In fact, the kind of programs neurogenomic methods are enabling neuroscientists to identify as realized in regions of the brain, hold out the prospects of *computational compositionality*, *systematicity*, and *productivity*. These are the very features of thought that constitute the best arguments for computationalism in cognitive science. Accordingly, these neural programs identified by genomic/proteonomic methods have the very features we should look for in processes that vindicate a significant part of computationalism about the mind.

Consider first the compositionality of synaptic structures in the hippocampus. If each such structure embodies a specific schedule of learning from inputs, output, and feedback, and if there are upward of a million or so of them in the three regions of the hippocampus about which we already know something, then as genomic and proteonomic programming adds and subtracts or temporarily blocks or opens connections between them, the combinatorial combinations of these synaptic patterns will add up to unimaginably large exponential powers of the numbers of basic synaptic structures that are to be found in a normal hippocampus. This probably gives us as much productivity as we require to explain the fact that actual patterns of synaptic structures are only a small proportion of possible ones and to show why the actual behaviors they eventuate in are only a small proportion of the repertoire of behaviors brain states can give rise to. A huge number of such basic synaptic structures operated on by even a small number of computational programs, encoded in somatic genomes and their protein products, will be just as powerful as a more complex computational program operating on a smaller number of highly structured propositional representations. The large number of basic dispositional knowledge how synaptic structures operated on by many iterations of the same relatively limited package of subprograms can produce the same output—indeed, can be the very realization of the higher level program operating on syntactically richer structures. This is just what goes on in the realization of higher level programs by assembly-level programs, by machine-language programs at the basement-level computations realized in the or-, and-, and not-gates of the microprocessors in a computer.

Because every synaptic network comes equipped with exactly the same set of structural and regulatory genes, prepared to respond to various signals, the synaptic structures will also show the systematicity that computationalism credits to the mind. The same syntactic structure can figure in a large number of different networks, depending on how changes in the neural inputs to it affect the switching on and off of genes and their neurotransmitters, which leave the initial structure intact but simply allow or establish connections to other such structures. It is as if each basic structure comes with a set of connectors that can be plugged into the connectors of other members of a large (but not infinite) set of structures that have the same or coordinated connectors. These connectors can be used to change the direction in which a structure sends signals, can coordinate the sending of signals with other structures, or when pulled apart stop sending signals in the same direction, and so on. What does the changing, coordinating, disaggregating? The obvious candidate is the general neurogenomic/proteonomic program laid down in the genome, carried by all the cells in the body but only switched on in the brain tissue cells by the operation of regulatory genes and environmental inputs in those very cells. Most of these programs, exploiting immediate early genes, are epigenetically switched on in all the brain cells, whereas other more specialized neurogenetic programs operate in each of the distinct regions of the brain, such as the CA1 or CA3 regions of the hippocampus.

8. COMPUTATIONALISM AND NEUROSCIENCE

It requires little argument to show that cognitive psychologists cannot uncover the programs that implement cognition by reverse engineering from behavior. Just trying to infer the programs of a much simpler system, such as a laptop computer's central processing unit, is too much to demand. Of course, there have been some successes reverse engineering the program that the visual cortex employs to solve the so-called inverse optics problem of inferring a three-dimensional environment from the two-dimensional array on the retina, and some advances in identifying the problem-solving heuristics employed by human cognitive agents instead of less convenient algorithms that ensure correct answers. But for many reasons, neither of these lines of research will vindicate computationalism. The comparative ease of discovering programs operated in the sensory modules is a reflection of their modularity and the relatively simple problems they have to solve, along with the significant constraints that make the range of alternative solutions relatively small. The problem-solving heuristics that have been uncovered are more in the nature of data that a computational theory would need to explain than they are advances in a computational research program for cognitive science.

The other main lines of research in cognitive neuroscience, especially those devoted to localization of distinctive cognitive function to particular areas of the brain and to the timing, temporal sequence, and duration of cognitive processes, that fMRI or other techniques provides is much too coarse-grained to tell us much about how the regions they identify do what they do, let alone the programs that are realized by processes in these regions. If anything, such studies are the necessary precursors to a neurogenomic approach, which first seeks differences in the timing and rates of gene expression between areas mapped by the coarse-grained anatomical studies to vindicate the taxonomies they suggest.[12] Then, if neurogenomic studies find these differences in gene and protein expression, it begins knockout studies to reverse engineer from deficits to the genomic/proteonomic programs and subprograms to these programs' computational structure.

What are the chances that the resulting computational neuroscience will vindicate a computational cognitive science? Computationalism as traditionally understood is the bet that top-down cognitive science can uncover programs operating over such *semantically* characterizable states in the brain. If we could do this, the next step in the research program would be cognitive neuroscience—the search for the physical nature of such computational processes and the physical composition of the semantically characterized states which these processes syntactically manipulate. Were computationalism to succeed, we should expect that it would meet bottom-up neuroscience in one or another smooth "reduction."[13]

It's hard to say whether bottom-up neuroscience will meet top-down cognitive science, because there really isn't any of the latter yet. In fact, the paucity of successful computationally motivated theory in cognitive science, in spite of its comparative antiquity, and the success of computational neuroscience in spite of its youth, may suggest that there is nothing much for a bottom-up science to meet. At most, so far computationally motivated cognitive science has identified the behavioral capacities a cognitive theory needs to explain and has placed some general constraints on any theory that does so: It should explain the productivity, systematicity, and creativity of thought as evinced in behavior.

The best-case scenario for a smooth link between some future cognitive science and neuroscience will be one in which a theory committed to representations is vindicated as a model to which the real nonrepresentational neural processes approximate or approach asymptotically. This would require two things: first, that representations required by computational cognitive science be approximated by independently individuated sets of synaptic structures that never represent any distinct propositions; and second, that the "high-level" computations that cognitive science identifies be shown to be constituted or closely approximated by sets of "lower level" computations over these sets of synaptic structures or subsets of them. The worst-case scenario for a cognitive science motivated by computationalism would be the conclusion that neither its representational states nor computations that operate over them are anything like sets of synaptic structures and the computations to which the genome/proteonome subjects them.

In the absence of any significant success of computationally inspired cognitive science, philosophers and cognitive scientists will offer a range of arguments familiar from other disciplines in favor of continuing a top-down research program. Such arguments conclude that if there are any interesting theories or models of computation at the level that approximates to semantically evaluable representations, then a bottom-up approach will miss them. When pressed to give examples of such higher level regularities from elsewhere in biology or the special sciences, exponents of this claim can at best cite some ceteris paribus generalizations that in fact describe the explananda of the science in question, not the explanantia, or else they cite mathematical models—necessary truths—whose explanatory power is limited and which a bottom-up approach is unlikely to miss in any case. On one hand, exponents of a bottom-up approach can claim a long history of vindication in the discovery of regularities; equally important, the bottom up results can explain both those explananda-describing ceteris paribus generalizations and the circumstances under which their ceteris paribus clauses must be invoked.

On the other hand, the best relevant example adduced in favor of bottom-up approaches is both powerful and highly relevant to the top-down/bottom-up dialectic in cognitive science. It is to be found in developmental molecular biology and its "evo-devo" applications. In the past 20 years, more than one Nobel Prize has been awarded for uncovering the genetic program that actually explains more than a century of descriptive regularities in the development of many species. Until these achievements of genomics in developmental biology, there were no real explanations, and a good deal of agreement about what such explanations had to explain (in particular, developmental recapitulation, serial homology, and phylogenetic novelty). These features bear important similarities to the productivity, systematicity, and creativity that computationalism demands any cognitive theory explain. The bottom-up approach of molecular developmental genetics has provided the required explanations in terms of computationally realizable programs of development. It has shown that there are no generalizations to be uncovered at the level of organismal development, only descriptions of phenomena that needed to be explained.

The precedent of molecular developmental biology and the conspicuous initial success of a computational neurogenomics are part of a strong case that the most promising line of research in cognitive science is bottom-up. If the best-case scenario is in the cards, then a bottom-up approach should vindicate it as the systems biology of the nervous system discovers motifs at successively higher levels of aggregation of synaptic structures. Such successes will suggest experiments in humans and infrahuman species that could narrow down the representational states to which the sets of synaptic structures approximate. If, on the other hand, no such vindication of a computationally inspired cognitive science is in the cards, time, money, and genius will not have been wasted trying to develop a top-down theory that does not exist.

NOTES

1. The study of the proteins the genes encode and of their interrelation on the model of genomics—the study of the genome, whence proteonomics, the study of the proteonome.

2. See Rosenberg (2006), chapters 2 and 3, for an introduction and Davidson (2006) for an advanced treatment.

3. There is some evidence that remote early memories in vertebrates are moved from the hippocampus to storage in the neocortex. But there is also evidence that the macromolecular processes obtaining in this area of the brain are substantially the same and involve the same genetic programs and the same neurotransmitters as those obtaining in the hippocampus and the sensory motor cortex. See Silva, Brown, Talton, and Wiltgen (2007).

4. See, for example, Bailey, Kandel, and Si (2004) and Yang Zhou et al. (2006).

5. Such receptors have recently been identified in the *Aplysia* ganglia. See Ha, Kohn, Bobkova, and Moroz (2006).

6. It is also worth pointing out that the similarity of molecular mechanism in these four different kinds of memory processes is entirely neutral with respect to any multiple realizability claims about the neuroanatomy of memory. Similarity of mechanism is not the same as identity of it. Moreover, none of the inferences drawn here from the similarity of mechanisms to the general nature of cognitive processes turn on whether there is substantial, some, slight, or no multiple realizability in the relationships in question.

7. Here, of course, one must be careful not to lapse into literal attribution of intentionality while explaining why there can be no such thing. "Treating signs as symbols" cannot mean bringing them under descriptions or any other activity whose description is referentially opaque. But this is a philosopher's problem, not a neuroscientist's.

8. Perhaps only when we think of a mathematical truth such as $2 + 2 = 4$ or first-person truths such as "I am here now," it will be reasonable to narrow down the class of propositions attributed to a unique one.

9. Suppose that after SN_1 has been established, treepies begin to show up regularly and SN_2 becomes established. That would lead us to revise our heuristic attribution to SN_1 of the proposition "raven here now" to "raven or treepie or jay or other member of the *Corvidea* family of birds here now," with no temptation to credit the bearer of SN_1 or SN_2 with acquaintance with Linnaean binomial nomenclature.

10. Why should the control be probabilistic: "Why not just respond in an all-or-none manner? The reason is that a circuit that generates probabilistic behavior leaves itself open to further modulation. The circuit involving AWC, AIY and AIB neurons is only a sub-circuit within a much larger, interconnected neuronal network" (Chasalani et al., 2007, p. 35). Inputs from this network could modulate the output of smaller subcircuits, allowing the organism to integrate information from several environmental sources and accordingly alter the probability of a response. Thus, a probabilistic network might cope better with uncertainty and unpredictability—characteristics of the real-world environment.

11. Chalasani et al. (2007) write: "The sensory responses of AWC neurons are similar to those of vertebrate rod and cone photoreceptors, which have tonic activity in the dark, are hyperpolarized by light, and are depolarized by the removal of light. Like AWC neurons, photoreceptors are non-spiking and have graded glutamate release. Molecular analogies also link AWC neurons with vertebrate photoreceptors: their sensory transduction pathways rely on G-protein-coupled receptors, G_i-like proteins, receptor-type guanylate

cyclases and cyclic GMP-gated channels, and their differentiation is controlled by Otx homeodomain proteins. The synaptic connections between AWC, AIY and AIB neurons are also reminiscent of those between vertebrate photoreceptors and their targets, the ON and OFF bipolar cells. In the retina, glutamate from photoreceptors is sensed by AMPA-type receptors on the OFF bipolar cell, a connection that is functionally and molecularly analogous to the AWC-to-AIB connection. The vertebrate ON bipolar cell is inhibited by glutamate, as are AIY neurons. In mammals, the ON bipolar cell is inhibited by a G-protein-coupled glutamate receptor and, in fish, by a glutamate-gated chloride channel that is functionally although not molecularly similar to *C. elegans* GLC-3. The parallel ON and OFF streams enhance contrast sensitivity in vertebrate vision; it is possible that the parallel AIY and AIB neurons have analogous functions in odour detection" (p. 68).

12. Timing and rates are everything in such studies, because there is good reason to believe that almost all the neural genes are expressed at some time or other in almost all the regions of the brain, See the online brain gene expression map at www.stjudebgem.org/web/mainPage/mainPage.

13. Using the term loosely enough, so that it includes ones that may leave important residual philosophical difficulties unanswered, such as those involved in the "reduction" of thermodynamics to statistical mechanics, and excludes eliminative explanations like the latter-day redescription of phlogiston chemistry's isolation of oxygen as a case of reduction.

REFERENCES

Alon, U. (2006). *Introduction to Systems Biology: Design Principles of Biological Circuits.* Boca Raton, Fla.: CRC.

Bailey, C., Kandel, E., and Si, H. (2004). The persistence of long term memory: A molecular approach to self-sustaining changes in learning-induced synaptic growth. *Neuron* 44: 49–57.

Brown, J. R., Ye, H., Bronson, R. T., Dikkes, P., and Greenberg, M. (1996). A defect in nurturing in mice lacking the immediate early gene fosB. *Cell* 86: 297–309.

Chalasani, S. H., Chronis, N., Tsunozaki, M., Gray, J. M., Ramot, D., Goodman M. B., et al. (2007). Dissecting a circuit for olfactory behaviour in *Caenorhabditis elegans*. *Nature* 450: 63–70.

Davidson, E. H. (2006). *The Regulatory Genome*. New York: Academic Press.

Fodor, J. (1991). *The Theory of Content*. Cambridge, Mass.: MIT Press.

Gingrich, J., and Hen, R. (2000). Commentary: The broken mouse: The role of development, plasticity and environment in the interpretation of phenotypic changes in knockout mice. *Current Opinion in Neurobiology* 10: 146–152.

Ha, T. J., Kohn, A. B., Bobkova, Y. V., and Moroz, L. L. (2006). Molecular characterization of NMDA-like receptors in *Aplysia* and *Lymnaea*: Relevance to memory mechanisms. *Biological Bulletin* 210: 255–270.

Kandel, E., Bailey, C., and Bartsch, S. (1996). Toward a molecular definition of long-term memory storage. *Proceedings of the National Academy of Science USA* 93: 13445–13452.

Nakazawa, K., Quirk, M. C., Chitwood, R. A., Watanabe, M., Yeckel, M. F., Sun, L. D., Kato, A., Carr, C. A., Johnston, D., Wilson, M. A., Tonegawa, S. (2002). Requirement for hippocampal CA3 NMDA receptors in associative memory recall. *Science* 297:211–218.

Rosenberg, A. (2006). *Darwinian Reductionism, or How to Stop Worrying and Love Molecular Biology*. Chicago: University of Chicago Press.

Ryle, G. (1949). *The Concept of Mind*. Hammersmith: Penguin.

Searle, J. (1980). Minds, brains, and programs. *Behavioral and Brain Sciences* 3: 417–424.

Silva, A., Brown, R., Talton, A., and Wiltgen, B. (2007). New circuits for old memories: The role of the neocortex in consolidation. *Neuron* 44: 101–108.

Swaney, W. T., Curley, J. P., Champagne, F., and Kevern, E. B. (2007). Genomic imprinting mediates sexual experience-dependent olfactory learning in male mice. *Proceedings of the National Academy of Sciences USA* 104(14): 6084–6089.

Yang Zhou, H. W., Li, S., Chen, Q., Cheng, X.-W., Zheng, J., Takemori, H., et al. (2006). Requirement of TORC1 for late-phase long-term potentiation in the hippocampus. *PLoS ONE* 1: e16. DOI: 10.1371/journal.pone.0000016.

CHAPTER 7

LEARNING, NEUROSCIENCE, AND THE RETURN OF BEHAVIORISM

PETER MACHAMER

1. INTRODUCTION: SOME PRESUPPOSITIONAL QUESTIONS

In recent years, learning and memory are among the topics that have occupied a great deal of research time in the neuroscience community. Some of the experimental tasks used to research these systems on human subjects, especially those who have suffered some sort of brain damage, are taken from "traditional" cognitive science experiments. However, in both cognitive neuroscience and neurobiology, most of the experimental tasks used to study humans and animals, to discover the underlying neural mechanisms, use very limited learning paradigms. In fact, they use the experimental designs identical to or much like those that were used by the behaviorists: repetition, classical conditioning, and operant or reward conditioning. The ubiquity of these paradigms ought to raise an important issue: Is behaviorism alive and well in neuroscience? Alternatively, did the cognitive revolution of the 1950s and after have no messages of importance for neuroscience, despite the fact that it radically changed the field of experimental psychology? This chapter proposes to examine a few aspects of these questions.

Presupposed by the framing of the questions, in terms of the relation of neuroscience to behaviorism, are certain background questions that need an answer. (1) What do we mean by *behaviorism*? (2) Are all experiments in learning and memory used by neuroscientists designed according to repetition (R), classical conditioning (CC), and stimulus-response-reward (SRR) paradigms? Or (2′) Are there any experimental paradigms used in cognitive neuroscience and neurobiology that are not instances of the behaviorist's big three (R, CC, SRR)? Finally (3), if, as suspected, classical conditioning and reward learning are the most prominent paradigms, can they be generalized in a way that allows explanations of all forms of memory encoding and learning that animals, and by implication humans, accomplish? This is a form of the question that was posed to the behaviorist program in the 1950s and 1960s. At that time, cognitive psychologists, and some linguists, answered it in the negative.

2. Some Brief Background

There were many forms of behaviorism. The most prominent have been associated with the names Clark Hull, Donald Hebb, B. F. Skinner, and Kenneth Spence. I do not go into the important yet subtle differences among these forms of behaviorism. Nor shall we offer much detail concerning the nature of different forms of classical conditioning (Pavlovian conditioning) and their relation to the reward or operant conditioning paradigms. However, we must say enough to begin to answer the presuppositional questions.

CC is where a naturally paired relation between an unconditioned stimulus (UCS) and a response, is augmented by pairing a newly introduced stimulus in close proximity with the UCS. After a number of trials, this new stimulus elicits the response, and becomes the conditioned stimulus (CS). Learning is taken to have occurred, when the CS elicits the same response as the UCS, without the UCS being present. In short, there is created an association between the UCS and the CS with respect to the response, which is why this is taken as a form of associative learning, with respect to eliciting a response. The classical example is Pavlov's dog, where food (UCS) elicits salivation (the response), and the food (UCS) gets paired with a bell ring (CS), so that learning occurs when the dog salivates to the bell's ringing alone.

In operant, instrumental, or reward conditioning, the basic pattern is that an organism emits a behavior (an operant) in a set of environmental conditions, which behavior may bring about consequences (by itself or in the form of another event) that may increase or decrease the probability that the same behavior will be emitted again in similar conditions. In learning, the probability of the behavior being emitted is increased. The reward, or later the expectation of a reward, is the associating of the consequences or other events or conditions that have, ex post facto, been shown to be rewarding. In theory, there is no assumption about what kinds of events or consequences are rewarding for the organism.

In Skinner's radical form of behaviorism, all variables that might be taken to intervene between a stimulus and an overt behavioral response were to be eschewed, particularly any mentalistic, functional, or internal state variables, because such intervening variables were unobservable. Skinner even dismisses the usefulness of physiological variables, because he believes that they could add nothing of relevance to the science of behavior. All one needed, for Skinner, were the environmental or stimulus conditions (including the deprivation state of the organism), the behavioral response, and the contingencies or conditions that led to reinforcement. In learning, the effect of reinforcement (positive or negative) was to increase the probability that the response being studied was emitted. Clearly in this radical Skinnerian sense, no neuroscientist could be a behaviorist, for they, by virtue of discipline, must discuss variables that are internal to the organism and irrelevant to a science of behavior.

Other behaviorists (Hull and Spence) countenanced the use of explanatory internal intervening variables to get "tighter" associative connections between the observable variables. Furthermore, some psychologists, like Hebb, even held that such intervening variables could refer to physiological or neurological processes or functions.

What is also true of behaviorist psychologists is that they were concerned with behaviors of the whole organism, organism-level (O-level) behaviors. In this sense, learning, even if the relevant behavior involves only some part of an organism (such as a certain arm movement or facial expression), is something that the organism as a whole accomplishes. Learning is not to be attributed to suborganism parts or systems, though by analogy some scientists might talk loosely about the visual system learning to detect or discriminate some variable it had not been able to attend to before or a limb being conditioned to behave in a specific fashion.

It should be clear then that to attribute a form of behaviorism to neuroscientists, we need to expand the general character of what counts as a behaviorist commitment. We could do this in three ways: (1) by extending the range of the domain of behaviors to be explained so that they include more than just O-level behaviors; (2) by characterizing behaviorism in terms of its methodological commitments to specific experimental paradigms, that is, those experimental designs that are definitive of behaviorist practice; or (3) by giving a more general account of behaviorism in terms of associationism.

Let me elaborate and explore this last point. Associationist psychology, and its underlying doctrine, holds that all forms of learning come about by forging (or strengthening) associations among independent elements that are the building blocks of what is to be learned. This view assumes that these elements are somehow basic atomic constituents that become linked together because of experience (or development). The origin of this association view probably lies in the sensationalist epistemology of the eighteenth century. It almost exactly parallels the phenomenalist program for constructing object perceptions out of sensations. What is striking is that all the forms of behaviorist learning are associationist. Repetition, classical conditioning, and reward conditioning are all theories whereby learning is taken to be constituted by the making or increasing the strength of connections among elements that are already somehow present in or accessible to an organism. So in Pavlov's famous dog experiment, the food is paired with salivation. It is of note that although this is a reflex and thus presumably a causal connection, this aspect is not important in the experiment. It is merely the way these two elements are paired in the first place. Then the bell ringing is introduced, paired with the food presentation. This association gets established. Of course, the conditioning (learning) occurs when the dog salivates only to the bell ringing (without food). That is, learning is the newly formed association between the bell and the salivation response.

In this case, it should be obvious that the dog had to be able to perceive (see and smell) the food and hear the bell. Salivation depended on their being a (reflex) mechanism from perceiving the food to the drooling response, so this association was already extant.

3. Prototypical Examples
of Neurobehaviorism

To establish my claim about the frequency of quasi behaviorist experimental paradigms in the contemporary neuroscience of learning and memory would be a major undertaking, if one were to attempt to review a major chunk of the recent literature. To make the task tractable, I propose to make a selection from the most often cited recent (1997–2007) learning and memory publications to analyze in some detail and briefly report on the rest. The citation index used is ISI Web of Knowledge (*Web of Science*, queried July 24, 2007). This is a fallible methodology, but the presumption that papers that are often cited are somehow representative of the field seems plausible. Here, then, is a list of the top 10 most cited papers.

1. LeDoux (2000). Times cited: 1,076.
2. Kandel (2001). Times cited: 534.
3. Yuste and Bonhoeffer (2001). Times cited: 259.
4. Gabrieli (1998). Times cited: 243.
5. Crawley and Paylor (1997). Times cited: 212.
6. Ohman and Mineka (2001). Times cited: 197.
7. D'Hooge and De Deyn (2001). Times cited: 175.
8. Vizi and Kiss (1998). Times cited: 172.
9. Bayer et al. (2001). Times cited: 169.
10. Lynch (2004). Times cited: 161.

A few properties of entries on this list are worth remarking. A citation search for "learning and memory," versus just for "learning," has at the number 10 spot: Goldstone (1998), times cited: 148, and deletes Ohman and Mineka (2001) from the foregoing list.

The first two papers are cited extensively, well above the remainder on the list, and the first, LeDoux (2000), stands alone statistically. Most of the publications, though in differing degrees, deal with the hippocampus and its function in learning and memory, which shows where a great amount of research interest has been focused. This shows that the major goal of such research has been to find the neurobiological substructures that are causally productive of certain behavioral (or cognitive) events (at the O-level).

Here, to begin the discussion, are some reasonably typical quotations from some of the top 10 papers. Only the last citation, from Gabrieli (1998), brings a putative challenge to the claim that behavioral experimental paradigms dominate the field.

From LeDoux (2000) we read:

> It has, in fact, been research on fear conditioning, and the progress that has been made on this topic, that has been largely responsible for the renaissance of interest of emotion within neuroscience. In this work, the fear system has been treated as a set of processing circuits that detect and respond to danger, rather than as a mechanism through which subjective states of fear are experienced. Through this approach, fear is operationalized, or made experimentally tractable.

As far as fear conditioning itself is typically characterized, it is standard classical conditioning: "Simply stated, Pavlovian fear conditioning involves learning that certain environmental stimuli predict aversive events—it is the mechanism whereby we learn to fear people, places, objects, and animals" (Maren 2001). Here is an example from Crawley and Paylor (1997):

> Abstract: Behavioral phenotyping of transgenic and knockout mice requires rigorous, formal analyses. Well-characterized paradigms can be chosen from the established behavioral neuroscience literature. This review describes...a series of specific behavioral paradigms, clustered by category. Included are multiple paradigms for each category, including learning and memory, feeding, analgesia, aggression, anxiety, depression, schizophrenia, and drug abuse models.

Kandel's work (2001) is somewhat typified by the following experimental design and mechanism tracing:

> We found that five spaced puffs of serotonin (simulating five spaced shocks to the tail) activate PKA, which in turn recruits the mitogen-activated protein kinase (MAPK). Both translocate to the nucleus, where they activate a transcriptional cascade beginning with the transcription factor CREB-1, the cAMP response binding protein 1, so called because it binds to a cAMP response elements (CRE) in the promoters of target genes. (p. 1033)

Howard Eichenbaum is one of the major memory researchers and so is good for our illustrative purposes. Although he is not in our top 10, his work is cited by many on that list. He has used many exemplary paradigms:

> Memories were viewed as mediated by a systematic organization of associations based on various relationships between items....To address these questions we developed an odor-guided version of the paired associate task for rats, and

we extended the learning requirement to include multiple stimulus-stimulus associations with overlapping stimulus elements. Exploiting rodents' natural foraging strategies that employ olfactory cues, animals were trained with stimuli that consisted of distinctive odors added to a mixture of ground rat chow and sand through which they dug to obtain buried cereal rewards. On each paired associate trial one of two sample odors initially presented was followed by two choice odors, each assigned as the "associate" of one of the samples and baited only when preceded by that sample. Following training on two sets of overlapping odor-odor associations, subsequent probe tests were used to characterize the extent to which learned representations supported two forms of flexible memory expression, transitivity, the ability to judge inferentially across stimulus pairs that share a common element, and symmetry, the ability to associate paired elements presented in the reverse of training order. (1997, pp. 553–555)

Efforts to delineate the anatomical structures involved in maintaining a memory trace have focused on the delayed nonmatch to sample (DNMS) task first developed for monkeys using three-dimensional junk objects that provide rich and salient cues for this species....In our own work on rats we developed a variant of the DNMS task that used odor cues....In this task a sequence of odor cues is presented, and subjects are rewarded for responding to a stimulus that is different from (a nonmatch with) the preceding cue, but they are not rewarded for responding to a stimulus that is the same as (a match with) the preceding odor. We compared the effects of selective ablation of the parahippocampal region versus that of damage to the hippocampus (fornix transection) and found that neither lesion affected the acquisition rate. In subsequent tests with longer memory delays, intact rats showed a gradual performance decline, but rats with damage to the parahippocampal region had an abnormally rapid memory decay, showing a severe deficit within several seconds. In contrast, rats with hippocampal damage were unimpaired across delays, showing the same gradual memory decay as intact rats. (1997, p. 560)

As mentioned, Gabrieli (1998) discusses some apparent nonbehavioral paradigms—cognitive skills, perceptual skills, repetition priming; then various forms of conditioning (delay, trace and discrimination reversal, fear):

Functional neuroimaging studies allow for the design of psychological experiments targeted at specific memory processes. (p. 88)

Skill learning, repetition priming, and conditioning are classes of implicit tests that often reveal procedural memory processes dissociable from declarative memory....(p. 90)

Lesions have revealed remarkable specificity in the cortical representation of long-term memories. Some patients with cortical lesions have shown category-specific inabilities to produce the names of objects (anomias). Thus, patients have shown selective deficits for retrieving the names of (a) people and other proper nouns...; (b) fruits and vegetables...; (c) living things such as animals...; and (d) manufactured things such as tools....These patients can demonstrate retention of knowledge about objects that they cannot name by, for example, selecting the names of such objects from multiple choices....(p. 93)

> In skill-learning tasks, subjects perform a challenging task on repeated trials in one or more sessions. The indirect or implicit measure of learning is the improvement in speed or accuracy achieved by a subject across trials and sessions. Preservation of sensorimotor, perceptual, and cognitive skill learning in amnesia indicates that such learning for some skills is not dependent upon declarative memory....Intact sensorimotor skill learning in amnesia is well documented for three tasks: mirror tracing, rotary pursuit, and serial reaction time (SRT). (p. 97)

In most of these examples, I think it is fairly obvious that we are dealing with behaviorist paradigms. In some of Gabrieli's examples, the behaviors elicited or tasks required are fairly complex, though they are still a pairing of a sensory input with a motor output, though unlike Pavlov's dog, the output or task in some cases had to be learned first, before the behavioral association with sensory input could be established. The question is, can this original learning be explained by a reward associationist mechanism? In lesion studies, one correlates lesions with impairments or inabilities to perform normal tasks, and sometimes with the inability to learn new information under the given experimental conditions. Lacking a mechanism for the functioning of the lesioned part of the brain and its associated deficit, we have just an association (or at best a mechanism sketch).

4. COMPUTATIONALISM: MODELING ASSOCIATIONIST LEARNING

The relation between neural network models of learning (PDP or Hebbian learning) and the conditioning paradigms is very tight. Neural nets (or whatever form is used to make the associationist connections) must connect nodes of the net. In some cases, they just increase connection strengths, like most LTP induction experiments. In other cases they work over representations. This latter case is most interesting. Representations have both form (structure) and content, and any initial learning or later changes in representation have to involve a type of learning that goes beyond strengthening a connection between two different representations. So in the visual system, whether or not you believe there are cognitively impenetrable basic elements, what is learned visually has to be some information (say, about the world) that gets represented in the system in a particular form that provides the basis, gives the original content, for whatever the network can do. Furthermore, modifications, say, top-down cognitive modifications, have to work on changing the content of the representation (at least in part.) This is kind of like how Susan Carey (1985) talks about changing kids' concepts of physics (though this may not be perceptual, of course).

Thus, to take a really good example of someone who uses reward conditioning in a strong way, when Richard Sutton and colleagues write their programs they take for granted such basics (fundamentals of structure and content):

We apply this strategy to Go by *creating over a million features based on templates for small fragments of the board*, and then use temporal difference learning and self-play. This method identifies hundreds of low level shapes with recognisable significance to expert Go players, and provides quantitative estimates of their values. (Silver, Sutton, and Mueller, 2007; emphasis added)

On another occasion: "This difference can be decisive in modern applications of reinforcement learning where the *use of a large number of features has proven to be an effective solution strategy*" (Geramifard, Bowling, and Sutton, 2006; emphasis added).

So how does one learn the features? We have accounts of learning visual features (albeit somewhat disparate accounts, e.g., for action vs. recognition), and this is a kind of learning that seems intractable by reward learning or just repetition. So how can one learn concepts on this model? In network talk, where does one get the node, and what is it a representation of? If you have the concept and it proves useful for acting (in some way) and is rewarded, and then comes to be expected, maybe it will be used more frequently to give rise to that action in the future.

Here's the best argument that I have come across for getting content out of connections.[1] Suppose the atomic elements (individual axon or dendrite processes, say) don't have content but respond differentially to different inputs connected directly or indirectly to environmental influences (e.g., light reflected from a tomato or retinal responses to it). There's no element that has a tomato content. It's just that various atoms turn on or off in the presence of tomatoes under certain common lighting and other conditions. Suppose connections between a number of atoms weaken or strengthen so as to produce a characteristic pattern of activity given repeated exposures to tomato influenced visual and other sensory inputs. The activity patterns among a fair number of axons and dendrites in different parts of the brain will produce what Haxby and colleagues call an activity landscape (see Courtney, Ungerleider, Keil, and Haxby, 1997). Suppose the associations among axons and dendrites developed during repeated tomato exposures result in a probabilistic connection between tomatoes and one or more characteristic activity landscapes. Assign tomato content to the landscapes by appeal to their causal roles (cognitive and behavioral). The idea is that association can take you from atoms with no content to action landscapes with content. Then think of memories as more or less permanent dispositions in neuronal populations to produce just those activity landscapes in the course of selected perceptual, cognitive, or behavioral goings on involving tomatoes.

This is just like phenomenalism except that sense data have content while nerve network atoms do not. Note that content can change if it's the content of activity landscapes—as the landscapes or their causal roles change under the influence of new experiences. It hopes to avoid the objection to people who think the atoms have content that their content can't be parlayed into the kind of content a tomato representation should have.

Even in this argument, content has to get into the system somehow. In the foregoing argument, it gets in by our assigning tomato content based on our taking the stimulus–atom causal association to be one of reference (or some such content-conveying relation). So the explanation of learning has to include the active pickup of information and learning to attend to the informational features present in the world. The only other way to think about content is to assume that the content is just the compete set of associations. This associationist theory of meaning was prevalent somewhat in the old days with people like Paul Feyerabend and the early Jerry Fodor. But I do not think anyone holds it now. It is a completely internalist theory of content or meaning with no acknowledgment of reference.

In terms of our earlier associationist picture, what gets associated, the "elements," must be learned before associations can be forged or strengthened. As noted earlier, this almost is the same strategy as was used in the phenomenalist theory of perception. There sensations had to be glued together to give object perceptions. But as Roderick Chisholm (1948) pointed out, any sense datum statement can be true when the relevant object statement is false unless the former is conjoined with an object statement that mentions observation conditions, or the condition of the observer. For example, you can have a red, round, bulgy, and so on tomato experience when there's no tomato if you look at a holograph, a wax fake, a hallucination, and so on, and a tomato can be there when you don't see red because you're blind, the lights are too dim, and so forth. So you have to add conditions about your eyesight, the lighting conditions, and so on, which themselves have to be replaced by sense data statements subject to the same difficulties. This was but one objection to the phenomenalist program. It is generally conceded that it is a failed program, in whatever form it occurred. Interestingly, Rick Grush (2000) provided an analogous argument against informational, causal, and covariational accounts of content. He calls it the *distility* problem.

In this same way, any form of the neural network program seems unable to address the question of how nodes in the net obtain content or representational information (parallel to object properties). It also is difficult to see how they can handle change of content.

This criticism of the associationist or behaviorist program is unlike the kind of criticisms that were leveled at behaviorism during the cognitive revolution. Classically, Jerry Fodor and Noam Chomsky criticized behaviorism on the grounds that one needed internal variables to explain learning (language) or certain forms of behavior (hearing words as segmented). These kinds of criticism were based on purely cognitive models and wanted no part in any claims about the brain or its function in learning. But more important for my purpose here, the cognitivist program often was just another form of associationism, introducing intervening variables to get tighter connections (or mappings) between inputs and outputs. Again, the problem of the content of the cognitive states was neglected until very late, after the revolution had been won. But the problem of content does require talking about the brain and representational capacities and modes of operation. As argued above, this cannot be explained or studied by the associationist or behaviorist principles (see Grush, 2000, for supporting arguments).

Here's another aspect of the nodes as representational problem. If each node has a content that represents something (say, in the world, or some internal state), then how would it be possible to change that content on the associationist picture?

Let us assume a content gets into the system by some mechanism that creates the representation in the brain. Then if there is any possibility of changing that content, it may be because the same mechanism or similar one operates to substitute one content for another. But this substitution cannot be explained by changing strengths of association among different representations. The problem gets worse, for if there is conceptual blending or any sort of assimilation or internal structural change to the representative content, then there must be a learning procedure that allows for such contentful changes. The alternative view would seem to require that each bit of content is atomic in some sense, and new content for representations can only arise of recombinatory strategies among the atomic bits, maybe with some additions (by whatever process) or deletions (maybe by extinction). But this collapses into the view that was already discussed.

5. THE UPSHOT

There is nothing wrong per se with behaviorist, associationist, or strict input-output mapping experiments and models. Indeed, it might be plausibly argued that in some cases, especially neurobiological cases, this is all we are able to do. But if anyone has so argued this, I do not know of it. What is assumed is much more tendentious, that such experiments and models are all we need. But if learning, memory, and knowledge themselves require more than just probabilistic input-output models, then there is a need for devising new and better experiments—experiments that will make clearer the external validity of the results and will help us understand learning and memory as they occur in humans in the real world. If there were world enough and time, and I were just a tad smarter, the next section of this chapter would go on to develop such a model. But there is not, and I am not.

NOTE

1. This argument was reconstructed by Jim Bogen, to whom I am most grateful.

REFERENCES

Bayer, K. U., De Koninck, P., Leonard, A. S., et al. (2001). Interaction with the NMDA receptor locks CaMKII in an active conformation. *Nature* 411: 801–805.
Carey, S. (1985). *Conceptual Change in Childhood*. Cambridge, Mass.: MIT Press.
Chisholm, R. (1948). The problem of empiricism. *Journal of Philosophy* 45: 512–517.

Courtney, S. M., Ungerleider, L. G., Keil, K., and Haxby, J. V. (1997). Transient and sustained activity in a distributed neural system for human working memory. *Nature* 386: 608–611.

Crawley, J. N., and Paylor, R. (1997). A proposed test battery and constellations of specific behavioral paradigms to investigate the behavioral phenotypes of transgenic and knockout mice. *Hormones and Behavior* 31: 197–211.

D'Hooge, R., and De Deyn, P. P. (2001). Applications of the Morris water maze in the study of learning and memory. *Brain Research Reviews* 36: 60–90.

Eichenbaum, H. (1997). Declarative memory: Insights from cognitive neurobiology. *Annual Review of Psychology* 48: 547–572.

Gabrieli, J. D. E. (1998). Cognitive neuroscience of human memory. *Annual Review of Psychology* 49: 87–115.

Geramifard, A., Bowling, M., and Sutton, R. S. (2006). Incremental least-squares temporal difference learning. In *Proceedings of the Twenty-First National Conference on Artificial Intelligence (AAAI-06)*: 356–361.

Goldstone, R. L. (1998). Perceptual learning. *Annual Review of Psychology* 49: 585–612.

Grush, R. (2000). Cognitive science. In P. Machamer and M. Silberstein (Eds.), *The Blackwell Guide to Philosophy of Science*. London: Blackwell.

Kandel, E. R. (2001). Neuroscience—the molecular biology of memory storage: A dialogue between genes and synapses. *Science* 294: 1030–1038.

LeDoux, J. E. (2000). Emotion circuits in the brain. *Annual Review of Neuroscience* 23: 155–184.

Lynch, M. A. (2004). Long-term potentiation and memory. *Physiological Review* 84: 87–136.

Maren, S. (2001) "Neurobiology of pavlovian fear conditioning." *Annual Review of Neuroscience* 24: 897–931.

Ohman, A., and Mineka, S. (2001). Fears, phobias, and preparedness: Toward an evolved module of fear and fear learning. *Psychological Review* 108: 483–522.

Silver, D., Sutton, R. S., and Mueller, M. (2007). Reinforcement learning of local shape in the game of Go. *Proceedings of the 20th International Joint Conference on Artificial Intelligence (IJCAI-07)*.

Vizi, E. S., and Kiss, J. P. (1998). Neurochemistry and pharmacology of the major hippocampal transmitter systems: Synaptic and nonsynaptic interactions. *Hippocampus* 8: 566–607.

Yuste, R., and Bonhoeffer, T. (2001). Morphological changes in dendritic spines associated with long-term synaptic plasticity. *Annual Review of Neuroscience* 24: 1071–1089.

PART III

SENSATION AND PERCEPTION

fMRI: A MODERN CEREBRASCOPE? THE CASE OF PAIN

VALERIE GRAY HARDCASTLE AND C. MATTHEW STEWART

1. THE BRIEF HISTORY OF fMRI

It has been popular since the 1950s for philosophers of mind and science to hypothesize the existence of a "cerebrascope," a machine that could read a brain's activity, which we could then presumably correlate (or not) with concomitant cognition. Philosophers use these hypothetical devices to help them reason about identity theories from the armchair. If we could access the firing patterns of our neurons, are we accessing the actual thoughts, the physical manifestation of thoughts, the physical parallel of thoughts, or something else entirely? If we compare cerebrascope outputs across individuals or of the same individual over time, can we see multiple manifestations of the same thought, or multiple manifestations of similar thoughts, or is each thought completely different from all others?

Until recently, the cerebrascope has been nothing more than a philosopher's fancy. But now, technology appears to have caught up with philosophy. Is functional magnetic resonance imaging (fMRI) the modern-day cerebrascope? fMRI can record changes in the flow of fluids or in the chemical composition in some region, which helps neuroscientists visualize patterns of activity in the brain. Can we use this technology to access our thoughts (or their instantiations)? If so, what do MRI data tell us about cognition? If not, then why not? What else would we need for philosophy to get its cerebrascope machine? This chapter tries to answer these questions by looking at one particular area of recent study in MRI, that of imaging pain.

Because MRIs are so ubiquitous these days, it is important to remember that this is still a very new technology. fMRI of the human brain is the latest incarnation in a field that came into existence only a quarter of a century ago.

It really began when Felix Bloch, at Stanford University, and Edward Purcell, at Harvard University, independently carried out the first successful nuclear magnetic resonance (NMR) experiments in 1946. They discovered that when certain nuclei were placed in a magnetic field, they absorbed energy in the radiofrequency range of the electromagnetic spectrum and then reemitted this energy when the nuclei transferred back to their original state. Both were awarded the Nobel Prize in 1952 for this research. Hence, NMR spectroscopy was born and soon became an important analytical method in the study of the composition of chemical compounds.

During the 1950s and 1960s, NMR spectroscopy became widely used in the noninvasive analysis of small samples. In the late 1960s and early 1970s, Raymond Damadian, at the State University of New York in Brooklyn, showed that the nuclear magnetic relaxation times of tissues and tumors differed in vitro, thus opening the possibility that magnetic resonance could be used to detect diseases. Then, in the spring of 1973, *Nature* published a short article by Paul Lauterbur, from the State University of New York at Stony Brook. This now seminal essay describes a new imaging technique, which Lauterbur called *zeugmatography* (from the Greek *zeugmo*, meaning a joining together), which joined a spatially uniform static magnetic field with a second, weaker magnetic field that varied with position in a controlled fashion. This created what is known as a magnetic field gradient and allowed for the first time spatial localization with magnetic imaging.

In 1975, Richard Ernst proposed using phase and frequency encoding and the Fourier transformation in magnetic resonance imaging. This technique, along with techniques borrowed from CT scans, forms the basis of current MRI protocols. Then, in 1977, Peter Mansfield developed what is known as the echo-planar imaging technique, which was later developed to create images at video rates.

Advances in high-speed computing and superconducting magnets enormously improved the sensitivity and resolution of MRI machines. By 1986, the time required to get an image had been reduced to about 5 seconds. But it was not until 1993 that functional MRI became possible, and the first MR images of pain processing in humans were only published in 1994 (Hirato et al., 1994).

So, this chapter looks at an experimental protocol that has only been around for a decade or so. Our comments should be taken with that in mind. We offer suggestions for how to improve fMRI experiments and their theoretical implications with the full knowledge that scientists are still figuring out how best to use these machines. Although we are critical of some of the work done to date, we also realize that we are asking a lot of neuroscientists to move beyond what they have been doing in fMRI experiments because they only just started doing the experiments at all. We celebrate the promise of MRI, while being mindful of its limitations, pitfalls, and overpromises.

2. OUR PAIN PROCESSING AND PAIN INHIBITING SYSTEMS

A long time ago, in 1911 to be exact, Head and Holmes proposed a dual system of afferent projections in our pain sensory system: an "epicritic" system that processes information regarding intensity and precise location, and a "protopathic" system that delivers the actual pain sensations. Eighty-plus years later, we believe their proposal is largely correct. Pain specialists typically divide our pain processing system into a "sensory discriminative" or "fast pain" subsystem, originating with the A-∂ fibers, that computes the location, intensity, duration, and nature (stabbing, burning, prickling) of stimuli, and an "affective-motivational" or "slow pain" subsystem, beginning with the well-known C-fibers, that supports the unpleasant part of painful sensations. Each subsystem has a set of neurons that resides in the dorsal root ganglion of the spinal column. These neurons extend their axons to whatever tissue they innervate and receive input there; they also have a second axon that projects across to the dorsal horn. Then our basic pain system continues up through cortex (see figure 8.1).

Roughly speaking, once pain information exits the dorsal horn, it travels either to the reticular formation in the brain stem or to the thalamus. Laminae I and V project to the lateral nuclei in the thalamus (Craig, Bushnell, Zhang, and Blomqvist, 1994), and laminae I, V, and VI project to the medial nuclei. Each type of nucleus underwrites a different sort of information; the lateral nuclei process sensory-discriminative information, and the medial nuclei and reticular connections process affective-motivational information. The two thalamic streams remain separate on their trip to cortex as well.

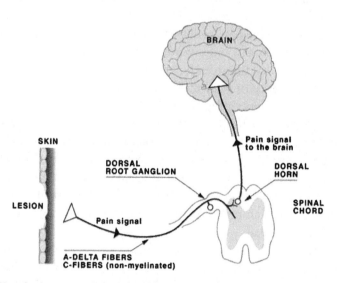

Figure 8.1. Simple diagram of the precortical pain processing system. Nociceptive information received via the A-∂ or the C-fibers travels in parallel from the periphery to the dorsal horn in the spinal cord and then on up to cortex.

Pain neurons in the lateral nuclei synapse in sensory cortex, which can then compute the location and characteristics of the pain; those in the medial nuclei synapse in the anterior cingulate gyrus in the frontal lobe, which figures in our emotional reactions to pain. The frontal lobe (and its connections) processes our actual suffering.

In general, current theories of pain hold that the robust feedback loops in our pain system inhibit, enhance, or distort incoming nociceptive information. There are additional ascending connections from the spinal cord to the brainstem, circular pathways from the spinal cord to other areas in the spinal cord itself, and descending feedback loops from the cortex, hypothalamus, and brainstem back to the spinal cord. Some portions of this theory have been worked out in considerable detail.

However, we have known for some time that many of the inhibitory streams are not just feedback loops in our ascending pain fibers—they are anatomically distinct from our pain processors. Three areas are primarily responsible for inhibiting pain information in the spinal column: the cortex, the thalamus, and the brainstem. The dorsal raphe probably is heavily involved as well. In addition, neocortex and hypothalamus project to periaqueductal gray region (PAG), which then sends projections to the reticular formation. The reticular nuclei then work to inhibit activity in the dorsal horn. This processing stream works by preventing a central cortical representation of pain from forming. Endogenous opioids, like PAG activity, dampen incoming information in the dorsal horn. These pain inhibition streams do not merely disrupt the transmission of pain information, they actively prevent it from occurring (see figure 8.2).

If we look at the connections of the inhibitory streams, we can see that they differ substantially from the incoming pain processing system. It would not be proper to call them sensory systems or subsystems, for they have no connections to the periphery. The pain inhibitory streams halt at the dorsal horn. Also, unlike the ascending pain streams, the hypothamalus and dorsal raphe nuclei receive massive inputs from cortical processors, which presumably could carry information about our goals and immediate plans, what else is occurring in the environment, our larger emotional context, and so forth. Our inhibitory systems have immediate access to information that the ascending pathways do not.

A two-system theory of pain makes good evolutionary sense. When we are under stress, it is often more adaptive to not feel pain than to be incapacitated by pain. If we are fighting or fleeing from an enemy, it would be preferable to do so unencumbered by the need to nurse or protect our limbs, even it this results in more nursing or protecting later (when we are presumably safe). It is important to know when damage is occurring in our bodies, but it is equally important to be able to shut that information out when circumstances demand. A dual system allows just such contingencies; we inhibit our pains as needed, but then feel them again when the danger is gone. A pain processing system and a pain inhibitory system then serve two different goals: The pain processing system keeps us informed regarding the status of our bodies. It monitors our tissues to maintain their intactness whenever possible. In contrast, the pain inhibitory shuts down the pain processing system when flight or fleeing is eminent, and then enhances the pain processing system response in moments of calm.

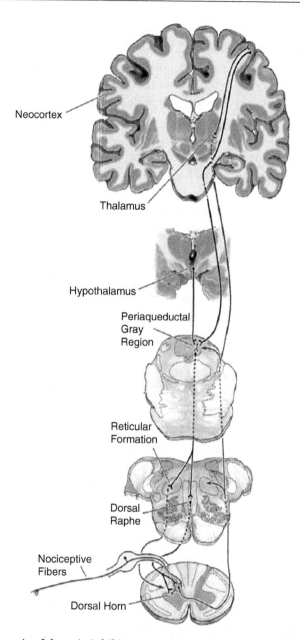

Neocortex

Thalamus

Hypothalamus

Periaqueductal
Gray
Region

Reticular
Formation

Dorsal
Raphe

Nociceptive
Fibers

Dorsal Horn

Figure 8.2. Schematic of the pain inhibitory system. Inhibitory signals travel from neocortex and hypothalamus to the periqueductal gray region and then on to the reticular nuclei. The reticular nuclei inhibit activity in the dorsal horn, thus preventing a cortical representation of pain from occurring.

The interactions of our pain processing and pain inhibitory systems mean that our sensations of pain are constructed on the fly, as it were. What a pain feels like, if it feels like anything at all, depends on how the nociceptive information is embedded in the environment in the brain—what the subjects believe, what they are paying attention to, the emotions they are feeling. It also depends on the environment of the organism—what the subject is doing and in what social and physical milieu.

For example, some lesions to the thalamus and cortex can result in the cessation of pain experiences, even though the peripheral neurons continue to operate normally, and stimulating the medial PAG, tectum, or thalamus directly gives us a painful experience (Davis, Tasker, Kiss, Hutchison, and Dostrovsky, 1995; Keay, Clement, Owler, Depaulis, and Bandelr, 1994). Placebos are notoriously helpful in relieving pain. (Interestingly enough, they relieve pain at half the rate of the real drug, regardless of the supposed strength of the drug; Evans, 1974.) Hypnosis allows some subjects to engage in what would otherwise be painful activities without being in pain. Stories of athletes and soldiers continuing to function without pain even though severely injured are legend. Indeed, about 40 percent of all ER patients reported feeling no pain at the time of injury; 40 percent more report greater pain that one would expect, leaving only 20 percent of all ER visitors having pains appropriate to their injuries (Melzack, Wall, and Ty, 1982). In fact, there is a poor correlation between nociception and pain perception (Wall, 1989; Wall and McMahon, 1985).

Considerations such as these have led the International Association for the Study of Pain (IASP) Subcommittee on Classification to conclude:

> Pain is always subjective.…Many people report pain in the absence of tissue damage or any pathophysiological cause; usually this happens for psychological reasons. There is usually no way to distinguish their experience from that due to tissue damage if we take the subjective report.… [Pain] is always a psychological state. (1986, p. 217)

Some take this perspective a bit too far and write as though just about any psychological event or any area of cortex has the potential of influencing the perception of pain, what Melzack calls a "neuromatrix" (Melzack, 1990, 1991, 1992; see also discussion in Canavaro, 1994). However, even though there are lots of feedback loops and other sorts of pain connections, not every area in the brain is sensitive to pain information. We believe the higher centers of pain are indeed centers, and they work together to influence, dampen, enhance, eliminate, and create our sensations and behaviors connected to pain.

Even though we know a lot about our basic pain processing and pain inhibitory systems, there are still many unanswered questions. Why is chronic pain chronic? What is a pain disorder? Why are there such apparent individual differences in pain reports/sensations? One hope is that recent advances in imaging technology will be able to shed some light on these puzzles. If we could peer into the active human brain as it is experiencing what from the outside appear to be abnormal responses, then perhaps we could understand what is going on. If only we had a cerebrascope.…

Is this hope misplaced? Before answering this question, let us first quickly review the principles behind functional magnetic imaging.

3. A BRIEF PRIMER ON FUNCTIONAL MAGNETIC IMAGING TECHNIQUES

Imaging technology does not record precise changes in brain activation or metabolism. Instead, an increase in a brain region's metabolic rate correlates with increased delivery of blood to that area. These local increases in blood flow and microvascular oxygenation are measured and later recorded as changes in pixel intensity in an image.

In particular, noninvasive MRI in high magnetic fields is sensitive to deoxygenated hemoglobin. MRI measures the rate of change in either proton spin phase coherence or local magnetic field homogeneity, both of which are modulated by amount of oxygen present in blood; hence, MRI is a "blood oxygenation level–dependent" (BOLD) measuring technique. Though both measurements are used in BOLD recordings, change in local magnetic field homogeneity creates effects that are 3 to 10 times larger than changes in the rate of change of proton spin phase coherence and so is the most widely used mechanism in MRI experiments. Scientists believe that changes in local magnetic field homogeneity reflect regional deoxygenation in the venous system.

Any substance in a magnetic field changes that field to some degree or other. Certain metals, such as gadolinium and dysprosium, have a naturally high magnetic moment relative to water or air and become extremely polarized when placed in a magnetic field. The degree of a substance's polarization is called its magnetic susceptibility. Even though the iron in hemoglobin has superb natural magnetic susceptibility, oxygenated blood, which contains oxygenated hemoglobin, is diamagnetic and has a small magnetic susceptibility. It cannot, therefore, significantly alter the regional magnetic field, and MRI cannot detect it in tissues.

However, the deoxygenation of hemoglobin produces deoxyhemoglobin, which is significantly more paramagnetic because it has four unpaired electrons. It does disturb local magnetic fields and therefore has large magnetic susceptibility. Changes in local concentrations of deoxygenated and oxygenated iron affect magnetic field homogeneity by changing local magnetic susceptibility.

Blood in arteries consists mostly of oxyhemoglobin, but as it passes through the capillary bed, its concentration of deoxyhemoglobin increases. Therefore, a gradient in magnetic field homogeneity exists across the vascular tree from a diamagnetic oxyhemoglobin-rich environment to a more "paramagnetic" deoxyhemoglobin-rich environment.[1]

The balance of deoxygenated to oxygenated hemoglobin in blood within a voxel (volume picture element) is the local measurement critical to MRI. Increasing the flow of oxygenated blood to a brain region or reducing its oxygen extraction increases its local, intravoxel, magnetic field homogeneity, which in turn increases image intensity.

The balance between deoxygenated and oxygenated hemoglobin is a function of local arterial autoregulation and vasodilation. An increase in local activation causes the arteries to deliver more oxygenated blood to that region, which then

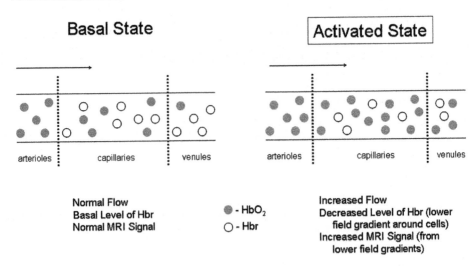

Figure 8.3. fMRI BOLD signals. Changes in the concentration of deoxygenated or oxygenated iron in an area alter the magnetic susceptibility in that area, which in turn affects magnetic field homogeneity. The relative concentration of oxyhemoglobin in arterial blood decreases as it passes through the capillary bed, as its concentration of deoxyhemoglobin increases. Hence, a gradient in magnetic field homogeneity exists across the vascular tree. Increasing the activation causes the arteries to deliver more oxygenated blood, which results in more oxygenated iron in the capillary and venous vascular beds, which then causes change in magnetic field homogeneity and a change in image intensity.

results in more oxygenated iron in the capillary and venous vascular beds, which then causes change in magnetic field homogeneity and a change in image intensity (see figure 8.3). In other words, the image intensity for a given voxel in the brain increases if more oxygenated blood enters this region and fills the venous bed. This happens when local activation increases. Scientists therefore rely on deoxygenated hemoglobin as an index for local activation.

Behind all these principles is the assumption that cortical activation causes local vasodilation with little or no concomitant increase in metabolizing oxygen. In addition, local image intensity increases will also depend heavily on the architecture of particular vessels (their radii, orientation, and relative vascular openness). Whether these two assumptions are well justified is a discussion we leave for another day.

4. DIFFICULTIES WITH IMAGING PAIN

However, even if we can agree that the architecture of our brains is such that we get vasodilation without an increase in oxygen metabolism and that the structure of our blood vessels promotes good MR images, there are still several problems remaining with using MRI as a tool for studying brain activity. These problems are exacerbated or compounded when it is used as a tool for studying brain activity associated with pain.

The first and most obvious difficulty is that the BOLD factors used in MRI are not the same thing as cognition. Changes in pixel intensity, proton spin phase coherence, local magnetic field homogeneity, blood oxygen levels, or even local brain activity are obviously not the same thing as thinking a thought or having a phenomenal experience. Although we assume tight linkages between thoughts and changes in nearby blood chemistry, what the connections really are in particular instances still has to be spelled out. Right now, we just assume the connection without any real data or detailed theory behind it.

Second, moving from measuring changes in proton spin phase coherence or local magnetic field homogeneity to drawing an increase in pixel intensity on top of a high-resolution brain image requires some serious data manipulation. Some would call it serious data creation. Regardless, there is an art to creating the pretty pictures associated with MRI scans and there is a further art to interpreting those pictures. Whether too much of the artist goes into making meaningful images is a question neuroscience still needs to address.

Third, using voxels as units of analysis is very artificial. Although this was not a difficulty when our measuring techniques were relatively crude, since changes in image intensity were smeared over a number of voxels, as our instruments have gotten better, the window for just-noticeable-differences has gotten smaller. Soon scientists will be able to measure significant differences in intensity between individual voxels. But a voxel is not tied to any unit of anything in particular in the brain; it does not carve Nature at her joints, as it were. It is simply the unit we use to track digital images. Hence, knowing that two voxels differ from each other may not tell us—indeed, probably does not tell us—anything of value about underlying brain activity.

Fourth, the time course in which MRI occurs is much too broad. Brain activity is fast. Action potentials occur in milliseconds. Potassium influx and efflux across cell walls takes only hundredths of milliseconds. But the best we can measure with our fastest imaging equipment is a few seconds, thus ensuring that images of the brain show activity "smeared" across time. As a result, we cannot use imaging studies to tell how much about the time progression or computation of cognition. We can only get snapshots of end results.

Finally, the commonly used subtraction method in fMRI can subtract out crucial data. When we use imaging technology to study some particular cognitive event, we compare averaged trials of that event with averaged trials of so-called neutral events. So we might compare seeing flashes of light with seeing nothing, or hearing English words with hearing white noise. We subtract the activity we find in the cognitive events from the activity we get with neutral events. The idea is that whatever activity is left over after subtraction is activity specifically devoted to solving the cognitive task: seeing a flash as opposed to just seeing in general, or processing a language as opposed to just hearing noise.

But in each so-called neutral comparison, it is not the case that the brain does nothing; it is still processing information about the world around it. It is entirely possible—indeed, highly likely—that some of the same brain areas are used to process flashing lights as to process seeing "nothing." If so, then subtracting the activity in one condition from the others in these regions would show zero net effect, instead of indicating that these regions are used in the task of interest. It is important to remember that the subtraction method will only reveal a portion of areas tied to particular brain functions; it will reveal only those not also used to process the neutral comparison events.

Similarly, the subtraction method creates problems for trying to localize functions in the brain. If an fMRI does not indicate all areas associated with a task, then it cannot indicate all locations relevant to the task as well. In addition, because the time course of the brain's response is significantly shorter than what MRI can measure, we cannot use MRI to determine the time course over which various areas process stimuli.

Moreover, on top of all these rather generic difficulties with using MRI to learn about the brain, there are additional problems when MRI is used to track pain processing. For example, pain processing or activating the pain inhibitory system causes a global decrease in cerebral blood flow. As a result, pain-related signals are statistically weaker, have a less consistent time course than, say, visual processing tasks, and decay before the end of the stimulus. The bottom line is that pain BOLD signals are attenuated by pain-induced cerebral blood flow decrease (Kurata, Thulborn, Gyulai, and Firestone, 2002).

In addition, the somatotopic organization of the primary sensory cortex means that pain processing causes only small focal activations, which are then degraded by anatomical variability in brains' sulci when recordings are averaged across subjects. Only small pockets of activation would be detected, even though larger areas may be contributing to the processing (Bushnell et al., 1999). This difficulty is compounded by the fact that we adapt quickly to pain, so it is hard to use protocols that require multiple instances of the target stimuli, as most imaging experiments do.

Moreover, nociceptive and tactile receptors are close to one another in cortex, so it is very difficult to separate genuine pain processing from activation of the tactile system or from cognition itself, because it is hard to create pain without also touching the body or without the subject thinking about the pain as it is happening (Treede, Apkarian, Bromm, Greenspan, and Lenz, 2000). These mixed signals would be further compounded by excitatory and inhibitory effects being disparately represented in different experimental paradigms (Bushnell et al., 1999) and with the significant individual variation we find in pain processing and perception across subjects (Davis, 2000).

Finally, subtraction methods may not be sensitive enough to image nociceptive cells, which are rather sparsely distributed in sensory cortex (Disbrow, Buonocore, Antognini, Carstens, and Rowley, 1998). Sparsely distributed cells, even if they are all strongly activated, will not change the activity level of a region of interest enough to show up in a final analysis.

The end result of all these difficulties is that we find conflicting results in corti-cal fMRI studies of pain as well as tremendous individual differences in the pain levels reported for the same stimuli. Despite these difficulties, can imaging studies of pain tell us anything at all useful about pain processing or painful experiences? We believe they can.

5. What Imaging Studies Tell Us about Pain

The first thing that becomes immediately clear when looking at imaging studies of pain is that even if we are capturing only a subset of the relevant activity, it is a highly distributed process. The structures that are most consistently active during pain processing include the contralateral insula, anterior cingulate cortex, thalamus, pre-motor cortex, and the cerebellar vermis. This activation varies parametrically with perceived pain intensity (Apkarian, 1995; Casey, 1999; see also Downar, Mikulis, and Davis, 2003). More specifically, we can see a central network for pain processing in imaging studies that runs from the thalamus to the primary and secondary sensory cortex (which probably code sensory-discriminative information and recognition, learning, and memory, respectively), the insula (which is connected with autonomic reactions and the affective aspects of learning and memory), and the anterior cin-gulate cortex (which is tied to the sensation of unpleasantness and appears to inte-grate intensity information, affect, cognition, and response selection) (Buchel et al., 2002; Chen, Ha, Bushnell, Pike, and Duncan, 2002; Ringler, Greiner, Kohlloeffel, Hnadwerker, and Forster, 2003; Schnitzler and Ploner, 2000; see also Alkire, White, Hsieh, and Haier, 2004). Then the information flows to prefrontal cortex (Treede, Kenshalo, Gracely, and Jones, 1999).

In the images of pain processing, we can see pretty quickly that the original simple dichotomy into sensory-discriminative and affective-motivational process-ing streams was too simple—our pain networks are too interconnected to identify two or even three separate processing streams. Indeed, conservation of intensity information across multiple areas suggests that we have a genuine pain processing network, and this possibility would help explain why patients can still experience pain after multiple lesions in their alleged pain processing streams (Coghill et al., 1994; Coghill, Sang, Maisog, and Iadarola, 1999; Treede et al., 1999).

In addition, the apparent simultaneous activation of contralateral primary and secondary sensory cortices suggests that thalamocortical nociceptive infor-mation is distributed in parallel. This anatomical arrangement contrasts with the serial cortical organization we find in tactile and visual processing in higher pri-mates. Instead, it corresponds to the parallel cortical organization we find in lower primates and nonprimates (Ploner, Schmitz, Freund, and Schnitzler, 1999; see also Price, 2000). This helps confirm what we already believe: Pain processing is an ancient system.

But more than learning about the general anatomy and physiology of our pain processing systems, we can now visualize the relationship between pain processing, pain inhibition, and beliefs, desires, and feelings. For example, the degree to which pain is perceived to be controllable affects pain tolerance, learning, motivation, and the ability to cope with intractable pain. In other words, the more we believe we are in control of our pains, the less they bother us. It also affects our neural responses. It turns out that the more we believe we control our pain, the more we get attenuated activation in anterior cingulate, the insula, and secondary sensory cortex (Salomons, Johnstone, Backonja, and Davidson, 2004). (This fact also suggests that these areas are modulated by cognition and therefore that pain studies might overestimate the degree to which the painful stimulus itself drives our responses and we can generalize pain responses across cognitive contexts.)

We know that both opioid and nonopioid mechanisms mediate pain attenuation by cognitive control. The greater the sense of self-efficacy one has, the more one's opioids are activated (Bandura, O'Leary, Taylor, Gauthier, and Gossard, 1987). We can see these effects in some detail in the level of activity in our pain processing networks.

We can see that attention and previous experience increase activation in the anterior cingulate and orbitofrontal cortex but modulate pain activity in the thalamus, insula, and primary sensory cortex (Bantick et al., 2002; Bushnell et al., 1999; Dowman, 2001). It appears that attention works through the frontal cortical areas to damp down activation in other regions of the brain. How one directs attention affects reaction time, accuracy, and perceived pain intensity and unpleasantness (Longe et al., 2001; Miron, Duncan, and Bushnell, 1989), which is what one would expect if activity diminishes in thalamus, insula, and primary sensory cortex, the very areas that appear to process pain intensity and its unpleasantness. Clearly, both nonspecific attention networks and selection/orienting networks are activated in pain processing, which may explain some of the variability we find in pain studies (Peyron et al., 1999).

When subjects expect a stimulus to be painful, they typically experience more pain than if they expect a stimulus to be pleasant or neutral. Indeed, expecting a stimulus to be painful also increases the perceived unpleasantness of innocuous stimuli. Anticipation of pain modulates our cortical systems involved in pain processing even without actual noxious inputs (Porro et al., 2002; see also Carlsson, Petrovic, Skare, Petersson, and Ingvar, 2000). We can correlate the expectation of a painful stimulus with enhanced brain responses to nonpainful stimuli in the anterior cingulate, the operculum, and the posterior insula (Sawamoto et al., 2000). Similarly, a negative emotional context modulates neural responses and perceived discomfort with nonpainful stimulation. We are more likely to read stimuli as painful, when they in fact may not be, when we are unhappy, depressed, sad, and the like (Phillips et al., 2003).

We can also get the opposite effect: Distraction from painful stimuli decreases pain sensations. This explains why football players can continue playing with broken bones and soldiers can continue on despite severe injuries. We can see these attentional effects in anterior cingulate as well (Frankenstein, Richter, McIntyre, and Remy, 2001). We also see increased activity in the PAG activity, which tells us that distraction or focusing one's attention away from pain activates our pain suppression system (Tracey et al., 2002).

6. WHAT HAVE WE LEARNED?

As you can see, despite all the problems with fMRI techniques in studying pain, there are many things that these techniques can still show us about pain, pain processing, and pain inhibition. However, our contention is that most of these studies are not telling scientists anything that they did not already know from traditional psychology and clinical investigations. Although we might have a better sense of where the pain networks are located in the brain and additional confirming evidence for how pain processing unfolds, we have not broken any significant conceptual or theoretical ground with these sorts of imaging studies.

We have not learned much about the time course of pain, both because of the inherent time limitations and because pain appears to be a primitive parallel system. We would need significantly more precise imaging technology to be able to trace the actual paths nociceptive information takes through our pain network. All we can detect now are the larger areas associated with pain processing and pain inhibition.

We have not learned that individual differences exist. One of the original impetuses for positing the pain inhibiting system was the existence of huge individual differences in pain reports and differences within the same individual in different circumstances. At the same time, fMRIs of pain highlight for us individual differences in pain processing, for we can clearly see differences in activation levels that correlate with differences in pain reports. Perhaps they do give us additional evidence that these differences are real and do not merely reflect individual's differing abilities to tolerate pain.

Similarly, we have not learned that attention and other distractors, beliefs, mood, and emotions affect pain processing. All of these things we knew before MRI studies on pain began. However, we can now see these effects on various areas in our pain network, which does give additional confirming evidence to the reality of the effects for those skeptical that cognition and affect influence experiences of pain. But being able to see these effects in the various brain areas does not tell us much about the details of what is happening, only that it is indeed happening.

In short, what we have are largely replications of previous psychological experiments, but now in color. Though we do not take up the larger point in this chapter, our persistent suspicion is that many fMRI experiments repeat what we already know. They just give us another window into the same theoretical room. It would perhaps be better if this relatively new technology would bring with it new ways of conceptualizing phenomena, but so far that has not happened.

Indeed, with this brief recitation of imaging results, one might be tempted to conclude that Jerry Fodor was right 30 years ago when he argued for a division of labor between neuroscience and psychology. Psychology would outline the "boxology" of cognitive process and then neuroscience would hunt for the underlying mechanisms that implemented the "boxes." Thus far, it appears that the imaging technology has not improved our theoretical understanding of cognition; it has merely given us vivid illustrations of the cognitive processes that psychology had already surmised were there. We are left wondering: What are fMRIs of pain processing really good for?

7. Why Bother with fMRIs
of Pain Processing?

While the previous section paints a rather dismal view of imaging studies, we do believe that they have distinct value in moving our understanding of pain processing forward. In particular, they allow for better understanding of pain disorders and other abnormal cases of pain processing or pain inhibition. In many cases, they illustrate what has gone wrong in the pain network's response to stimuli, something psychologists and neurologists could not ascertain prior to imaging these patients. Imaging studies of pain, therefore, have a crucial role to play in diagnosing pain disorders as well as advancing our theoretical framework for explaining them. (In some cases, they also will help demonstrate the reality of some pain disorders, as opposed to relegating them to a by-product of other mental disorders that the putative pain patient allegedly has.)

For example, chronic pain appears to modify the cortex of its sufferers (Wiech, Preissl, and Birbaumer, 2001). Although phasic pains are keyed to increased activity in areas of the limbic system, anterior cingulate, frontal cortex, thalamus, and primary and secondary sensory cortex, chronic pains are correlated with increased activity in cingulate and frontal cortex, as well as sometimes with insular cortex, hypothalamus, and PAG (see discussion and references in Apkarian, 1995). In addition, we can see differences in how the ipsilateral and contralateral thalamus responds to chronic pain as opposed to acute pain (Coghill et al., 1999). We do not yet know what these differences in brain response mean in terms of why chronic pain persists; however, just knowing that the differences are there gives neurologists something more specific to investigate in chronic pain patients.

Hyperalgesia, a condition such that stimuli that would normally induce small discomfort cause significant pain, is correlated with increased activity in contralateral prefrontal cortex and in all areas in sensory cortex, though without additional activity in the anterior cingulate (Baron, Baron, Disbrow, and Roberts, 1999; Verne et al., 2003). These data lead one to suspect that hyperalgesia is related to increased afferent processing as nociceptive information ascends into the higher areas of the brain.

Patients with fibromyalgia, a widespread musculoskeletal pain and fatigue disorder characterized by pain in the muscles, ligaments, and tendons, show greater pain activation levels to both painful and nonpainful stimuli all across the pain network (Cook et al., 2004). This tells us that fibromyalgia patients really do have more pain than normal subjects, though the reasons for these responses are still unknown.

Allodynia, a condition in which patients experience pain from stimuli that are not normally painful, also can be indexed using MRIs. In patients with allodynia, innocuous rubbing showed up on the MR image as a pattern of activation similar to one if the patient given a genuine painful stimulus. The only difference is that the activity is in contralateral cingulate gyrus. This difference may help account for the strange pain sensations associated with allodynia (Peyron et al., 1998; Peyron, Laurent, and Garcia-Larrea, 2000), in which patients report often feeling nauseated with the pain sensation.

Patients with temporomandibular joint (TMJ) disorders, a group of conditions that cause pain and dysfunction in the jaw and the muscles that control jaw movement, show less activation and report less pain when stimulated on the painful side of their jaw muscle. It is not clear why one would get these responses. In addition, cortical and brainstem nociceptive responses were attenuated, which suggests that at least some instances of chronic TMJ pain may be related to a malfunctioning trigeminal nociceptive system (Timmermann et al., 2001).

We can also use fMRI of pain processing to index other, more common abnormalities in pain response. Patients with chronic migraine, as opposed to other types of headache, showed no attentional distraction effects on the MR image (DeTommaso et al., 2003). Subjects under hypnosis who are instructed to change their sensation of pain show altered activation levels in the anterior cingulate (Faymoville et al., 2000). Subjects who empathize with pain show activity in the anterior cingulate and anterior insula but not in the sensory neurons themselves. We can literally feel another's pain.

In each of these cases, the MR scan told us something about a pain process that we did not know before; it told us how a process differed from normal, which we can then correlate with differences in pain reports and other pain indicators. As a result, they each open up new avenues for investigating why we get an abnormal pain response. Taken together, they illustrate that our pain network is extremely nuanced and complicated, that individual variation makes a tremendous difference in resultant pain sensations, and that there are genuine differences in processing between pain patients and normal subjects.

8. What Are fMRIs Contributing Theoretically?

If we are right and imaging studies of pain do have a significant role to play in our diagnosis and understanding of abnormal pain processing, then it must be the case that imaging techniques can shape our theoretical understanding of pain processing. How might they be doing this?

First and foremost, it is clear that the simple boxology theories of the past are no longer tenable. Pain is not a two-pathway set of serial circuits. Instead, it is a parallel network that taps into significant portions of the brain. What happens in the cortex in pain processing is quite complicated, and the earlier theories are simply no longer up to the task of accounting for the data we have.

This point becomes especially clear when we consider the variations in processing found in pain disorders. Any theory of pain will have to allow not only for the pain inhibitory system but also for differences in the actual computations the brain performs and differences in the areas used or emphasized under different processing conditions. Information flow in pain processing is not a simple matter of moving inputs through a set of passive modules. Just about everything appears to influence everything else.

Second, imaging studies of pain tell us that individual variation is as important as commonalities across subjects. How pain affects individuals varies significantly, and we put ourselves at a theoretical disadvantage if we do not take those differences as important data to be explained. As a result, imaging studies of pain, especially those of abnormal pain responses, have shifted explanatory emphases away from larger generalizations and toward specific details. Focusing on individuals and individual cases of pain also help diminish some of the methodological difficulties with imaging studies mentioned earlier.

This renewed focus on details entails that "theories" in neuroscience will not look like those in the physical sciences, where the focus is on generalizations that are applicable across many different sets of circumstances. Neuroscience, instead, must put its focus in describing how differences in anatomy and physiology result in differences in cognition and experience. Although a larger theoretical framework that is common across individual variation should remain as important scaffolding to support explanations of individuals, it will not drive explanation and investigation the same way it does in other sciences.

Finally, imaging studies of pain are shifting the definitions of pain itself. The IASP definition of pain as being "always subjective . . . always a psychological state" claims that we should identify pain by what people report and not by any physical condition they have. If someone claims to be in pain, then that person is in pain, regardless of how the nociceptors or the brain is activated.

In contrast, in 2004, the National Research Council of Canada, Institute for Biodiagnostics, indicated that its ultimate goal in supporting imaging studies of pain process "is to develop a clinical MR tool that will allow a clinician to assess . . . whether or not a patient is truly experiencing pain (either intermittent acute or chronic)."

Pain has switched from being purely subjective to something purely physical. This agency suggests that ideally, we should determine whether people are in pain by what is happening in their brains and not by what they claim to be experiencing.

This change in approach represents a complete transformation in how we are to think about pain and is a change due largely or solely in part to advances in imaging technology. We have gone from a purely mentalistic description of pain (pain is a sensation) to one that is purely physical (pain is brain activity). This change obviously should have enormous implications for how pain patients are evaluated and treated, for saying that you feel pain and acting as though you are in pain would no longer be sufficient for getting treated.

It also has large implications for philosophy. Historically, philosophers have long believed that there is no appearance-reality distinction relative to pain. Pain just is the experience of pain—the appearance of pain is its reality. (In contrast, a red apple is not the same thing as our experience of a red apple—the appearance of the apple is not the same thing as its reality.) As Saul Kripke reminds us:

> To be in the same epistemic situation that would obtain if one had a pain *is* to have a pain; to be in the same epistemic situation that would obtain in the absence of pain *is* not to have a pain. . . . [Pain] is not picked out by one of its accidental properties; rather, it is picked out by its immediate phenomenological quality. . . . If any phenomenon is picked out in exactly the same way as we pick out pain, then that phenomenon *is* pain. (1980, pp. 152–153)

To define pain in terms of brain activity, and not in terms of phenomenological feel, flies in the face of decades of philosophical tradition and argumentation. We leave it for another day to discuss whether discontinuing this philosophical tradition and making pain into a brain response are wise decisions. We can say that they will likely be disruptive.

Let us return now to our original question of whether fMRI is neuroscience's answer to the philosopher's desire for a cerebrascope. On one hand, limitations in MRI's ability to record in the time scale of neural activity preclude it from being a true recorder of cognitive processes in the brain. On the other hand, it does give us a way to watch some brain activity, as the philosophers dreamed. What we find most telling is how the promise of imaging pain is shifting the way clinicians and regulatory and funding agencies think about pain itself. This tool has changed how pain is understood and approached. Being able to image pain in almost–real time means, for the neuroscientists at least, that we can indeed look at cognition by looking at brain activity. They appear to believe that the age of the cerebrascope has arrived.

NOTE

1. Linus Pauling and Charles D. Coryll, then both at the California Institute of Technology, first described the magnetic properties of hemoglobin in an article published in 1936. They noted that the magnetic susceptibility of fully oxygenated arterial blood

differed by as much as 20 percent from that of fully deoxygenated venous blood. However, the breakthrough that led to fMRI had to wait until the early 1980s, when George Radda, at the University of Oxford, discovered that MRI could register changes in the level of oxygen in the blood, which in turn could be used to track physiological activity. Then in 1990, Seiji Ogawa, working at AT&T's Bell Laboratories using live animals, reported that, when placed in a magnetic field, deoxygenated hemoglobin would increase the strength of the field in its vicinity, whereas oxygenated hemoglobin would not. Ogawa demonstrated that a region containing a lot of deoxygenated hemoglobin will slightly distort the magnetic field surrounding the blood vessel and that a magnetic resonance image can record this distortion.

REFERENCES

Alkire, M. T., White, N. S., Hsieh, R., and Haier, R. J. (2004). Dissociable brain activation responses to 5-Hz electrical pain stimulation: A high-field functional magnetic imaging study. *Anesthesiology* 100: 939–946.

Apkarian, A. V. (1995) Functional imaging of pain, new insights regarding the role of the cerebral cortex in human pain perception. *Seminars in the Neurosciences* 7: 279–293.

Bandura, A., O'Leary, A., Taylor, C. B., Gauthier, J., and Gossard, D. (1987). Perceived self-efficacy and pain control: Opioid and nonopioid mechanisms. *Journal of Personal and Social Psychology* 53: 563–571.

Bantick, S. J., Wise, R. G., Ploghaus, A., Clare, S., Smith, P., and Tracey, I. (2002). Imagining how attention modulates pain in humans using functional MRI. *Brain* 125: 310–319.

Baron, R., Baron, Y., Disbrow, E., and Roberts, T. P. (1999). Brain processing of capsaicin-induced secondary hyperalgesia: A functional MRI study. *Neurology* 53: 548–557.

Buchel, C., Bornhovd, K., Quante, M., Glauche, V., Bromm, B., and Weller, C. (2002). Dissociable neural responses related to pain intensity, stimulus intensity, and stimulus awareness within the anterior cingulated cortex: A parametric single-trial laser functional magnetic resonance imaging study. *Journal of Neuroscience* 22: 970–976.

Bushnell, M. C., Duncan, G. H., Hofbauer, R. K., Ha, B., Chen, J. I., and Carrier, B. (1999). Pain perception: Is there a role for primary sensory cortex? *Proceedings of the National Academy of Science USA* 96: 7705–7709.

Canavaro, S. (1994) Dynamic reverberation, a unified mechanism for central and phantom pain. *Medical Hypotheses* 42: 203–207.

Carlsson, K., Petrovic, P., Skare, S., Petersson, K. M., and Ingvar, M. (2000. Tickling expectations: Neural processing in anticipation of a sensory stimulus. *Journal of Cognitive Neuroscience* 12: 691–703.

Casey, K. L. (1999). Forebrain mechanisms of nociception and pain: Analysis through imagining. *Proceedings of the National Academy of Science USA* 96: 7668–7674.

Chen, J. I., Ha, B., Bushnell, M. C., Pike, B., and Duncan, G. H. (2002). Differentiating noxious- and innocuous-related activation of human sensory cortices using temporal analysis of FMRI. *Journal of Neurophysiology* 88: 464–474.

Coghill, R. C., Talbot, J. D., Evans, A. C., Meyer, E., Gjedde, A., Bushnell, M. C., et al. (1994). Distributed processing of pain and vibration by the human brain. *Journal of Neuroscience* 14: 4095–4108.

Coghill, R. C., Sang, C. N., Maisog, J. M., and Iadarola, M. J. (1999). Pain intensity processing within the human brain: A bilateral, distributed mechanism. *Journal of Neurophysiology* 82: 1934–1943.

Cook, D. B., Lange, G., Ciccone, D. S., Liu, W. C, Steffener, J., and Natelson, B. H. (2004). Functional imagining of pain in patients with primary fibromyalgia. *Journal of Rheumatology* 2: 364–378.

Craig, A. D., Bushnell, M. C., Zhang, E.-T., and Blomqvist, A. (1994). A thalamic nucleus specific for pain and temperature sensation. *Nature* 372: 770–773.

Davis, K. D. (2000). The neural circuitry of pain as explored with functional MRI. *Neurology Research* 22: 313–317.

Davis, K. D., Tasker, R. R., Kiss, Z. H. T., Hutchison, W. D., and Dostrovsky, J. O. (1995). Visceral pain evoked by thalamic microstimulation in humans. *Neuroreport* 6: 369–374.

DeTommaso, M., Valeriani, M., Guido, M., Libro, G., Specchio, L. M., Tonali, P., et al. (2003). Abnormal brain processing of cutaneous pain in patients with chronic migraine. *Pain* 101: 25–32.

Disbrow, E., Buonocore, M., Antognini, J., Carstens, E., and Rowley, H. A. (1998). Sensory cortex: A comparison of the response to noxious thermal, mechanical, and electrical stimuli using functional magnetic resonance imagining. *Human Brain Mapping* 6: 150–159.

Dowman, R. (2001). Attentional set effects on spinal and supraspinal spinal responses to pain. *Psychophysiology* 38: 451–464.

Downar, J., Mikulis, D. J., and Davis, D. K. (2003). Neural correlates of the prolonged salience of painful stimulation. *Neuroimage* 20: 1540–1551.

Evans, F. J. (1974) The placebo response in pain reduction. In J. J. Bonica (Ed.), *International Symposium on Pain, Advances in Neurology*, vol. 4. New York: Raven Press, 289–296.

Faymoville, M. E., Laureys, S., Degueldre, C., DelFiore, G., Luxen, A., Frannck, G., et al. (2000). Neural mechanisms of antinociceptive effects of hypnosis. *Anesthesiology* 92: 1257–1267.

Frankenstein, U. N., Richter, W., McIntyre, M. C., and Rémy, F. (2001). Distraction modulates anterior cingulate gyrus activations during the cold pressor test. *Neuroimage* 14: 827–836.

Hirato, M., Watanabe, K., Takahashi, A., Hayase, N., Horikoshi, S., Shibaskaki, T., et al. (1994). Pathophysiology of central (thalamic) pain: combined change of sensory thalamus with cerebral cortex around central sulcus. *Stereotactic and Functional Neurosurgery* 62: 300–303.

Head, H., and Holmes, G. (1911) Sensory disturbances from cerebral lesions. *Brain* 34: 102–254.

International Association for the Study of Pain (IASP) Subcommittee on Classification. (1986). Pain terms, a current list with definitions and notes on usage. *Pain* 3 (supplement): 216–221.

Keay, K. A., Clement, C. I., Owler, B., Depaulis, A., and Bandelr, R. (1994). Convergence of deep somatic and visceral nociceptive-information onto a discrete ventrolateral midbrain periaqueductal gray region. *Neuroscience* 61: 727–732.

Kripke, S. (1980). *Naming and Necessity*. Cambridge, Mass.: Harvard University Press.

Kurata, J., Thulborn, K. R., Gyulai, F. E., and Firestone, L. L. (2002). Early decay of pain-related cerebral activation in functional magnetic resonance imaging: Comparison with visual and motor tasks. *Anesthesiology* 96: 35–44.

Longe, S. E., Wise, R., Bantik, S., Lloyd, D., Johansen-Berg, H., McGlone, F., et al. (2001). Counter-stimulatory effects on pain perception and processing are significantly altered by attention: An fMRI study. *Neuroreport* 12: 2021–2025.

Melzack, R. (1990) Phantom limbs and the concept of a neuromatrix. *Trends in Neuroscience* 13: 88–92.

Melzack, R. (1991) Central pain syndromes and theories of pain. In E. L. Casey (Ed.), *Pain and Central Nervous Disease, The Central Pain Syndromes*. New York: Raven Press, 59–64.

Melzack, R. (1992) Phantom limbs. *Scientific American* 266: 90–96.

Melzack, R., Wall, P. D., and Ty, T. C. (1982) Acute pain in an emergency clinic, latency of onset and descriptor patterns related to different injuries. *Pain* 14: 33–43.

Miron, D., Duncan, G. H., and Bushnell, M. C. (1989). Effects of attention on the intensity and unpleasantness of thermal pain. *Pain* 39: 345–352.

National Research Council of Canada. (2004). Institute for Biodiagnostics. Available at: ibd.nrc-cnrc.gc.ca/main_e.html.

Peyron, R., Garcia-Larrea, L., Gregoire, M. C., Convers, P., Lavenne, F., Veyre, L., et al. (1998). Allodynia after lateral-medullary (Wallenberg) infarct. A PET study. *Brain* 121: 345–356.

Peyron, R., Garcia-Larrea, L. Gregoire, M. C., Costes, N., Convers, P., Lavenne, F., et al. (1999). Haemodynamic brain responses to acute pain in humans: Sensory and attentional networks. *Brain* 9: 1765–1780.

Peyron, R., Laurent, B., and Garcia-Larrea, L. (2000). Functional imaging of brain responses to pain. A review and meta-analysis. *Neurophysiological Clinic* 30: 263–288.

Phillips, M. L., Gregory, L. J., Cullen, S., Coen, S., Ng, V., Andrew, C., Giampietro, V., et al. (2003). The effect of negative emotional context on neural and behavioral responses to oesophageal stimulation. *Brain* 126: 669–684.

Ploner, M., Schmitz, F., Freund, H. J., and Schnitzler, A. (1999). Parallel activation of primary and secondary sensory cortices in human pain processing. *Journal of Neurophysiology* 81: 3100–3104.

Porro, C. A., Baraldi, P., Pagnoni, G., Serafini, M., Facchin, P., Maieron, M., et al. (2002). Does anticipation of pain affect cortical nociceptive systems? *Journal of Neuroscience* 22: 3206–3214.

Price, D. D. (2000). Psychological and neural mechanisms of the affective dimension of pain. *Science* 288: 1769–1772.

Ringler, R., Greiner, M., Kohlloeffel, L., Hnadwerker, H. O., and Forster, C. (2003). BOLD effects in different areas of the cerebral cortex during painful mechanical stimulation. *Pain* 105: 445–453.

Salomons, T. V., Johnstone, T., Backonja, N. M., and Davidson, R. J. (2004). Perceived controllability modulates the neural response to pain. *Journal of Neuroscience* 32: 7199–7203.

Sawamoto, N., Honda, M., Okada, T., Hanakawa, T., Kanda, M., Fukuyama, H., et al. (2000). Expectation of pain enhances responses to nonpainful sensory stimulation in the anterior cingulated cortex and parietal operculum/posterior insula: An event-related functional magnetic resonance imagine study. *Journal of Neuroscience* 20: 7438–7445.

Schnitzler, A., and Ploner, M. (2000). Neurophysiology and functional neuroanatomy of pain perception. *Journal of Clinical Neurophysiology* 17: 592–603.

Timmermann, L., Ploner, M., Haucke, K., Schmitz, F., Baltissen, R., and Schnitzler, A. (2001). Differential coding of pain intensity in human primary and secondary sensory cortex. *Journal of Neurophysiology* 86: 1499–1503.

Tracey, I., Ploghaus, A., Gati, J. S., Clare, S., Smith, S., Menon, R. S., et al. (2002). Imaging attentional modulation of pain in the periaqueductal gray in humans. *Journal of Neuroscience* 22: 2748–2752.

Treede, R. D., Kenshalo, D. R., Gracely, R. H., and Jones, A. K. (1999). The cortical representation of pain. *Pain* 79: 105–111.

Treede, R. D., Apkarian, A. V., Bromm, B., Greenspan, J. D., and Lenz, F. A. (2000). Cortical representation of pain: Functional characterization of nociceptive areas near the lateral sulcus. *Pain* 87: 113–119.

Verne, G. N., Himes, N. C., Robinson, E., Gopinath, K. S., Briggs, R. W., Crosson, B., et al. (2003). Central representation of visceral and cutaneous hypersensitivity in the irritable bowel syndrome. *Pain* 103: 99–110.

Wall, P. D. (1989). The dorsal horn. In P. D. Wall and R. Melzack (Eds.), *Textbook of Pain*. New York: Churchill Livingstone, 102–111.

Wall, P. D., and McMahon, S. B. (1985) Microneuronography and its relation to perceived sensation. *Pain* 21: 209–229.

Wiech, K., Preissl, H., and Birbaumer, N. (2001). Neural networks and pain processing: New insights from imaging techniques. *Anaesthesist* 50: 2–12.

CHAPTER 9

THE EMBEDDED NEURON, THE ENACTIVE FIELD?

MAZVIITA CHIRIMUUTA AND IAN GOLD

1. INTRODUCTION

One role for the philosopher of neuroscience is to examine issues raised by the central concepts of neuroscience (Gold and Roskies, in press), just as philosophy of biology does for biology and philosophy of physics for physics. In this chapter, we make an attempt to explore one issue around the concept of the *receptive field* (RF) of visual neurons. Fundamentally, the RF of a neuron represents "how a cell responds when a point of light falls in a position of space (or time)" (Rapela, Mendel, and Grzywacz, 2006, p. 464). It also describes the kind of stimulus that activates a neuron—a moving bar, a red patch, or whatever. The phrase "receptive field" was coined by American neurophysiologist and Nobel laureate Haldan K. Hartline (1903–1983), in 1938 (Hartline, 1938); Barlow (1953; see Lettvin, Maturana, McCulloch, and Pitts, 1968) and, in particular, Hubel and Weisel (e.g., Hubel and Wiesel, 1959) developed the concept; and it has become the central way of characterizing neurons in the visual system and elsewhere. Currently, as Rapela et al. (2006, p. 464) say, "receptive fields are the main theoretical framework to represent functional properties of visual cells."

However, recent findings in the neurophysiology of neurons in primary visual cortex (V1) are at odds with the "classical" conception of the RF (Albright and Stoner, 2002), and it is possible that the concept of the visual RF is in transition. Our aim here, therefore, is to examine the concept of the RF and explore the possible consequences of these data for neurophysiology and computational vision. We are not concerned with arguing for a particular view about the status of the concept but rather beginning to articulate some of the options. We make some anodyne remarks at the end of the chapter about which of the options we think are most promising, but our purpose here is merely to contribute to the beginning of a discussion about the issues.

We introduce the concept of visual RFs by discussing the classical picture of V1 physiology, most associated with the work of Hubel and Wiesel (section 2). We then turn to the psychophysics and computational vision of contrast discrimination to place the visual neurophysiology in context (section 3). We then review the recent data that have raised questions about the classical conception of the RF (section 4). We turn to consider some of the options available for absorbing the data into visual theory (section 5). We conclude with some remarks on the relevance of these data for thinking about the role of the environment in visual theory (section 6).

2. THE CLASSICAL RECEPTIVE FIELD

The simplest picture or model of visual processing is of a one-way flow of information from the photoreceptors of the eye, via successively more complex information transformations in the retina, thalamus, and the visual cortex, toward integration with other functions in the higher cortical areas. Most likely owing to its simplicity, it has long been the picture most appealing to scientists confronted with the daunting complexity of the visual brain. Indeed, this "bottom-up" picture has held sway even though neuroanatomy has shown, for example, that "top-down" neuronal connections from visual cortex to the thalamus outnumber bottom-up connections from the retina (see Sherman and Guillery, 2002). The hierarchical scheme is illustrated in figure 9.1a, which shows the key anatomical loci of the human visual system up to and including primary visual cortex. These brain structures are shared by higher mammals, and for this reason studies on cat, ferret, and other mammals aside from primates have been considered important steps toward an understanding human vision.

Figure 9.1, b and c, illustrates Hubel and Wiesel's famous hierarchical model of RFs in primary visual cortex, where the elongated RFs of V1 simple and complex cells are taken to be the result of the arrangement of cells lower down in the visual pathway that synapse onto them. The modern era of study of the RF begins with the work of Hubel and Wiesel, and we will, for the purposes of this chapter, take theirs to be the standard conception of the RF. However, we note that the work of many other scientists is of equal importance. In particular, Hubel and Wiesel's studies were of a largely qualitative nature, so almost all quantitative measurement understanding of RF properties is due to the efforts of other laboratories.

Much of the basic understanding of the visual neurons that inspired the traditional picture came from extracellular electrode recordings in the cat. In such experiments, various stimuli would be presented to the eyes of anaesthetized animals

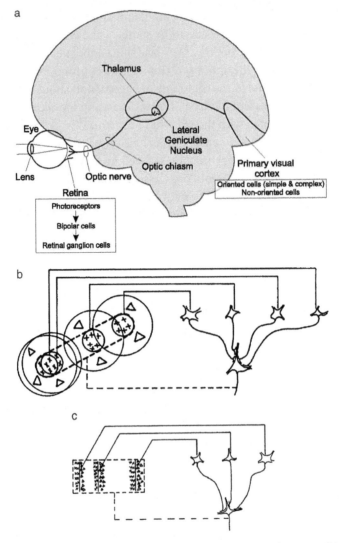

Figure 9.1. (a) The main structures of the early mammalian visual system. (b) From Hubel and Wiesel (1962), the explanation of simple cell elongated receptive fields in terms of the rectangular arrangement of LGN input cells which have circular RFs (left). (c) From Hubel and Wiesel (1962), complex cells were classified as having responses indifferent to the phase (black or white polarity) of the stimulus. This property was explained by their having simple cell inputs with various phase tunings (left).

while electrodes measured neuronal responses in the cortex in terms of spikes per second. A crucial finding of Hubel and Wiesel (1959) was that neurons in the cat visual cortex respond well to moving or flashing bars of a particular orientation, width, and location (see Hubel and Wiesel, 1998, for a historical overview of their work, including the "accidental" discovery of elongated RFs). This suggested that in contrast to the neurons of the retina and lateral geniculate nucleus (LGN) which had been found to have circular RFs (Kuffler, 1953), V1 RFs were elongated and orientation specific. Hubel and Wiesel mapped these RFs by flashing small spots of light in the visual field. As in earlier studies, any area in space in which flashing a light elicited an increase in neuronal firing rate was defined as part of the ON portion of the RF, and any adjacent area in which a black spot (i.e., a decrease in luminance relative to the background) elicited firing was taken to constitute part of the OFF area. Figure 9.2a illustrates a receptive field mapped in this way by Hubel and Wiesel (1959). Hubel and Wiesel (1962) also made a distinction between *simple* and *complex* cells, the first type apparently exhibiting *predictable linear spatial summation* and the second type not. In effect, only simple cell RFs had clearly defined ON and OFF regions and could be mapped with localized spots of light.[1]

In contrast, complex cells showed unpredictable *nonlinear* spatial summation and were indifferent to the phase of a bar or grating stimulus (see figure 9.3). In the absence of defined ON and OFF regions, the complex cell response would be the same whatever the precise position of the white and dark portions of the stimulus with respect to the RF. These findings motivated the hierarchical model represented

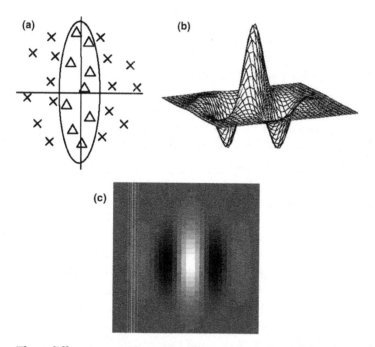

Figure 9.2. Three different sorts of receptive field maps of a V1 simple cell. (a) A qualitative map of the type used by Hubel and Wiesel (1959). Triangles and crosses represent ON and OFF regions, respectively. (b) A quantitative map, as used by Jones, Stepnowski, and Palmer (1987). The height of the surface at each point is proportional to the strength of the cell's response to stimulation at that point, with positive values indicating ON responses and negative values indicating OFF responses. (c) A quantitative map of the type used by De Angelis, Ohzawa, and Freeman (1993). The brightness at each point is proportional to the strength of the cell's response at that point; mid-gray indicates zero response, brighter shades indicate ON responses, and darker shades indicate OFF responses.

b

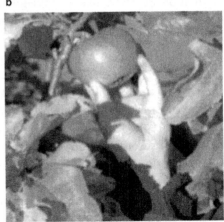

a

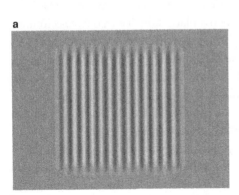

Figure 9.3. Examples of images used as stimuli in neurophysiological and psychophysical experiments. (a) A standard sinusoidal grating. In neurophysiological work gratings are normally presented "drifting" across the phase of the sinusoid, rather than static. (b) Natural image.

in figure 9.1b. An obvious explanation for the structure of the simple cell RF is that a small number of LGN cells whose RFs occur in a row in visual space all synapse onto one simple cell. Likewise, an obvious explanation for phase invariance of the complex cells is that these neurons receive input from a small number of simple cells whose RFs overlap but are of different ON-OFF polarity in space.

Other researchers went on to make more detailed studies of simple and complex cells to quantify, for example, the linearity of spatial summation. These studies often used sinusoidal grating stimuli rather than spots of light or bars (see figure 9.3a). One important reason for using sinusoids was that physiologists were engaged in performing a *systems analysis* of primary visual cortex (see Albrecht, Geisler, and Crane, 2003). On the assumption that V1 neurons are linear analyzers, these methods, borrowed from the physical sciences and engineering, show how the response of such linear neurons to sinusoids can then be used to predict the responses to any image. Recordings were made both in the cat (see, e.g., Henry, 1977; Jones and Palmer, 1987; Jones, Stepnowski, and Palmer, 1987; Li, Peterson, and Freeman, 2003; Movshon, Thompson, and Tolhurst, 1978a, 1978b, 1978c) and monkey (e.g., Hawken and Parker, 1987; Hubel and Wiesel, 1968; Parker and Hawken, 1988; Ringach, 2002). Figure 9.2, b and c, shows further examples of simple cell receptive field maps, similar to those presented by Jones et al. (1987) and De Angelis, Ohzawa, and Freeman (1993), respectively. These studies revealed properties of V1 neurons that significantly challenge the classical picture. Indeed, Hubel and Wiesel's original hierarchical model was soon found to be inconsistent with quantitative measurement of simple and complex cell responses implicating some role for top-down or lateral connections in shaping RF properties. Discussion of these later studies, and the extent to which they undermine the classical conception of the RF, is the subject of sections 4 and 5. In the next section we examine the influence of the classical conception in the other disciplines of visual neuroscience, notably psychophysics and computation.

3. Psychophysics, Computational Modeling, and the Classical RF

3.1. Psychophysics

Psychophysics is a subdiscipline of visual neuroscience in which detailed, quantitative measurements are made of assumed basic visual responses or percepts. For example, classic psychophysical studies measured absolute detection thresholds for dim spots of light, and also for sinusoidal gratings of different spatial frequencies. Historically, much research on the physiology of vision has been motivated by psychophysical findings.[2] A major subject of psychophysical investigation has been the supposed properties of *spatial frequency* and *orientation channels* (Blakemore and Campbell, 1969; Campbell and Robson, 1968). A corresponding target for physiologists has been to find a neural explanation for these results (e.g., Campbell, Cooper, and Enroth-Cugell, 1969; Maffei and Fiorentini, 1973). The idea of a channel is basically that of a spatial frequency or orientation selective filter (Braddick, Campbell, and Atkinson, 1978; Graham, 1989), such a filter being the result of the operation of one or more structures in the visual system. Just as any continuous, intensity-varying signal, such as a sound wave, can be described as a set of sinusoidal Fourier components of different amplitudes, frequencies, and phases with respect to one another, any visual image can be analyzed as a two-dimensional Fourier transform (Robson, 1980; Westheimer, 2001). The channel theory of vision was therefore the working hypothesis that the visual system itself breaks down images roughly into its Fourier components, by way of its channels, and that for each channel, there is a sinusoidal stimulus of a particular spatial frequency and orientation to which the channel gives its optimal response (Campbell and Robson, 1968).

On Hubel and Wiesel's description of visual cortex, neuronal response properties are fixed and dependent solely on the response properties of the upstream neurons, which provide their input. A number of authors (e.g., Blakemore and Campbell, 1969; Campbell et al., 1969; Maffei and Fiorentini, 1973) were therefore prompted to equate these cortical properties with the properties of the psychophysical channels. However, as Marr and Hildreth (1980) pointed out, these physiological and psychophysical theories of cortical processing are rather different in that the psychophysical channels are said to perform something akin to a Fourier transform of the visual image, which is a *nonlocal* analysis of frequency; the simple cells of Hubel and Wiesel, on the other hand, operate as detectors of *localized* contrast features, such as edges. Still, the channel hypothesis is now established, in so far as it is generally accepted that the key mechanisms in the visual system revealed by psychophysics are spatial frequency and orientation selective, rather than broad-band (Majaj, Pelli, Kurshan, and Palomares, 2002).

At the same time, channel models have evolved. Originally, it was not thought that the response of one channel should alter the output of another channel (but see Tolhurst, 1972). But in response to more recent neurophysiological work (see section 4.1) and to better account for psychophysical data, some psychophysicists have rejected the *independent*-channels hypothesis, developing models in which channels are dynamically effected by the responses of other channels (e.g., Foley, 1994). The convergence of psychophysics and neurophysiology has also been given a helping hand in recent years with the advancement of scanning techniques. In particular, with functional magnetic resonance imaging (fMRI), it is possible for experimenters to track areas of increased neural activity while observers perform traditional psychophysical tasks. Boynton, Demb, Glover, and Heeger (1999) argue that observers' contrast discrimination functions (detection of an increase in grating contrast as a function of background contrast) can be predicted by fMRI signals in V1 and V2, implicating these areas as critical for setting thresholds in this task. This result gave new support to psychophysicists' attempts to account for their data in terms of V1 physiology (Chirimuuta and Tolhurst, 2005; Foley, 1994).

3.2. Computational Models of V1 RFs

As noted in section 2, Hubel and Wiesel's work was largely qualitative, but scientists following them aimed to get a mathematically precise grasp of V1 physiology. A powerful tool here was the computational modeling of RFs. A computational model of an RF is supposed to capture the key functional properties of the RF, such that it can be used to predict how a neuron will respond to any hypothetical stimulus. With the intense research on V1 following Hubel and Wiesel, there soon grew to be a large body of data on response properties, and some of these data sets gave conflicting evidence on key questions, such as whether there really are two classes of simple and complex cells. One way of usefully integrating this large amount of data was to develop computational models of cortical receptive fields and measure the goodness of fit with the data: If the fit is good, it may be inferred that the mathematical principle operational in the model (e.g., linear vs. nonlinear contrast response) captures the key properties of the neuron.

A large number of simple cell models have been developed since the 1980s. One that has achieved notable popularity is the Gabor model. The Gabor function is the product of a sinusoid and a Gaussian envelope, giving a localized sinusoidal modulation. The one-dimensional Gabor function was first developed by Dennis Gabor (1946) for use in communications engineering, and it is a particularly useful coding function because it minimizes joint uncertainty about time and temporal frequency (Gabor-Heisenberg-Weyl uncertainty). In the case of visual analysis, the function minimizes joint uncertainty about location and spatial frequency, enabling one to perform local Fourier analysis (see section 3.1). The function was introduced to vision science by Marcelja (1980).

With the Gabor model comes the implication that simple cells are essentially linear fixed filters whose job it is to analyze any given visual scene into simple bar- or blob-like components. Thus, the Gabor model shares a common fate with a particular conception of the RF. Over the past two decades, the appropriateness of the Gabor as a model for V1 neurons has been researched intensively, and given the significant nonlinearities reported, it seems a fair summary of the findings to say that the Gabor model can account for roughly half of the response behavior of simple cells in anaesthetized animals (Tolhurst, personal communication; see Carandini et al., 2005, for a recent assessment of the standard RF models). In section 4 we discuss some of these reported nonlinearities, and in section 5 we discuss neuroscientists' responses to the reported discrepancies between the data and the linear model.

3.3. Computer Vision

The field of computer vision, as opposed to the development of computational techniques in neurophysiology, attempts to reproduce useful visual function in computers or robots. Perhaps the most influential figure in computer vision is David Marr. His project was to develop mechanisms that were equivalent to the biological ones and could operate in artificial systems (Marr, 1982). Crucial to his methodology was the distinction between *algorithm* and *implementation*, or "software" and "hardware." This distinction allowed him to argue that a process in the visual system, for example, making a selective response to vertical edges, could be exactly equivalent to a computational process such as convolution with vertical filters, even though the processes are realized in very different physical substrates. Marr hoped to find algorithms that could carry out processes useful to machine vision, such as edge extraction for the purpose of object recognition (Marr and Hildreth, 1980). Still, what is shared by computer vision and the computational modeling discussed in section 3.2 is the assumption that the processing that takes place in the visual system can also be implemented in a digital computer. Marr's work was not especially inspired by detailed physiology, but later researchers have taken this line further. For example, John Daugman's algorithm for iris scanning is a convergence of ideas from computer vision, statistics, V1 physiology, and computational modeling of V1 (see Daugman, 2003).

4. RECENT FINDINGS IN V1 PHYSIOLOGY

Hubel and Wiesel's conception of the RF is known as the classical RF because later investigation of V1 physiology revealed that a given neuron's response could be modified by stimulation of the neuron in visual field regions that would not in themselves elicit a response or by presentation of stimuli to which the neuron was apparently unresponsive. Such findings challenged the picture of the visual system as feedforward and hierarchical, with little or no modulation of responses due to interaction between neurons at the same level of the hierarchy or from higher levels. Another assumption of the classical picture was that RFs are fixed properties of neurons. This has also been challenged by recent work. This section reviews some key findings in the extensive literature on the visual cortex.

In passing, it is worth asking to what extent these discoveries have been made possible with new techniques unavailable in the 1950s and 1960s. For example, the advent of intracellular recording allowed researchers to record directly inhibitory input to V1 neurons, now taken to be a critical factor behind RF tuning properties. It has also been argued that recordings from awake-behaving animals have revealed nonlinearities not apparent in the traditional anesthetized preparation (Lamme, 2004). On the other hand, it is worth considering the idea that complex nonlinear behavior is receiving more attention now because scientists' conception of V1 function and RFs has altered, making more salient complex behaviors which might previously have been put down to noise in the system (see section 4.4).

4.1. Inhibitory Networks and Surround Effects in V1

Later neurophysiological investigation did not bear out the conjecture of Hubel and Wiesel's (1962) hierarchical model, according to which response properties of cortical neurons can be explained in terms of summation of upstream neurons that have simpler RFs. For example, the intracellular recordings of Hirsch, Alonso, Reid, and Martinez (1998) found that cortical neurons receive a significant amount of inhibitory and excitatory input from within the cortex, as well as the excitatory geniculate input mentioned by the hierarchical model. Furthermore, computational studies (Lauritzen, Krukowski, and Miller, 2001; Troyer, Krukowski, Priebe, and Miller, 1998; Wielaard, Shelley, McLaughlin, and Shapley, 2001) have shown that the inhibitory input is necessary for keeping tuning bandwidth invariant with stimulus contrast, as is approximately the case in V1 (Sclar and Freeman, 1982; Skottun, Bradley, Sclar, Ohzawa, and Freeman, 1987).

It follows from these findings that cortical response properties cannot be independent of the activity of neighboring neurons (Blakemore and Tobin, 1972). An important example is the work of Bonds (1989), which showed that simultaneous stimulation with an optimal stimulus and a superimposed mask at a different orientation or spatial frequency will cause the neuron's responses to drop below its response level to the optimal stimulus alone. Because the neuron is not thought to be directly (i.e., by way of excitatory geniculate input) affected by the mask to which it is poorly tuned, the implication is that the neuron is receiving inhibition from neurons that *do* respond to the mask.

Another line of research which has challenged the "discrete" receptive fields picture is the investigation of the effects of stimulating beyond the spatial extent of the classical RF. Hubel and Wiesel (1962) defined the RF as the area over which a neuron responds to small spots of light.[3] However, it has been shown that V1 neurons often produce a greater response if a stimulus is extended beyond this area, even if stimulation in this area alone is not able to drive the neuron. The maximum extent of the area that causes progressive excitation is known as the summation field. Stimulation beyond the summation field often causes a decline in response, and the area over which one observes this inhibition is known as the suppressive surround. Examples of different surround effects can be found in the work of, among others, Blakemore and Tobin (1972), Maffei and Fiorentini (1976), Nelson and Frost (1978), Gilbert and Wiesel (1990), De Angelis, Freeman, and Ohzawa (1994), Jones, Grieve, Wang, and Sillito (2001), Cavanaugh, Bair, and Movshon (2002a, 2002b), and Levitt and Lund (2002); see Albright and Stoner (2002) and Tucker and Fitzpatrick (2003) for reviews.

The existence of a suppressive surround means that neurons are affected by parts of the image adjacent to their receptive fields, and so, in an ecological context where there will be complex image structure around the RF (rather than blank gray screen), it will be difficult to predict the responses to any particular stimulus. There has been much speculation over the purpose of the surround in ecological vision. Marcus and van Essen (2002) suggest that the surround may aid scene segmentation in primate V1 and V2; similarly, Li and Gilbert (2002) and Sugita (1999) suggest a role in contour integration and grouping problems (see Lamme, 2004, for a review). Following such results, another new concept that has been added to that of the RF is that of the association field (Kapadia, Westheimer, and Gilbert, 2000). It was a term first introduced in psychophysics (Field, Hayes, and Hess, 1993), but in neurophysiology the association field maps the amount of modulation invoked by different stimuli surrounding an optimal stimulus for any given RF.

To conclude this subsection, we note that the finding of the interdependence of neurons' RF properties raises questions about what level of analysis—single neuron or population—is best for experimental work in the visual cortex, an issue we raise again in section 5.

4.2. The Dynamic RF

As already noted, the traditional concept of a RF is of a fixed filter—that is, of a unit that signals the presence of its preferred stimulus, its preference unaffected by recent history of stimulation or by the activity of other units. This notion is tied up with the idea that visual neurons represent the features to which they are responsive, or that they perform pattern recognition (Craik, 1966). The physiological findings we review in this section cast doubt on the assumption that RF properties are fixed. As Tucker and Fitzpatrick (2003) recently put it, "the cortical RF has become a dynamic entity, one in which context and history play significant roles in shaping its boundaries and altering its properties."

We begin a discussion of this literature with one of the most robust reports on how RF size is readily modified by stimulus contrast. A number of different research groups reported at around the same time that the RF is found to be larger if the neuron is stimulated with low-contrast gratings (Kapadia, Westheimer, and Gilbert, 1999; Levitt and Lund, 1997; Polat, Mizobe, Pettet, Kasamatsu, and Norcia, 1998; Sceniak, Ringach, Hawken, and Shapley, 1999). Explanations for this phenomenon suggest that it is a means of increasing sensitivity at low contrasts, analogous to the way photoreceptors and other cells in the retina show increased pooling of signals between neighboring neurons in dim light conditions. The conceptual interest of this result is simply that it means one cannot speak of an RF as having a fixed size; size must always be given relative to the contrast at which the neurons was tested, and this complicates the traditional model of the RF.

A comparable result to this is the finding that RF size is also dependent on the neuron's recent history of stimulation. "Artificial scotoma" is the term given to a blank stimulus presented in the RF center that suppresses response activity. Gilbert and Wiesel (1992), Kapadia, Gilbert, and Westheimer (1994), and Pettet and Gilbert (1992) have shown that presentation of an artificial scotoma for a number of minutes causes the RF of cortical neurons to grow to several times their original size. The effect is reversible by subsequent presentation of stimuli to which the neuron is responsive and is thought to be mediated by horizontal connections between neurons in the same cortical layer (Tucker and Fitzpatrick, 2003). Indeed, fast plasticity of horizontal connections and of top-down connections from higher cortical areas are commonly put forward as the physiological explanation of RF dynamism and of the surround and cross stimulus effects already discussed, though the details of such mechanisms remain an area of contention.

One striking demonstration of the dynamism of visual neuronal properties can be seen in the work of Bair and Movshon (2004) on direction-selective (DS) neurons in V1 and motion area MT/V5 of the macaque monkey. Such neurons have been modeled extensively as linear filters that are oriented in space-time to give directional sensitivity, and in such models RFs are taken to be stable. However, these authors note many psychophysical reports showing that, at a perceptual level, the temporal profile of motion integration—the time course or pattern of motion analysis undertaken by the visual system—is variable with stimulus speed, spatial frequency, and contrast. So the aim of the investigation was to find out if this variability is a property that arises at a population level, while the profiles of individual neurons are fixed, or if the basis of the variability can be shown at the level of individual neurons whose RFs are dependent on stimulus properties.

Bair and Movshon showed convincingly that the latter is the case. For example, neurons extend their integration time (i.e., the time window in which a spiking response signifies the presence of a stimulus moving in the preferred direction) for slowly moving gratings. They call this adaptive temporal integration, because such a stimulus-dependent shift is advantageous, improving the signal-to-noise ratio of the response to slowly moving objects. They conclude that "it is possible that no single RF profile can be attributed to a cortical cell. This implies that models relying on a fixed filter to endow component neurons with their tuning properties could be highly inaccurate, in general" (p. 7320).

4.3. Natural Images

All of the studies mentioned so far have used artificial stimuli, but since the 1990s, studies using natural stimuli—photographs or video clips taken in the outside world—have become increasingly central to vision science (see figure 9.3b). The reason for this interest in natural stimuli is that the visual system evolved in the natural environment, and presumably many of its features are adaptations to the peculiarities of natural visual information. Of particular interest is the view that properties of simple cell RFs are special adaptations to the informational "redundancies" of natural images,[4] in that they minimize both the correlations between neurons' responses and level of activity of individual neurons; this is known as sparse coding (Baddeley and Hancock, 1991; Olshausen and Field, 1997; van Hateren and van der Schaaf, 1998; Vinje and Gallant, 2000; Willmore and Tolhurst, 2001).

A key question is whether the cortex shows radically different physiological properties under natural and artificial stimulation. Two studies (Ringach, Hawken, and Shapley, 2002; Smyth, Willmore, Baker, Thompson, and Tolhurst, 2003) have shown that RF maps generated from responses to natural images resemble the elongated, oriented fields derived from the classic grating experiments. In contrast, David, Vinje, and Gallant (2004) have made the case that RF models generated by stimulation with natural stimuli give significantly better predictions of responses to novel natural stimuli than do RF models generated by stimulation with gratings. Likewise, the predictions of responses to novel grating stimuli were superior if the RF model had been constructed from the correlations of responses to gratings. If V1 neurons were linear filters, this would not be the case; RF models would generalize between classes of stimuli. This stimulus-specificity of the RF points to a more dynamic notion of RF than was originally conceived.

4.4. Science and Simplicity

The introduction to this section raised the question of whether the increase in attention physiologists now give to the complex nonlinear properties of RFs can be put down to the advent of new techniques to reveal such properties, or if a changing conception of the RF has made such properties now more salient to scientists. The answer is probably both. Anecdotally, it is worth noting that Kuffler (1953) presented a messier picture of the responses of visual neurons than either Hartline before him or Hubel and Wiesel after him. In fact, his description of the physiology of the ganglion cells in the cat retina sounds more like the picture emerging from the recent results that we have discussed in this section. For example, he notes that these neurons' response patterns vary with overall illumination changes; that "the most outstanding feature in the present analysis is the flexibility and fluidity of the discharge patterns arising in each RF" (p. 61); and that "there seems to exist a very great variability between individual RFs and therefore a detailed classification cannot be made at present" (p. 62).

Thus, there may not be anything so new after all in the idea of the dynamic RF that has been presented as the result of novel findings. Aside from data made accessible by new technologies, such observations were available to physiologists in the early days of visual neuroscience. This is not to condemn the scientists who put forward the simpler picture of the RF, for it should be appreciated that the most promising route for any new science has always been to seek out any underlying simplicity in what appears to be a formidably complex and unpredictable object of investigation. Indeed, one wonders if work on the visual cortex would have expanded and flourished the way that it did had Hubel and Wiesel not presented such an attractively neat picture of its physiology. The challenge raised by the recent work discussed in this section is whether these simplifying assumptions ultimately defeated the aim of understanding V1 function by disregarding as noise the very neuronal properties that make our visual system work in the real world.

5. OPTIONS

In this section we consider a number of ways the stimulus-dependence data could be integrated into visual neuroscience and cognitive theory. Our aim is to map out some theoretical strategies rather than defend one in particular. It is premature to be defending one theoretical option when considerably more empirical work is necessary to confirm that the classical conception of the RF is in fact untenable. The job for the philosopher of neuroscience—at least at this stage—is to consider the pros and cons of various ideas as a way of beginning the debate. We consider five options, in order of increasing radicalness.

5.1. Option 1: Expanding the Classical RF

The data reviewed before show that the classical conception of the RF is no longer compelling, but that is not yet to say that the concept of the RF is dead. If the concept can be altered or expanded to accommodate the new data, this might be the most appropriate strategy to adopt. Because the concept of the RF has proven so useful up to now, it's better to stretch the concept than dispense with it. The central issue to be decided is whether the data would require us to stretch the concept to the point where it would no longer be recognizable. Can we revise the concept of the RF, or must we eliminate it?

Elegant and conservative extensions of the classical RF may be available. An example is David Heeger's normalization model of visual neurons. Heeger (1992) notes that the linear model of V1 fails to account for all of the physiological data. Rather than rejecting the linear model outright, Heeger's model includes divisive normalization. This is the idea that every neuron's response is divided by a term reflecting the combined activity of all of its neighbors. Thus, the local activity is accounted for in a model of the single neuron by means of an equation that summarizes the effects of the circuit, without specifically parametizing other neurons. The model does not include biological detail, though it has been noted that the division could be implemented in the brain by what is known as shunting inhibition (Carandini, Heeger, and Movshon, 1997; but see Carandini, Heeger, and Senn, 2002; Freeman, Durand, Kiper, and Carandini, 2002; Meier and Carandini, 2002). The normalization model preserves a linear conception of the RF and successfully predicts a good deal of neurophysiological data, including the shape of the contrast response curve, especially response saturation (Albrecht and Hamilton, 1982; Maffei and Fiorentini, 1973; Sclar, Maunsell, and Lennie, 1990), cross-orientation masking (Bonds, 1989), and surround suppression (reviewed in Fitzpatrick, 2000). Heeger's approach has been particularly influential in subsequent psychophysical models, an important example being Foley's (1994) model of contrast discrimination.

Despite the successes of Heeger's normalization model in accounting for a number of surround inhibition effects, it by no means assimilates all of the problematic findings discussed here. In particular, the normalization model cannot explain findings of surround enhancement (Gilbert and Wiesel, 1990; Maffei and Fiorentini, 1976), an effect equivalent to the presence of a summation field beyond the classical RF.

5.2. Option 2: Piecemeal Solutions

Option 1 does not tackle head-on the problem of stimulus dependence. It may be that a sophisticated extension of the classical RF model will eventually be able to predict that an individual neuron will demonstrate different response properties under natural as opposed to artificial stimulation or as a result of different surround input. On the other hand, no such "universal model" may be forthcoming. Even if the RF changes with categories of stimulus and with visual tasks, it is nonetheless possible to produce models for particular stimulus–task pairs or classes of pairs. One could give up on the idea of a single model of V1 suitable for all stimuli and visual tasks and focus attention on piecemeal solutions to visual problems. This option would allow one to preserve the procedure for modeling visual circuits by treating neurons as fixed (i.e., not stimulus-dependent) components, but the modeling would be relativized to stimulus class, visual task, or both.

This solution might be criticized as inelegant and ad hoc, but piecemeal solutions are, in a sense, the norm in visual neuroscience, where RF models are usually devised to account for specific data sets (a particular animal responding to a particular sort of stimulus). It is usually hoped that the model will generalize to novel data, but expectations are that the fit will worsen.

A deeper worry is that by relativizing RFs to stimulus classes or visual tasks, we are ignoring some of the significant dynamic features of neurons—precisely those features that are responsive to stimulus or visual task. It would be counterproductive at best to retain the classical RF at the expense of ignoring the neuron's dynamic properties.

5.3. Option 3: Natural Stimuli

Another possible answer to the problem of the stimulus dependency of RFs might be to choose a canonical stimulus. In this case, natural stimuli are the prime candidate for two reasons: first, because our ultimate goal is to understand vision in the real world, and second, there is evidence that richer neural responses are revealed by natural stimuli. The prospect of refiguring all of visual neuroscience using natural scenes as canonical stimuli, however, is daunting to say the least because it would require that much of the work of the past 40 years be repeated with natural stimuli instead of sinusoids and the like.

Moreover, the idea that RF properties can only be fully revealed by natural stimuli is radical. It is sometimes suggested (e.g., David et al., 2004) that the RFs revealed by natural stimuli are so complex that a natural image-derived model is only good at predicting responses to other natural stimuli. Adopting natural images as canonical stimuli thus entails giving up on the idea that once one fully characterizes a neuron's RF, the characterization can then be used to predict responses to *any* stimulus. As Rust and Movshon (2005) put it, "ultimately, one hopes to integrate all these models into a single theory that can predict neuronal and population responses to any arbitrary stimulus" (p. 1647). Even the piecemeal option optimistically leaves open the possibility that all of the partially successful models might be integrated into a powerful general model. To choose natural scenes as canonical stimuli is to give up on this hope.

5.4. Option 4: The Primacy of Circuitry

The last two options were presented as only fairly radical. Yet there is a case to be made that the notion of generality is so crucial to the concept of the RF that to give up on it is to change the concept beyond recognition. If we are poised to do mortal damage to the idea of the RF, a natural question to consider is whether we could dispense with the concept altogether. One way of doing this would be to attempt to model the circuitry of V1 as a whole and hope that the information contained in the RF will emerge or be replaced by something equally informative in the circuit model. The success of Hubel and Weisel's model of V1 was one of the decisive factors that moved vision science in the direction of single-unit (rather than network) analysis (Churchland and Sejnowski, 1992). Perhaps a return to the network level is the way forward.

In particular, if we model V1 at the level of its circuitry, it is possible that the uniformity that would be lost by relativizing RFs to stimulus and task would be recovered. This would be the case if the RF of a particular neuron was altered due to predictable responses of other V1 neurons in response to the stimulus or task. In other words, if the dynamic nature of the RF could be explained by static features of other V1 neurons and the connections among them, then it is plausible that a single model of V1 could be developed that would have dynamic RFs as a consequence. Perhaps this is what Bair (2005, p. 463) has in mind when he predicts that "the primacy of the RF as a concept for embodying the function of V1 neurons will be replaced by a set of circuits and synaptic mechanisms as our computational models begin to explain ever more response properties. The RF can then be understood as an emergent property that changes with the statistics of the input." Whether this is the case, of course, is an empirical question. There is no guarantee that V1 circuitry will not itself be affected by feedback from other visual areas and, as a result, prove as dynamic as the RFs of V1 neurons.

Even if we could produce a model of this kind, however, it is worth considering whether it might not be preferable to continue to analyze visual function at the level of individual neurons whose RFs are dynamic rather than to move up to the level of circuitry. Barlow (1972) adapted the phrase "neuron doctrine" (originally the name for the view that the brain is composed of discrete cells rather than being a single continuous structure) to express the view that brain function is best understood at the level of individual neural activity. One motivation for retaining the notion of a dynamic RF might be to hold on to the neuron doctrine as a general methodological principle of neuroscience. If we reject the notion of a dynamic RF in favor of network- or circuit-level explanation of function, we must abandon the neuron doctrine in favor of a "higher" level of explanation. Although this might turn out to be a beneficial break from the past, it will require a dramatic rethinking of neural computation. We turn to this issue in the next section.

5.5 Option 5: Decoupling Computer Vision from Neurophysiology

The last option considered amounts to an elimination of the concept of the RF, so we must ask what visual neuroscience would look like without it. We don't know the answer to this question, but it seems certain that it would require a significant shift in neurophysiological theory and would have consequences for computational approaches to vision. Analysis by fixed filters is a very natural way to think about vision, and it is straightforward to implement artificially. Without the simplifying assumptions behind traditional V1 physiology, the problem of vision begins to look intractable.

In addition, even if one could model a dynamic RF, it is a further question whether it could easily be incorporated into robot vision. We have claimed that at least in some branches of the discipline computational vision and visual neurophysiology have been developed with an eye to linking the two (Teller, 1984) or understanding how visual computations are implemented by neurophysiological mechanisms. One virtue of the classical RF is that it is a natural way to begin to see neurons as elements in these implementations. As we have seen, modeling early visual processes and the neurophysiology of V1 both conceive of vision as composed of a circuit composed of a small number of simple feedforward mechanisms, and the history of the study of contrast perception provides ample evidence of the coevolution of the two disciplines. However, the loss of a fixed RF might lead to a break between the theories of neuronal and artificial vision. One might, therefore, be concerned by the consequences for computational vision of radically altering or giving up the classical conception of the RF. If neurophysiology does not provide computational modeling with the basic units needed, then it is more difficult to model early vision, or at any rate, to model it realistically.

With this kind of worry in mind, one theoretical option would be to give up the idea of an isomorphism between the elements of computational modeling and neurophysiology. On this view, the task of computational modeling remains to provide a theoretical framework for early vision, and the task of visual neurophysiology remains to describe the properties of the neurons and circuits that implement this computation. However, in this view, it is no longer an assumption that the building blocks of the implementation are individual neurons. Although this may be a significant departure from current practice, the idea that individual neurons implement the basic computational processes is a methodological assumption rather than a substantiated doctrine—though not an arbitrary one. If we give up the neuron doctrine, however, then we need not assume that the abstract organization of visual computation has to be implemented by individual neurons that behave as the computational components do. Linear feedforward models of visual computation need not be implemented by linear feedforward visual neurons.

5.6. Which Option?

Which of the foregoing options should we choose? That question is an empirical one, but only in part. Some of these paths are likely to be less fruitful than others, so it is worth thinking about which one to choose prior to investing a lot of time in any of them. We suspect that more than one option ought to be pursued and others are worth setting to one side for the time being. In this section, we make some remarks about how to choose among the options.

Option 1—redescribing or expanding the concept of the RF so as to retain a large part of the classical conception—is clearly worth pursuing. As we noted, the work of Heeger (1992) shows that there are mathematical techniques that might make this possible. Heeger's work cannot handle all the data, and it is an empirical question whether a single model will do the job, but this is clearly an option that ought to be explored on the grounds of conservatism.

As we remarked with respect to Option 2 of piecemeal solutions to visual modeling, we think this is an option that is not only inelegant but would leave quite a bit of visual functioning unexplained. We want to know *why* neurons respond in different ways to different stimuli. If we know that, then it's unlikely that piecemeal solutions will remain piecemeal. If we understand how visual neurons change their state and why, then the models of function that are specific to different classes of stimuli will presumably form part of a single unified theory. Although piecemeal exploration is an indispensable dimension of scientific practice, it should not, in our view, be a methodological ideal.

It would be hard to deny that more work with natural stimuli is a crucial requirement of future experiments, and there is already a lot of work being done along these lines. One important question for this work is whether there are a number of clearly distinguishable classes of natural stimuli that produce categorially different neural responses and, if so, how these classes ought to be characterized. We suggested that 40 years of visual neurophysiology might have to be repeated, but that is a worst-case scenario. It is possible that the use of natural stimuli would produce data that would lead to different ways of conceiving of V1 neurons—and other visual neurons—and generate rapid progress. Nonetheless, it seems quite likely that working with natural stimuli will still require that we think about how to understand the RF in a new way.

Option 4 of exploring circuitry is likely to be fruitful. We suspect this option has not been more fully explored because it is both technically and mathematically complex. It is also possible that a bias in favor of single-unit explanations has also influenced the course of research. Dealing with the complexity of the problem is empirical, and the encouragement of philosophy is neither necessary nor particularly helpful. In contrast, we think that philosophers *can* argue for calling the neuron doctrine into question and making room for the possibility of circuit-level explanations. Whether such explanations will be successful remains to be seen, and we should not allow the success of single-unit neurophysiology to discourage visual neuroscience from thinking of the RF as a derivative (or, as Bair puts it, as an "emergent") property.

We are also in favor of disengaging computation from neurophysiology to some extent. It is a truism that one of the essential features of a computational theory of any kind is that it is implementable by neurons. This constraint has become more important in modeling over the years in part (we suspect) as a result of a backlash against the sort of computational theory that saw the brain as an afterthought—as a matter of "mere" implementation. This is a positive development. However, at this stage, we know so little about how the visual system implements visual computation that we should not let this constraint exert too much force on computational modeling. By trying to maintain an isomorphism between computation and neurophysiology, computational theory is restricted. In turn, this restriction reduces the ways of thinking about how visual neurons might implement the computation. Different styles of computational modeling might suggest ways of thinking of circuits as the unit of implementation, and this might lead to different ways of doing the neurophysiology.

This suggests that the option of changing computational vision to mirror the new data coming from neurophysiology may be one best left to one side for the present as well. Visual modeling might get some ideas from neurophysiology, but we should not make an isomorphism between the two de rigueur. When we know more at both the physiological and modeling levels, the question of implementation can more fruitfully be pursued.

6. Perception and Environment

We noted that we do not yet know the mechanism that underlies stimulus dependence of V1 cells. One possibility is that changes in neural state or responsiveness are a kind of adaptation. It is well known that neurons change their behavior when the visual stimulus changes substantially. When one moves from conditions of low light levels to bright sunshine, for example, a relatively quick process of adaptation to the light level occurs in which the activity of visual neurons is dampened. The same sort of thing happens with color. If you put on rose-colored glasses, the world looks pink for a while but soon resumes its chromatic range. Or if you look at a waterfall, and then look at a stationary scene, the stationary scene seems to move as an after-effect of the adaptation of motion-sensitive neurons to the downward movement of the water. The same holds true of many other phenomena.

Adaptation is important in perception because by altering the state of the visual system, or some part of it, the system is able to function across a greater range of stimuli than would otherwise be possible. A change in neural state or responsiveness to the *statistics* of the visual stimulus might represent a complex version of adaptation (Balboa and Grzywacz, 2002) that would expand the repertoire of the visual system and allow it to function effectively in different kinds of natural environments. If something like this is correct, then stimulus dependence, though surprising, may not be a qualitatively new phenomenon. It does, however, allow us to think somewhat differently about the role of the environment in modulating perception.

There is a long-standing tension between two traditions in the philosophy of perception. One tradition, favored by analytic philosophy, takes mental representations as central to perception. The perceptual action is all in the mind of the perceiver. In the other tradition, favored by continental philosophy, perception is more a matter of action than of representation, and, for this reason, the environment in which perception occurs is essential to understanding perception. Merleau-Ponty (1962) is perhaps the most important figure associated with this view.

In recent years, there has been a rapprochement between these traditions. Gareth Evans's solution to the Molyneux problem (Evans, 1996) makes use of something much like Merleau-Ponty's framework for perception. More recent work, such as that of Clark (1998), has emphasized the importance of the environment in understanding perception. More important, neuroscience may be in the process of resolving the debate. The work of Milner and Goodale (2006) has provided evidence that there are two distinct but interacting visual systems, one responsible for representing the way the world looks and the other responsible for providing information about how to interact with the objects visually perceived. As Ennen (2003) notes in a different context, the difference between analytic and continental philosophy of perception may be a difference in subject matter (i.e., which of the two visual systems one is of greatest interest) and not in theory.

A recent attempt to reconcile the two traditions in the context of color perception is due to Thompson, Palacios, and Varela (1992). They emphasize the importance of environmental features in developing a theory of color perception, and they develop an ontological theory of color that takes color to be a relation between perceiver and environment. Summarizing Levins and Lewontin (1985), they say:

> (1) Organisms determine in and through their interactions what in the physical environment constitutes their relative environments; (2) organisms alter the world external to them as they interact with it; (3) organisms transduce the physical signals that reach them, and so the significance of these signals depends on the structure of the organism; (4) organisms transform the statistical pattern of environmental variation in the world external to them; and (5) the organism-environment relationship defines the "traits" selected for in evolution (cf. Oyama, 1985). (p. 21)

They go on to say: "We must encompass both the extradermal world conceived as the animal's environment and the sensory-motor structure of the animal in any adequate theory of perception" (p. 22). This view, though attractive, is rather programmatic. The notion of stimulus dependence as adaptation provides one concrete way of thinking about one narrow aspect of visual perception and its relation to the environment. If the mechanism of stimulus dependence is a kind of adaptation, then the environment can modulate the visual system in a complex way by means of a familiar type of mechanism. The statistics of the visual stimulus can alter the way the visual system processes the information it is receiving, and this shows that the statistical properties of the environment are an ineliminable part of a theory of visual perception. V_1 neurons may thus give us the beginnings of a theory of the complex interactions between perceiver and environment.

ACKNOWLEDGMENT

We thank Ben Willmore for permission to use figures 9.1a and 9.2, and David Tolhurst and Wyeth Bair for discussion and comments on the manuscript.

NOTES

1. See Mechler and Ringach (2002) for the case against the simple-complex dichotomy. The classification has faced severe scrutiny but is still in play in the physiology

literature. Because this debate is not crucial to our discussion of RFs, it is not discussed further here.

2. This is more true of the British than the American school of visual neuroscience (Lennie and Movshon, 2005).

3. See Barlow, Blakemore, and Pettigrew (1967). This, however, is just one way of measuring the size of the classical RF; it measures the minimum response field (MRF). Another method is to stimulate the neuron with a grating of increasing size to find the optimal stimulus dimensions for its RF, measuring the grating summation field (GSF) (DeAngelis et al., 1994; Sceniak et al., 1999). The first method tends to give smaller estimates of RF size than the other; see Cavanaugh et al. (2002a).

4. Attneave (1954) and Barlow (1960) introduced the idea of redundancy reduction as a design principle of sensory systems. Redundancy reduction may explain why there are so many nonlinearities in V1 responses: "Linear operations can only partially exploit the statistical redundancies of natural scenes, and nonlinear operations are ubiquitous in visual cortex. However, neither the detailed function of the nonlinearities nor the higher-order image statistics are yet fully understood" (Zetzsche and Nuding, 2005, p. 191).

REFERENCES

Albrecht, D. G., and Hamilton, D. B. (1982). Striate cortex of monkey and cat: contrast response function. *Journal of Neurophysiology* 48: 217–237.

Albrecht, D. G., Geisler, W. S., and Crane, A. M. (2003). Nonlinear properties of visual cortex neurons: Temporal dynamics, stimulus selectivity, neural performance. In L. Chalupa and J. Werner (Eds.), *The Visual Neurosciences*. Boston: MIT Press, 747–764.

Albright, T. D., and Stoner, G. R. (2002). Contextual influences on visual processing. *Annual Review of Neuroscience* 25: 339–379.

Attneave, F. (1954). Some informational aspects of visual perception, *Psychological Review* 61: 183–193.

Baddeley, R. J., and Hancock, P. J. (1991). A statistical analysis of natural images matches psychophysically derived orientation tuning curves. *Proceedings of the Royal Society of London B* 246: 219–223.

Bair, W. (2005). Visual receptive field organization. *Current Opinion in Neurobiology* 15: 459–464.

Bair, W., and Movshon, J. A. (2004). Adaptive temporal integration of motion in direction-selective neurons in macaque visual cortex. *Journal of Neuroscience* 24: 7305–7323.

Balboa, R. M., and Grzywacz, N. M. (2002). A Bayesian framework for sensory adaptation. *Neural Computation* 14: 543–559.

Barlow, H. B. (1953). Summation and inhibition in the frog's retina. *Journal of Physiology* 119: 69–88.

Barlow, H. B. (1960). The coding of sensory messages. In W. H. Thorpe and O. L. Zangwill (Eds.), *Current Problems in Animal Behaviour*. Cambridge: Cambridge University Press.

Barlow, H. B. (1972). Single units and sensation: A neuron doctrine for perceptual psychology. *Perception* 1: 371–394.

Barlow, H. B., Blakemore, C., and Pettigrew, J. D. (1967). The neural mechanism of binocular depth discrimination. *Journal of Physiology* 193: 327–342.

Blakemore, C., and Campbell, F. W. (1969). On the existence of neurons in the human visual system selectively sensitive to the orientation and size of retinal images. *Journal of Physiology* 203: 237–260.

Blakemore, C., and Tobin, E. A. (1972). Lateral inhibition between orientation detectors in the cat's visual cortex. *Experimental Brain Research* 15: 439–440.

Bonds, A. B. (1989). Role of inhibition in the specification of orientation selectivity of cells in the cat striate cortex. *Visual Neuroscience* 2: 41–55.

Boynton, G. M., Demb, J. B., Glover, G. H., and Heeger, D. J. (1999). Neuronal basis of contrast discrimination. *Vision Research* 39: 257–269.

Braddick, O. J., Campbell, F. W., and Atkinson, J. (1978). Channels in vision: Basic aspects. In R. Held, H. Leibowitz, and H. Teuber (Eds.), *Handbook of Sensory Physiology, vol. 8 (Perception)*. Heidelberg: Springer, 1–38.

Campbell, F. W., Cooper, G. F., and Enroth-Cugell, C. (1969). The spatial selectivity of the visual cells of the cat. *Journal of Physiology* 203: 223–225.

Campbell, F. W., and Robson, J. G. (1968). Application of Fourier analysis to the visibility of gratings *Journal of Physiology* 197: 551–566.

Carandini, M., Heeger D. J., and Movshon, J. A. (1997). Linearity and normalization in simple cells of the macaque primary visual cortex. *Journal of Neuroscience* 17: 8621–8644.

Carandini, M., Heeger D. J., and Senn, W. (2002). A synaptic explanation of suppression in visual cortex. *Journal of Neuroscience* 22: 10053–10065.

Carandini, M., Demb, J. B., Mante, V., Tolhurst, D. J., Dan, Y., Olshausen, B. A., et al. (2005). Do we know what the early visual system does? *Journal of Neuroscience* 25: 10577–10597.

Cavanaugh, J. R., Bair, W., and Movshon, J. A. (2002a). Nature and interaction of signals from the receptive field center and surround in macaque V1 neurons. *Journal of Neurophysiology* 88: 2530–2546.

Cavanaugh J. R., Bair, W., and Movshon, J. A. (2002b). Selectivity and spatial distribution of signals from the receptive field surround in macaque v1 neurons. *Journal of Neurophysiology* 88: 2547–2556.

Chirimuuta, M., and Tolhurst, D. J. (2005). Does a Bayesian model of V1 contrast coding offer a neurophysiological account of human contrast discrimination? *Vision Research* 45: 2943–2959.

Churchland, P. S., and Sejnowski, T. (1992). *The Computational Brain*. Cambridge, Mass.: MIT Press.

Clark, A. (1998). *Being There*. Cambridge, Mass.: MIT Press.

Craik, K. J. W. (1966). *The Nature of Psychology*. Cambridge: Cambridge University Press.

Daugman, J. (2003). The importance of being random: Statistical principles of iris recognition. *Pattern Recognition* 36: 279–291.

David, S. V., Vinje, W. E., and Gallant, J. L. (2004). Natural stimulus statistics alter the receptive field structure of V1 neurons. *Journal of Neuroscience* 24: 6991–7006.

De Angelis, G. C., Freeman, R. D., and Ohzawa, I. (1994). Length and width tuning in the cat's primary visual cortex. *Journal of Neurophysiology* 71: 347–374.

De Angelis, G. C., Ohzawa, I., and Freeman, R. D. (1993). Spatiotemporal organization of simple-cell receptive fields in the cat's striate cortex. I. General characteristics and postnatal development. *Journal of Neurophysiology* 69: 1091–1117.

Ennen, E. (2003). Phenomenological coping skills and the striatal memory system. *Phenomenology and the Cognitive Sciences* 2: 299–325.

Evans, G. (1996). Molyneux's question. In *Collected Papers*. New York: Oxford University Press.

Field, D. J., Hayes, A., and Hess, R. (1993). Contour integration by the human visual system: Evidence for a local "association field." *Vision Research* 33: 173–193.

Fitzpatrick, D. (2000). Seeing beyond the receptive field in primary visual cortex. *Current Opinion in Neurobiology* 10: 438–443.

Foley, J. M. (1994). Human luminance pattern-vision mechanisms: Masking experiments require a new model. *Journal of the Optical Society of America A* 11: 1710–1719.

Freeman, T. C. B., Durand, S., Kiper, D. C., and Carandini, M. (2002). Suppression without inhibition in visual cortex. *Neuron* 35: 759–771.

Gabor, D. (1946). Theory of communication. *Journal of the Institution of Electrical Engineers* 93: 429–459.

Gilbert, C. D., and Wiesel, T. N. (1990). The influence of contextual stimuli on the orientation selectivity of cells in primary visual cortex of the cat. *Vision Research* 30: 1689–1701.

Gilbert, C. D., and Wiesel, T. N. (1992) Receptive field dynamics in adult primary visual cortex. *Nature* 356: 150–152.

Gold, I., and Roskies, A. (in press). Philosophy of neuroscience. In M. Ruse (Ed.), *Oxford Handbook of Philosophy of Biology*. New York: Oxford University Press.

Graham, N. (1989). *Visual Pattern Analyzers*. Oxford: Clarendon Press.

Hartline, H. K. (1938). The response of single optic nerve fibers of the vertebrate eye to illumination of the retina. *American Journal of Physiology* 121: 400–415.

Hawken, M. J., and Parker, A. J. (1987). Spatial properties of neurons in the monkey striate cortex. *Proceedings of the Royal Society of London B* 231: 251–288.

Heeger, D. J. (1992). Normalization of cell responses in cat striate cortex. *Visual Neuroscience* 9: 181–197.

Henry, G. H. (1977). Receptive field classes of cells in the striate cortex of the cat. *Brain Research* 133: 1–28.

Hirsch, J. A., Alonso, J., Reid, R. C., and Martinez, L. M. (1998). Synaptic integration in striate cortical simple cells. *Journal of Neuroscience* 18: 9517–9528.

Hubel, D. H., and Wiesel, T. N. (1959). Receptive fields of single neurons in the cat's striate cortex. *Journal of Physiology* 148: 574–591.

Hubel, D. H., and Wiesel, T. N. (1962). Receptive fields, binocular interaction and functional architecture in the cat's visual cortex. *Journal of Physiology* 160: 106–154.

Hubel, D. H., and Wiesel, T. N. (1968). Receptive fields and functional architecture of monkey striate cortex. *Journal of Physiology* 195: 215–244.

Hubel, D. H., and Wiesel, T. N. (1998). Early exploration of the visual cortex. *Neuron* 20: 401–412.

Jones, H. E, Grieve, K. L., Wang, W., and Sillito, A. M. (2001). Surround suppression in primate V1. *Journal of Neurophysiology* 86: 2011–2028.

Jones, J. P., and Palmer, L. A. (1987). An evaluation of the two-dimensional Gabor filter model of simple receptive fields in cat striate cortex. *Journal of Neurophysiology* 58: 1233–1258.

Jones, J. P., Stepnowski, A., and Palmer, L. A. (1987). The two-dimensional spectral structure of simple receptive fields in cat striate cortex. *Journal of Neurophysiology* 58: 1212–1232.

Kapadia, M. K., Gilbert, C. D., and Westheimer, G. (1994). A quantitative measure for short-term cortical plasticity in human vision. *Journal of Neuroscience* 14: 451–457.

Kapadia, M. K., Westheimer, G., and Gilbert, C. D. (1999). Dynamics of spatial summation in primary visual cortex of alert monkeys. *Proceedings of the National Academy of Sciences USA* 96: 12073–12078.

Kapadia, M. K., Westheimer, G., and Gilbert, C. D. (2000). The spatial distribution of contextual interactions in primary visual cortex and in human perception. *Journal of Neurophysiology* 84: 2048–2062.

Kuffler, S. W. (1953). Discharge patterns and functional organization of mammalian retina. *Journal of Neurophysiology* 16: 37–68.

Lamme, V. A. F. (2004). Separate neural definitions of visual consciousness and visual attention. *Neural Networks* 17: 861–872.

Lauritzen, J. S., Krukowski, A. E., and Miller, K. D. (2001). Local correlation-based circuitry can account for responses to multi-grating stimuli in a model of cat V1. *Journal of Neurophysiology* 86: 1803–1815.

Lennie, P., and Movshon, J. A. (2005). Coding of color and form in the geniculostriate visual pathway. *Journal of the Optical Society of America A* 22: 2013–2033.

Lettvin, J. Y., Maturana, H. R., McCulloch, W. S., and Pitts, W. H. (1968). What the frog's eye tells the frog's brain. In W. C. Corning and M. Balaban (Eds.), *The Mind: Biological Approaches to its Functions,* New York: Interscience, 233–258.

Levins, R., and Lewontin, R. (1985). *The Dialectical Biologist.* Cambridge, Mass.: Harvard University Press.

Levitt, J. B., and Lund, J. S. (1997). Contrast dependence of contextual effects in primate visual cortex. *Nature* 387: 73–76.

Levitt, J. B., and Lund, J. (2002). The spatial extent over which neurons in macaque striate cortex pool visual signals. *Visual Neuroscience* 19: 439–452.

Li, B., Peterson, M. R., and Freeman, R. D. (2003). Oblique effect: A neural basis in the visual cortex. *Journal of Neurophysiology* 90: 204–217.

Li, W., and Gilbert, C D. (2002). Global contour saliency and local colinear interactions. *Journal of Neurophysiology* 88: 2864–2856.

Maffei, L., and Fiorentini, A. (1973). The visual cortex as a spatial-frequency analyzer. *Vision Research* 13: 1255–1267.

Maffei, L., and Fiorentini, A. (1976). The unresponsive regions of visual cortical receptive fields. *Vision Research* 16: 1131–1139.

Majaj, N. J., Pelli, D. G., Kurshan, P., and Palomares, M. (2002). The role of spatial channels in letter identification. *Vision Research* 42: 1165–1184.

Marcelja, S. (1980). Mathematical description of the responses of simple cortical cells. *Journal of the Optical Society of America* 70: 1297–1300.

Marcus, D. S., and van Essen, D. C. (2002). Scene segmentation and attention in primate cortical areas V1 and V2. *Journal of Neurophysiology* 88: 2648–2658.

Marr, D. (1982). *Vision.* San Francisco: Freeman.

Marr, D., and Hildreth, E. (1980). Theory of edge detection. *Proceedings of the Royal Society of London B* 207: 187–217.

Mechler, F., and Ringach, D. L. (2002). On the classification of simple and complex cells. *Vision Research* 42: 1017–1033.

Merleau-Ponty, M. (1962). *Phenomenology of Perception.* London: Routledge and Kegan Paul.

Meier, L., and Carandini, M. (2002). Masking by fast gratings. *Journal of Vision* 2: 293–301.

Milner, D., and Goodale, M. (2006). *The Visual Brain in Action,* 2nd ed. New York: Oxford University Press.

Movshon, J. A., Thompson, I. D., and Tolhurst, D. J. (1978a). Spatial summation in the receptive fields of simple cells in the cat's striate cortex. *Journal of Physiology* 283: 53–77.

Movshon, J. A., Thompson, I. D., and Tolhurst, D. J. (1978b). Receptive field organization of complex cells in the cat's striate cortex. *Journal of Physiology* 283: 79–99.

Movshon, J. A., Thompson, I. D., and Tolhurst, D. J. (1978c). Spatial and temporal contrast sensitivity of neurons in areas 17 and 18 of the cat's visual cortex. *Journal of Physiology* 283: 101–120.

Nelson, J. I., and Frost, B. (1978). Orientation selective inhibition from beyond the classical receptive field. *Brain Research* 139: 359–365.

Olshausen, B. A., and Field, D. J. (1997). Sparse coding with an overcomplete basis set: A strategy employed by v1? *Vision Research* 37: 3311–3325.

Oyama, S. (1985). *The Ontogeny of Information.* New York: Cambridge University Press.

Parker, A. J., and Hawken, M. J. (1987). Two-dimensional spatial structure of receptive fields in monkey striate cortex. *Journal of the Optical Society of America A* 6: 598–605.

Pettet, M. W., and Gilbert, C. D. (1992). Dynamic changes in receptive-field size in cat primary visual cortex. *Proceedings of the National Academy of Sciences USA* 89: 8366–8370.

Polat, U., Mizobe, K., Pettet, M. W., Kasamatsu, T., and Norcia, A. M. (1998). Collinear stimuli regulate visual responses depending on cell's contrast threshold. *Nature* 391: 580–584.

Rapela, J., Mendel, J. M., and Grzywacz, N. M. (2006). Estimating nonlinear receptive fields from natural images. *Journal of Vision* 6: 441–474.

Ringach, D. L. (2002). Spatial structure and symmetry of simple-cell receptive fields in macaque primary visual cortex. *Journal of Neurophysiology* 88: 455–463.

Ringach, D. L., Hawken, M. J., and Shapley, R. (2002). Receptive field structure of neurons in monkey primary visual cortex revealed by stimulation with natural image sequences. *Journal of Vision* 2: 12–24.

Robson, J. G. (1980). Neural images: The physiological basis of spatial vision. In C. Harris (Ed.), *Visual Coding and Adaptability.* Hillsdale, N.J.: Erlbaum, 177–214.

Rust, N., and Movshon, J. A. (2005). In praise of artifice. *Nature Neuroscience* 8: 1647–1650.

Sceniak, M. P., Ringach, D. L., Hawken, M. J., and Shapley, R. M. (1999). Contrast's effect on spatial summation by macaque V1 neurons. *Nature Neuroscience* 2: 733–739.

Sclar, G., and Freeman, R. (1982). Orientation selectivity in the cat's striate cortex is invariant with stimulus contrast. *Experimental Brain Research* 46: 457–461.

Sclar, G., Maunsell, J. H. R., and Lennie, P. (1990). Coding of image contrast in central visual pathways of the macaque monkey. *Vision Research* 30: 1–10.

Sherman, S. M., and Guillery, R. W. (2002). The role of the thalamus in the flow of information to the cortex. *Philosophical Transactions of the Royal Society of London, B: Biological Sciences* 357: 1643–1894.

Skottun, B. C., Bradley, A., Sclar, G., Ohzawa, I., and Freeman, R. D. (1987). The effects of contrast on visual orientation and spatial frequency discrimination: A comparison of single cells and behaviour. *Journal of Neurophysiology* 57: 773–786.

Smyth, D., Willmore, B., Baker, G. E., Thompson, I. D., and Tolhurst, D. J. (2003). The receptive field organization of simple cells in primary visual cortex of ferrets under natural scene stimulation. *Journal of Neuroscience* 23: 4746–4759.

Sugita, Y. (1999). Grouping of image fragments in primary visual cortex. *Nature* 401: 269–272.

Teller, D. Y. (1984). Linking propositions. *Vision Research* 24: 1233–1246.

Thompson, E., Palacios, A., and Varela, F. J. (1992) Ways of coloring: Comparative color vision as a case study for cognitive science. *Behavioral and Brain Sciences* 15: 1–26.

Tolhurst, D. J. (1972). On the possible existence of edge detector neurons in the human visual system. *Vision Research* 12: 797–804.

Troyer, T. W., Krukowski, A. E., Priebe, N., and Miller, K. D. (1998). Contrast-invariant orientation tuning in cat visual cortex: Thalamocortical input tuning and correlation-based intracortical connectivity. *Journal of Neuroscience* 18: 5908–5927.

Tucker, T. R., and Fitzpatrick, D. (2003). Contributions of vertical and horizontal circuits to the response properties of neurons in primary visual cortex. In L. M. Chalupa and J. S. Werner (Eds.), *The Visual Neurosciences*. Cambridge, Mass.: MIT Press.

van Hateren, J. H., and van der Schaaf, A. (1998). Independent component filters of natural images compared with simple cells in primary visual cortex. *Proceedings of the Royal Society of London B* 256: 359–366.

Vinje, W. E., and Gallant, J. L. (2000). Sparse coding and decorrelation in primary visual cortex during natural vision. *Science* 287: 1273–1276.

Westheimer, G. (2001). The Fourier theory of vision. *Perception* 30: 531–541.

Wielaard, D. J., Shelley, M., McLaughlin, D., and Shapley, R. M. (2001). How simple cells are made in a nonlinear network model of the visual cortex. *Journal of Neuroscience* 21: 5203–5211.

Willmore, B., and Tolhurst, D. J. (2001). Characterizing the sparseness of neural codes. *Network* 12: 255–270.

Zetzsche, C., and Nuding, U. (2005). Nonlinear and higher-order approaches to the encoding of natural scenes. *Network: Computation in Neural Systems* 16: 191–221.

CHAPTER 10

THE ROLE OF NEUROBIOLOGY IN DIFFERENTIATING THE SENSES

BRIAN L. KEELEY

For one who is convinced that progress in psychology
depends upon the security of the biological foundations
upon which it rests, and that these alone afford the crucial
criteria of the truth of data derived from introspection
and other methods of approach little amenable directly to
scientific discipline, perception is of unique importance. It is
the bridge which spans the gap—if indeed it be more than an
illusory gap—between nerve processes and consciousness.

—Sir John Parsons, *An Introduction
to the Theory of Perception*

1. INTRODUCTION

It is my thesis that neurobiological facts are necessary for the attribution of an important
understanding of a sensory modality. In Western-influenced culture, at least, a commonsense understanding of the senses and how many separate senses there are intimately

involves the number of apparent sensory organs.[1] We commonly number the senses at five—sight, hearing, smell, taste, and touch—in parallel with the number of obvious sensory organs—the eyes, ears, nose, tongue, and skin, respectively. Although there is undoubtedly more to a folk theory of the senses than this, it does not seem implausible that an "organ criterion" plays at the very least a strong heuristic role in commonsense differentiation of the senses.

This commonsense organ criterion of the senses can be found in contemporary scientific understandings of the senses in the form that I have previously called a "neurobiological criterion": "The character of the putative sense organs and their modes of connection with the brain" (Keeley, 2002, p. 13).[2] For example, during the twentieth century, biologists attempting to determine whether certain fishes possessed a distinct "electric sense" did not consider their task to be done until the neurobiological basis of this sense—its organ—had been discovered (Keeley, 1999). My philosophical reading of this scientific practice, as well as of folk psychology, is that the existence of an identifiable neurobiological substrate is a necessary condition for positing a sensory modality.

However, such a criterion, especially taken as a *necessary* condition for a sense, is not without its critics. An interesting, contemporary line of criticism has been developed against it, taking its cue from a distinctly *psychological* starting point. This line—currently championed by Alva Noë—derives from ecological psychology and phenomenological influences on philosophy of mind (Noë, 2002, 2004). The upshot of this account is that, although they are heuristically helpful, neurobiological facts are not essential for the differentiation of the senses. That is to say, a sense is not a matter of what organ you have; it is entirely a matter of what you can do.

As it happens, this contemporary debate has its origins in earlier proposals at the genesis of modern neuroscience; specifically, concerning the "Law of Specific Nerve Energies" articulated and defended in the early nineteenth century by Johannes Müller. I propose that the debate over the role of a neurobiological criterion in the differentiation of the senses is a fundamental choice point concerning how one ought to theorize in the sciences of the mind. Just as Sir John Parsons indicates in the epigraph (Parsons, 1927, p. v), the study of perception is a bridge between the domains of neuroscience and psychology. Extending that metaphor, this chapter's goal is to better understand the principles of construction of such a bridge.

In section 2, I present the Aristotelian account of the senses. This account is important because, as the first sustained exploration of the question of how to differentiate the senses, it establishes the terms of the discussion. Many of the criteria Aristotle originally proposed still live with us, albeit often transformed. From the Aristotelian account, I extract the beginnings of the neurobiological criterion. Next, in section 3, I present the view against which I defend the neurobiological criterion, namely, that psychological facts alone are sufficient to account for the different senses, or at least that organ criterion is far less important than some have argued. In section 4, I return to some somewhat more recent history, Müller's nineteenth-century neurophysiological characterization of the senses. This historical discussion lays the foundation of my defense of the neurobiological criterion in section 5. My hope is that even if I do not convince you of the ultimate correctness of my view, I at least remind us all that the current debates in the philosophy of perception have a rich (often unrecognized) history that we would do well to appreciate more fully. As Santayana famously warned us, the danger of historical ignorance is needless repetition.

2. ARISTOTELIAN BEGINNINGS

In the Western tradition, the earliest sustained account of the number and nature of the senses can be found in the work of Aristotle (384–322 B.C.E.). It is traditional to attribute to "the Philosopher" the common assertion that there are five senses, based on the accounts he gives in his works *De Anima* and *De Sensu*. Therefore, it is reasonable to start a discussion of the senses with him, although Aristotle was not the first to speak of the senses in the Western tradition. For example, one of the so-called pre-Socratic philosophers, Democritus, also counted exactly five senses.[3] However, all we have now of many such earlier philosophers are fragments and secondhand discussions of their work, whereas for Aristotle we have a large corpus of extant works that represent one of the earliest attempts to give a comprehensive account of the nature of the universe, including the role of the senses in it.

Aristotle's predecessor and mentor, Plato, also presented a relatively comprehensive account of the nature of the universe, of course. However, in Plato's work, relatively little attention is paid to the processes of perception. Platonic philosophy— with its primary focus on the realm of the immaterial forms at the expense of the pedestrian world of physical things—wastes little time describing how organisms come to experience the physical world of objects. There is some discussion of perception (*aesthesis*; "perception" or perhaps better, "sensation and sense perception," or sometimes even "sense organ") in his late dialogue *Timeaus*, but that's largely the extent of it. Platonic philosophy, then, offers a comprehensive philosophical worldview, but one in which the senses are relatively unimportant, and hence not high on the list of phenomena requiring understanding.[4]

Aristotle's approach to these matters is different. In his *Intellectual History of Psychology*, Daniel Robinson argues that unlike his predecessors, Aristotle advanced a "*psychobiological* theory of the perceptual and rational faculties. While [Aristotle's] own version of Empiricism did not go so far as to submit scientific truths merely to confirmation by the senses, it did establish the validity and importance of the world of sense. In the process, *Aristotle presented the senses themselves as objects of study*" (Robinson, 1976, p. 95; emphasis added). Furthermore, according to Robinson's reading of the history,

> No predecessor could possibly or plausibly lay claim to the title of an early physiological psychologist, and this is precisely the title we may assign to Aristotle. He was the first authority to delineate a domain specifically embracing the subject matter of psychology, and within that domain, to confine his explanations to principles of a biological sort. That the entire body of Aristotelian philosophy

does not fit into a materialist mold is clear;[5] the philosopher himself goes to some lengths to make it clear. But on the narrower issues of learning, memory, sleep and dreams, routine perceptions, animal behavior, emotion, and motivation, Aristotle's approach is naturalistic, physiological, and empirical. (1976, p. 83)

So in Aristotle, we find a philosophical stance that stresses the importance of the physical, biological world. If Plato is a highly metaphysical—even mystical, at times—philosopher, Aristotle is a down-to-earth, worldly thinker. As a result, Aristotle felt called on to give a thorough account of the phenomena of the natural world, including the nature of the senses whereby we are acquainted with it. As a result, we find in his work a systematic account of the nature of the senses embedded within a larger framework accounting for all aspects of natural phenomena.

To begin the account, according to Aristotle, the fundamental characteristic of the physical world is motion ("change" seems a better term to me), of which there are three kinds: locomotion, alteration, and increase/decrease. *Sensation* is a subtype of alteration, that is, "qualitative change." According to Aristotle, when an organism perceives, something in the world outside of the organism brings about a change (a motion) within the organism.

Question: *What* is it that is changed in perception? Answer: A *sense organ*; more specifically, the medium contained within a sense organ. In the eye, this is the transparent medium (presumably, what we now call the vitreous humor, the "eye jelly"). In the case of the ear, this medium is air trapped within the inner ear. For each sense organ, there is its medium that is the locus of change. (At least, this is the initial change within the organism. The action on the sense organ is then transmitted further into the organism.)

In Aristotle's account, it is the organism's ability to be changed in just this way that is the essential feature of animate life. In Aristotelian parlance, the process of perception is one in which some *actual* thing in the world causes a change in the sense organ of an organism; that sense organ previously existing in a state of *potentiality*. In other words, in perception, the sense organ undergoes a change (an alteration, a qualitative change) from a state of potentiality to one of actuality as a result of the causal activity of the object being perceived. It is this capacity of animals that make them unique and different from everything else in the universe (Baltussen, 2000, pp. 74–75; see also Hamlyn, 1993, p. x). The animate can undergo all of the motion of inanimate entities, but not vice versa (in virtue of the fact that the inanimate is incapable of sensation). The close connection Aristotle draws between sentience and the defining feature of animals underscores the *biological* emphasis of his theory.

Returning to the details of the process: Question: What is it that brings about this change of the medium of a sense organ from potential to actual? Answer: The special object of the particular mode of perception in question. For example, a *sound* can make a change in the ear (as transmitted to it from the originating thing in the world via the motion of the air). A *color* makes a change within the eye (as transmitted to it via light), and so on (with some complications) for the other senses.

We are now in a position to characterize two important components of Aristotle's (1931) account:

> (A) By a "sense" is meant what has the power of receiving into itself the sensible forms of things without the matter.[6] This must be conceived of as taking place in the way in which a piece of wax takes on the impress of a signet-ring without the iron or gold; we say that what produces the impression is a signet of bronze or gold, but its particular metallic constitution makes no difference: in a similar way the sense is affected by what is coloured or flavoured or sounding, but it is indifferent what in each case the *substance* is; what alone matters is what *quality* it has, i.e., what *ratio* its constituents are combined.
>
>   (B) By "an organ of sense" is meant that in which ultimately such a power is seated. (424a16–24)

According to Aristotle's account in the *De Anima*, there are three categories of objects of sense, two of which are essential to perception and one that is incidental. The first type of object is the one just mentioned. According to Aristotle (1931, p. 2),

> I call by the name of special object [or "proper object"] of this or that sense that which cannot be perceived by any other sense than that one and in respect of which no error is possible; in this sense colour is the special object of sight, sound of hearing, flavour of taste. Touch, indeed, discriminates more than one set of different qualities. Each sense has one kind of object which it discerns, and never errs in reporting that what is before it is colour or sound (though it may err as to what it is that is coloured or where that is, or what it is that sounding or where that is).[7]

As just noted, this power is to be found in the sensory organs. (The concept of proper objects has a starring role in the Aristotelian story about what differentiates the senses, so I return to it later. For the moment, let us continue the current discussion of the different objects of sensation.)

The second type of sense object involves those that can be directly apprehended by more than one sense. Because they are common to multiple senses, they are called the "common sensibles" (*koina*). In Book II of *De Anima*, Aristotle lists them as "movement, rest, number, figure, [and] magnitude" (418a17). Later, at *De Anima* (424a16), "unity" is added to the list. In *De Memoria* (451a17, 452b7–9), he adds "time" to the list. Aristotle (1931) explains that "these are not peculiar to any one sense, but are common to all" (418a18). Color or flavor can only be perceived via a single sense, but the *number* of cows before one, say, can be seen, heard, and perhaps even smelled. Aristotle apparently did not have an explicit opinion concerning where the perception of common sense occurred, although it seems safe to infer that he would have put it where he thought all intellectual activity occurred: the heart.[8]

Aristotle gives no name to the third type of object beyond referring to it as an "incidental object of sense":

> We speak of an incidental object of sense where, e.g., the white object which we see is the son of Diares; here because "being the son of Diares" is incidental to the directly visible white patch we speak of the son of Diares as being (incidentally) perceived or seen by us. Because this is only incidentally an object of sense, it in no way as such affects the senses. (418a20–23)

Aristotle's precise meaning is a bit obscure here, but he seems to have in mind the notion of perception where we say we perceive that something comes under a particular conceptual description or belongs to some category. This may map on to the contemporary distinction within the philosophy of perception between *perceiving simpliciter* and *perceiving as*. There is not only the "raw" perception, say, that of being in the presence of something white, but also a perceptual interpretation— this white something I see is the son of Diares, dressed in a robe, for instance. Being "incidental," this third object is even further removed from a role in differentiation of the senses than are the common sensibles.

If Hamlyn (1961) is right, then in the case of the pre-Socratics, we have an exclusive preoccupation with raw *sensation* rather than the more involved, success term of *perception*.[9] In any case, with Aristotle, we have the full-blown modern distinction in his description of the three kinds of sense-objects. The first—the proper object—is unique to each individual sense (in the pre-Socratic sense, I want to say), the second—the common sensible—is essentially sensory (it needs a sense) but is not special to any one sense. The last object is incidental. This is the judgment or conceptualization of what is sensed. This is the "perceiving as" notion of perception, as when I "see the son of Diares."

In Aristotle's theory, we have a two-part account of the senses, pairing something independent of the perceiver, the proper objects of sense, with something that is part of the perceiver, namely, a sense organ with the capacity to be uniquely affected by the proper object, perhaps like a lock capable of being opened only by keys of a particular type. There is one important thing to keep in mind about Aristotle's theory here: Although there are *three* different objects of the senses, *only* the proper objects have the role of differentiating the senses, because they are the objects of sense that most directly and uniquely interact with the sensory organs. As Sorabji puts it, "the so-called proper objects of the senses, are the things to which the very being of each sense is naturally related" (1971, p. 56). That said, that intimate connection between sensory organs and the proper objects to which they are uniquely attuned—and only through which we human perceivers have any access at all to them—continues to play a role in some of our more modern accounts of the senses. The account I favor agrees with the Aristotelian account insofar as it makes for an essential role for both the sensory organ as well as that which interacts with the organ. However, not all contemporary accounts of the senses agree, and the discussion of one such theory is the next item on our agenda.

3. A Contemporary Case against Organs

There are a number of plausible objections to any account that lays too much stress on the organs of sense. I want to take a closer look at a contemporary line of criticism, which I argue suffers a common, deep confusion about the nature of the senses. Noë's *enactive approach* to the senses derives from his interest in ecological psychology, most famously presented in the work of James J. Gibson (1979), but Noë's account is also filtered through the lens of Merleau-Ponty's (1962) phenomenology and the interdisciplinary cognitive science of Francisco Varela and colleagues (Varela, Thompson, and Rosch, 1991).

Noë's account makes much of our status as "embodied agents" with a sensorimotor understanding of the world with which we daily engage; the different senses are defined by the differing ways they enable our bodies' ability to act on and in the world. Although Noë has been developing his account over the past several years through collaboration with a number of authors, I concentrate on the recent comprehensive presentation in his book *Action in Perception* (Noë, 2004). In the theory recounted there, Noë rejects accounts of perception that rely entirely on the passive reception of the world through the various senses. Instead, he stresses the essentially active elements of perception. We don't just passively see, we actively *look*—we move our eyes, crane our necks, and visually explore our environments by the skillful deployment of our bodies. This active role of perception is most obvious in a sense such as touch, in which the most natural deployment of the sense is to feel by physically running our hands over surfaces or rubbing the soft flannel of a blanket over our faces.[10]

This resituating of perception as part of an active sensorimotor process gives us the resources for differentiating the senses, Noë argues:

> What differentiates the senses, on the enactive approach, is that they are each modes of awareness...of different structured *appearance* spaces....Sensory modalities may in this way be individuated by means of their corresponding appearance structures (or objects). That is to say, we can endorse Aristotle's view that each of the senses has proper objects. The proper object of each sense is the type of appearance (looks, sounds, etc.) that is made available uniquely to that sense. (2004, p. 107)

However, Noë follows this with the warning not to "overdo the significance" of this endorsement of Aristotle: "For at the ground of our encounter with these different objects—appearances in one modality or another—is sensorimotor skill" (2004, p. 107). What he wants to avoid is the connotation of passivity in Aristotle's theory, with the sensory organs passively awaiting the impress of a given proper object, as warm wax awaits the impress of the signet ring.

One might conclude that all Noë does here is update Aristotle with a more modern psychological theory. Instead of speaking of the rather obscure "proper objects," he instead replaces them with his structured appearance spaces that play the same role in the individuation of sensory modalities. Though this is a tempting interpretation of the relationship between Aristotle and Noë on the senses, it is mistaken. Rather, on closer inspection, it results in an incoherent account of the senses. But it will take me a moment before I can make good on that provocative charge.

Noë is extremely clear that he believes a qualia-based approach to perception and the senses is a nonstarter. He argues that to try to figure out what qualia an organism has—that is, an organism's introspectibly accessible qualitative experiences—just doesn't get us anywhere.[11] He rejects the idea that H. P. Grice presented thus: "It might be suggested that two senses, for example seeing and smelling, are to be distinguished by the special introspectible character of the experiences of seeing and smelling; that is, disregarding the differences between the characteristics we learn about by sight and smell, we are entitled to say that seeing is itself different in character from smelling" (1962/1989, p. 250).[12] The problem is that although he is at pains to avoid this conscious experiential component in an account of sensory differentiation, I don't think his account successfully does this.

Noë is also clear that the presence of an organ—even one that has a clear effect on the behavior of an organism—ought not to lead us to talk about a sensory modality. He notes that on his account of "the nature of sensory modalities, the senses are not merely channels by which information about the environment reaches the central nervous system, as argued recently by Keeley (2002). This view is too liberal in what it counts as a sense" (2004, p. 110). He then goes on make that charge of liberality concrete by taking issue with my discussion of the vomeronasal system as a sensory modality. This is a case that could be described (in humans at least, pace the future course of empirical discoveries) as a sense—and a sense organ—without qualia. Noë rejects the notion that the vomeronasal system represents a distinct sense; yet despite his avowed rejection of the qualia approach to the senses, in the end that seems to be what his rejection of it amounts to. Hence, the incoherence I accuse him of. On the one hand, he rejects a role for introspectibly accessible quality of experience in individuating the senses. On the other, where the rubber meets the road—in rejecting a putative human vomeronasal sense—he falls back on exactly this criterion.

Before continuing, let me say a bit about the case here, so that Noë's and my disagreement might make a little more sense. In a very large number of tetrapods (four-legged vertebrates) there is not one but two separate olfactory senses. The first is the more familiar system mediated by the sensory organ known as the olfactory bulb, a system that often has an important role in the evaluation of food. (One's strong reaction to sticking one's nose in a carton of spoiled milk is this sensory system at work.) The second is a system mediated by the vomeronasal organ (VNO; also called Jacobson's organ) and reacts to the presence of pheromones. The VNO plays a role in a variety of reproduction-related behavior: identification of conspecifics and evaluation of their suitability for reproduction, among related phenomena. The existence of a vomeronasal sense in humans is currently a matter of some controversy. In many nonhuman animals, there is a clearly defined organ; there doesn't seem to be one in humans (although it is surprising just how bad human neuroanatomy can be, so we ought to hold off on drawing too firm a conclusion here). However, there are a number of behaviors in humans that have been identified—behaviors that in nonhuman animals have been laid squarely at the feet of a vomeronasal system.

It might seem a bit odd to the reader that I use human vomeronasal abilities in support of a *neurobiological* account of the senses, given that the presence of an organ is currently undetermined. To the contrary, I argue that this is exactly the kind of case that shows why this seemingly esoteric philosophical question about how to count the number of senses is actually quite important and relevant. There is an open question, I claim, on exactly what scientists need to do to establish the existence of a vomeronasal sense in humans. My proposal is that the jury is out until we have a clearer understanding of the route pheromone information takes getting into human subjects (if, indeed, that turns out to be the best way to understand the empirical facts of human behavior). It is important to the sensory story we tell, I argue, whether that putative information is coming in through an anatomically distinct neurobiological system, as it apparently does in other mammals. Noë, on the other hand, argues that we need not wait for the neuroanatomical witness to testify; he argues that we already have enough information to render a decision. I suspect that human vomeronasal perceptual scientists are going to continue to do whatever they want to do, regardless of this philosophical debate, but philosophers would not be doing our job in trying to explain how to interpret the importance of that scientific work if we failed to have this discussion.

As I just noted, Noë denies that the vomeronasal system is a sense. What's his problem with this sense? There are, he says, three considerations that lead him to this conclusion. Let me lay them out here and label them for clearer identification.

1. "Consider, first, that <u>there are no vomeronasal appearances</u>, in the way that there are visual and tactile appearances. Vomeronasal information may make it more likely, for example, that an animal finds another physically attractive. But the animal does not find the other attractive *vomeronasally* (i.e., in a vomeronasal respect). Vomeronasal states may influence our feelings, attitudes, actions, and so forth, but they do not inform perceivers as to how things stand in the environment."

2. "To concede all this, however, and this is a second point, is to concede that <u>there are no vomeronasal experiences</u>. There is no activity of exploring how things are as mediated by one's encounter with how the vomeronasally appear."

3. "As a consequence of the first two considerations, even animals in whom the vomeronasal system is highly effective <u>do not master patterns of vomeronasal motor contingencies</u> that mediate their causal influence. That is, there is nothing analogous to knowing how to position one's nose to pick up a good scent, or the better to smell something, in the domain of vomeronasal information." (2004, pp. 110–111; underscored emphasis added, italicized emphasis in original)

These are rich passages, and it is difficult to figure out where to begin, as there are both empirical and conceptual problems reflected in what Noë says. Let's start with the third, which is supposed to be a consequence of the other two considerations: that animals do not "master patterns of vomeronasal motor contingencies that mediate their causal influence." This empirical claim is simply false as a general rule. To give only two examples among many, first, we've all seen images of elephants grabbing things with their trunks and bringing them to their mouths. It is also common in courtship situations for them to bring chemosensory stimuli to their VNOs (located at the roof of their mouths). That is, courting elephants will use their trunks to very deftly explore the vomeronasal dimensions of their partner. Here's a second example: There is a behavioral response in a wide range of mammals—most prominently the hoofed mammals—that is so common that it has a name: the flehmen response. In it, a horse or a goat, say, pulls its lips back in what looks to the uninitiated as a kind of grimace; in fact, it is a facial posture that better exposes the VNO to airborne pheromones. In some species, the tongue is also extended and curved to better direct the airflow across the opening of the VNO. This behavior also involves the positioning of the head and changes to breathing (not to mention the animal ceasing to perform other behaviors, e.g., grazing).

Given these facts of animal behavior, we would need to hear a lot more before concluding, as Noë does, that nonhuman animal sensorimotor behavior with respect to the vomeronasal system is relevantly different from their behavior with respect to the olfactory system, say. If a goat pausing and performing a flehmen response in response to a whiff of something caught on the wind doesn't indicate the existence of a vomeronal sense, it's unclear why a prairie dog stopping and rearing up on its rear legs and craning her neck in response to noticing a possible ground-based predator should be taken as evidence for her having a sense of vision.

What then of the two considerations that Noë believes implies the third? Is it the case that there are no vomeronasal experiences and vomeronasal appearances? The flip answer is: The heck if we know! One confusion in the Noë passage is that he mixes up the human and the nonhuman cases. My original (2002) purpose in bringing up this case is that the vomeronasal system is unarguably a sense in many nonhuman animals; the interesting question is whether it is a sense *in humans*. Although Noë seems to be throwing it into doubt, there is not much motivation in the biological literature for treating a nonhuman sense of pheromones any differently than other well-established nonhuman senses—an infrared sense in snakes; a magnetic sense in sharks, skates, and rays; an electric sense in certain fish, and so on.

The problem raised by the vomeronasal sense is that the neurobiological basis of such a sense *in humans* is currently extremely unclear. It seems pretty clear that we don't have a spatially distinct VNO as other animals do; perhaps pheromone-sensitive cells are mixed in with other sensory cells in the olfactory bulb. VNO-type cells might be a distinct subset of chemosensory cells in the human olfactory bulb. As I already mentioned, human neuroanatomy still harbors many mysteries. What *is* clear is that however vomeronasal information is getting into human nervous systems, we don't have distinctive conscious awareness of it. There are no vomeronasal experiences and no conscious vomeronasal appearances...*in humans*.[13] Determining the presence and character of conscious sensory qualities in nonhuman or nonlinguistic organisms is not an easy thing to do, to say the least. In fact, this difficulty is one of the reasons I was motivated to find a way to individuate modalities that does not involve recourse to talk of introspectible sensory qualities (qualia). Perhaps we are just forced, by the philosophical situation, to figure out whether weakly electric fish have electrical qualia as a precondition to talking about a legitimate, nonhuman electrical sense—but if we could avoid that necessity, that would make for an easier row to hoe.

But isn't this all a little unfair to Noë? All right, so perhaps he failed to take into account the empirical details of animal behavior; nonhuman animals, in fact, exhibit the kinds of sensorimotor skills that his account requires. And perhaps he is a bit too anthropocentric in his characterization of "what it is like" to have a robust vomeronasal system. Why isn't this a reasonable conclusion: If I've here correctly characterized the scientific facts, Noë *ought to have said* that a nonhuman vomeronasal sense exists. However, the case would still be different, on his account, in humans. After all, surely he is right that *humans* do not "master patterns of vomeronasal motor contingencies that mediate their causal influence." And, that *in humans*, "there is nothing analogous to knowing how to position one's nose to pick up a good scent, or the better to smell something, in the domain of vomeronasal information." Furthermore, this is because *in humans* (the one case we can be sure of), there are no vomeronasal experiences; there are no vomeronasal appearance spaces. Surely, this is right?

Again, I think this is wrong, and again, I think what's wrong has both an empirical and philosophical dimension.

First, on the more empirical side, it is not at all clear that humans do not exhibit behaviors that reflect a mastery of motor contingencies related to the acquisition of vomeronasal stimuli. This may come as a surprise, but remember: Putatively, we're dealing with an *unconscious* sense here, so it may well be guiding our behavior in all sorts of ways of which we are unaware. For example, if I were to come into close physical proximity of a gender-appropriate conspecific[14] who possessed a vomeronasal chemical signature that my nervous system rated highly, without any conscious awareness on my part, I might stand just a little closer to her, flare my nostrils or start breathing though my mouth, take slightly deeper breaths, and so on—effectively allowing me to explore her vomeronasal aspects all the more fully. If this situation were to continue in one particular way—she responds to my vomeronasal profile in a similar fashion, plus untold other social and biological intricacies, we might end up conducting all sorts of species-specific reproductive behavior later in the evening (much of which, as with the example of the elephants discussed earlier, might be well described in terms of exploring one another's vomeronasal dimensions, whether or not we were conscious of that).

Consider that to an extraterrestrial ethologist from another solar system observing my behavior, and the behavior of other humans, my pheromone-mediated behavior might look no different in kind than my photon- and olfactory-mediated behaviors. Though it's true that we don't verbally report conscious experiences of the vomeronasal aspect of our perception, such an alien ethologist would stand in the same relationship to us as we stand to the male goat curling its lips back in a flehmen response to an approaching female goat in estrus. Furthermore, there's a deeper philosophy of language issue here concerning the indeterminacy of translation. It's not clear to me at all that when the alien ethologist records my (extremely boorish) verbal report, "My, she's extremely cute. I'd like to have sex with her," an appropriate translation of that into the alien's language wouldn't be "Subject finds the conspecific's pheromone profile to be vomeronasally attractive, among other things." This could be parallel with its translation of my verbal report, "She has a cute nose," as "Subject finds the conspecific's facial profile to be visually appealing."[15]

This brings me to the philosophical difficulty I see in Noë's account. Despite his disavowal of the qualia theory with respect to differentiating the senses, this is exactly what his theory boils down to, as revealed by his rejection of the vomeronasal system as a sense. Because if we set aside everything else in the long passage quoted before, we are still left with the sentence that I believe represents the nub of the issue here: "Vomeronasal states may *influence* our feelings, attitudes, actions, and so forth, but they do not *inform* perceivers as to how things stand in the environment" (2004, p. 110; emphasis added). There is an important sense in which what he says here is true. This is another way of saying that whatever vomeronasal information is to humans, it does not come to us with the special introspectible quality that visual, auditory, and other sensory experiences have. Putative vomeronasal information is not something we consciously perceive and then *act* on, even if it is does play a role in what *happens* to us. However, what's not clear is why this is relevant to the issues at hand, especially as it seems like we can, in principle, have all the other parts of Noë's theory (in particular, the mastery of sensorimotor skills with respect to the alleged modality). All we seem to need for a coherent account of the senses is *influence*, not the more tricked-out *information*. To ask for more, as Noë wants, is to needlessly fall back into a qualia-based account, something that Noë says he wants to avoid.

Although I believe that Noë falls into the qualia trap when rejecting a human vomeronasal sense, the situation is different when he considers a case in which his rejection of the neurobiological criterion is clearest: his endorsement of a visual sense in blind individuals equipped with prosthetic visual systems. For several decades now, scientists and engineers have been studying ways to help sensory-disabled individuals with prosthetic devices that bring about sensory substitution (Marks, 1978). Perhaps the most famous of these systems is the tactile-visual substitution system (TVSS) developed by Paul Bach-y-Rita (for a review, see Bach-y-Rita and Kercel, 2002). Noë succinctly describes it:

> The subject is outfitted with a head-mounted camera that is wired up to electrodes (say, on the tongue) in such a way that visual information presented to the camera produces patterns of activation on the tongue. For subjects who are active (who control the information received by the camera by manipulations of themselves and the camera), it becomes possible, in a matter of hours, to make quasi-visual perceptual judgments. For example, subjects can report the number,

size, spatial arrangement, and so forth of objects at a distance from themselves across the room. On the basis of this perception, they are enabled to reach out and grasp, to make swatting or grabbing movements of the hand. In addition, Bach-y-Rita reports that these subjects experience certain well-known visual illusions such as the waterfall illusion. (2004, p. 111)

The important role of sensorimotor engagement in the successful deployment of the TVSS system is what excites Noë about this example. Just sitting on your butt with the TVSS system hooked up doesn't result in anything interesting. However, when someone who is congenitally blind engages the world by using the TVSS system to perceptually explore their environment, remarkable things happen: She can operate in a visual world for the first time. This is a great example for supporting Noë's enactive approach to sensory modalities:

> In what does the *visual* character, such as it is, of these perceptual experiences consist?...First, we might notice that TVSS enables perception of *visual* qualities, that is, of looks. One can track perspectival visible features such as the way the apparent size changes as one moves with respect to the object. But second, this account in terms of the space of visual appearances is grounded on the more basic fact that the laws of sensorimotor contingency governing the quasi-vision of TVSS are like those of normal vision, at least to some substantial degree (e.g., at the appropriate level of abstraction). (2004, pp. 111–112)

Noë characterizes the example like this: "TVSS is a mode of quasi-seeing without any involvement of eyes or visual cortex" (2004, p. 111). It is not clear why he hedges and refers to "quasi-seeing" instead of just coming out and claiming that a TVSS-equipped and trained formerly blind person is now sighted and has vision. He might speak of "quasi-seeing" because the range of looks made available through the TVSS system is significantly impoverished relative to normal human vision. If this is correct, then the TVSS subject has quasi-vision in the same way we might say that a person afflicted with severe cataracts—but who can still make out some visual features of her world—has a mode of quasi-seeing.

However, I argue that referring to quasi-seeing is closer to accurate than Noë might like. On my account, the result of TVSS is literally "quasi-seeing" in the Latin etymological sense of "almost" or "as if" seeing. In the case of TVSS, the mode of connection to the world is still tactile, even if the information conveyed is ultimately visual in nature. In Aristotelian terms, the TVSS system converts the proper objects of one sense—here the visual sense—into the proper objects of another—in this case, touch. Although the information that the TVSS subject deals with was originally visual in nature, his or her mode of contact with it in the end is via touch.

This is an amazing thing, no doubt. If I were blind, I would probably want such a system myself; in answer to the kind of question that motivates us here, this system truly gives one quasi-vision.[16] I believe it is too quick to conclude from such examples, as Noë does, that "Perceptual modalities...are autonomous of the physical systems (the organs) in which they are embodied" (2004, p. 112). In the next section, I consider an account which runs counter to Noë's proposal, after which we return to what I believe he is getting wrong in all of this.

4. MÜLLER AND THE LAW OF SPECIFIC NERVE ENERGIES

The nineteenth century was a period of tremendous development of our understanding of physiology. It wouldn't be an exaggeration to say that what we now think of as "neurophysiology" began in that century. Perhaps *the* key figure in this development was Johannes Petrus Müller (1801–1858), due to his scientific contributions and landmark publications, but even more important were those scientists he influenced directly as a teacher and a mentor.[17] The list of his students and lab members is a "who's who" list of neurophysiological founding fathers: Emil du Bois-Reymond (discovered the action potential; first experimental electrophysiologist), Carl Ludwig (contributed to our understanding of the physiology of the secretory system), Ernst Wilhelm von Brücke (like Müller, a physiological polymath with contributions too numerous to list),[18] Rudolph Virchow (founded comparative pathology; first to identify leukemia and embolism), Theodor Schwann (articulated contemporary cell theory, discovered Schwann cells, coined the term *metabolism*), and likely most famous of all was Hermann Helmholtz (articulated the principle of conservation of energy in physics, invented the ophthalmoscope, and made numerous contributions to sensory physiology, particularly visual and auditory).[19]

The theoretical doctrine most closely associated with Müller is the law of specific nerve energies (LSNE), which articulates his view on the nature of the senses and addresses the same kind of questions with which Aristotle grappled. Our understanding of the physiology of the nervous system more generally, and perception in specific, had developed much in the two millennia that have passed since Aristotle had thought about these issues. For example, it had been discovered that the sensory organs were connected to the brain via bundles of fibers—the nerves. Surprisingly to those who studied these things, the nerves that connected the eye to the brain looked pretty much exactly like those that connected the tongue to the brain. Even more surprising, these nerves were largely indistinguishable from those that connected the brain to the various muscles of the body. Although such physiological data were quite sparse and uncertain at the time, the activity of these differently situated nerves showed no apparent difference either, whether one was investigating nerves underlying vision, hearing, or muscular contraction. That the remarkable difference in psychological function was matched with an apparent complete lack of difference the nervous substrate represented a remarkable conundrum for these scientists.[20]

Here's how the question is posed, and Müller's response characterized, in a physiological textbook:

> Despite the fact that we experience...different modalities of sensation, nerve fibers transmit only impulses. Therefore, how is it that different nerve fibers transmit different modalities of sensation? The answer to this is that each nerve tract terminates at a specific point in the central nervous system, and the type of sensation felt when a nerve fiber is stimulated is determined by the specific area in the nervous system to which the fiber leads. For instance,...if a touch fiber

is stimulated by exciting a touch receptor electrically or in any other way, the person perceives touch because touch fibers lead to specific touch areas in the brain. Similarly, fibers from the retina of the eye terminate in the vision areas of the brain, fibers from the ear terminate in the auditory areas of the brain, and temperature fibers terminate in the temperature areas.... This specificity of nerve fibers for transmitting only one modality of sensation is called the *law of specific nerve energies*. (Guyton, 1976, p. 20)[21]

The intuition embodied in the LSNE does not originate with Müller, although he deserves credit for fully articulating it in such a clear fashion and marshaling the data of the day in support of it. Hamlyn (1961, p. 147) credits David Hartley (in his 1749 *Observations on Man, His Frame, His Duty, and His Expectations*) with the idea that "each nerve [associated with a sense organ] vibrates in a characteristic way," although Hamlyn deems this "pure speculation" on Hartley's part. The notion is clearly also indicated in the famous work of both Charles Bell and François Magendie in localizing the motor and sensory components of psychological function to the ventral and dorsal portions of the spinal nerves, respectively (the Bell-Magendie law). Bell (1811) clearly prefigures the LSNE when he writes that

> it is most essential to observe that while each organ of sense is provided with a capacity for receiving certain changes to be played upon it, as it were, yet each is utterly incapable of receiving the impression destined for another organ of sensation. It is also very remarkable that an impression made on two different nerves of sense, though with the same instrument, will produce two distinct sensations; and the ideas resulting will only have relation to the organ affected. (1811, p. 9)

So, the general idea of neural specificity was in play prior to Müller's formulation of it.[22] However, he does present the idea in a clear and detailed fashion. His law is presented by him in the form of 10 parts—it makes some sense to call them "axioms"—in Book the Fifth, "Of the Senses," of his 1838 *Handbuch der Physiologie des Menschen*.[23] We'll consider these in turn, to see how this incipient neurophysiologist attempts to bridge the gap between biology and psychology.

I.   In the first place, it must be kept in mind that external agencies can give rise to no kind of sensation which cannot also be produced by internal causes, exciting changes in the condition of our nerves.

Here, Müller is reminding us that our sensory biology is the necessary intermediary between our central nervous system (and our mind) and the external world. The world outside of us can have no influence on us directly, except in line with how our sensory system can influence us. As he explains,

> sensations are constantly being produced by internal causes in all parts of our body endowed with sensitive nerves; they may also be excited by causes acting from without, but external agencies are not capable of adding any new element to their nature. The sensations of the nerves of touch are therefore states or qualities proper to themselves, and merely rendered manifest by exciting causes external or internal. (1843/2003, p. 1060)

II. The same internal cause excites in the different senses different sensations—in each sense the sensations peculiar to it.

III. The same external cause also gives rise to different sensations in each sense, according to the special endowments of its nerve.

IV. The peculiar sensations of each nerve of sense can be excited by several distinct causes internal and external.

These three axioms embody the core idea—the notion expressed by Hartley and Bell—that each sensory organ gives rise to its own peculiar sensation or quality, and that it is the activity of the specific nerves—not the nature of the causative agent on that nerve—that tracks the quality sensed.

These three axioms exhibit how Aristotle's account has been modified. The problem with the proper objects account is that by the late eighteenth century, it had become clear that although sensory organs are remarkably fine-tuned in their sensitivities, they are not perfectly so tuned. Mechanical pressure might be considered a proper object of touch, but Müller reminds us that when you have spent some time in a completely dark room and press the edge of your eyeball, the eye responds to this pressure with a sensation of *light*. The same goes for the rather gruesome example, commonly discussed at the time, of lancing the retina with a needle. Again, this elicits a *visual* response in the subject. As Bell notes, the sensation elicited by a given stimulus is not a function of the stimulus—as the proper object account would lead us to expect—but rather of the organ stimulated.

Also, as these three axioms advert to, by the early nineteenth century, a number of very different stimuli had been discovered to elicit responses from most of the sensory systems. For example, chemical stimulation, applied either *externally* to the surface of an organ or *internally* (e.g., via the bloodstream, as in the case of narcotics), had been shown to elicit responses from the stimulated organs (Müller, 1843/2003, p. 1063). Also, by this time, the relatively new phenomenon of "galvanism" (direct electrical stimulation) had been quite extensively applied to the study of sensory physiology (Müller, 1843/2003, pp. 1062–1063).

The striking regularity observed in all of these situations is that the quality sensed in a case of stimulation was a function, not of the causative agent, but rather of the organ so stimulated. For example, galvanic stimulation of the tongue gives rise to a sensation of taste, galvanic stimulation of the eye gives rise to a sensation of light, galvanic stimulation of the ear gives rise to sound, and so on. As in the Aristotelian account, sensation is explained by reference to both stimuli and specifically receptive organs, but the LSNE shifts the balance of importance more in the direction of the organs.

V. Sensation consists in the sensorium receiving through the medium of the nerves, and as the result of the action of an external cause, a knowledge of certain qualities or conditions, not of external bodies, but of the nerves of sense themselves; and these qualities of the nerves of sense are in all different, the nerve of each sense having its own peculiar quality or energy.

At this point, some special terminology begins to appear. First, *sensorium* is defined by Colman as, "Any area of the brain responsible for receiving and analysing information from the sense organs; also the apparatus of perception considered as a whole. [From Latin *sensorius* 'of the senses,' from *sensus* 'felt,' from *sentire* 'to sense']" (2001, p. 666).[24] Second, the term *energy* here is *not* the term commonly associated with physics ("*energie*") (as noted by Brazier, 1988, p. 56). The German original is *Spezifische Sinnesenergien*—literally, "specific sense-energy."[25] Precisely what this axiom commits us to, with respect to this "energy," is unclear. Müller's own reading of it was in line with the vitalist theory to which he subscribed: "The hypothesis of a specific irritability of the nerves of the senses for certain stimuli, is therefore insufficient; and we are compelled to ascribe, with Aristotle, peculiar energies to each nerve,—energies which are vital qualities of the nerve, just as contractility is the vital property of muscle" (1843/2003, p. 1065).

Reading Müller on these specific nerve energies reminds one of contemporary discussions of the irreducibility of consciousness (see Chalmers, 1996; McGinn, 1999). When one reads passages of Müller, such as the following, one cannot help but suspect that Owen Flanagan got it slightly wrong when he referred to the "New Mysterians"—the "New Vitalists" might be closer to the mark:

> The essential nature of these conditions of the nerves, by virtue of which they see light and hear sound,—the essential nature of sound as a property of the auditory nerve, and of light as a property of the optic nerve, of taste, of smell, and of feeling,—remains, like the ultimate causes of natural phenomena generally, a problem incapable of solution. Respecting the nature of the sensation of the colour "blue," for example, we can reason no farther; it is one of the many facts which mark the limits of our powers of mind. (Müller, 1843/2003, p. 1067)

> VI. The nerve of each sense seems to be capable of one determinate kind of sensation only, and not of those proper to the other organs of sense; hence one nerve of sense cannot take the place and perform the function of the nerve of another sense.

Here we have the crux of Müller's rejection of the kind of analysis Noë gives us of the TVSS-equipped blind individuals. Müller, of course, could not imagine the complicated sensory substitution systems scientists would develop in the century following his own, but he was well aware of the crude attempts the sensory-disabled have made since time immemorial. He knew that the blind became exceedingly skilled at the use of their remaining senses in coping with their worlds. And that, in turn, led him to the conclusion that as sensitive as touch, say, might become in a blind person, it would not lead to the restoration of even the tiniest amount of vision: "Among the well-attested facts of physiology, again, there is not one to support the belief that one nerve of sense can assume the functions of another. The exaggeration of the sense of touch in the blind will not in these days be called seeing with the fingers" (Müller, 1843/2003, p. 1071).

Having presented six constitutive features of the relationship between the LSNE and the senses, Müller next turns to an obvious question about his account—a question on which he must admit that the evidence of the day does not provide an answer.

> VII. It is not known whether the essential cause of the peculiar "energy" of each nerve of sense is seated in the nerve itself, or in the parts of the brain and spinal cord with which it is connected; but it is certain that the central portions of the nerves included in the encephalon are susceptible of their peculiar sensations, independently of the more peripheral portion of the nervous cords which form the means of communication with the external organs of sense.

Müller is honest about the ignorance of the scientists of his time on the question of whether the seat of the detected quality rests in the nerves themselves or in the cortical areas to which they project, or some combination of the two. That he does not tie his account exclusively to the sensory organs is something that is occasionally overlooked. For example, in her *History of Neurophysiology in the 19th Century,* Mary Brazier (1988), discusses the 1853 work of A. Vulpian and J. M. Philipeaux, in which they surgically crossed motor and sensory nerves. Doing this, they were able to use sensory nerves to elicit contraction in muscle tissue. According to Brazier, this is exactly the wrong result predicted by Müller's LSNE and she goes on to claim that "the work of Vulpian...essentially destroyed the theory of 'specific nerve energies'" (1998, p. 58). But there is some confusion here (as evidenced by the fact that currently, we still find positive discussions of this "destroyed" theory). Far from "destroying" the LSNE, results such as these can be welcomed as alleviating some of the ignorance that Müller notes in axiom VII. These findings suggest that the projection site of the nerves plays a more important role than we previously understood.

Finally, the account of the LSNE ends with three additional axioms that seem to have less to do with defining the position itself and more with how Müller believes that this framework addresses questions of contemporary interest in early nineteenth-century perceptual psychology. Although they seem to be less pertinent to the question of how to differentiate the senses, I include discussion of them here for the sake of completeness.

> VIII. The immediate objects of the perception of our senses are merely particular states induced in the nerves, and felt as sensations either by the nerves themselves or by the sensorium; but inasmuch as the nerves of the senses are material bodies, and therefore participate in the properties of matter generally occupying space, being susceptible of vibratory motion, and capable of being changed chemically as well as by the action of heat and electricity, they make known to the sensorium, by virtue of the changes thus produced in them by external causes, not merely their own condition, but also properties and changes of condition of external bodies. The information thus obtained by the senses concerning external nature, varies in each sense, having a relation to the qualities or energies of the nerve.
>
> IX. That sensations are referred from their proper seat towards the exterior, is owing, not to anything in the nature of the nerves themselves, but to the accompanying idea derived from experience.

For early twenty-first-century readers, Müller's discussion of these two axioms is the most obscure of all 10. However, the issue with which he is grappling is simply stated: On the theory developed here, what an organism senses is entirely a function of the local state of its nerves (or its sensorium, given the unanswered question of axiom VII). Yet despite that, our perceptual experience is of a three-dimensional, spatially extended world. We experience objects as being "out there," beyond our bodies—not smack up against our sensory organs. Somehow, the state of our sensory organs allows us to perceive a world in spatially extended terms. Furthermore, the different senses differ in the sense of "extension" that they provide us. Vision (ultimately, retinal stimulation) presents us with a highly extended perceptual world. Hearing (ultimately, cochlear stimulation) provides with almost none.[26] The question of how we come to perceive a spatially extended world via our apparently impoverished senses was a topic of much discussion at the time of Müller's *Handbook,* and here he proposes that it might be explained in terms of the LSNE.[27]

Incidentally, Noë's enactive account might be well suited, in my opinion, to explain this perceptual phenomenon, and I believe Müller could have assented to it.

> X. The mind not only perceives the sensations and interprets them according to ideas previously obtained, but it has a direct influence upon them, imparting to them intensity. This influence of the mind, in the cast of the senses which have the power of distinguishing the property of extension in objects, may be confined to definite parts of the sentient organ; in the sense gifted with the power of distinguishing with delicacy intervals of time, it may be confined to particular acts of sensation. It also has the power of giving to one sense a predominant activity.

Here, Müller is speaking of the psychological phenomenon of *attention.* One can attend to sensations of one sense; heightening our notice of what it provides us to the relative diminishment of the others. Similarly, within a given sense, one can single out a particular element being perceived for more intense consideration.

So concludes my discussion of the details of Müller's LSNE. It is significant in that although Müller and Noë disagree in important ways concerning the senses, both point favorably to Aristotle's account. In the next section, I make some sense of these different theories and figure out what ought to be the role of neurobiology in differentiating the senses.

5. Discussion

How are we best to understand what is at issue between Aristotle, Müller, and Noë with respect to their different but related accounts of the senses? Recall that on Aristotle's account, the way we ought to differentiate the senses from one another is in terms of the necessary interplay between the proper objects of sensation and the organs that are endowed with the capacity to be transformed by those proper objects. In other words, you need both because the two elements are inextricably linked. You need a description of proper objects to define the sense organs in the first place, and the only way that we know that such proper objects exist is by virtue of having appropriately constituted sense organs.

Müller takes this basic Aristotelian theory and modifies it in response to the empirical discovery that the sensory organs in fact respond to a much larger variety of stimuli than Aristotle ever imagined. However, he recognizes that Aristotle's theory is still basically sound; one just has to reformulate proper objects as the individualized *products* of the interaction of sense organs and physical stimuli. The sensory organs and their unusual affinities to stimulation (or perhaps now the organ and its concomitant cortical brain areas) are still essential to differentiating the senses, but the story is now more complex.

Turning now to Noë, the proper objects have been transformed yet again. With Müller, he sees them as the products of the interaction of stimuli with sensory organs, but instead of speaking of "proper objects," or "specific nerve energies," his products are "appearances" or "structured appearance spaces." Furthermore, they are not so much products of the organs as they are products of the sensorimotor *use* of those organs in the exploration of the world. These structured appearance spaces are not a result of what the organs are made of (which seems to be what Aristotle and Müller have in mind) but the results of what the engaged agent does with those organs.

However, I suspect that Aristotle and Müller would argue that Noë's account of the senses has swung the balance between organs and that with which they interact much too far away from the organs, such that he can claim that "Perceptual modalities... are autonomous of the physical systems (the organs) in which they are embodied" (Noë, 2004, p. 112).

What Noë's account does, I argue, is forget the original Aristotelian distinction between the three different objects of sense: proper objects, common sensibles, and incidental objects. Recall that in Aristotle's account, there *is* an aspect of sensation that is properly described as being "autonomous of the physical systems (the organs) in which they are embodied" and this is the incidental objects of sense. As I glossed it previously, this is our capacity to perceive what we perceive under some description; *perception as* such and such. There is a strong sense in which that is autonomous of the particular sense organ(s) involved. Furthermore, I propose that this is why it sounds correct to speak of the results of the TVSS system as quasi-seeing. As a result of this special equipment and training, the blind individual is now capable of coming to incidental "visual" knowledge of the world via the tactile system.

The question of how to differentiate the senses from one another is vexed, as illustrated by the large number of years separating the proponents discussed in this paper (Aristotle, Müller, Noë). Despite the obviousness that a lot of folks detect in the answer to the question, spelling out in a detailed and coherent fashion precisely how to understand the differences between the senses is far from easy. In this chapter, I tried to demonstrate the necessity of understanding the neurobiological substrate of the senses to this question. Making use of this criterion is not always easy, but as I tried to show with Noë's attempt to detour around it, it is more difficult to develop a coherent account that does not avail itself of a necessary role for neurobiology.

ACKNOWLEDGMENT

My thanks to John Bickle, Eric Brown, Carrie Figdor, Michael Griffin, David Lundmark, Peter Ross, Chuck Young, and the members of the Claremont Colleges' Philosophy Work-in-Progress seminar for useful feedback on this chapter.

NOTES

1. I speak of "Western-influenced common sense" because it is far from clear exactly how culturally universal such a posit of folk psychology is, despite the assumptions of some Anglo-American philosophers (e.g., Nudds, 2004). For example, the Anlo-Ewe–speaking people of southeastern Ghana speak of balance as one of the basic senses, despite the lack of any obvious organ (Geurts, 2002). The anthropology of senses is currently rather underdeveloped, although this is beginning to change (see Howes, 1991, 2005).

2. As I noted in my original publication, the wording here derives from Coady (1974).

3. For the sake of fairness, it should be noted that contrary to traditional practice, Democritus should not be categorized among the pre-Socratics at all, as he was a contemporary of Socrates. While trying to make sense of the intellectual history I am discussing here, David Hamlyn's (1961) observation should be kept in mind: "The history of thought is never so tidy as one would wish. Philosophical thought, even in relation to a restricted field, tends to be drawn into side issues and to adopt lines of development for extraneous reasons" (p. x).

4. "Perception for Aristotle is not to be viewed as a rudimentary reaction with little content, as is suggested by Plato. Nor on the other hand is it the work of reason and thought (*dianoia, noein, nous*), as was claimed by Aristotle's rebellious successor Strato. It is a half-way house between the two" (Sorabji, 1992, p. 195).

5. The anachronistic incoherence of fitting Aristotle into the modern philosophical category of "materialist" is also discussed in the introduction of Magee (2003).

6. One presumes that this is the difference between sensation and digestion, the latter being a change in the organism that *does* receive into itself the matter of the object digested.

7. Reading Aristotle as claiming a strict incorrigibility with respect to a given sense's apprehension of its object is probably too strong (as well as likely anachronistic, such concern with epistemic certainly being the stuff of modern philosophy). It would be more charitable to read Aristotle as claiming a *relative* incorrigibility here. The eye is far less

likely to err about the presence of something white than it is identifying *what it is* that is white. In any case, nothing essential in the current discussion rides on issues of epistemic certainty.

8. Sorabji (1971, p. 57) concurs, citing Aristotle's *De Sensu* (449a16–20) and *De Somno* (455a21–22). See Beare (1906, pp. 329–333) for more on this.

9. Beare (1906, 202–203), concurs on this assessment, suggesting that the question can only meaningfully arise within ancient psychology with the positing of the *sensus communis*, as attributed to Aristotle.

10. A historical note: Noë's account of the differentiation of the senses closely resembles that discussed by Armstrong (1968, pp. 211–213) in his *Materialist Theory of the Mind,* citing an earlier proposal by Anthony Kenny. Armstrong explores the possibility of differentiating the senses via the determination of sensory organs identified by their use. That is, genuine sensory organs are those that are actively used by an organism perceptually to explore its environment. However, Armstrong notes that this account is problematic for a case such as the vestibular sense (our sense of local gravitational forces as mediated by the semicircular canals of the inner ear). Prima facie, it would seem to be a sense (and, as I noted in note 1, there are cultures that do speak of it as a basic sense), but it is odd to think of us actively using the organs of the inner ear to "explore" the ever-present gravitational forces acting on us. Although Noë cites other passages of Armstrong (1968), he doesn't explicitly discuss Armstrong's related proposal. There is more to say about Armstrong's line of argument, but it would take me too far astray from the current discussion (although see Keeley, 2002, pp. 13–14).

11. Noë states this pretty explicitly in note 21, p. 243: "I agree…that the senses cannot be individuated in terms of qualia."

12. In Keeley (2002), I called this the "sensation criterion," and, like Noë, I agree that it's a nonstarter, despite how tempting it is. However, disliking it and successfully avoiding it are two very different things. (This is one of the lessons of Grice, 1962/1989.) One way of characterizing my critique of Noë is that invoking a sensorimotor criterion does not, in the end, avoid recourse to qualia, and that I believe that invoking neurobiology might.

13. In *adult* humans, would probably be more accurate. As it happens, there is evidence—anatomical reports from the early twentieth century—that human infants have a VNO that disappears later in development. The speculation is that this organ plays a role in the bonding process between a nursing child and the mother. As I am with nonhuman animals, I am unclear on what it takes to establish the existence of vomeronasal experiences in infants of nursing age.

14. Unfortunately, I am tripping over the heteronormative limitations of English here. We don't have a good nonheterocentric term in English for somebody deemed to be an appropriate candidate for sexual contact. For me, a largely heterosexual male (to my conscious knowledge), a "gender-appropriate conspecific" would be a human female. As it would be for a homosexual woman, and so on, for the panoply of human sexuality.

15. By invoking the standpoint of an intelligent, sentient alien, I intend to harken back to Grice's (1962/1989) extraterrestrials, who are discussed more fully in Coady's (1974) "The Senses of Martians." Grice asks us how we should understand alien verbal reports about the nature of their senses and shows how difficult a task this is. However, a more appropriate—and more real-world—example would be Oliver Sacks's "Anthropologist from Mars," the high-functioning autistic individual Temple Grandin (Sacks, 1995).

16. In Keeley (1999), I spell out a distinction used by neuroethologists between "-reception" and "-detection." The former suffix refers to a genuine modality that an organism has evolved or developed to possess, whereas the latter describes a case in

which an organ developed for the purpose of one sense is in some way used to convey information proper to a different sense. This distinction allows us to make what seems to be a relevant distinction between animals, such as electric fish, that have a genuine electrical sense, and those that can use a different sense to detect the presence or absence of electricity, such as when a human touches a 9-volt battery to his tongue to see whether it is "dead." In the case of electric fish, neuroethologists would say that they have an "electroreceptive" sense, whereas humans would be described as having the ability to "electrodetect." Using this terminology, an appropriately equipped and trained TVSS possessor would thereby have the ability to visually detect aspects of his or her   ·   environment.

17. Pat Churchland reminds us that Müller is often called "the father of modern physiology" and she passes on the legend of his prolificacy, "allegedly producing a paper every seven weeks from the age of nineteen until his death" (1986, p. 21).

18. Brücke had students of his own, including a medical student in the 1870s who performed neurophysiological studies on male eels before going on to do a few other things: Sigmund Freud.

19. Helmholtz had his own who's who list of students: Heinrich Hertz, Albert Michelson, Wilhelm Wundt, and William James.

20. The theoretical difficulty here is the same as that which motivates any attempt to localize psychological phenomena in a material substrate. The same intuition is invoked by Gall and Spurzheim when motivating their attempt to localize cerebral function: "It would be quite inconceivable that a single organ absolutely homogenous throughout could present phenomena so different and give rise to manifestation of moral qualities and intellectual faculties so various and so dissimilar" (quoted in Clarke and O'Malley, 1996, p. 477).

21. This passage is taken from the 5th edition of this standard medical physiology textbook. Notably, by the 10th edition (Guyton and Hall, 2000), this discussion has been deleted, leaving medical students with no account at all concerning the seemingly interesting question concerning what ultimately distinguishes the various senses from one another. I'll refrain from making jokes about the intellectual differences between M.D.s and Ph.D.s.

22. As indicated by the quotation given in note 20, Gall and Spurzheim's early nineteenth-century phrenological work was driven by a very similar intuition. To my knowledge, Müller himself did not make any strong claims to having discovered the Law. For example, in an undated passage of Müller's given by Brazier (1988, p. 57), he describes the kind of regularities just mentioned by Bell and notes that "These considerations have induced physiologists to ascribe to the individual nerves of the senses a special sensibility to certain impressions, by which they are supposed to be rendered conductors of certain qualities of bodies, and not of others." This passage suggests that even Müller believes he is simply putting a name to a regularity that previous physiologists have observed.

23. Translated into English in 1840–1843 by William Baly as *Elements of Physiology*. Recently, Nicholas Wade has been overseeing the republication of important nineteenth-century works in the history of neuroscience, including classic English translations of Müller's key works. The Baly translation is what I cite here. See Müller (1843/2003) and Müller (2000). The 10 axioms that follow are direct quotations from the Baly translation, pp. 1059–1087.

24. "Sensorium" then is the descendent of the Aristotelian concept of the "common sense," the location within the psychological architecture where the various senses come together, and where intermodal perceptual judgments are made.

25. My thanks to Verena Gottschling for helping me with the ambiguities of German.

26. Or so Müller clearly claims: "The sense of hearing is almost totally incapable of perceiving the quality of extension; and for this reason, that the organ of hearing has no perception of its own extension. The cause of this difference between the senses is not known" (1843/2003, p. 1075). I don't know how well the phenomenon of echolocation was understood in the early nineteenth century.

27. It is worth noting that it is over exactly this point—whether our experience of a spatially extended world is created by our mind or is a property of the external world that our senses passively received—that Müller's most prominent contemporary critic took issue. Lotze (1842) advocated a "local sign" theory of spatial perception and debate over this issue continued for a century, with Müller's student Helmholtz being a prominent participant. It would take us too far astray to go into the debate, but see Hamlyn (1961), James (1879), and Cabot (1878).

REFERENCES

Aristotle. (1931). *De anima*. In *The Works of Aristotle*, Trans. J. A. Smith, General Ed. W. D. Ross, vol. 3. Oxford: Clarendon Press.

Armstrong, D. M. (1968). *A Materialist Theory of the Mind*. New York: Routledge.

Bach-y-Rita, P., and Kercel, S. (2002). Sensory substitution and augmentation: Incorporating humans-in-the-loop. *Intellectica* 2 (35): 287–297.

Baltussen, H. (2000). "Theophrastus against the Presocratics and Plato: Peripatetic Dialectic in the De Sensibus." In J. Mansfeld, D. T. Runia, and J. C. M. van Winden (Eds.), *Philosophia Antiqua: A Series of Studies on Ancient Philosophy, vol.* 86. Leiden: Brill.

Beare, J. I. (1906). *Greek Theories of Elementary Cognition from Alcmaeon to Aristotle*. Oxford: Clarendon Press.

Bell, C. (1811). *Idea of a New Anatomy of the Brain: Submitted for the Observations of his Friends*. London: Strahan and Preson.

Brazier, M. A. B. (1988). *A History of Neurophysiology in the 19th Century*. New York: Raven Press.

Cabot, J. E. (1878). Some considerations on the notion of space. *Journal of Speculative Philosophy* 12: 225–236.

Chalmers, D. J. (1996). *The Conscious Mind: In Search of a Fundamental Theory*. New York: Oxford University Press.

Churchland, P. S. (1986). *Neurophilosophy: Toward a Unified Science of the Mind/Brain*. Cambridge, Mass.: MIT Press.

Clarke, E., and O'Malley, C. D. (Eds.). (1996). *The Human Brain and Spinal Cord: A Historical Study Illustrated by Writings from Antiquity to the Twentieth Century*, 2nd ed. San Francisco: Norman.

Coady, C. A. J. (1974). The senses of Martians. *Philosophical Review* 83: 107–125.

Colman, A. M. (2001). *A Dictionary of Psychology*. Oxford: Oxford University Press.

Geurts, K. L. (2002). *Culture and the Senses: Bodily Ways of Knowing in an African Community*. Berkeley: University of California Press.

Gibson, J. J. (1979). *The Ecological Approach to Visual Perception*. Hillsdale, N.J.: Erlbaum.

Grice, H. P. (1962/1989). Some remarks about the senses. In R. J. Butler (Ed.), *Analytical Philosophy*, Series I. Oxford: Oxford University Press.

Guyton, A. C. (1976). *Textbook of Medical Physiology*, 5th ed. Philadelphia: Saunders.

Guyton, A. C., and Hall, J. E. (2000). *Textbook of Medical Physiology*, 10th ed. Philadelphia: Saunders.

Hamlyn, D. W. (1961). *Sensation and Perception: A History of the Philosophy of Perception*. London: Routledge and Kegan Paul.

Hamlyn, D. W. (1993). *De Anima, books II and III with Passages from Book I/Aristotle; translated with introduction and notes by D. W. Hamlyn; with a report on recent work and a revised bibliography by Christopher Shields*. J. L. Ackrill and L. Judson (Eds.), Clarendon Aristotle series. Oxford: Clarendon Press.

Howes, D. (Ed.). (1991). *The Varieties of Sensory Experience: A Sourcebook in the Anthropology of the Senses*. Toronto: University of Toronto Press.

Howes, D. (Ed.). (2005). *Empire of the Senses: The Sensual Culture Reader*. Oxford: Berg.

James, W. (1879). The spatial *quale*. *Journal of Speculative Philosophy* 13: 64–87.

Keeley, B. L. (1999). Fixing content and function in neurobiological systems: The neuroethology of electroreception. *Biology and Philosophy* 14: 395–430.

Keeley, B. L. (2002). Making sense of the senses: Individuating modalities in humans and other animals. *Journal of Philosophy* 99: 5–28.

Lotze, R. H. (1842). *Allgemeine Pathologie und Therapie als Mechanische Naturwissenschaften*. Leipzig: Weidmann'sche Buchhandlung.

Magee, J. M. (2003). *Unmixing the Intellect: Aristotle on Cognitive Powers and Bodily Organs*. Westport, Conn.: Greenwood Press.

Marks, L. E. (1978). *The Unity of the Senses: Interrelations among the Modalities*. New York: Academic Press.

McGinn, C. (1999). *The Mysterious Flame: Conscious Minds in a Material World*. New York: Basic Books.

Merleau-Ponty, M. (1962). *The Phenomenology of Perception*. Trans. C. Smith. London and Henley: Routledge and Kegan Paul.

Müller, J. (1843/2003). *Müller's Elements of Physiology*. Trans. W. Baly. Bristol: Thoemmes Press.

Müller, J. (2000). Physiology of the nerve. In N. J. Wade (Ed.), *The Emergence of Neuroscience in the Nineteenth Century*. London: Routledge/Thoemmes Press.

Noë, A. (2002). On what we see. *Pacific Philosophical Quarterly* 83: 57–80.

Noë, A. (2004). *Action in Perception*. Cambridge, Mass.: MIT Press.

Nudds, M. (2004). The significance of the senses. *Proceedings of the Aristotelian Society* 104: 31–51.

Parsons, J. H. (1927). *An Introduction to the Theory of Perception*. New York: Macmillan.

Robinson, D. N. (1976). *An Intellectual History of Psychology*. New York: Macmillan.

Sacks, O. (1995). *An Anthropologist on Mars: Seven Paradoxical Tales*. New York: Knopf.

Sorabji, R. (1971). Aristotle on demarcating the five senses. *Philosophical Review* 80: 55–79.

Sorabji, R. (1992). Intentionality and physiological processes: Aristotle's theory of sense-perception. In M. C. Nussbaum and A. O. Rorty (Eds.), *Essays on Aristotle's De Anima*. Oxford: Clarendon Press.

Varela, F. J., Thompson, E., and Rosch, E. (1991). *The Embodied Mind*. Cambridge, Mass.: MIT Press.

CHAPTER 11

....

ENACTIVISM'S VISION: NEUROCOGNITIVE BASIS OR NEUROCOGNITIVELY BASELESS?

....

CHARLES WALLIS AND WAYNE WRIGHT

1. INTRODUCTION

....

Researchers across a number of fields have increasingly turned to explorations of vision's connections to action, with particular emphasis on motor planning and execution, memory, and attention (Cavina-Pratesi et al., 2006; Churchland, Ramachandran, Sejnowski, Koch, and Davis, 1994; Findlay and Gilchrist, 2003; Rensink, 2000). Although several lines of reasoning fuel this trend, a growing dissatisfaction with established "passive" approaches to the study of vision—those that are primarily concerned with inverse optics, covert attention, tachistoscopic presentations, and the like—heads the list. This dissatisfaction stems largely from two sources. First, despite its past contributions, many question the passive approach's potential to yield new and significant advances in the study of visual processing. In particular, concerns have emerged regarding passive vision research's chances of offering insights into complex, highly interactive visual processing. Some researchers view such interactive visual processing as paradigmatic of vision "outside the laboratory" and portray the idealized and highly constrained visual tasks typical of laboratory research as blunt, maladapted investigatory instruments providing little basis for theoretical insight into interactive vision. Second, laboratory tasks involving, inter alia, change detection, reading, and visual search prompt doubts about the passive approach's potential to understand the role of saccades, memory, and attention in vision (Findlay and Gilchrist, 2003; Gilchrist, Brown, and Findlay, 1997; Rensink, 2000, 2002).

Vision research has not heretofore proceeded incognizant of the numerous movements routinely made by sighted creatures as a part of their normal, everyday use of their visual equipment. However, "active" vision researchers claim that the passive framework's experiments and theories improperly marginalize such movements. Therefore, much of the research falling under the heading of active vision aims to avoid the perceived shortcomings of the passive tradition by rejecting or revising many of its fundamental assumptions. For instance, active vision researchers reject the notion that the fundamental purpose of vision is to construct highly detailed, picture-like internal representations of the scene before the eyes from the confounded retinal input through a cumulative series of computationally and representationally intensive operations (Churchland et al., 1994; Goodale, 1998; Rensick, 2000, 2002). Arguably, something like the inner picture model of perception has been presupposed in most perception research throughout the history of the field.[1]

Conjoined with the rejection of the inner picture view is an accentuation of the role of movement—of the eyes, head, or entire body—in many visual accomplishments. Active vision researchers stress the perceivers' ability to selectively sample the environment over time, thereby reducing the representational and computational resources required to use visually acquired information in the unfolding of complex behaviors. Although we believe greater environmental interaction can simplify tasks, we note later that active perception can pose complications of its own, and thus one should not view interaction as a panacea for representational or computational complexity.

Enactivism represents a radical development in the flight from passive approaches. Enactivists advocate a complete reconceptualization of perception with a complementary refocusing of perception research in the light of profound interdependencies between perception and action. Besides challenging the idea that perception is a process of creating internal models of the environment, enactivists hold that action—in the form of skillful, body-involving exercise of sensorimotor knowledge—plays a *constitutive* role in perceptual content, contending that scientists should understand perceptual systems in terms of the behaving organism. Leading enactivists are quite clear—even excited—about the revolutionary nature of their view and its consequences for neuroscientific and psychological investigations of perception. For example, J. Kevin O'Regan and Alva Noë (O&N) argue that their view reveals the much-discussed binding problem to be a pseudo-problem, based on a mistaken conception of perception (2001, p. 967). O&N go on to proclaim that the "solution to the puzzle of understanding how consciousness arises in the brain is to realize that consciousness does not in fact arise in the brain!" (2001, p. 970). Similarly, Noë states that a "neuroscience of perceptual consciousness must be…a neuroscience of embodied activity, rather than a neuroscience of brain activity" (2004, p. 227).

This chapter seeks to clarify the central commitments as well as claimed advantages of enactivism, examine empirical findings relevant to the plausibility of enactivism, and assess what genuine contribution enactivism might make to the study of perception. We organize the body of the text into five major sections; claims and commitments, conceptual issues, empirical evidence cited in support of enactivism, enactivist responses to empirical evidence cited as posing difficulties for enactivism as well as alternative research programs, and areas of neuroscience we deem highly relevant but that remain unconsidered by enactivism.

2. Basic Enactivism: Commitments and Claims

The core view of enactivism as advocated by Hurley, Noë, and O'Regan consists in the assertion that perception is neither brain-based, primarily representational, nor passively receptive (Hurley and Noë, 2003a, 2003b; Noë, 2002, 2004, 2005, 2006a, 2006b; Noë and Hurley, 2003; Noë and O'Regan, 2000, 2002; Noë and Thompson, 2004; O'Regan and Noë, 2001; Philipona and O'Regan, 2006; Philipona, O'Regan, and Nadal, 2003). Rather, as Noë asserts, "perception is not something that happens to us, or in us. It is something we do" (2004, p. 1).

What follows from rejecting brain-based notions of perception in favor of the thesis that action and the body play a constitutive role in perception? Consider Noë's remarks that to "perceive like us…you must have a body like us" (2004, p. 25) and that a correct model of vision must include "the animate body and the world" (2004, p. 30). Enactivists suppose these consequences follow from reconceptualizing perception as a kind of skillful activity on the part of the entire creature, including its body and motor capacities (as opposed to a potentially disembodied processing of mental representations). Clearly, enactivism differs considerably from mainstream scientific thinking about perception. Enactivists differ even from other recent researchers who disavow traditional passive approaches in favor of giving greater weight to the role of action in perception in that these other active vision researchers continue to suppose that the brain alone is the ultimate locus of perception (Block, 2003, 2005). Enactivists do not merely seek to remind mainstream (non-Gibsonian) researchers that perceivers can move their eyes, heads, and bodies. Rather, enactivists contend that mainstream researchers are grossly mistaken in their conception of the fundamental object of study: the isolated, inert perceiver and his or her inner model of the world.

Taking vision as an example, enactivists claim that "vision is a mode of exploration of the world that is mediated by knowledge, on the part of the perceiver, of what we call sensorimotor contingencies" (O'Regan and Noë, 2001, p. 940) Knowledge of sensorimotor contingencies consists of nonpropositional know-how rather than propositional knowledge. Thus, one's possession of the relevant knowledge lies in one's mastery of the relationships between one's movements and the resulting transformations in the patterns of stimulation to which those movements give rise. In short, sensorimotor contingencies (SMCs) are "the *structure of the rules* governing the sensory changes produced by various motor actions" (O'Regan and Noë, 2001, p. 941). Perception and perceptual content supposedly consists in exercising one's capacity for skillful manipulation of SMCs during environmental explorations. For example, the "visual quality of shape is precisely the set of all potential distortions that the shape undergoes when it is moved relative to us, or when we move relative to it" (O'Regan and Noë, 2001, p. 942).

O&N (Noë and O'Regan, 2002; O'Regan and Noë, 2001) further divide the traditional notion of vision into two capacities: "visual sensitivity" and "visual awareness." Visual sensitivity is "the perceptual coupling of animal and environment that consists in the animal's access to environmental detail thanks to its mastery of the relevant sensorimotor contingencies." (Noë and O'Regan, 2002, p. 569). To have the capacity for visual awareness, the animal must "integrate its coupling behavior with its broader capacities for thought and rationally guided action" (ibid.) Exercise of the capacity for visual sensation, while facilitating an animal's interactions with its environment, constitutes neither seeing nor conscious perception for O&N. Exercise of the capacity for visual awareness, on the other hand, results in both seeing and (transitive) perceptual consciousness.

It follows that without a mastery of SMCs, one cannot even be sensate. Likewise, without integration of one's knowledge of SMCs with one's capacities for thought and rational action, one would, in a very real sense, be blind. Enactivists see this striking commitment as a boon to the development of their view. Indeed, nearly all the conceptual (philosophical) claims and alleged empirical support for enactivism are tied to the capacity for visual awareness and the consequences of its absence. For instance, enactivists claim that empirical evidence supports their prediction that a lack of sensorimotor knowledge or a disruption thereto results in an absence of perceptual experience (i.e., visual awareness), while the traditional view of perception predicts that dissociating action from perception does no harm to the latter (see Noë, 2004, p. 4). We consider enactivists' claims about experiential blindness later in the chapter. Likewise, we evaluate enactivists' claims about the essential role of sensorimotor know-how for perception in the light of the neurophysiological and behavioral evidence from the literature on learning and memory.

Just as enactivists posit two perceptual capacities, they posit two classes of SMCs, each playing a different role in perception. On the one hand, one class—the sensory modality-related SMCs—provide the basis for individuation between the senses. According to O&N, neither activity inherent in a neuron, nor modality-specific neuronal interconnectivity can explain why certain inputs result in visual rather than tactile experience (O'Regan and Noë, 2001, p. 940). The enactivist alternative distinguishes, say, vision from olfaction exclusively in terms of the unique and invariant modality-related SMCs. Modality-related SMCs differentiate the various senses precisely because sensory content is dictated by the nature of the modality-specific perceptual apparatus and the structure of the environments that apparatus is (or might be) used to explore. On the other hand, another class—attribute-related SMCs—guide perception of attributes within a modality so as to distinguish objects from one another. For instance, as one moves relative to a red object, X (or it moves relative to a perceiver), sensory input varies in law-governed ways. Sensory input variation from a green object, Y, differs from X's motion-generated input, even for comparable movements. These attribute-related SMCs can have strong connections to other sense modalities as a result of the brain's abstracting the appropriate nomic correlations from one's sense-specific experiences. SMC-based differentiation of senses and perceptual attributes supposedly offers the enactivist a means of explaining phenomena such as synesthesia and the tactile-vision substitution studied by Paul Bach y Rita and colleagues (Bach y Rita, 1983, 1984), phenomena that seem difficult to accommodate within a "specific nerve energies" framework (see Hurley and Noë, 2003b, esp. pp. 139–148).[2]

3. Conceptual Issues

In our view, enactivism involves two interrelated conceptual issues. On one hand, enactivists seek to change scientific and philosophic conceptions of perception and perceptual consciousness. On the other hand, enactivists argue against representationalist treatments of perception. We consider the enactivists' arguments for each of their desired reconceptualizations, ending the section by considering whether enactivism's reconceptualizations are or need be as radical as one might at first suppose.

3.1. Perceptual Consciousness

The first issue we consider is how to conceptualize consciousness and how to understand consciousness as an unproblematic physical phenomenon. Many researchers, especially philosophers, raise doubts about the possibility of a complete scientific explanation of conscious, qualitative experience. These doubts find expression as the well-known explanatory gap (Levine, 1983) or hard problem (Chalmers, 1996). In brief, advocates of the hard problem allege that scientific research provides no means by which to understand how brain states come to have qualitative properties—much less some specific qualitative property rather than some other. Enactivists allege that understanding perceptual awareness in terms of a mastery of SMCs integrated with capacities for thought and rationally guided action provides a basis from which to dispel doubts raised by philosophers. In fact, O&N state that "the most important claim in [their] article was that the sensorimotor approach allows [them] to address the problem of the explanatory gap" (O'Regan and Noë, 2001, p. 1020). Enactivists argue that qualia become unproblematic within their new conceptual framework. Specifically, recognizing the constitutive role of action in perception reveals the category mistake involved in attributing qualia to experiences.

Philosophers tend to conceive of qualia as intrinsic, qualitative properties of experiential states through which those states manifest a felt character. A natural physical interpretation of the philosopher's conception understands a subject's conscious states as nothing more than the subject's brain states, and qualia as nothing more than properties of those states. On the enactivist conception, in contrast, perceptual experiences consist in the temporally extended activity of exploring the environment through the rational exercise of one's mastery of SMCs (O'Regan and Noë, 2001, p. 961). Thus, one can no longer reduce experiences to states of the subject's brain at any one moment and in isolation from the body and environment, that is, to temporally isolated patterns of neural firing. The extended temporal scale of perceptual experience also prevents researchers from fruitfully studying it with presentations "in a flash." Experiences, in consequence, are the wrong kind of thing for bearing qualia; only states can have qualia, but experiences are not states.

If the explanatory gap proves recalcitrant, science cannot explain how the brain states to which researchers reduce experiences can have qualitative properties. But for O&N, one cannot reduce experiences to brain states, thus one need not explain how experiences can have qualia—there is no real explanatory gap. Indeed, O&N tell readers that "qualia are an illusion" (O'Regan and Noë, 2001), a conceptual artifact of the attempt to explain perception and perceptual experience from within a faulty paradigm.

O&N's diagnosis—that qualia are fictions, posited to explain consciousness within a fundamentally flawed theory of perception—seems quite radical. However, several commentators suggest that enactivism amounts to nothing more than an alternative functionalism about qualitative perceptual consciousness (Gray, 2003; Manzotti, 2001). Noë and Hurley's (2003) response to these comments seems to tacitly acknowledge enactivism's functionalist nature. They object only to the possible implications that enactivism constitutes an a priori analysis of qualitative perceptual experiences, and that behaviors constitute the sole functional relata of enactivism (Noë and Hurley, 2003, p. 195) Similarly, O&N respond to commentators by asserting:

> Our view thus allows for the judgment that creatures with radically different kinds of physical make up can enjoy an experience which is, to an important degree, the same in content and quality. But it also allows for the possibility (indeed, the necessity) that where there are physical differences, there are also qualitative differences. To this extent, our proposal deviates from classical functionalism. That is, we are rejecting a certain way of thinking about the multiple-realizability of functional systems. (O'Regan and Noë, 2001, p. 1013)

However, as a form of functionalism, enactivists face the familiar problem of why functional relations give rise to experience at all (see Harnad, 2001; Kurthen, 2001; Manzotti, 2001; Oberauer, 2001), as well as the two problems—chauvinism and liberalism—so well illustrated by Ned Block (Block, 1993).[3] Indeed, enactivists reject charges that their view allows (1) functionally equivalent zombies (absent qualia/liberalism) (see Block, 2001; Clark and Toribio, 2001); (2) creatures who lack the appropriate functional relations but still plausibly have qualitative conscious experiences (chauvinism—see following) (see Goodale, 2001; Koch, 2004; Revonsuo, 2001);[4] (3) creatures whose physical bodies and SMCs are type-identical but whose experiences differ qualitatively (inversion/type-identity cases); and (4) the difficulties of determining type-identity across large and small functional differences (see Clark and Toribio, 2001).

Even if one grants the enactivist argument banishing the conception of qualia as intrinsic properties of experiential states, one does not thereby excise the qualitative dimension of experience. Nor do enactivists deny or downplay the phenomenal aspects of experiences. In fact, they go to great pains to point out that they are not behaviorists, despite similarities between their position and behavioristic treatments of perception, and they attempt to draw support for their view from phenomenological reflection. However, neither appeal to rationally guided skillful manipulation of SMCs, the temporally extended nature of experience, nor any other resource of the enactivist position satisfactorily explains the qualitative dimension of experience (on the understanding of explanation typically at work in the consciousness debates). That is, the enactivist position seems to neither rule out nor answer the questions: Why should an extended sequence of perceptual exploration guided by knowledge of SMCs result in any phenomenology at all? Is it not possible that you and I could be absolutely alike along all the relevant enactivist criteria while having systematically inverted qualitative experiences? Thus, one can recast all the familiar intuitions about the conceivability of zombies and inverted qualia in terms that make them applicable to enactivism.

O&N clearly recognize the difficulty these questions pose, and they struggle to work out a complete response (see their remarks in O'Regan and Noë, 2001, pp. 1011–1012). Ultimately, many enactivists appear to abandon the pursuit of a solution to the hard problem in favor of lesser problems in that neighborhood. For example, Hurley and Noë (2003a) claim that they have a story about "comparative explanatory gaps," but they think it is a further question whether enactivism says anything helpful about the "absolute explanatory gap" (2003a, p. 132). An inability to explain the individuation of the senses or the individuation of perceived attributes within a modality results in a comparative explanatory gap, whereas an inability to explain why there is any experience at all results in the absolute explanatory gap.

We have only briefly discussed the enactivists' account of intermodal and attribute individuation. Perhaps enactivism is on the right track about intermodal and attribute individuation—that is up for further examination. However, the absolute explanatory gap about consciousness agitates many philosophers and scientists. Moreover, comparative explanatory gaps, one might argue, are what Chalmers (1996) labels "easy problems" of consciousness. According to Chalmers, one ought not assume that answers to the easy problems provide any inroads into the truly hard problem of consciousness, that is, the absolute explanatory gap. Indeed, Noë remarks that he has "to take a *little bit* of consciousness for granted" (2004, p. 230) in developing his enactivist theory, indicating that he does not take enactivism to offer a solution to the absolute explanatory gap.[5] Thus, despite O&N's (2001) bold claims and O'Regan's more recent comments (Philapona and O'Regan, 2006, p. 338), we find no reason to suppose that enactivism either solves or significantly advances thinking on the tough core of the problem of consciousness.

Even if one has sympathies with enactivism's criticisms of brain-based approaches to consciousness, one need not turn to enactivism as the sole alternative. The enactivist's strategy for addressing the explanatory gap—that is, as arising from misconceived worries about the connection between brain states and the qualitative character of experience—has much in common with the work of externalist representationalists about consciousness (see Dretske, 1995; Lycan, 2001; Tye, 2000). For example, Michael Tye writes: "Peer as hard as you like at the neurons. Probe deeper and deeper into the structure of the brain. According to the PANIC theory [Tye's externalist representationalist theory of phenomenal consciousness], you will not find any phenomenology. It simply is not there" (1995, p. 162). By tracing the genesis of phenomenology to factors outside the head, both externalist representationalists and enactivists offer similar explanations of the persistent shortcomings of brain-based accounts of consciousness: Brain-based research is searching in the wrong place. One must look beyond brain activity to discover what kind of experience a creature is having.

Of course, while both representationalists and enactivists reject the notion of qualia as intrinsic properties of experiences, there are crucial differences between the views. Representationalists retain the more traditional model of conscious states as brain states and felt qualities as properties of those states—specifically, a species of representational content. Representationalists deviate from brain-based views in advocating externalist theories of content that individuate content and phenomenal character through a subject's causal interactions with the environment. In contrast, enactivists insist that conscious experience emerges from ongoing, body-involving, skillful interaction with the environment—demoting the brain to one of many elements in an ongoing process. Although the status of phenomenal representationalism goes well beyond the scope of this chapter, its significance here lies in the fact that one can attempt to abandon the idea that the felt qualities of experience are intrinsic properties of experiences, without altogether forsaking talk of representations and going down the enactivists' neo-Gibsonian route. Thus, even if one ranks solving or disposing of the hard problem very high when evaluating competing theories, there is no reason to assume that enactivism has an "only game in town" advantage on that score. Of course, enactivists will also argue that there are certain important phenomena that can be explained only on their approach. Nevertheless, the availability of alternative explanations as well as the standard challenges for functionalist accounts compromises the enactivists' basis for claiming that their view successfully deals with issues of consciousness on which other approaches necessarily stumble.

3.2. The Denial of Representations

The second conceptual strength claimed for enactivism by its advocates is simplicity of explanation. As noted in the introduction, one can construe passive vision research as structuring all visual tasks in terms of a highly detailed, picture-like internal representation of the distal scene that the subject first constructs from retinal input through a cumulative series of computationally and representationally intensive operations. This approach faces difficulties in terms of the sheer resource demands such a construction places on the subject, even in performing the simplest task. Other difficulties emerge in so far as subjects seem to lack the sort of information or abilities passive vision predicts. Many active vision theorists suggest that a perceiver's actions—as opposed to elaborate, picture-like internal representations—can greatly simplify or even dispel such problems.

However, enactivists appear to use the potential simplicity of action-based explanations of various specific phenomena to argue against the existence of all—or nearly all—representations in perception:

> The answer to these [passive vision] questions, I have claimed here, is that
> they need not be posed at all. Like the concept of the "ether" in physics at the
> beginning of the century, the questions evaporate if we abandon the idea that
> "seeing" involves passively contemplating an internal representation of the world
> that has metric properties like a photograph or scale model. (O'Regan, 1992,
> p. 485)
>
> Under the present theory, visual experience does not arise because an
> internal representation of the world is activated in some brain area.... Indeed,
> there is no "re"-presentation of the world inside the brain: the only pictorial or
> 3D version required is the real outside version. (O'Regan and Noë, 2001,
> p. 946)
>
> We break with the orthodox view by proposing a framework within
> which vision, rather than being a process whereby the brain produces detailed
> representations of what is experienced, is taken to be an activity of exploring the
> environment drawing on sensorimotor skills. (Noë, 2005, p. 218)

The heart of the enactivist argument against representations lies in the supposition that "seeing constitutes an active process of probing the external environment as though it were a continuously available *external memory*" (O'Regan, 1992, p. 487). Sampling the environment can facilitate or simplify cognitive tasks. For example, consistent visual feedback via the dentate and lateral interposed deep cerebellar nuclei facilitates both the learning and execution of motor movements, such as aiming movements (Cheng, Tremblay, and Luis, 2007; Georgopoulos et al., 2000; Goodkin and Thach, 2003a, 2003b; Grierson and Elliott, 2007; Sober and Sabes, 2005; Xing and Andersen, 2000). However, to effectively use the world as an external memory, a cognizer must have some internal index of that environment. Absent such an internally represented index of the external memory, the cognizer would have to resort to random search of its external memory. The idea that "the world functions in cognition as continuously available *external memory*" provides no comfort to someone who has lost her keys. Likewise, perceivers must represent contingent features important to the task. As Singh and Hoffman note:

Consider the perceptually guided task of playing professional basketball. One must keep track of one's four teammates, the five opponents, two baskets, the ball, the coach, and a stand full of noisy fans. The burden is on advocates of the activity-based approach to show how this task can be accomplished with minimal representations. (1998, p. 771)

Additional difficulties for enactivism's across-the-board rejection of representation emerge when one contemplates tasks in which skillful exploration of the perceptual environment does not appear to facilitate performance. For instance, one of the hallmarks of object recognition is that cognizers regularly and reliably recognize objects from a single viewpoint, across different rotations and distances, in cases of partial occlusion, and despite considerable signal noise, such as blurring or shading. Moreover, the two prominent views of object recognition, structural-description (Biederman, 1987) and image-description (Riesenhuber and Poggio, 1999) models, though both heavily representational, have real-time, computationally tractable models (Hummel, 1994; Hummel and Biederman, 1992; Serre et al., 2007).

To invoke action in otherwise static object recognition, enactivists must resort to saccades. However, appealing to saccades introduces nothing new or revelatory into object recognition theories. For instance, more than twenty years ago Gouras compared saccades to "a hand which rubs across the contours in order to enhance their contrast" (1984, p. 229). Worse still, to handle object recognition from single, static viewpoints, enactivists must build all the needed information about rotation, object occlusion, and signal noise required for object recognition into nonrepresentational knowledge of SMCs.

Such enactivist object recognition proposals raise two difficulties. First, since O&N define sensorimotor contingencies as "the *structure of the rules* governing the sensory changes produced by various motor actions" (2001, p. 941), SMCs do not seem to be the proper sort of knowledge needed in cases like object recognition where more often than not there is no motor actions and no sensory changes. For example, the "visual quality of shape is precisely the set of all potential distortions that the shape undergoes when it is moved relative to us, or when we move relative to it" (O'Regan and Noë, 2001, p. 942) seems of little help in detecting shapes absent movement. Second, enactivists belie the basis of their claimed explanatory simplicity by requiring large amounts of stored know-how in the brain. That is, the enactivists' antirepresentationalist argument declares all such knowledge stores unnecessary in that "seeing constitutes an active process of probing the external environment as though it were a continuously available *external memory*" (O'Regan, 1992, p. 487).

One might suspect that we treat the enactivist unfairly above. However, O'Regan's (1992) discussion of object recognition employs both saccades as actions and knowledge of SMCs as the mechanisms for recognition. In fact, O'Regan's proposal for pattern and object recognition seems to require that subjects know a great deal of SMCs, and structures object recognition in a manner derivative on Biederman's (1987) R-B-C theory:

> For discriminating patterns therefore, only a small battery of simple components
> or features may suffice in most cases, and providing these have been learnt
> at many retinal positions and in many sizes and orientations, then most
> new patterns can be classified by using these features, and by noting in what
> approximate spatial relationships they lie. (1992, p. 485)

Thus, we suggest that without further details, there appears to be no reason to grant assessments of relative simplicity (or originality) to O'Regan's enactivist object recognition account when compared to current representational theories.

So the enactivist's apparent rejection of representational accounts of perceptual task performance in favor of an external memory account seems to run afoul of two problems. First, using the world as an external memory can only simplify perceptual tasks in so far as memory utilization is neither random nor itself a significant representationally and computationally intensive cognitive task. Second, appeals to nonrepresentational know-how of SMCs will not necessarily simplify cognitive tasks nor offer significant new insights into the performance of such tasks.

3.3. Reconceptualizing the Reconceptualizations

We claim that enactivists "appear" to reject the idea that representations play an integral role in visual (and other) perception because their statements of their view on representations strike us as tergiversatory. For instance, against the backdrop of the explicit antirepresentational quotes in the last section, one also finds the following sorts of modest/ambiguous statements:

> We argue not that there are no representations, but that the category
> "representation" should be demoted within the context of visual theory.....Do
> subjects experience this represented detail, as some have suggested? Empirical and
> conceptual progress is needed to answer this question. (Noë, 2005, p. 218)

We suspect that the contrast between these quotations and those in the previous section derives largely from the difficulties faced by enactivism in explaining a wide array of visual phenomena without appeal to representations. Indeed, another general area of concern in understanding and evaluating enactivist claims regarding their reconceptualization of perception and perceptual consciousness is the apparent inconsistency with which various advocates of enactivism sometimes characterize their view.

On some ways of understanding enactivism—certainly the most headline-grabbing way of putting things, and one that (if true) would be the basis for a massive rethinking of perception research—perceptual experience is constituted by skilled, body-involving activity. Other passages suggest that sensorimotor skills, though essential to perceptual experience, can be exercised in ways not involving bodily activity, implying that enactivism is not quite as radical as its proponents proclaim. Yet other statements seem consistent with the idea that perceptual experience is neither body-involving nor temporally extended, but can be affected by one's sensorimotor know-how. If enactivism amounts to the latter view, there is little to recommend it as revolutionary. Getting clear on enactivism's actual commitments, or conversely, recognizing whether enactivists have constructed a moving target—one sure to frustrate any attempt at constructive critical engagement with their view—is central to a full appraisal of the enactivist challenge to mainstream perception research.

Readers can begin to appreciate the variation in enactivists' statements about the role of sensorimotor skills in perceptual experience by considering the following quotes.

- "However, sensorimotor theories of perception suggest that, on the contrary, the transformations created by action in the sensory input are a necessary condition for all perception" (Bompas and O'Regan, 2006, p. 65).
- "To model vision correctly...we must model it not as something that takes place inside the animal's brain, but as something that directly involves not only the brain but also the animate body and the world" (Noë, 2004, p. 30).
- "[We] have taken the bolder step of actually identifying color *experience* with the exercise of these laws [of sensorimotor contingency], or, more precisely, with activity carried out in accord with the laws and based on knowledge of the laws" (O'Regan and Noë, 2001, p. 952; emphasis in original).
- "According to the dynamic sensorimotor view, perceptual experience *is a skillful activity*, in part constituted by such practical know-how" (Hurley and Noë, 2003a, p. 146; emphasis in original).
- "What determines the perceived quality of sensations...are intrinsic features of the overall constraints imposed on the interaction of the organism with its environment" (Philapona and O'Regan, 2006, p. 338).
- "Seeing an object consists precisely in the knowledge of the relevant SMCs— that is, in being able to exercise mastery" (O'Regan and Noë, 2001, p. 968).
- "The work of the enactive approach is done by perceivers' *expectations* of the sensory effects of movement" (Noë, 2004, p. 119; emphasis in original).

Although perhaps not perfectly arranged in terms of a decreasing commitment to the role of the body and action in perceptual experience, these passages epitomize the inconstant manner in which enactivists communicate their view. We contend that one source of the disconsonant elements in the enactivist literature stems from enactivism's uneasy relationship with certain empirical findings, none of which offer clear support for the most extreme characterizations of the view, and several of which are deeply at odds with such characterizations. These tensions should emerge at various points in the following sections.

4. EVIDENCE CITED IN SUPPORT OF ENACTIVISM

Enactivists have coopted a long list of empirical findings to support their theories. In this section, we consider just three cases: prismatic adaptation, visual development, and color perception. Our choice of examples is driven largely by the fact that we feel we have novel contributions to make in these cases. We encourage readers to look at the many commentaries on other empirical evidence cited by enactivists. For example, we view Simons and Rensink's (2005a, 2005b) papers on change blindness as excellent discussions of that topic.

4.1. Prismatic Adaptation

Some of the most widely discussed claims of empirical support for enactivism concern the enactivists' interpretation of a select subset of experiments from the literature on visual adaptation and development (Bompas and O'Regan, 2006; Noë, 2004; O'Regan and Noë, 2001). Indeed, Noë (2004) asserts that prismatic adaptation constitutes an uncontentious crucial experiment verifying enactivism. Specifically, prismatic adaptation produces experiential blindness—a phenomenon predicted by enactivism and in direct contradiction to traditional views of visual perception (Noë, 2004). Though often repeated, these claims represent to us perhaps the most disappointing enactivist contributions to the debate on perception. We find two general difficulties with enactivist research in this area. First, the enactivist interpretation of the experimental data strikes us a deeply flawed. Second, the SMC account enactivists offer for experiential blindness in prismatic adaptation seems to falter both with regard to the specific features of prismatic adaptation, as well as a wide variety of much more mundane cases of analogous perceptual alterations.

Noë begins one discussion of prismatic inversion by claiming that "The initial effect of inverting glasses of this sort is not an inversion of the content of experience (an inversion of what is seen) but rather a partial disruption of seeing itself" (2004, pp. 7–8). He concludes this discussion saying:

> To summarize, experiential blindness exists and is important for two reasons. First, it lends support for the enactive view. Genuine perceptual experience depends not only on the character and quality of stimulation, but on our exercise of sensorimotor knowledge.... For mere sensory stimulation to constitute perceptual experience—that is, for it to have genuine world-presenting content—the perceiver must possess and make use of *sensorimotor knowledge*. (2004, p. 10)

We see no obvious way to reconcile either of the two quoted claims—particularly the second one's tacit admission that individuals continue to have qualitative experiences in inversion—with earlier quoted claims that "the qualitative character of experience" or "visual sensitivity" arises only through making use of sensorimotor knowledge. Worse still, the debate regarding this issue improperly focuses upon a small handful of articles (primarily Kohler 1951), largely ignoring the body of literature on prismatic adaptation since Taylor's 1962 book (Bedford, 1999; Guigon and Baraduc, 2002; Kohler, 1963; Redding, Rossetti, and Wallace, 2005; Redding and Wallace, 2006a, 2006b; Stratton, 1897; Taylor, 1962; Wolgin, Hein, and Teitelbaum, 1980). The prismatic literature clearly notes that one can disrupt one's sensorimotor knowledge in systematic ways without affecting the qualitative nature of experience. For instance, Bedford (2007, personal communication) comments that "if the question is *must one* have visual distortions/spatial problems/conscious awareness [with prismatic goggles], the answer is definitely no." Redding likewise indicates that

> prismatic displacement has no effect on the experience of objects or their relationships. . . . Subjects usually do not have conscious experience of the displacement and unless or until they bump into a wall or miss reach for an object they do not know anything has changed. Even then, virtually no subject I have ever tested in a free ranging situation can say exactly what the prisms do without prompting. They do sometimes notice some other minor effects of the prisms like "rainbows" along contrast lines and small shearing of shapes as they move their head.
>
> These comments extend to the adapted condition after having worn the prisms for some time and with the prisms still on. Subjects only know that they don't make the same behavioral errors. Their conscious visual experiences are normal in every way. Similarly, when the prisms are removed the short lived aftereffects are only experienced via performance errors. (2007, personal communication)

Of equal importance, O&N's claims regarding inversion represent an inference from the fact that a visual distortion of *some kind* occurs to some significant degree of verification for enactivism. However, enactivism—even in its current schematic state—makes quite specific predictions regarding the nature of experiential blindness that do not seem to be verified by the experiments O&N cite. Because one's qualitative experiences supposedly arise from using one's sensorimotor knowledge, disruptions to specific elements of that knowledge should result in at least a failure of the corresponding specific aspects of qualitative experiences. For instance, inversion belies all or nearly all sensorimotor knowledge guiding vertical movement. Enactivism thus predicts total loss—at least severe impairment of—qualitative experiences of vertical spatial relations. But this does not happen.

One needn't don prismatic goggles to experience dramatic spatial transpositions invalidating aspects of one's sensorimotor knowledge, and thus judge for oneself whether O&N accurately characterize the consequences thereof. The same sorts of spatial transpositions—left for right—are experienced by people every day when they look into mirrors. One might suppose that one has the relevant sensorimotor knowledge for mirrors, but try holding some text up to the mirror. One has a great deal of trouble reading the text, so one presumably lacks some sensorimotor knowledge. Yet the qualitative experiences of the spatial relations in the text remain unaffected. Moreover, one can learn to read, draw, and so on, using mirror images, but one does not thereby switch the dimensional qualities of one's perceptions of mirrored images and text. Nor does one experience total failure of letter and word recognition when one turns this text upside down (both vertical and horizontal transpositions).

In fact, O&N's SMC hypothesis appears impotent to explain the apparent robust perceptual experiences in such relatively common but comparable SMC-violating perceptual situations, such as funhouse mirrors, standing on one's hands, and so on. Thus, O&N's enactivist hypothesis seems to make false predictions—even given their incorrect interpretation of the prismatic adaptation data. Furthermore, O&N's enactivist hypothesis cannot explain related perceptual alteration phenomena. I may have difficulties shuffling cards or mixing drinks while hanging in gravity boots, but I'm not experientially blind.

Finally, in none of their discussions do O&N consider any alternative explanations of any of the vaguely specified visual distortions they cite, nor do they consider the explanations on offer in the literature for prismatic adaptation. For instance, their treatment ignores the fact that prismatic goggles—especially the inversion goggles they discuss—distort the image presented to the subject. O&N likewise fail to note that the generally accepted findings of prismatic studies are that recalibration is not phenomenal, nor are subjects necessarily consciously aware of recalibration. O&N also fail to acknowledge the widely accepted general theory of prismatic adaptation that supposes that after a period of cognitively adapting to the goggles (i.e., consciously reasoning if I want to reach "up," I have to move my hand down) spatial information explicitly represented in one modality is used to recalibrate spatial maps in another modality. That is, perceptual representations from one modality are used to recalibrate the perceptual representations of another.

For example, Bedford tells readers that "research has suggested that there is a preference for changes in space perception that shift space rigidly everywhere, that shrink or expand space uniformly, and that preserve the one-to-one relationship between modalities. (1999, p. 4). Bedford explains these change preference facts by positing two things. (1) Innate knowledge of certain constraints on objects which likewise constrain perception within a modality. Objects can only be in one place at one time—to take a case. (2) When systematic, relatively coherent experiences in one modality (vision) misrepresent the world in ways detectable in another modality (touch), that is, by violating these innate constraints, then the brain uses information from the latter modality to recalibrate the representational schema of the former modality.

4.2. Visual Development

Similar difficulties of interpretation infect O&N's discussions of Held and Hein's (1963) kittens. Susan Blackmore (2001) suggests that O&N's theory predicts that dissociating vision from sensorimotor activity results in blindness in the sense of a failure of qualitative perceptual experiences. O&N agree, citing a single paper by Held and Hein as a case where a limited version of this "blindness" occurs (O'Regan and Noë, 2001, p. 1020). Discussion of the kitten case in the literature seems to accept O&N's assertion and never cites any other experiments within this paradigm (which is within the same area of research as prismatic adaptation) (Bauer and Held, 1975; Block, 2005; Edelman, 2006; Hein and Diamond, 1971, 1972; Hein and Held, 1967; Hein, Held, and Gower, 1970; Held and Bauer, 1967, 1974; Held and Hein, 1963; Jacobson, 2007; Prinz, 2006). Prinz (2006), for instance, claims that the experiments were never reproduced. O&N appear to interpret Held and Hein's experiment as demonstrating a failure of depth perception resulting from a failure to have qualitative experiences of depth. But Held and Hein never claim that the kittens are blind to depth or lack qualitative depth experiences. In fact, the hypothesis they are testing is that the kittens need to coordinate their existing perceptual spatial maps with motor maps by being active. This is certainly true of Held's later monkey work and Hein's later kitten work (op. cit. plus Blakemore, Van Sluyters, Peck, and Hein, 1975). Moreover, Held and Hein note that eye blink and paw placement—both indicators of depth perception—are manifested by kittens in the passive experimental group (no self-movement, only visual stimulation) after approximately 31 hours in the apparatus. Because the only data presented by Held and Hein (1963) that is suggestive of lack of depth perception is the visual cliff, O&N need the visual cliff to represent a clear-cut test of depth perception. However, work with children has shown that avoidance of the visual cliff takes place as a function of developing a fear of heights and after developing depth perception (Campos, Hiatt, Ramsay, Henderson, and Svejda, 1978; Campos et al., 2000; Witherington, Campos, Anderson, Lejeune, and Seah, 2005). Moreover, depth perception in infants appears to emerge in response to object properties that do not require movement of the subject (like object motion relative to background, size constancy), and prior to 7 months when infants usually learn to crawl (Imura et al., 2006; Welchman, Deubelius, Conrad, Bülthoff, and Kourtzi, 2005; Yonas and Granrud, 2006). Held's work with monkeys leads him to claim "that sight of the moving hand is responsible for calibrating the metrical relation between the space of vision and that of reaching" (Bauer and Held, 1975, p. 307). Finally, work by Walk, Shepherd, and Miller (1988) seems to suggest attention to the environment—not self-produced motion—is the key factor in depth perception in kittens.

We conclude, therefore, that the claims of support for enactivism in both prismatic adaptation and visual development data are unfounded. In fact, the enactivist claims represent deeply flawed interpretations of the scientific literature, ignorance of vast amounts of that literature, failure to consider alternative explanations of cited results—including the widely accepted theories within the literature—and a failure to correctly characterize the predications of enactivism to properly evaluate support for the theory—even given O&N's flawed interpretation of the data. We end this section by discussing a more recent enactivist attempt to support their theory using color perception.

4.3. Color and What's in the Light

The use of sensory terms in many of the quoted enactivist statements threatens circularity for the view. Clearly, if those terms are understood in their natural way, as involving or being equivalent to experience, the account is viciously circular: We would have before us an account of the content of one's current experience in terms of other experiences one might have, which would need to be accounted for in terms of yet other potential experiences, and so on. As Ned Block notes, Noë (2004) is aware of the potential circularity and has in mind a technical understanding of terms such as *look* and *appearance*, one on which they are objective (see, for example, Noë, 2004, p. 85). Additionally, many of the passages discussing sensorimotor knowledge quoted before are stated in terms of sensory stimulation or sensory input, providing ample room for enactivists to avoid charges of circularity. What is required, however, is an account of sensory input that fits the bill. In particular, it will provide for the various relations of similarity and difference, including constancy and contrast phenomena, between perceptual qualities that play such a central role in the discussion of discriminatory abilities, without being pitched at the level of experience.

Using color as an example to study this issue, Noë contends that color is neither a purely subjective property (i.e., one that exists only as a property of or encountered in experiences) nor a purely physical property of objects (i.e., one that is typeidentifiable with a structure specified in terms of kinds drawn from physical theory). Rather, color is a relational property that is defined by the interaction between objects and their environments. The particularly Gibsonian nature of this account emerges when Noë writes that "colors are ways objects act on the ambient optic array, namely, the light-filled, structured environment" (2004, p. 155). In keeping with much ecological theorizing about perception, Noë (2004, pp. 155–156) tells readers that environments consist not simply of configurations of the physical world alone but are also determined by a creature's standpoint on the world—the perspective dictated by the creature's sensory, cognitive, and motor capacities. Thus the world contains multiple, variously overlapping environments corresponding to the nonequivalent viewpoints of different kinds of creatures. So, applied to color, the idea in a nutshell is this: Colors exist as part of one's environment, and to the extent that one employs mastery of the ways that movement of objects or oneself (the perceiver) would alter certain properties of the light, one experiences the colors of things.

Although Noë has little more to say about the particulars of the relationship between objects, perceivers, and the effects of action on the light given our various capacities, O'Regan, in collaboration with David Philipona (Philipona and O'Regan, 2006, henceforth P&O), offers an account of various color phenomena. P&O ground their account entirely in "accessible information" in the light, to the exclusion of neural processing beyond the retina; that is, they explicitly deny the brain basis of the color phenomena treated. For P&O (2006, p. 332), the accessible information "about a light [is] the restricted information about the spectral composition of that light which is accessible through an organism's photopigment set"; in the case of normal human color perceivers, the long-, medium, and short- wavelength cones. P&O are quite clear that their focus is the cone quantum catch and not something dependent on subsequent neural coding or processing (2006, p. 332), and they make statements about their account's prospects for banishing the standard explanatory concerns about consciousness very similar to those found throughout the enactivist literature (2006, p. 338).

The mathematical details of P&O's account are quite complex and deserving of extended discussion elsewhere (see Johnson and Wright, 2008). But for our present purposes we focus on P&O's argument that there is a linear relationship between information about the illuminant and the information about the light reflected by a surface. Simplifying their mathematical treatment, surfaces turn out to have properties of reflecting light at each of three noninteracting "components" of the light. Because of the linear relationship between the accessible information about the reflected light and that of the illuminant, once both are known, it is a simple matter to solve for (i.e., recover) the surface's properties of reflecting light at those three components—in P&O's framework, its "reflectance coefficients." The color experience elicited when viewing a surface is tied to the surface's pattern of reflectance along the three dimensions of the light (2006, p. 338). To have a certain color experience, it seems, requires that one possess and exercise mastery of how changes in the arrangement between the currently viewed surface, the illuminant, or one's sensory equipment alter the accessible information in the light.

Crucially, P&O claim that although most surfaces reflect light along all three directions of the accessible information space, certain surfaces reflect light along only one or two directions. These latter surfaces score highly on P&O's "singularity index." A surface's singularity index is computed by first ordering its three reflection coefficients from highest to lowest and then taking the maximum from the ratios of the highest to the middle and the middle to the lowest (2006, p. 334). As special cases, surfaces with high singularity scores figure prominently in explanations of a wide range of data, with considerable emphasis placed on color naming. That all this could be achieved without invoking cortical representations would be a significant boost to the enactivist program, although it would not by itself entail that enactivists are right about the brain not being the ultimate locus of experience.

A plot of the singularity index values for the Munsell chips used as the stimulus array in the World Color Survey (WCS) bears a resemblance to a plot of data from the WCS (see figure 11.1).

A few clarifying remarks are in order. The WCS followed up on a far greater scale the color naming research of Berlin and Kay (1969), studying in the field 110 unwritten languages in nonindustrialized societies (see Cook, Kay, and Regier, 2005). The Munsell chips are a set of colored papers, organized around the concepts of hue, value, and chroma, and they are used in industrial, artistic, and scientific settings; the WCS stimulus array employs only a fraction of the chips included in the full Munsell set. P&O describe their plot of WCS data in terms of the number of speakers who have a name for a chip, which might suggest a color naming task. In the WCS color naming task (which differs from that of the original Berlin and Kay, 1969, study), subjects were presented each of the 330 Munsell chips in the stimulus array (40 equally spaced hues at eight levels of lightness, plus ten achromatic chips) one by one and were instructed to name each chip with as simple an expression as possible. Field workers determined "basic color terms" from the naming responses. A language's basic color terms form the smallest set of simple terms that could be used to name any color. In the focal choice task, for each of their language's basic

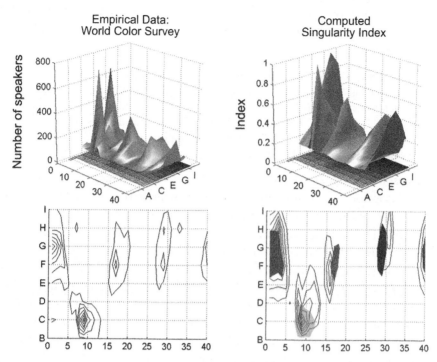

Figure 11.1. Plots of WCS focal choice data (left) and calculated singularity index scores for the Munsell chips used as the WCS stimulus array (right). On the axes representing the stimulus array, letters correspond to levels of lightness and numbers correspond to hue steps. Each contour in the WCS plot represents an increment of 100 speakers who selected a particular chip as a best exemplar of one of his or her basic color terms. The scale of the contours in the singularity index plot is not provided by Philipona and O'Regan. *Source:* Philipona and O'Regan (2006), figure 3, p. 335.

color terms, participants were to select a particular chip as being the best exemplar of that term. Although P&O do not specify in their text the source of the WCS plot in their figure, since their contour plot for the WCS data looks just like (aside from the order of the labels on the lightness axis and sizing differences) plots of WCS focus color data (e.g., figure 2 of Regier, 2007) and differs from plots of WCS color naming data (e.g., figure 4 of Kay and Regier, 2003), it is safe to say that the plot they are working with is of focal choice data.

About the relationship between the WCS focal choice data and the singularity index scores for the WCS stimuli, P&O write:

> The chips most often given a name by widely separated human cultures... and which we call "red", "yellow", "green", and "blue"' in English, can be seen to be within one chip of those having maximally singular reflecting properties.... It could thus be argued that the reason the colors "red", "yellow", "green", and "blue" are so often singled out among all other colors as being worth giving a name, is that surfaces of these colors have the particularity that they alter incoming light in a simpler way than other surfaces. (2006, pp. 335–336)

One problem that immediately arises comes from Kimberly Jameson's (in press) discussion of Rolf Kuehni's (2005) study of WCS focal color data and unique hue ranges:

> [Only] 38 out of 110 WCS languages had the linguistic glosses needed for comparison against the four unique hue ranges. In some of these 38 languages, however, more than one distinct linguistic gloss was found for unique hue categories.... In 76% of [those] 38 languages [Kuehni] considered, some participants "...had distinctly different interpretations of a given color name, as demonstrated with their choice of focal color."

Jameson also remarks in a note that "of the WCS languages that lacked linguistic glosses for one or more of the Hering primaries [i.e., red, green, blue, and yellow] many of these exhibit distinct terms for color categories considered [nonfundamental]...according to the received view." Importantly, many languages have a basic color term that covers both green and blue ("grue" terms; see Lindsey and Brown, 2002). Whatever else might be explained or suggested by the similarities between WCS focal choice data and P&O's singularity index calculations, cross-cultural color naming patterns are unlikely to be on the list. If P&O are right about the special, universal (for human color experience) nature of the Hering primaries, a lot remains to be explained about why so few languages in the WCS have basic color names that neatly match up with all four of them.

Inspection of the full WCS focal choice data presented in Cook, Kay, and Regier (2005) and Regier, Kay, and Cook (2005) raises further questions. Approximately 2,640 total speakers took part in the WCS. The peaks of the focal choice distribution, along with the number of participants who selected a particular Munsell chip as a best exemplar of one of his or her language's basic color terms are as follows.

A0: 2,048
J0: 1,988
G1: 668
C9: 752
F17: 351
F29: 253

Chips A0 and J0 are at the extreme ends of the range of achromatic Munsell chips used in the WCS and correspond to best exemplars of English "white" and "black," respectively. The remaining chips (G1, C9, F17, and F29) align well with averaged focal points for English "red," "yellow," "green," and "blue," respectively (see Cook, Kay, and Regier, 2005). As P&O (2006, p. 335) mention, the WCS focal choice peaks line up nicely with the chips having the highest scores on their singularity index: G2, C9, F16, and H31. Note, however, that H31 is two chips—and four "city blocks"—away from F29, not just one, as P&O claim.

So fewer than 30 percent of participants pick chips with singularity scores near the maximum value of 1.0 (G2 and C9) as a best exemplar. Fewer than 15 percent of participants select as best exemplars chips with singularity values in the middle of the scale (F16 and H31). Because P&O do not offer a metric to use as a standard of comparison between the WCS data and the singularities they identify, it is difficult to know what to make of this pattern or any others that might be discovered. By simply looking at reflectance coefficients and singularity index scores, there is no obvious reason why achromatic focal choices should find agreement amongst over 75 percent of participants while chromatic chips with high singularity scores have only about 15–30 percent of participants picking them as a best exemplar. In trying to understand what color naming phenomenon P&O target and assess their success, the reader is forced to rely on eyeballing the contour plots, as the similarities between the plots they provide carries a great deal of their argumentative burden. See figure 11.1. Such inspection is, of course, an unreliable guide in quantitative evaluation. It will naturally lead one to latch on to conspicuous features (such as similarities in contour peaks) and overlook more subtle or complex but perhaps crucial characteristics, such as differences in the range and slope of the contour clusters. These concerns are at the core of determining whether P&O have struck on a promising new way of doing perception research, one that—by avoiding consideration of neural pathways and cortical representations—is radically different than current mainstream approaches.

5. Enactivist Responses to Troublesome Empirical Data and Alternative Proposals

In addition to worries regarding several classes of empirical results that enactivists cite as supporting their view, we also have concerns regarding the enactivists' responses to alternative research perspectives and additional data that have emerged in the literature. In this section we consider two cases that we find troublesome both for enactivism's theoretical perspective and its methodological development.

5.1. The Sense of Coherence and Detail, and Two Visual Systems

Consider an issue that has been a focus of much recent discussion: the apparent unity of visual experience, which includes a sense of stability and awareness of the entire scene before one's eyes, over relatively long stretches of time (on the order of several seconds). It is remarkable that a sense of unity emerges despite, for example, our susceptibility to blindness for unattended large-scale changes in the visual scene, the rapid diminishing of visual acuity as eccentricity from the fovea increases, the existence of a receptorless region where the optic nerve exits the eye, the approximately 20,000 eye blinks per day, and fixation changes about three times per second. Noë includes the sense of rich detail and coherence arising under such chaotic circumstances in his characterization of "the puzzle of perceptual presence" (2004, p. 33), and he takes enactivism's solution to this puzzle as one if its virtues. Enactivists are likely correct, though by no means unique, in urging that action has a role to play in explaining the emergence a seemingly coherent and highly detailed perceptual experience. However, no matter how fascinating one finds perceptual presence, no matter how great its importance to vision research, and no matter how significant one takes action's role to be in addressing perceptual presence, perceptual presence in itself does not license one to build action into the content of all perceptual experience. Enactivists propose an account of the seeming coherence and detail of visual experience, but an alternative explanation of these aspects of vision is emerging in the literature, one with which enactivists have had very little constructive interaction.

A promising start toward accounting for our sense of "picture-like" experience can be gathered from a diverse body of work on attention, memory, visual processing, and scene perception. First, visual information acquisition is driven by the interests and needs of the perceiver and is dominated by a "fixate and saccade" strategy. We cycle through periods of stationary viewing (typically, around 300 ms) followed by brief eye movements (typically, less than 50 ms) to a different location for another period of stationary viewing; movements of the head and body can also be used to fixate relevant scene elements (see Land and Nilson). Second, preattentive processing provides abstract information about semantic and structural aspects of the scene (e.g., gist, spatial layout) that can be used to guide attention to locations or objects that are relevant to the task at hand. Third, only those elements of the visual scene that receive attention are incorporated in a spatially coherent, temporally durable representation that can be placed into visual short-term memory (VSTM). VSTM has a very limited capacity; different researchers claim it holds anywhere from one to six objects. Representations in VSTM decay, collapse, or are moved to a much larger capacity visual long-term memory (VLTM), after the withdrawal of attention from the represented scene element. Fourth, the objects in VSTM either exhaust the representation of the visual scene (see Noë, 2004; O'Regan and Noë, 2001; Rensick, 2000) or enjoy a recency advantage over representations in VLTM that might also play a role in determining the content of scene perception.[6] Fifth, because overt attention is typically engaged in natural viewing,[7] the features that are stored in memory will tend to be represented with a high degree of detail. Sixth, elements of the visual scene that do not receive attention are forgotten.

Visual experience seems so coherent and highly detailed because what we are aware of is represented in considerable detail, what we don't attend to is forgotten, we have available abstract information about the nature of the scene before our eyes (and possibly visual information about some objects and features retained even after attention is withdrawn from them), and we fixate different areas of that scene several times a second.

Regardless of the further details of how it might be developed, action is vitally important to this proposal. It enables us to usefully extend in time the process of visually acquiring information, thereby simplifying the processing load while extracting useful information about the stimulus scene. This surely has consequences for how certain aspects of vision should be understood and researched. However, it would be a mistake to conclude from research into attention, memory, and scene perception that the proper object of study in vision science is the entire organism and that brain-based approaches to studying vision are fundamentally mistaken.

Noë (2004, p. 218) commits just this mistake, claiming that because "mature human experience" is by its very nature temporally extended and dependent on dynamic access to the world, "a neural duplicate of me now, at a moment in time, won't by dint of being my duplicate, have *any* experience at all." The further implication of this and numerous other enactivist statements is that vision cannot be fruitfully studied in a disembodied way. Why should one make such a leap? It is one thing to observe that our everyday visual experience depends on temporally extended dynamic access, that our ecological success routinely hangs on how such factors shape our experience, and that conceptions of vision as exclusively passive and static hinder vision research. It is something else altogether to use those observations as the basis for a sweeping conclusion about the essential nature of visual experience and how it should be studied. Furthermore, to establish that the ultimate basis of experience lies outside the brain requires substantial argument drawn from empirical data. That is, the enactivist needs to establish not just that bodily movement is importantly implicated in visual processing; they need to demonstrate the insufficiency of certain kinds of activity in, say, motor, sensorimotor, and procedural memory brain areas alone to underpin the "active" contribution to perception.

One reason Noë (2004) offers for the rejection of the brain-based framework is the failure to this point of neuroscientists to produce anything but very primitive experiences through cortical stimulation. Not only is the alleged failure irrelevant (for one thing, it runs together issues about the admittedly quite crude current state of scientific knowledge and technology with the facts of the matter), it is false. Visual states such as illusory motion, objects, and faces can be elicited by cortical stimulation (Cohen and Newsome, 2004; Edelman, 2006; Lee, Hong, Seo, Tae, and Hong, 2000; Liu and Newsome, 2000; Puce, Allison, and McCarthy, 1999).

Regarding the enactivist's concerns about traditional perception research, *of course* natural viewing is different from presentations "in a flash." But it does not follow that laboratory findings stemming from the latter lack ecological validity and that only more natural, active settings could produce ecologically valid results. What does follow is that one must be cautious about drawing wide-ranging conclusions from reductionistic experiments. The same goes for experiments involving more natural stimuli. A great deal of work will be needed to weave together the results of such studies with research employing, for example, free viewing of complex scenes, in a way that facilitates progress on broader, more complicated issues (McCrone, 2004).[8] As Julian Hochberg notes, we "need to study successful and unsuccessful viewing…over multiple glances, just as we need research on effects of stimulus information within a single presentation" (2002, p. 108). We find it unproblematic to set as a long-range goal of vision science the development of an account of vision's role in everyday life vastly more complex than accounts of anything encountered in the laboratory. However, it is common practice for scientists across a range of disciplines to begin their assault on problems of such great scale by studying simple phenomena in highly controlled settings until those phenomena become well understood. Once researchers achieve the prerequisite understanding of these causally isolated simple phenomena through achievements like success in constructing predictive mathematical models and in controlling the target system, synthesis can begin (Regan, 2000, p. 4, n. 1).[9] The accumulation of such successes enables researchers to tackle increasingly complex phenomena through the combined insights gained through the mastery of their component elements. One benefit of such a step-wise approach lies in its division of labor. Typically, separate groups of researchers investigate different "simple" aspects of the system of interest. Vision research currently exhibits just such a fragmentation (Simons and Rensink, 2005a, 2005b; Velichkovsky, Joos, Helmert, and Pannasch, 2005). As simpler cases become well understood, researchers taking on more complex phenomena can further elaborate existing models to capture greater complexity or combine models of multiple simple elements to guide their research, for example, to generate quantitative predictions about the behavior of a more complex phenomenon. This is not to say that such an approach guarantees useful combinations of models will emerge without considerable effort. We suggest only that such practices maximize the chances of a steady (if slow) increase in our knowledge.

5.2. Enactivism and the Dual Systems Hypothesis

One example of the cumulative model building[10] approach in the empirical literature is the dual visual systems hypothesis of Melvyn Goodale and A. David Milner (2005) that has been much discussed in relation to enactivism. In brief, the dual systems hypothesis claims that the anatomically separate ventral and dorsal streams of visual processing are also functionally separate; the former underlies conscious visual experience, and the latter handles visuomotor processing (see figure 11.2). Milner and Goodale's hypothesis draws heavily on their work with subjects who have suffered injuries to either the ventral or dorsal visual systems, and whose resulting behavior exhibits a dissociation between "vision for perception" and "vision for action."

For example, subjects who suffer ventral stream damage can develop visual form agnosia. Such agnosic subjects manifest a severely compromised ability to visually discriminate and identify objects, shapes, and patterns. Despite a profound deficit in their conscious visual experience, some visual form agnosics, such as Milner and Goodale's subject DF, exhibit surprisingly well-preserved visuomotor abilities. DF exhibits severely impaired visual object recognition and cannot even reliably report the size, orientation, shape, or relative position of different objects in allocentric space. Nevertheless, DF exhibits fluent visually guided prehension and obstacle avoidance during locomotion (Carey, Dijkerman, Murphy, Goodale, and Milner, 2006; Goodale, 1998, 2001; Goodale, Jakobson, and Keillor, 1994; Goodale and Milner, 2005; James, Culham, Humphrey, Milner, and Goodale, 2003; Murphy, Racicot, and Goodale, 1996; Palta and Goodale, 1996). Conversely, optic ataxics, like IG, suffer unilateral or bilateral dorsal stream damage. As a result, ataxics exhibit decreased or altered performance in visuomotor tasks. For instance, ataxics exhibit deficits in visually guided reaching and grasping using the contralesional hand (the "hand effect") as well as visually guided reaching or grasping for targets in the contralesional visual field (the "field effect") using either hand. Some evidence suggests that ataxics exhibit deficits in spatial integration of proprioceptive information from the contralesional arm. In clinical settings optic ataxics exhibit a range of visuomotor deficits ranging from somewhat mild problems—like increased action initiation latency, abnormal hand trajectories, increased variability in motion endpoints, tendency to reach to one side, and abnormal grip force—to more dramatic problems, such as dissociations of distance and direction control (Blangero et al., 2007; Goodale and Milner, 2005; Milner et al., 2001). Despite their deficits in visually guided prehension and locomotion, ataxic subjects are capable of making quite accurate judgments about object features such as orientation, shape, and object category in their contralesional visual field on the basis of visual experience. For example, an ataxic subject may well be capable of identifying a pencil in her contralesional visual field and describing its shape and orientation, yet prove incapable of accurately using her conscious visual experiences to guide the contralesional hand to grasp the pencil or even correctly adjust finger position, and so on, during movement to reflect the metric properties of the pencil.

Some researchers take the dissociability of visual experience from visuomotor activity exhibited by agnosic subjects like DF and ataxic subjects like IG to completely undercut enactivism (Block, 2005; Goodale, 2001). We agree that the

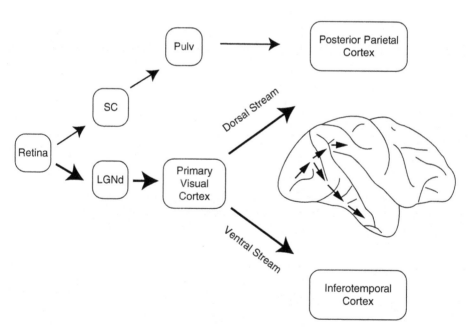

Figure 11.2. Schematic diagram of the major pathways from the retina to the inferotemporal and posterior parietal cortices in a macaque brain. SC = superior colliculus, Pulv = Pulvinar, LGNd = lateral geniculate nucleus, pars dorsalis. *Source:* Milner and Goodale (1995), figure 3.1, p. 68.

experimental findings create formidable difficulties in consistently adhering to the more provocative forms of enactivism. There are, however, weaker claims to which the enactivist can retreat.

For instance, consider the following comments on visual form agnosia and optic ataxia by O&N:

> [We are led] to doubt...Milner and Goodale's claim that what the visual agnosia patient DF...lacks is visual awareness....According to the view developed here...*people are aware of what they see to the extent that they have control over that information for the purposes of guiding action and thought.*...DF is thus a case of what would seem to be partial awareness. She is unable to describe what she sees, but she is otherwise able to use it for the purpose of guiding action. (O'Regan and Noë, 2001, p. 969; emphasis added)
>
> [From] the fact that a patient suffers optic ataxia, it doesn't follow that he or she lacks relevant sensorimotor knowledge. (Noë, 2004, p. 12)

O&N's suggestion that the agnosic DF is "partially visually aware" falsely supposes that DF's deficit is limited to object naming and that her deficit has no wider implications for the integration of her knowledge of SMCs within her broader capacities for thought and rationally guided action. Such a suggestion couldn't be farther from the truth. Likewise, Noë's claim that ataxics like IG may have the relevant sensorimotor knowledge despite visuomotor deficits proves inadequate to underwrite the robust phenomenal and cognitive experiences of ataxics. It is true that ataxics often exhibit appropriate prehensile movements in pantomime and related memory-based reaching and grasping tasks (Milner et al., 2001). However, such subtleties seem inadequate to fulfill enactivist requirements that visual sensitivity consist in "the perceptual coupling of animal and environment that consists in the animal's access to environmental detail thanks to its mastery of the relevant sensorimotor contingencies" (Noë and O'Regan, 2002, p. 569) Moreover, memory-based abilities do nothing to satisfy the requirement that visual awareness "integrate [the subject's] coupling behavior with its broader capacities for thought and rationally guided action" (ibid.).

It is tempting to suppose that either the various deficiencies of environmentally coupled or cognitively integrated visuomotor skills exhibited by optic ataxics and visual form agnosics have a constitutive role in visual experience and content, or they do not. On such a view of things, it certainly looks like O&N want to have it both ways. Noë's further remarks around this issue are of no help, as he claims: "What would undercut the enactive approach would be the existence of perception in the absence of bodily skills and sensorimotor knowledge, which, on the enactive view, are constitutive of the ability to perceive. Could there be an entirely inactive, an *inert*, perceiver?" (2004, p. 12). This simply is not to the point. Optic ataxics have certain failures in visually guiding action, but accurate visual experience, with respect to the same object features. The visual form agnosic has an impressive range of preserved control of visual information for purposes of guiding action, but a visual phenomenology that does not match that in terms of its quality. Recalling at least some of the quotes offered previously and the discussion of how perceptual attributes are to be individuated, sensorimotor know-how is not just constitutive of the ability to perceive, it is constitutive of the *content* of perceptual experience. For the enactivist, there needs to be a *match* of some sort between the content of perceptual experience and the sensorimotor skills exercised in exploring and interacting with the environment. Note too that Noë (2004, p. 86) explains misperception in terms of a subject drawing on the wrong sensorimotor skills and expectations. Such an account of misperception fits poorly both with optic ataxics' success in visual object recognition despite sometimes highly inadequate sensorimotor skills and expectations, and with the agnosic's apt sensorimotor skills despite deficits in visual object recognition. Optic ataxia and visual form agnosia belie enactivist demands for a close match between one's coupled and integrated sensorimotor knowledge and the content and nature of one's perceptual experiences.

There is a strategy for addressing this problem available for the enactivist, one that will sound familiar to those who have encountered Mrs. T (Stich, 1983). However, this maneuver pretty quickly guts enactivism of its radical claims about the essential role of action in perception and the need to study perception at the level of the environmentally embedded organism. We noted earlier that enactivism seems to be an instance of functionalism—albeit one not spelled out in terms of states and properties of states. Functionalists face severe difficulties in differentiating states in cases where only some of the typical functional roles associated with a state are present. For instance, Stich uses Mrs. T to run a paradox of the heap on functionalists, slowly removing individual beliefs or inferences until one reaches the case where Mrs. T still claims to know that McKinley was assassinated, but does not know if McKinley was murdered. As Stich notes, functionalists tend to respond to such cases by adjusting their requirements for functional differentiation—making some subset of the agent's overall functional connections necessary for differentiation. So one might claim that Mrs. T's loss of beliefs or inferences do not affect belief differentiation until she loses those beliefs or inferences constitutive of what it is to be McKinley and what it is to be assassinated.

The hard line enactivist position defines visual sensitivity in terms of the coupling of the agent and environment through a mastery of the relevant sensorimotor contingencies. They then define visual awareness in terms of the integration of that coupling with higher order thinking and rationality. Because visual form agnosia and optic ataxia violate aspects of both agent environment coupling and the integration of that coupling with thinking and rationality, enactivists can choose to adjust the extent or nature of those forms of functional connections that are necessary for perceptual experience and content. Because agent–environment coupling is the central idea of enactivism and is necessary for both visual sensitivity and visual awareness, whereas higher order integration is less central and necessary only for visual awareness, visual form agnosia seems the most amenable to the revisionist strategy. Indeed, by deprecating the significance of DF's descriptive deficits, O&N appear to be adopting just such a strategy.

We are skeptical of the enactivists' ability to cleanly separate integration from coupling in agnosia, thereby preserving coupling in such cases. Regardless, it is clear that in cases of ataxia no such coupling-sparing is possible. Here enactivists must back away from their strong claims about perception as ongoing, skilled, dynamic, bodily interaction with the environment. In fact, Noë's quote (2004, p. 12) looks very much like such a retreat. However, we don't view such a retreat as the abandonment or utter defeat of the enactivist position—though it does move perception and perceptual experience back into the head. The gist of this understanding of enactivism lies in the claim that the know-how grounding perception and perceptual content has to do with one's expectations of how *sensory input* would change, were one to move about the environment or the environment itself to change (Noë, 2004, p. 119); no demand is made that one manipulate, explore, or otherwise engage with things in one's environment. This way of putting the enactivist thesis accords well with some of the quotes listed before, but is distant from the more radical claims equating perception and perceptual experience with ongoing, skilled, dynamic, bodily interaction with the environment.

Plausibly, employing these expectations about changes in sensory input does not require that one actually move, nor that one's movements faithfully match up with the content of one's experience. Hurley and Noë (2007) explicitly adopt this sort of position, stating that perceptual experience should not be understood in terms of action mediated by dorsal stream activity and that it is not the case that "you need to move or act in order to see....We do claim that the ability to see is partly constituted by implicit knowledge of the sensory effects of movement, and that an experience is inextricably linked to understanding of the ways experience would change were one to act in various ways."

Looking back at the initial characterization of SMCs, it is clear that this sort of view is all to which the modest enactivist need be committed. The appearance of conflict with the dual systems hypothesis, and perhaps other empirical findings connected to a dissociability between perception and action, is an unfortunate artifact of remarks by enactivists themselves that go well beyond the actual substance of their position. By putting things in these more modest terms, the sensorimotor skills that can be dissociated from visual experience on the dual systems hypothesis are not the same sort of sensorimotor skills that concern enactivists. The enactivist can claim that due to her brain lesion, DF lacks or is otherwise incapable of using expectations related to object form, despite her preserved visuomotor abilities, and that optic ataxics do have access to the relevant expectations, despite the visuomotor deficits they suffer as a result of their brain lesions.

This is a far cry from slogans such as "the experience lies in the doing" (O'Regan and Noë, 2001, p. 968) and flat-footed claims about visual consciousness being a "kind of skillful activity on the part of the animal as a whole" (Noë, 2004, p. 2) strewn across the enactivist literature. Perceptual experience turns out to be far less active and body-involving than enactivists often make it out to be, because perceivers do not need to "act out" their perceptual content when exercising their expectations. In fact, it is not clear why perceivers would have to possess a body at all to acquire and make use of this sort of sensorimotor know-how. Why wouldn't patterns of brain stimulation alone—likely not just in the canonical visual system—suffice for forming and bringing to bear the relevant expectations? The resulting enactivist view looks to be centrally composed of the idea that the content of perceptual experience is entirely conceptual in nature, with the relevant perceptual concepts rooted in one's ability to anticipate changes in appearance that would result from perceiver- or object-initiated movement. This is precisely the view that Noë develops (2004, chap. 6). The plausibility of this position is largely an empirical matter, depending on whether the appropriate systems exist for facilitating this sort of conceptual contribution to perceptual experience. We address this empirical commitment later in the next section.

6. Unconsidered Neuroscience

In this section, we turn to several cases of neurological data that we feel are of significant importance to enactivism but haven't been raised with regard to enactivism. We begin with a discussion of brain-based experiences, particularly out-of-body experiences, which seem to dissociate the tight link between embodiment and perceptual experience. We then turn to considering neurological systems that might subserve enactivism's theory of perception. Specifically, we look at several candidates for systems that might provide the neural mechanism for the learning and deployment in perceptual processing of a subject's nonpropositional knowledge of SMCs. We consider the absence of any clearly articulated neurological model for this aspect of the enactivist's view an unfortunate and highly significant feature of the position some 6 years after O'Regan and Noë (2001).

6.1. Out-of-Body and Other Brain-Based Experiences

One might feel that a discussion of brain-based experiences belongs in section 5, as an instance of troublesome empirical data for enactivism. However, we argue that O&N's treatment of such cases never actually discusses the neurological evidence (O'Regan and Noë, 2001, p. 947). Indeed, we suggest that O&N's discussion commits a double equivocation: First, they mention electrical stimulation of cortical surfaces in the inferior temporal lobe and the resulting vivid experiences, but their response deals only with dreaming. Second, even their treatment of dreaming falsely equates an objection alleging chauvinism on the part of enactivism based on exclusively brain-based conscious experiences with the claim that dreaming is both pictorial and involves "pictures in the head":

We have already noted that it does not follow from the fact that dreams are pictorial that, when we dream, there are pictures in the head.... Just as we have observed that the idea that seeing is pictorial reflects a kind of naïve phenomenology of vision, it may very well be that the claim that dreaming is pictorial is similarly ill-founded phenomenologically. Certainly it is not the case that when we dream, it is as if we were looking at pictures. (O'Regan and Noë, 2001, p. 947)

In fact, there is a well-established and widely recognized empirical record of diverse and vivid, conscious perceptual experiences resulting from electrical stimulation of cortical surfaces in the inferior temporal lobe (Cohen and Newsome, 2004; Lee et al., 2000; Liu and Newsome, 2000; Mullan and Penfield, 1959; Penfield, 1955a, 1955b, 1959; Puce et al., 1999; Salzman, Britten, and Newsome, 1990). In 1938, Penfield performed neurosurgeries to remove scar tissue to alleviate the symptoms of focal epilepsy in patients. Patients remain conscious during neurosurgery and require no general anesthesia so they can accurately report their conscious experiences during such operations. To minimize collateral damage of healthy tissue, Penfield administered electrical stimulation directly to small areas of the cortical surface of the temporal lobe. He then used the verbal feedback of his patients as to effects of the stimulation to map the cortex prior to tissue removal. Penfield's surgical practice allowed him to explore and map large regions of the neocortex, particularly the temporal lobe. He observed and reported that electrical stimulation during neurosurgery generated psychical hallucinations, memories, and religious visions that patients perceived as actually occurring. One striking aspect of this work was Penfield's discovery that temporal lobe stimulation elicited sensations of memories proceeding forward at a normal temporal progression. Electrical stimuli elicited only a single memory at a time, and manipulating the stimulus allowed Penfield to stop and replay the sensations almost like a videotape of one's life experiences.[11]

Perhaps the most troubling (for enactivism) of the empirical findings involving cortical stimulation are vivid experiences of either one's body and the world from a location outside one's body (OBE) or of a parasomatic image of one's own body called autoscopy (AS). Not only do OBE and AS experiences seem to be conscious perceptual experiences occurring without skillful interaction with the environment, they also seem to be cases of perception that radically violate the experient's SMCs. Blanke describes the two experiences, OBEs and AS, as follows: "During an out-of-body experience (OBE), the experient seems to be awake and to see his body and the world from a location outside the physical body. A closely related experience is autoscopy (AS), which is characterized by the experience of seeing one's body in extrapersonal space" (Blanke, Landis, Spinelli, and Seeck, 2004, p. 243).

OBEs are actually quite common and have a number of causes. Blackmore lists dreams, daydreams, memories, relaxing and falling asleep, meditation, epilepsy, anoxic seizures, electrical stimulation of the right angular gyrus (temporal limbic system), migraine, anesthetic, and recreational drugs like LSD, to which one

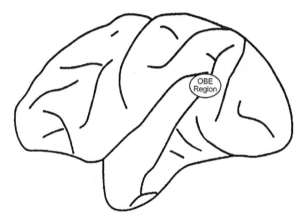

Figure 11.3. Shematic diagram indicating the location in the temporal-parietal junction associated with out-of-body experiences using mean lesion overlap analysis of six patients. *Source*: Blanke et al. (2004), based on figure 4, p. 252.

ought add sleep paralysis (Blackmore, 1991, 2002). Buzzi (2002) notes similar experiences under the influences of surgical general anesthesia. Ehrsson (2007) reports the induction of OBEs using virtual reality to provide correlated bodily visual and tactile information.

Moreover, OBEs and ASs are actually well understood. Blanke, Ortigue, Landis, and Seeck (2002) originally found that electrical stimulation of the right angular gyrus induced OBEs. Like Penfield, Blanke and his team made the serendipitous discovery during electrostimulatory brain mapping of an epileptic. They found that repeated stimuli generate repeated OBEs. Since that time, Blanke has gone on to localize both OBE and AS experiences in healthy and brain-damaged subjects in posterior part of the superior and middle temporal gyri and the angular gyrus in the right hemisphere as shown in figure 11.3 (Blanke, 2004; Blanke and Mohr, 2005; Blanke et al., 2004; Blanke et al., 2005). The right angular gyrus integrates information from the vestibular system regarding position and motion of the head and information about the position of the body and limbs from the somatosensory system used in spatial cognition tasks involving body and space awareness, and logical sequencing.

We conclude that there exists robust and widely documented evidence of conscious perceptual experiences absent skillful interaction with the environment as well as OBEs and ASs, which prima facie violate the perceiver's SMCs in addition to occurring absent skillful interaction with the environment. All of these experiences remain problematic for enactivism.

6.2. Neural Substrates

The most central and influential theses of enactivism are their characterizations of perception as form of skillful, body-involving exercise of sensorimotor knowledge and transient conscious perceptual experience as "the perceptual coupling of animal and environment that consists in the animal's access to environmental detail thanks to its mastery of the relevant sensorimotor contingencies…[integrated with] its broader capacities for thought and rationally guided action" (Noë and O'Regan, 2000, p. 569). Clearly, if SMCs guide all perception and integrate it with the broader capacities for thought and rational action, then a significant neural system subserving the learning and mastery of SMCs and facilitating SMC-driven perception in a manner integrating the perceptual process with capacities for thought and rational action must exist. Therefore, we find it remarkable that enactivists have never suggested a candidate neuronal substrate for a subject's knowledge of SMCs, or even evaluated the general neurological plausibility of this crucial aspect of their theory. The absence of critical comments on enactivism's inadequate exposition of potential mechanisms underlying the central concepts of their theoretical framework seems equally heteroclite in our view. We propose to explore five candidates for such an enactivist neural mechanism. Specifically, we examine the prima facie plausibility given current neuroscientific knowledge that any one of the following five systems could provide a mechanism for the proposed role of SMCs: (1) components of the primary visual pathway (and likewise for each sensory modality); (2) the mirror neuron system connecting elements of the parietal, frontal, and temporal cortex; (3) either system of long-term memory encoding, storage, and retrieval for declarative memory; (4) any of the systems of long-term memory encoding, storage, and retrieval for nondeclarative memory; and (5) the oculomotor system controlling saccades.

We adopt the following criteria for evaluating each candidate system.

1. Can the system as currently understood plausibly encode both modality-related and attribute-related SMCs as characterized by enactivists? We assume that an affirmative answer to this first question can only be given if the system encodes nonrepresentational knowledge that is not readily accessible to consciousness. Additionally, the system must be capable of encoding the unique and invariant modality-specific information of sensory modality-related SMCs as well as the general multimodal information of attribute-related SMCs. We call this the SMC-encoding criteria.

2. Can the system as currently understood plausibly support the constitutive role of SMC knowledge in both visual sensitivity and visual awareness (and the other corresponding modality-specific sensitivity and awareness capacities) as characterized by enactivists? We assume that an affirmative answer to this second question can only be given if the system is known to have significant connectivity to brain areas associated with very early sensory processing for each modality. For instance, in the case of visual processing, it seems reasonable to suppose that a candidate system ought to have significant connectivity at least as early as the lateral geniculate nucleus. We call this the SMC-processing criteria.

3. Can the system as currently understood plausibly support the integration of knowledge of SMCs with higher order thought and rationally guided action as required for the capacity of visual awareness? We assume that an affirmative answer to this third question can only be given if the system has significant connectivity to brain areas associated with these higher order capacities. We call this the SMC-integration criteria.

We do not assert that the foregoing criteria are exhaustive or immune from revision. We claim only that these criteria seem important and quite reasonable in light of our best understanding of the details of the enactivist view.

The neural components of the various sensory systems seem an obvious candidate for an enactivist SMC mechanism. In the case of vision, for example, one might find the neuronal mechanisms of SMC learning and perceptual processing in the components of the primary visual pathway. However, there are three general problems with sensory-specific neural mechanisms. First, different sensory modalities have different neural substrates. As a result, sensory-specific neural mechanisms only seem plausible candidates for modality-related SMCs. Recall that the nature of the perceptual apparatus together with the structure of actual and potential environments of exploration dictates the content of modality-related SMCs. The fact that attribute-related SMCs guide perception of attributes within a modality so as to distinguish objects from one another—as well as the fact that attribute-related SMCs are often intermodal—renders sensory modality-specific neural substrates improbable candidate mechanisms for a both classes of SMCs. Second, researchers have extensively explored the functioning of, for instance, the neurons in the primary visual pathway without finding evidence requiring the supposition of either class of SMCs (Hecht, Shlaer, and Pirenne, 1941, 1942; Hubel and Wiesel, 1959, 1962; Walls, 1934, 1942, 1953). Third, early sensory systems operate largely independently of higher order thinking and rational action. For instance, knowledge of the illusory nature of such illusions the Ames room in which differential size perception results from false depth cues does nothing to mitigate differential size perception. Thus, we conclude that sensory modality-specific neural substrates cannot provide enactivists with the necessary mechanisms required by their theory in that these systems appear unable to satisfy the SMC-encoding criteria (1) and the SMC-integration criteria (3).

The failure of modality-specific sensory systems to provide a plausible neural basis satisfying the SMC-encoding criteria (1) and the SMC-integration criteria, naturally suggests consideration of systems of sensorimotor integration. A cortical system of sensorimotor integration that has recently attracted a great deal interest and might appear attractive as a neural substrate for enactivism is the mirror neuron system. The term *mirror neurons*, has come to designate a group of interconnected neurons that fire (differentially) for the observation, execution, and (in humans but not in monkeys) imitation of goal-directed motor behaviors involving objects. Specifically, cell recordings in human homolog areas of the macaque brain (ventral premotor cortex, also known as F5, and posterior parietal areas PF/PFG) indicate that visual stimuli traceable to a biological agent's (hand or mouth) movements involving an object result in firing by mirror neurons (Gallese, Fadiga, Fogassi, and Rizzolatti, 1996; Iacoboni, 2006; Rizzolatti, 2001, 2004; Rizzolatti, Fadiga, Gallese, and Fogassi, 1996; Rizzolatti, Fogassi, and Gallese, 1997. Mirror neurons do not fire for mimicked actions, actions not involving an object, actions by nonbiological agents, or the presence of an object without agent actions. Thus, in macaque brains researchers distinguish mirror neurons from canonical neurons, in that the latter respond to the presentation of graspable objects of specific size, shape, and orientation.

Research consistently implicates three main brain areas bilaterally in a richer human sensorimotor mirroring function: the pars opercularis of the posterior inferior frontal gyrus (IFG), rostral inferior parietal lobule (IPL), and the posterior sector of the superior temporal sulcus (STS). See figure 11.4.

The STS provides the IFG and IPL with visual input specific to general bodily motion, motion of facial features (i.e., eye gaze, lip movements, etc.), and hand movements (grasping motions). The IPG and IPL are functionally and anatomically heterogeneous sensory-motor association areas. In addition to the relatively small number of cells exhibiting mirroring responses, cell recordings and intracortical electrical microstimulation in human homolog areas of the macaque suggest that the IPL contains cells processing visual, auditory, and motor information as well as cells providing sensorimotor integration (Gentilucci, Fogassi, Luppino, and Matelli, 1989; Rizzolatti, Scandolara, Matelli, and Gentilucci, 1981a, 1981b). Likewise, the IFG—also known as Brodmann's area 44 (part of Broca's area along with BA 45)—exhibits a similar functional and anatomical heterogeneity. The IFG is strongly associated with generation of motor control of vocal organs. The dorsal areas of the IFG are implicated in computing the syntactic structure of sentences, whereas

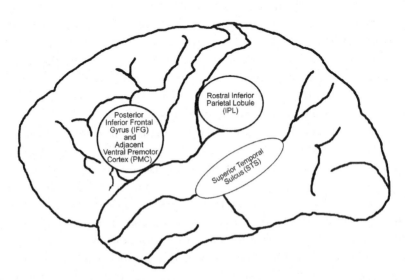

Figure 11.4. Schematic diagram of the core mirror neuron network anatomy based on Puce, Allison, & McCarthy (2000) and Iacaboni & Depretto (2006).

the ventral areas are implicated in semantic processing. Some debate exists in the literature as to the relative roles—motor control versus goal orientation aspects of actions—of the mirror cells in the IPL and the IFG (Carr, Iacoboni, Dubeau, Mazziotta, and Lenzi, 2003; Hamilton and Grafton, 2006, 2008; Iacoboni et al., 2005; Iacoboni, 2006). However, the majority of evidence in the mirror neuron literature supports the IFG as encoding the goal-orientation aspects of action and the IPL as encoding kinesthetic information.

Recent in vivo diffusion tensor magnetic resonance imaging tractography studies further clarify direct and indirect arcuate fasciculus subcortical pathways connecting the IPL, IFG, and STS in each hemisphere. The splenial portion of the corpus callosum connects the circuits bilaterally (Catani, Jones, and Ffytche, 2005; Iacoboni, 2006). The combined connectivity creates recurrent circuits communicating bilaterally and expressing some differentiation of specialization. See figure 11.5.

One can understand motor action imitation underwritten by the mirror neuron system in terms of the combined functioning of an action recognition sequence and a motor initiation sequence. In one account of mirror neuron functioning (Iacoboni, 2006), action recognition starts with observing, for example, the actions of another agent in performing a goal-oriented motor task. The observation triggers firing of the relevant neuronal encoding of a visual depiction of the action in the STS. STS information triggers firing of neurons in the IPL encoding a kinesthetic representation of the action. This information causes the firing of IFC neurons encoding motor-related goals. From this representation, the cognizer comes to recognize the other agent's actions as the performance of a goal-directed motor task

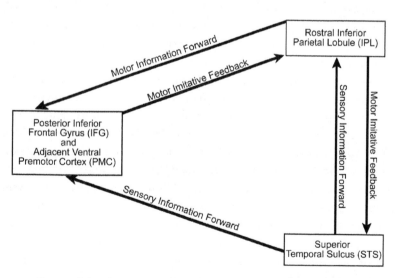

Figure 11.5. Connectivity between core mirror neuron network elements mediated through the direct and indirect arcuate fasciculus subcortical pathways Based on Baird, Colvin, Vanhorn, Inati, & Gazzaniga (2005); Catani, Jones, & Ffytche (2005); Allison, Puce, & McCarthy (2000); Iacoboni & Depretto (2006). Bilateral interconnectivity through the splenial portion of the corpus callosum not depicted here.

on the part of that agent. Note that any "mentalizing" or "adopting the intentional stance" toward another agent involves an indirectly connected cortical system in which the anterior paracingulate cortex appears to play an important role (Blair, 2005; Gallagher and Frith, 2003; Singer, 2006). When a cognizer performs a goal-directed motor task, the very same mirror neurons in the IFC and IPL fire to represent the cognizer's goal as well as the pattern of motor actions required to achieve the goal. The representation of goal and motor actions then guides the cognizer's movements through the primary and secondary motor cortices. Feedback from the STS allows fine-tuning of motor actions as they unfold. Imitation involves the recognition sequence creating IFC and IPL representations matched to the STS representation. IFC and IPL representations then guide the motor initiation sequence, and continued STS information serves to fine-tune imitation.

The mirror neuron system integrates sensory information from multiple modalities with goal-directed action and thus looks attractive as a potential neural substrate for enactivism. However, the directionality of information flow runs from late sensory processing to motor action. As with the previously considered neuronal systems, no evidence currently available supports the role of mirror neurons in sensory processing. Thus, although mirror neurons could potentially satisfy the SMC-encoding criteria (1) and the SMC-integration criteria (3), the system fails to satisfy the SMC-processing criterion (2).

Failing sensory-modality-specific and sensorimotor integrative cortical areas as neural substrates, the next, most obvious candidates for enactivist SMC mechanisms are the systems of the brain specifically associated with long-term memory functions. Unfortunately, a brief survey of long-term memory systems reveals that long-term memory systems cut across enactivist categories in ways that render all memory systems of the brain highly problematic as neural substrates for SMCs. We start with a brief survey of long-term memory systems, note the difficulties that emerge for each class of systems, and conclude by considering the specific case of the procedural memory system.

Recent memory research draws on data concerning function, neural anatomy, type of information, and type of encoding to distinguish two broad classes of long-term memory systems—declarative and nondeclarative (Alcaro, Huber, and Panksepp, 2007; Bayley, Frascino, and Squire, 2005; Bayley and Squire, 2005; Doya, 2000; Grillner, Wallen, Saitoh, Kozlov, and Robertson, in press; Kandel, Kupfermann, and Iverson, 2000; Marín, Wilhelmus, and González, 1998; Mogenson and Yim, 1980; Smeets and Gonzalez, 2000; Smith, Clark, Manns, and Squire, 2005; Smith and Squire, 2005; Squire, 2004, 2007; Squire, Wixted, and Clark, 2007; Tulving, 2002a, 2002b; Wheeler, Stuss, and Tulving, 1997). Each broad class encompasses more specialized systems. The specialized systems, their associated anatomical structure, and information specializations are given in figure 11.6, adapted from Squire, Kandel, and colleagues (Kandel et al., 2000; Squire, 2004).

Declarative memory systems share a common functional characterization and a significantly overlapping neural substrate. At the functional level, researchers consider declarative memory systems to be representational and to encode factual information (i.e., people, places, things, and times) as well as the significance of

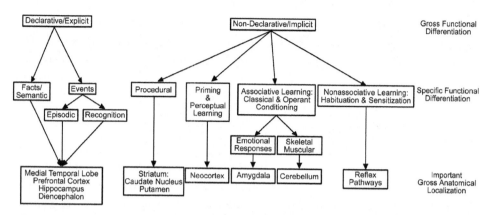

Figure 11.6. Schematic diagram depicting the long-term memory systems of the brain separated horizontally into declarative (left) and nondeclarative (right). The second vertical level indicates memory type, while the third vertical level indicates the primary neuronal structure. Diagram adapted from Kandel et al. (2000); Squire (2004).

such information. Though not necessarily propositionally encoded, normal subjects can express information stored in declarative memory through linguistic or graphic mediums with sufficient precision to warrant its evaluation for veridicality—most often truth functionality. Declarative memory systems encode information from many cognitive systems in a manner that is both associative and versatile in its application and elicitation of stored memories. Encoding of declarative memories depends on conscious attention. Recall likewise requires conscious effort.

Declarative memory encompasses two widely acknowledged systems first differentiated by Tulving (1972, 1983) into semantic and episodic memory. Semantic memory encodes factual and conceptual information in a relatively objective and atemporal format. Thus, semantic memory encodes such information as "prime numbers are numbers divisible only by one and themselves" and "Hitler was not a vegetarian." As characterized by Tulving, the episodic memory system "is a recently evolved [from semantic memory], late-developing, and early-deteriorating past-oriented memory system, more vulnerable than other memory systems to neuronal dysfunction, and probably unique to humans" (2002, p. 5). Episodic memory differs from semantic memory (and all other memory systems) in that it encodes personal experiences for retrieval through ecphoric autonoetic chronesthesia. *Autonoesis* refers to conscious self-awareness, whereas *chronesthesia* refers conscious awareness structured through one's subjective temporal metric. In other words, episodic memories are reexperienced as one's own experiences in the context of one's own past, present, and future (Schacter, 1989; Squire, 2004; Tulving, 1972, 1983, 1985a, 1985b, 2002; Tulving and Schacter, 1990; Tulving et al., 2002; Wheeler et al., 1997).

Semantic and episodic memory systems share a common subsystem for initial encoding and consolidation, and both declarative memory systems employ unimodal and polymodal association cortices for long-term storage and retrieval. Whereas episodic memory involves the prefrontal cortices, semantic memory involves the temporal and parietal cortices. However, most people think of the declarative memory system in terms of the neuronal structures used for initial encoding and consolidation of information—particularly the hippocampus. The fame of the hippocampal subsystem, of course, came about exactly because encoding and consolidation are dissociated from storage and retrieval of existing long-term memory in patients like H.M. Figures 11.7 and 11.8 show, respectively, hippocampal encoding and consolidating structures and the integration of those structures into the episodic memory system.

Nondeclarative memory systems share a general functional characterization but have distinct neural substrates. Nondeclarative memory systems do not have subsystems for encoding/consolidation and storage/retrieval. Rather, encoding occurs as modifications throughout the system over the course of many repetitions, and retrieval consists of automatic reactivation of the system expressed as performance. Nondeclarative memory systems do not depend on conscious attention for storage or retrieval, and these processes often occur without conscious awareness or effort. The information encoded in nondeclarative memory is usually unavailable to consciousness, difficult to express verbally, and not amenable to truth-functional analysis in that it governs operations and procedures (e.g., motor skills), low-level or nonconceptual associations (e.g., classical and operant conditioning), or reactive associations and dissociations (e.g., habituation and sensitization). Likewise,

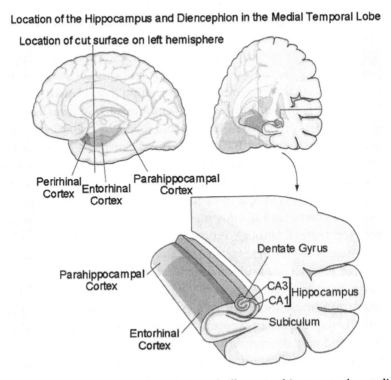

Figure 11.7. Diagram from Kandel et al. (2000) illustrates hippocampal encoding and consolidation structures of declarative memory in both right (medial) hemisphere bisection and in ventral bisection of the right hemisphere.

Schematic Diagram of the Episodic Memory System

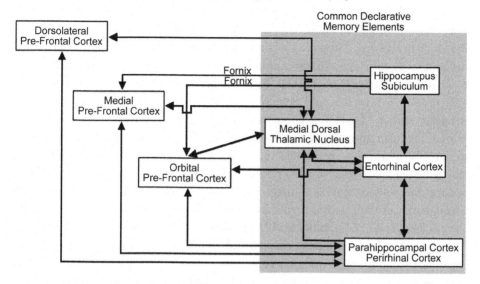

Figure 11.8. Schematic diagram of connectivity implicated in the episodic memory system of declarative/explicit memory. Recognition and other factual memory functions involve projections primarily to neocortical areas running from the anterior lateral temporal lobe to the posterior temporal/anterior inferior parietal cortex.

nondeclarative memory, unlike declarative memory, tends to be much more highly constrained by task, learning context, and modality.

Even in considering these two broad types of memory systems at a relatively high level of abstraction, one can begin to appreciate the difficulties faced by enactivists seeking to find the neural substrate of SMCs. Declarative memory looks attractive in that enactivists assert that attribute-specific SMCs are intermodal, and in that declarative memory constitutes the only memory class that would allow for the integration of SMCs with higher order thought and rational action. Such properties look promising regarding the SMC-encoding criteria and the SMC integration criteria—(1) and (3) from our list. However, declarative memory looks highly problematic overall with regard to the SMC-encoding criteria in that enactivists hold that knowledge of SMCs is both nonrepresentational and not consciously accessible. Furthermore, enactivists understand modality-specific SMCs as highly specialized to modalities in ways unsuited to the general-purpose, highly flexible declarative memory systems. Likewise, declarative memory fails to satisfy SMC-processing criteria (2) in that its only connections to perceptual processing centers are the very late processing centers of the unimodal and polymodal association areas.

One might then turn to nondeclarative memory. Nondeclarative memory is neither representational nor consciously accessible. Moreover, information encoded in nondeclarative memory is relatively modal-specific. Such features seem promising for SMC-encoding criteria (1). Unfortunately, nondeclarative memory is relatively rigid in ways that do not look promising for attribute-specific SMCs—violating the SMC-encoding criteria. Likewise, nondeclarative memory has little if any integration with higher order thinking and rational action—bad news for the SMC-integration criteria (3). Nondeclarative memory holds little promise for satisfying the SMC-processing criteria (2). With the exception of the reflex pathways, no nondeclarative memory system has output connectivity to early sensory processing.

Because enactivists often portray knowledge of SMCs in terms of sensorimotor skill and know-how, it would be remiss not to consider the cortical-basal ganglia-thalamic-cortical (CBTC) skeletomotor circuit of procedural memory. Patients like HM suffer from an inability to encode new declarative memories, but their nondeclarative memories are usually relatively unimpaired. Thus, memory research slowly teased apart what is often referred to as "the basal ganglia system" or "procedural memory system." The basal ganglia are a collection of nuclei deep in the white matter of the cerebral cortex, including the ventral striatum (which includes the nucleus accumbens), caudate nucleus, putamen (often collectively referred to as the striatum), globus pallidus (also called the pallidum), substantia nigra (consisting of the pars reticulata and pars compacta), and subthalamic nucleus. Researchers continue to discover new connections, but one can diagram the major known connections constituting the CBTC skeletomotor circuit as follows (DeLong, 2000) (figure 11.9).

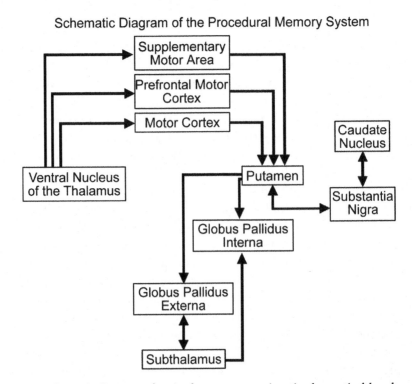

Figure 11.9. Schematic diagram of major known connections in the cortical-basal-ganglia-thalamic-cortical skeletomotor circuit, i.e, the basal ganglia or procedural memory system.

The CBTC skeletomotor circuit has long been recognized as subserving the learning and retention of habits and skills. Riding a bike, for instance, involves procedural memory. However, the basal ganglia system is not limited to motor skill learning. For example, researchers have linked improvements in more seemingly contemplative skills, such as the ability to solve the Tower of Hanoi puzzle or play checkers to the basal ganglia system. Because the operations of this memory system remain largely inaccessible to consciousness, it has also been described as "tacit knowledge" or "implicit knowledge."

The CBTC skeletomotor circuit encodes procedural knowledge by modification of systematic excitatory and inhibitory connections. The collective bodies of the striatum act as a gateway, receiving glutamatergic projections from cortical areas and dopaminergic projections from the substantia nigra and ventral tegmental areas and connecting to other bodies through GABAergic projections. In the circuit, output from the basal system inhibits areas of the ventral thalamus projecting to the cortex. As a motor plan develops, cortical input and internal activity alter the basal system output to the thalamus to selectively disinhibit thalamic projections to the motor cortex, which then trigger the execution of selected motor movements by the primary and supplementary motor areas (DeLong, 2000; Doya, 2000; Monchi, Petrides, Strafella, Worsley, and Doyon, 2006; Sesack et al., 2004). Motor learning occurs by modification of the connectivity within this system.

For the purposes of enactivism, it is important to note that the CBTC skeletomotor circuit has no direct output to sensory processing, and all sensory input to it comes very late in visual processing, providing no obvious manner for satisfying the SMC-processing criterion (2). Sensory information appears to be exclusively somatosensory, thereby making the encoding of general multimodal information via attribute-related SMCs unlikely—violating the SMC-encoding criteria (1). This pattern of connectivity is typical of nondeclarative memory systems. Likewise, the SMC-integration criterion (3) looks unsatisfied by the CBTC skeletomotor circuit, which demonstrates little if any integration of higher order thinking and rational action with the information encoded by the system.

The CBTC skeletomotor circuit is one of five known cortical-basal-ganglia-cortical circuits. These circuits all work to modulate cortical activity through inhibition and encompass skeletomotor, oculomotor, cognitive, and emotional functions. However, it is important to note that though the structures in the basal ganglia comprise the principal subcortical components of these circuits, the circuits are nevertheless almost entirely dissociated from one another in structure and function. As DeLong notes: "These circuits are largely segregated, both structurally and functionally. Each circuit originates in a specific area of the cerebral cortex and engages different portions of the basal ganglia and thalamus" (2000, p. 858).

We end this section by considering an important basal ganglia system for active vision generally—the oculomotor circuit controlling saccades (see figure 11.10). Cortical components of the circuit include the frontal (FEF) and supplementary eye fields (SEF) and the lateral intraparietal area (LIP). The FEF receives input from the SEF and has reciprocal interconnection with the LIP. Both the FEF and LIP have

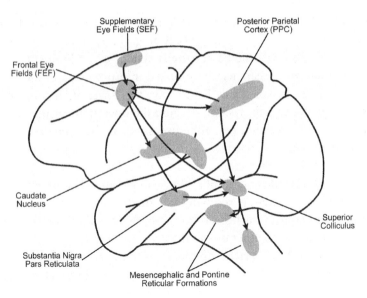

Figure 11.10. The oculomotor circuit for saccade control. *Source*: Adapted with permission from Goldberg (2000, p. 793).

direct connections to the superior colliculus. The FEF also has an indirect pathway to the superior colliculus through the caudate nucleus and the substantia nigra pars reticulata. The superior colliculus has input from the optic nerve (approximately 10 percent of the fibers). The superior colliculus projects to the mesencephalic and pontine reticular formations. The mesencephalic reticular formation controls vertical saccadic action, and the pontine reticular formation controls horizontal eye movements. The basal ganglia component of the oculomotor circuit works as an inhibitory gate on the superior colliculus. Excitatory stimulus from the FEF to the caudate nucleus causes it to inhibit substantia nigra pars reticulata which in turn disinhibits the superior colliculus. (For details, see Bullier, Schall, and Morel, 1996; Edelman, Kristjánsson, and Nakayama, 2007; Goldberg, 2000; Gottlieb and Goldberg, 1999; Gottlieb, Kusunoki, and Goldberg, 1998, 2005; Schall, 2002; Schall, Parker, Derrington, and Blakemore, 2003; Umeno and Goldberg, 2001).

Whereas the oculomotor circuit obviously contributes to early vision in that it directs foveation, it is actually driven by information from late visual processing. Input to both the FEF and the LIP appears to come from the STS and the dorsal and ventral prestriate areas. In other words, one cannot saccade without considerable visual information processing on which to base saccade targets. Thus, saccades, rather than being constitutive of vision, appear to be based on visual information. Further evidence that saccades are not constitutive of vision comes from individuals with Balint's syndrome (Clavagnier, Fruhmann Berger, Klockgether, Moskau, and Karnath, 2006; Goldberg, 2000). Until subjects recover from their deficits, Balint's syndrome patients have dramatically diminished saccadic function due to lesions in the posterior parietal and prestriate cortex. The lesions manifests in both optic ataxia and visual simultanagnosia (the inability to perceive a visual scene). Despite an inability to shift attention from their fixed fovea target, they nevertheless retain visual consciousness and normal descriptive/discriminatory capacities for objects within their foveal field.

We conclude from the review in this subsection that current neuroscientific knowledge eliminates the more obvious candidates for neuronal mechanisms of the enactivist approach to perception and consciousness. Nothing in our conclusion demonstrates that no such mechanism will emerge from future research, but we see no grounds for optimism. We end this section by considering other challenges raised by cortical-basal ganglia–related dysfunction.

6.3. Experiential Blindness and the Basal Ganglia

In clarifying his account of the specific role of sensorimotor knowledge in experience, Noë remarks, "To see the color of an object—to experience which color it has—… is to grasp how its appearance changes or would change as color-critical conditions change. To experience something as red, then, is to experience not merely how it looks here and now, but how it would look as color-critical conditions vary" (2004, p. 132). He goes on to add, "To perceive something as looking red, here and now, say, is to perceive it as standing in a complex set of relationships of similarity and difference. To perceive such a quality, therefore, is already to be in possession of and to be able to exercise a range of discriminatory capacities" (2004, p. 138). By portraying sensorimotor knowledge, discriminatory abilities, and the like as essential to perceptual experience, Noë (2004, p. 194) and other enactivists reject an understanding of experience in which experience temporally and causally proceeds discrimination, in that the former enables the latter. Two crucial points emerge in connection with the enactivist's understanding of experience.

The first has to do with the connection between this understanding of experience and the enactivists' earlier noted aims of addressing the hard problem of consciousness. Enactivists note that views marking a distinction between experience and discriminatory abilities invite concerns about the conceivability of inverted and absent qualia. It seems possible that two creatures identical with respect to the discriminations they make regarding their occurrent perceptual episodes differ when it comes to the qualitative aspects of those episodes. The enactivist strategy of equating discriminatory abilities and perceptual qualities entails that inversion and absent qualia are metaphysically impossible—thereby eliminating such concerns. The problem with this maneuver, however, is that it appears possible for qualitative episodes to take place in the absence of relevant sensorimotor knowledge. Noë (2004, pp. 4–7) himself discusses such cases, namely, those of previously blind subjects who have had their sight surgically restored. Such patients report that their postoperative vision is at first swirling and blurred and cannot in any sense be taken to represent the world in a way that would enable successful interaction, object recognition, and the like. The problem, as Noë sees it, is that these patients altogether lack practical understanding of the visual input; they have no understanding of how the visual input will change as they move or as external things move, and no grasp of what sort of opportunities for action are afforded by the distal causes of their visual episodes. Noë contends that in these cases, visual *sensation* has been restored, but visual *experience* is lacking; these subjects are *experientially blind*. While not wanting to get mired in a terminological dispute, whatever an enactivist might want to call such episodes, the subjects' reports make it very plausible to suppose that they have qualitative aspects, even though these aspects (in an important respect) do not make sense to their subjects. The subjects undergo "dramatic and robust visual impressions or sensations" (Noë, 2004, p. 5) and offer descriptions such as, "There was light, there was movement, there was color" (quoted in Noë, 2004, p. 5). If that is so, it is evidence that enactivism really is not addressing the central concerns of the hard problem and, as is often alleged by those preoccupied with the hard problem, the topic has simply been changed: Instead of getting an account of the metaphysical basis of the qualitative aspect of mentality, enactivists present an account of what it is for perceptual episodes to be meaningful for a subject.

Second, there is a question of how to interpret the source of the "meaningless-ness" of these patients' visual episodes. Sarah Creem-Regehr (2005) suggests that rather than motor integration, cataract surgery patients seem to be agnosic and to suffer from a failure of semantic or feature integration. That is, they are in a position akin to that of Milner and Goodale's subject DF. Given the preoperative history of these patients, there is good reason to suppose that their visual systems did not develop normally due to the absence of retinal input for extended periods of time or at critical junctures, resulting in visual (not just visuomotor) areas being unprepared to properly organize the input that is suddenly arriving. The earlier discussion of the enactivists' need to retreat from stronger versions of the doctrine becomes critical at this point. Part of what is needed to fully evaluate both the previously noted more modest enactivist explanation of DF's situation and the interpretation of patients who have had visual input restored by cataract surgery, is an account of what underlies the expectations about changes in sensory input. The following questions naturally emerge.

- Are those expectations stored in brain regions within or in close communication with the ventral system, the dorsal system, or both?
- What patterns of deficits and preserved abilities might be expected, were communication with areas in which the relevant expectations are housed disrupted or destroyed?
- How do those expectations normally develop in perceivers?

Unfortunately, a review of the enactivist literature does not suggest any specific candidate answers.

Although we do not wish to speculate too much on behalf of enactivists, a plausible answer to these questions from their perspective would seem to implicate one or more of the basal ganglia structures in one or more of the cortical-basal ganglia circuits, as those structures and circuits are among the structures at work in acquiring and maintaining skills, they receive input from and have reciprocal connections to both the dorsal and the ventral systems, damage to them can compromise the control of eye movements, and it is thought that they contribute to visual object cognition and visual spatial cognition (see Jongmans, Mercuri, Henderson, and de Vries, 2006; Koch, 2004, pp. 193–194; Lawrence, Watkins, Sahakian, Hodges, and Robbins, 2000, pp. 1349–1350; Mercuri et al., 1997). Particularly relevant is that dopamine, produced by the substantia nigra of the basal ganglia, plays a critical role in motor control and the prediction of reward and punishment, and thus in both learning and the selection of new actions in the light of changes in either sensory input or internal goals (Gazzaniga, Ivry, and Mangun, 1998; Langston, 1985; Langston and Palfreman, 1995). However, as engagingly discussed by J. William Langston and Jon Palfreman (1995) and cited by Christof Koch (2004, p. 130, n. 24), cases exist that seem to provide evidence against radical enactivist claims about the necessity of a motor contribution for consciousness. Destruction of the substantia nigra through the ingestion of MPTP-tainted synthetic heroin, which brought on an inability to move or speak, did not extinguish consciousness in six unfortunate drug addicts.

Of course, for the more modest enactivism sketched previously, the patients' inability to move while retaining consciousness is by itself not necessarily problematic. There is a question, nevertheless, of whether there is the right sort of match between any preserved expectations about changes in sensory input the victims of basal ganglia damage might have and the content of their conscious experiences. Studies of the effects on vision of Huntington's (HD) and Parkinson's (PD) disease, which attack basal ganglia structures, prove suggestive here. HD patients suffer impairments in selective attention, in selecting appropriate responses in visual spatial (but not object) tasks, in tasks requiring the integration of object recognition and spatial location information, and in visually recognizing facial expressions (particularly expressions of emotions such as disgust, anger, and fear). However, the pattern of deficits does not seem to be genuinely perceptual in nature, as HD patients show good choice accuracy (but considerable increase in latency of response as set size increases) in a visual search task (Lawrence et al., 2000, pp. 1352, 1355–1356) and little impairment in their ability to discriminate between male and female faces, sad and happy expressions, and the faces of Cary Grant and Humphrey Bogart (Sprengelmeyer et al., 2006). Additionally, experimental findings in a study of PD and HD patients indicate that in a throwing task, basal ganglia damage does not affect the rate and magnitude of visuomotor adaptation to lateral displacement induced by donning lenses with special prisms (Fernandez-Ruiz et al., 2003, p. 691). A significant difference was found, though, in the aftereffect of prism adaptation in PD and HD patients. Both as both groups showed considerably less overcorrection of their throws in the direction opposite of the prismatic displacement than control subjects, once the prisms were removed (ibid., pp. 691–692). Fernandez-Ruiz et al. (2003, p. 693) offer an explanation of the prism adaptation findings suggesting that the basal ganglia damage of PD and HD patients impairs their ability to more generally coordinate and remap different perceptual representations (e.g., visual and proprioceptive), forcing patients to rely on task-dependent motor adjustments; the former has been found to engender larger aftereffects than the latter. If any real substance is to be given to enactivists' claims about the role of expectations and other sensorimotor phenomena in perceptual experience, enactivists must account for—or better predict—patterns of preserved and impaired abilities like those just described.

7. CONCLUSION

In this chapter, we provide the reader with a broad and fair assessment of enactivism. In service of that assessment we call attention to both strong and weak versions of enactivism to separate what we view as core enactivist commitments from inconsistent and exaggerated claims in the literature. As with many other researchers, we find the most extreme forms of enactivism confused or false. Moreover, we view many of their treatments of empirical research as conceptually and methodologically flawed. Thus, we find no compelling reason to embrace either the enactivists' aim of completely revolutionizing vision science or their understanding of the character of that new vision science.

We remain, nevertheless, sympathetic with some of the basic issues driving enactivist research, particularly with respect to concerns about appeals to intense computational and representational resources. Additionally, we recognize the need to understand the complex relationship between vision and other capacities, such as action. However, we find numerous serious empirical and conceptual problems for even the more modest enactivism sketched in the chapter. Despite our pessimistic appraisal of the current state of enactivist research, we are interested to see what contributions the movement might be able to make in helping shape the development of perception research as it grows increasingly sensitive to the dependence of perception on action and action on perception.

NOTES

1. While Marr (1982) is rightly cited as a principal champion of passive research, it is important not to overlook his claims that "Vision is a process that produces from images of the external world a description that is useful to the viewer and not cluttered with irrelevant information" (p. 31) and "The usefulness of a representation depends on how well suited it is to the purpose for which it is used" (p. 32). Such statements fit well with the basic concerns driving active vision research.

2. For a detailed discussion of these issues, see chapter 10 in this volume.

3. Interestingly, Block focuses on O&N's rejection of the brain basis of consciousness and brands them behaviorists. Nonetheless, Block's counterexample to O&N's view is an alleged liberalism of qualitative conscious experience.

4. Koch bases his discussion on Langston and Palfreman (1995). Langston's academic works on the subject begin with Langston (1985), Irwin and Langston (1985), and Stern and Langston (1985). Similar cases due to encephalitis lethargica are documented in Sacks (1995).

5. Although we do not pursue the issue further, we do note the indefiniteness of *a little bit* of consciousness.

6. See Hollingworth (2003, 2004) and Hollingworth and Henderson (2002). Henderson and Hollingworth are clear that their VLTM account is not an account of visual phenomenology (see Hollingworth, 2003, p. 400). That does not preclude their account playing a role in an account of how we might misconstrue the actual phenomenology of experience. Given that introspection is not as reliable as we naively take it to be and that it is not common for people to recognize that there is more to vision than visual experience, perceivers might confound retrieved VLTM representations (and perhaps abstract information about gist and spatial layout) with what is actually present in their visual experience, thereby reinforcing a sense of rich and coherent experience of the entire visual scene.

7. Overt attention involves saccades to and fixations of items in or areas of the visual scene. Covert attention enables one to mentally focus on at item or area without fixating it.

8. As an example of this, consider attempts to develop models of eye scanning that would allow for accurate predictions of the timing and direction of saccades. Gaze shifts can be driven by both automatic processes (e.g., involuntary saccades directed to transients in the visual field) and top-down influences (e.g., the plans and knowledge of the perceiver). Absolutely central to how either factor plays a role in determining (1) when one fixation is terminated and a redirection of gaze to another location or object is initiated, and (2) what location or object is the target of the next fixation, is what information is obtained during a single fixation; see Findlay and Gilchrist (2003, p. 5 and pp. 129–149). The tools and methods of passive vision research are well-suited to studying those single fixations (Fei-Fei, Iyer, Koch, and Perona, 2007).

9. Interesting to note here are the remarks of Singh and Hoffman (1998) regarding the emphasis of Pessoa et al. (1998) on the entire active organism as the proper object of study in perception research. Singh and Hoffman call into question the idea that study of the active organism needs to be opposed to the representation-based approach, arguing that such a way of putting the choices before us relies on a gross oversimplification or distortion of what is needed by both approaches. Rather than being in competition, they are best seen as complementary: attributions of representations often turn on consideration of tasks performed at the level of the entire organism. Likewise, a creature's skillful performance of tasks looks to be explicable only by appeal to representations the creature has of relevant features of its environment and its own state.

10. Milner and Goodale's work builds on a tradition of research dating back to anatomical studies and recordings of the photoelectric response in the retina by, for instance, Waller (1909) and speculation as to retinal cell function in vision by researchers like Schanz (1923), Hopkins (1927), and Walls (1928). Researchers such as Brouwer (1934) and Clark and Penman (1934) extended research to the LGN and striate cortex. Hubel and Wiesel (1959, 1962), among others, carefully outlined the processing in the striate cortex, and researchers such as Karamyan, Zagorul'ko, Belekhova, and Kosareva (1968), Karamyan, Belekhova, and Veselkin (1969), Schneider (1969), Brody, Ungerleider, and Pribram (1977), Ungerleider and Pribruam (1977), and Mishkin and Ungerleider (1982) extended the functional and evolutionary understanding of the visual processing to the dorsal and ventral streams, along with their nonprimate analogs.

11. Robertson (1997) reports that the antidepressant fluoxetine can cause similar experiences.

REFERENCES

Alcaro, A., Huber, R., and Panksepp, J. (2007). Behavioral functions of the mesolimbic dopaminergic system: An affective neuroethological perspective. *Brain Research Reviews* 56: 283–321.

Bach y Rita, P. (1983). Tactile vision substitution: Past and future. *International Journal of Neuroscience* 19: 26–36.

Bach y Rita, P. (1984). The relationship between motor processes and cognition in tactile vision substitution. In A. F. Sanders and W. Prinz (Eds.), *Cognition and Motor Processes*. Berlin: Springer, 150–159.

Bauer, J., and Held, R. (1975). Comparison of visually guided reaching in normal and deprived infant monkeys. *Journal of Experimental Psychology: Animal Behavior Processes* 1: 298–308.

Bayley, P. J., Frascino, J. C., and Squire, L. R. (2005). Robust habit learning in the absence of awareness and independent of the medial temporal lobe. *Nature* 436: 550–553.

Bayley, P. J., and Squire, L. R. (2005). Failure to acquire new semantic knowledge in patients with large medial temporal lobe lesions. *Hippocampus* 15: 273–280.

Bedford, F. L. (1999). Keeping perception accurate. *Trends in Cognitive Sciences* 3: 4–11.

Berlin, B., and Kay, P. (1969). *Basic Color Terms: Their Universality and Evolution*. Berkeley: University of California Press.

Biederman, I. (1987). Recognition-by-components: A theory of human image understanding. *Psychological Review* 94: 115–117.

Blackmore, S. (1991). Near-death experiences: In or out of the body? *Skeptical Inquirer* 16.

Blackmore, S. (2001). Three experiments to test the sensorimotor theory of vision. *Behavioral and Brain Sciences* 24: 977.

Blackmore, S. (2002). Near-death experiences. In M. Shermer (Ed.), *The Skeptic Encyclopedia of Pseudoscience*. Santa Barbara, Calif.: ABC-CLIO, 152–157.

Blair, R. J. R. (2005). Responding to the emotions of others: Dissociating forms of empathy through the study of typical and psychiatric populations. *Consciousness and Cognition* 14: 698–718.

Blakemore, C., Van Sluyters, R. C., Peck, C. K., and Hein, A. (1975). Development of cat visual cortex following rotation of one eye. *Nature* 257: 584–586.

Blangero, A., Ota, H., Delporte, L., Revol, P., Vindras, P., Rode, G., et al. (2007). Optic ataxia is not only "optic": Impaired spatial integration of proprioceptive information. *Neuroimage* 36: T61–T68.

Blanke, O. (2004). Out of body experiences and their neural basis. *British Medical Journal* 329: 1414–1415.

Blanke, O., Landis, T., Spinelli, L., and Seeck, M. (2004). Out-of-body experience and autoscopy of neurological origin. *Brain: A Journal of Neurology* 127: 243–258.

Blanke, O., and Mohr, C. (2005). Out-of-body experience, heautoscopy, and autoscopic hallucination of neurological origin. implications for neurocognitive mechanisms of corporeal awareness and self-consciousness. *Brain Research Reviews* 50: 184–199.

Blanke, O., Ortigue, S., Landis, T., and Seeck, M. (2002). Stimulating illusory own-body perceptions: The part of the brain that can induce out-of-body experiences has been located. *Nature* 419: 269–270.

Blanke, O., Mohr, C., Michel, C. M., Pascual-Leone, A., Brugger, P., Seeck, M., et al. (2005). Linking out-of-body experience and self processing to mental own-body imagery at the temporoparietal junction. *Journal of Neuroscience* 25: 550–557.

Block, N. (2001). Behaviorism revisited. *Behavioral and Brain Sciences* 24: 977–978.

Block, N. (2003). Spatial perception via tactile sensation. *Trends in Cognitive Sciences* 7: 285–286.

Block, N. (2005). Review of Alva Noë, *Action in Perception. Journal of Philosophy* 102: 259–72.

Block, N. (1993). *Troubles with Functionalism*. Cambridge, Mass.: MIT Press.

Bompas, A., and O'Regan, J. K. (2006). Evidence for a role of action in colour perception. *Perception* 35: 65–78.

Brody, B. A., Ungerleider, L. G., and Pribram, K. H. (1977). The effects of instability of the visual display on pattern discrimination learning by monkeys: Dissociation produced after resections of frontal and inferotemporal cortex. *Neuropsychologia* 15: 439–448.

Brouwer, B. (1934). Projection of the retina on the cortex in man. *Proceedings Association for Research in Nervous and Mental Diseases* 13: 529–534.

Bullier, J., Schall, J. D., and Morel, A. (1996). Functional streams in occipito-frontal connections in the monkey. *Behavioural Brain Research* 76: 89–97.

Buzzi, G. (2002). Near-death experiences. *Lancet* 21: 2116–2117.

Campos, J. J., Anderson, D. I., Barbu-Roth, M. A., Hubbard, E. M., Hertenstein, M. J., and Witherington, D. (2000). Travel broadens the mind. *Infancy* 1: 149–219.

Campos, J. J., Hiatt, S., Ramsay, D., Henderson, C., and Svejda, M. (1978). The emergence of fear on the visual cliff. In M. K. L. Rosenblum (Ed.), *The Development of Affect*. New York: Plenum Press, 149–182.

Carey, D. P., Dijkerman, H. C., Murphy, K. J., Goodale, M. A., and Milner, A. D. (2006). Pointing to places and spaces in a patient with visual form agnosia. *Neuropsychologia* 44: 1584–1594.

Carr, L., Iacoboni, M., Dubeau, M., Mazziotta, J., and Lenzi, G. (2003). Neural mechanisms of empathy in humans: A relay from neural systems for imitation to limbic areas. *Proceedings of the National Academy of Sciences* 100: 5497–5502.

Catani, M., Jones, D. K., and Ffytche, D. H. (2005). Perisylvian language networks of the human brain. *Annals of Neurology* 57: 8–16.

Cavina-Pratesi, C., Valyear, K. F., Culham, J. C., Köhler, S., Obhi, S. S., Marzi, C. A., et al. (2006). Dissociating arbitrary stimulus-response mapping from movement planning during preparatory period: Evidence from event-related functional magnetic resonance imaging. *Journal of Neuroscience* 26: 2704–2713.

Chalmers, D. (1996). *The Conscious Mind*. New York: Oxford University Press.

Cheng, D., Tremblay, L., and Luis, M. (2007). The trial-by-trial effects of visual feedback uncertainty in manual aiming. *Journal of Sport and Exercise Psychology* 29: S60–S61.

Churchland, P. S., Ramachandran, V. S., Sejnowski, T. J., Koch, C., and Davis, J. L. (1994). *A Critique of Pure Vision*. Cambridge, Mass.: MIT Press.

Clark, A., and Toribio, J. (2001). Sensorimotor chauvinism? *Behavioral and Brain Sciences* 24: 979–980.

Clark, W. E. L., and Penman, G. G. (1934). The projection of the retina in the lateral geniculate body. *Proceedings Royal Society of London* 114: 291–313.

Clavagnier, S., Fruhmann Berger, M., Klockgether, T., Moskau, S., and Karnath, H.-O. (2006). Restricted ocular exploration does not seem to explain simultanagnosia. *Neuropsychologia* 44: 2330–2336.

Cohen, M. R., and Newsome, W. T. (2004). What electrical microstimulation has revealed about the neural basis of cognition. *Current Opinion in Neurobiology* 14: 169–177.

Cook, R., Kay, P., and Regier, T. (2005). The World Color Survey database. In H. Cohen and C. Lefebvre (Eds.), *Handbook of Categorization in the Cognitive Sciences*. Amsterdam: Elsevier.

Creem-Regehr, S. (2005). Perception by action versus perception for action. *Trends in Cognitive Sciences* 5: 510–511.

DeLong, M. (2000). The basal ganglia. In E. R. Kandel, J. H. Schwartz, and T. M. Jessel (Eds.), *Principles of Neural Science*. New York: McGraw-Hill, 851–867.

Doya, K. (2000). Complementary roles of basal ganglia and cerebellum in learning and motor control. *Current Opinion in Neurobiology* 10: 732–739.

Dretske, F. (1995). *Naturalizing the Mind*. Cambridge, Mass.: MIT Press.

Edelman, J. A., Kristjánsson, Á., and Nakayama, K. (2007). The influence of object-relative visuomotor set on express saccades. *Journal of Vision* 7: 1–13.

Edelman, S. (2006). Mostly harmless. *Artificial Life* 12: 183–186.

Ehrsson, H. H. (2007). The experimental induction of out-of-body experiences. *Science* 317: 1048.

Fei-Fei, L., Iyer, A., Koch, C., and Perona, P. (2007). What do we perceive in a glance of a real-world scene? *Journal of Vision* 7: 1–29.

Fernandez-Ruiz, J., Diaz, R., Hall-Haro, C., Vergara, P., Mischner, J., Nuñez, L., et al. (2003). Normal prism adaptation but reduced after-effect in basal ganglia disorders using a throwing task. *European Journal of Neuroscience* 18: 689–694.

Findlay, J. M., and Gilchrist, I. D. (2003) *Active Vision: The Psychology of Looking and Seeing*. New York: Oxford University Press.

Gallagher, H. L., and Frith, C. D. (2003). Functional imaging of "theory of mind." *Trends in Cognitive Sciences* 7: 77–83.

Gallese, V., Fadiga, L., Fogassi, L., and Rizzolatti, G. (1996). Action recognition in the premotor cortex. *Brain* 119: 593–609.

Gazzaniga, M., Ivry, R., and Mangun, G. R. (Eds.). (1998). *Cognitive Neuroscience*. New York: Norton.

Gentilucci, M., Fogassi, L., Luppino, G., and Matelli, M. (1989). Somatotopic representation in inferior area 6 of the macaque monkey. *Brain, Behavior and Evolution* 33: 118–121.

Georgopoulos, A. P. (2000). Neural mechanisms of motor cognitive processes: Functional MRI and neurophysiological studies. In Michael S. Gazzaniga (Ed.), *The New Cognitive Neurosciences*. MIT Press: Cambridge, MA, 525–538.

Gilchrist, I. D., Brown, V., and Findlay, J. M. (1997). Saccades without eye movements. *Nature* 390: 130–131.

Goldberg, M. E. (2000). The control of gaze. In E. R. Kandel, J. H. Schwartz, and T. M. Jessel (Eds.), *Principles of Neural Science*. New York: McGraw-Hill, 782–799.

Goodale, M. A. (2001). Real action in a virtual world. *Behavioral and Brain Sciences* 24: 984–985.

Goodale, M. A., Jakobson, L. S., and Keillor, J. M. (1994). Differences in the visual control of pantomimed and natural grasping movements. *Neuropsychologia* 32: 1159–1178.

Goodale, M. A., and Milner, A. D. (2005). *Sight Unseen*. New York: Oxford University Press.

Goodale, M. H. K. (1998). The objects of action and perception. *Cognition* 67: 181–207.

Goodkin, H. P., and Thach, W. T. (2003a). Cerebellar control of constrained and unconstrained movements. I: Nuclear inactivation. *Journal of Neurophysiology* 89: 884–895.

Goodkin, H. P., and Thach, W. T. (2003b) Cerebellar control of constrained and unconstrained movements. II: EMG and nuclear activity. *Journal of Neurophysiology* 89: 896–908.

Gottlieb, J., and Goldberg, M. E. (1999). Activity of neurons in the lateral intraparietal area of the monkey during an antisaccade task. *Nature Neuroscience* 2: 906.

Gottlieb, J. P., Kusunoki, M., and Goldberg, M. E. (1998). The representation of visual salience in monkey parietal cortex. *Nature* 391: 481.

Gottlieb, J., Kusunoki, M., and Goldberg, M. E. (2005). Simultaneous representation of saccade targets and visual onsets in monkey lateral intraparietal area. *Cerebral Cortex* 15: 1198–1206.

Gouras, P. (1984). Color vision. In N. Osborn and J. Chader (Eds.), *Progress in Retinal Research*, vol. 3. London: Pergamon Press.

Gray, J. (2003). How are qualia coupled to functions? *Trends in Cognitive Sciences* 7: 192–194.

Grierson, L. E., and Elliott, D. (2007). Goal-directed aiming and the relative contribution of two online control processes. *Journal of Sport and Exercise Psychology* 29: S79–S79.

Grillner, S., Wallen, P., Saitoh, K., Kozlov, A., and Robertson, B. (In press). Neural bases of goal-directed locomotion in vertebrates—an overview. *Brain Research Reviews*.

Guigon, E., and Baraduc, P. (2002). A neural model of perceptual-motor alignment. *Journal of Cognitive Neuroscience* 14: 538–549.

Hamilton, A., and Grafton, S. (2006). Goal representation in human anterior intraparietal sulcus. *Journal of Neuroscience* 26: 1133–1137.

Hamilton, A., and Grafton, S. (2008). The motor hierarchy: From kinematics to goals and intentions. In P. Haggard, Y. Rossetti, and M. Kawato (Eds.), *Sensorimotor Foundations of Higher Cognition (Attention and Performance)*. Oxford: Oxford University Press.

Harnad, S. (2001). Editorial comment. *Behavioral and Brain Sciences* 24: 973–974.

Hecht, S., Shlaer, S., and Pirenne, M. H. (1941). Energy at the threshold of vision. *Science* 93: 585–587.

Hecht, S., Shlaer, S., and Pirenne, M. H. (1942). Energy, quanta, and vision. *Journal of General Physiology* 25: 819–840.

Hein, A., and Diamond, R. M. (1971). Contrasting development of visually triggered and guided movements in kittens with respect to interocular and interlimb equivalence. *Journal of Comparative and Physiological Psychology* 76: 219–224.

Hein, A., and Diamond, R. M. (1972). Locomotory space as a prerequisite for acquiring visually guided reaching in kittens. *Journal of Comparative and Physiological Psychology* 81: 394–398.

Hein, A., and Held, R. (1967). Dissociation of the visual placing response into elicited and guided components. *Science* 158: 390–392.

Hein, A., Held, R., and Gower, E. C. (1970). Development and segmentation of visually controlled movement by selective exposure during rearing. *Journal of Comparative and Physiological Psychology* 73: 181–187.

Held, R., and Bauer, J. A. Jr. (1967). Visually guided reaching in infant monkeys after restricted rearing. *Science* 155: 718–720.

Held, R., and Bauer, J. A. (1974). Development of sensorially-guided reaching in infant monkeys. *Brain Research* 71: 247–248.

Held, R., and Hein, A. (1963). Movement-produced stimulation in the development of visually guided behavior. *Journal of Comparative and Physiological Psychology* 56: 872–876.

Hochberg, J. (2002). Direct information on the cutting room floor. *Behavioral and Brain Sciences* 25: 107–108.

Hollingworth, A. (2003). Failures of retrieval and comparison constrain change detection in natural scenes. *Journal of Experimental Psychology: Human Perception and Performance* 29: 388–403.

Hollingworth, A. (2004). Constructing visual representations of natural scenes: The roles of short- and long-term visual memory. *Journal of Experimental Psychology: Human Perception and Performance* 30: 519–537.

Hollingworth, A., and Henderson, J. (2002). Accurate visual memory for previously attended objects in natural scenes. *Visual Cognition* 7: 213–235.

Hopkins, A. E. (1927). Experiments on color vision in mice in relation to the duplicity theory. *Zeitschrift fur Vergleichende Physiologie* 6: 299–344.

Hubel, D. H., and Wiesel, T. N. (1959). Receptive fields of single neurones in the cat's striate cortex. *Journal of Physiology* 148: 574–591.

Hubel, D. H., and Wiesel, T. N. (1962). Receptive fields, binocular interaction and functional architecture in the cat's visual cortex. *Journal of Physiology (London)* 160: 106–154.

Hummel, J. E. (1994). Reference frames and relations in computational models of object recognition. *Current Directions in Psychological Science* 3: 111–116.

Hummel, J. E., and Biederman, I. (1992). Dynamic binding in a neural network for shape recognition. *Psychological Review* 99: 480–517.

Hurley, S., and Noë, A. (2003a). Neural plasticity and consciousness. *Biology and Philosophy* 18: 131–168.

Hurley, S., and Noë, A. (2003b). Neural plasticity and consciousness: Reply to Block. *Trends in Cognitive Sciences* 7: 342–342.

Hurley, S., and Noë, A. (2007). Can hunter-gatherers hear color? In G. Brennen, R. Goodin, F. Jackson, and M. Sith (Eds.), *Common Minds: Essays in Honor of Philip Pettit*. Oxford: Oxford University Press.

Iacoboni, M., Molnar-Szakacs, I., Gallese, V., Buccino, G., Mazziotta, J., and Rizzolatti, G. (2005). Grasping the intentions of others with one's own mirror neuron system. *PLoS Biology* 3: 529–535.

Iacoboni, M. (2006). The mirror neuron system and the consequences of its dysfunction. *Nature Reviews: Neuroscience* 7: 942–951.

Imura, T., Yamaguchi, M. K., Kanazawa, S., Shirai, N., Otsuka, Y., Tomonaga, M., et al. (2006). Perception of motion trajectory of object from the moving cast shadow in infants. *Vision Research* 46: 652–657.

Irwin, I., and Langston, J. W. (1985). Selective accumulation of MPP+ in the substantia nigra: A key to neurotoxicity? *Life Sciences* 36: 207–212.

Jacobson, A. (2007). Properly functioning vision: On Block on Noë? Presented at the 81st Annual American Philosophical Association Pacific Division Meeting, San Francisco.

James, T. W., Culham, J., Humphrey, G. K., Milner, A. D., and Goodale, M. A. (2003). Ventral occipital lesions impair object recognition but not object-directed grasping: An fMRI study. *Brain: A Journal of Neurology* 126: 2463–2475.

Jameson, K. (In press). Where in the world color surveys is the support for the Hering primaries as the basis for color categorization? In J. Cohen and M. Matthen (Eds.), *Color Ontology and Color Science*. Cambridge, Mass.: MIT Press.

Johnson, K., and Wright, W. (2008). Reply to Philipona and O'Regan. *Visual Neuroscience* 25: 221–224.

Jongmans, M., Mercuri, E., Henderson, S., and de Vries, L. (1996). Visual function of prematurely born children with and without perceptual-motor difficulties. *Early Human Development* 45: 73–82.

Kandel, E., Kupfermann, I., and Iverson, S. (2000). Learning and memory. In E. R. Kandel, J. H. Schwartz, and T. M. Jessel (Eds.), *Principles of Neural Science*. New York: McGraw-Hill, 1227–1246.

Karamyan, A. I., Zagorul'ko, A. A., Belekhova, M. G., and Kosareva, A. A. (1968). Morphofunctional features of cortico-subcortical interrelationships in premammalian vertebrates. In S. P. Narikashvili (Ed.), *Korkovaya regulyatsiya deyatel'nosti podkorkovykh obrazovanii golovnogo mozga* [Cortical regulation of the Activity of the Subcortical Formations of the Brain]. Oxford: Izd-vo Metsniereba.

Karamyan, A. I., Belekhova, M. G., and Veselkin, N. P. (1969). On the similarity and difference of the thalamotelencephalic system of the amphibian and reptilian brain. *Fiziologicheskii Zhurnal SSSR* 55: 977–986.

Kay, P., and Regier, T. (2003). Resolving the question of color naming universals. *Proceedings of the National Academy of Sciences USA* 100: 9085.

Koch, C. (2004). *The Quest for Consciousness*. Greenwood Village, Colo.: Roberts.

Kohler, I. (1951). *Über Aufbau und Wandlungen der Wahrnehmungswelt; Insbesondere Über 'bedingte Empfindungen.'* [Construction and Alteration in the World of Perception; Especially of "Conditional Sensations."] Oxford, England: Rudolph M. Rohrer.

Kohler, I. (1963). The formation and transformation of the perceptual world. *Psychological Issues* 3: 1–173.

Kuehni, R. G. (2005). Focal color variability and unique hue stimulus variability. *Journal of Cognition and Culture* 5: 409–426.

Kurthen, M. (2001). Consciousness as action: The eliminativist sirens are calling. *Behavioral and Brain Sciences* 24: 990–991.

Land, M., and Nilsson, D.E. (2002). *Animal Eyes*. Oxford: Oxford University Press.

Langston, J. W. (1985). MPTP neurotoxicity: An overview and characterization of phases of toxicity. *Life Sciences* 36: 201–206.

Langston, J. W., and Palfreman, J. (1995). *The Case of the Frozen Addicts*. New York: Pantheon Press.

Lawrence, A. D., Watkins, L. H. A., Sahakian, B. J., Hodges, J. R., and Robbins, T. W. (2000). Visual object and visuospatial cognition in Huntington's disease: Implications for information processing in corticostriatal circuits. *Brain: A Journal of Neurology* 123: 1349–1364.

Lee, H. W., Hong, S. B., Seo, D. W., Tae, W. S., and Hong, S. C. (2000). Mapping of functional organization in human visual cortex: Electrical cortical stimulation. *Neurology* 54: 849–854.

Levine, J. (1983). Materialism and qualia: the explanatory gap. *Pacific Philosophical Quarterly* 64: 354–361.

Lindsey, D. T., and Brown, A. M. (2002). Color naming and the phototoxic effects of sunlight on the eye. *Psychological Science* 13: 506–512.

Liu, J., and Newsome, W. T. (2000). Somatosensation: Touching the mind's fingers. *Current Biology* 10: R598–R600.

Lycan, W. (2001). The case for phenomenal externalism. *Noûs Supplemental: Philosophical Perspectives* 15: 17–35.

Manzotti, R. S. G. (2001). Does functionalism really deal with the phenomenal side of experience? *Behavioral and Brain Sciences* 24: 993–994.

Marín, O., Wilhelmus, J., and González, A. (1998). Evolution of the basal ganglia in tetrapods: A new perspective based on recent studies in amphibians. *Trends in Neuroscience* 21: 487–494.

Marr, D. (1982). *Vision*. New York: Freeman.

McCrone, J. (2004). Review of J. Findlay and I. Gilchrist's *Active Vision. Journal of Consciousness Studies* 11: 180–181.

Mercuri, E., Philpot, J., Atkinson, J., Grueter-Andrew, J., Sewry, C. A., Dubowitz, V., et al. (1997). Normal visual function in children with pure congenital muscular dystrophy. *Neuromuscular Disorders* 7: 433–434.

Milner, A. D., Dijkerman, H. C., Pisella, L., McIntosh, R. D., Tilikete, C., Vighetto, A., et al. (2001). Grasping the past: Delay can improve visuomotor performance. *Current Biology* 11: 1896–1901.

Mishkin, M., and Ungerleider, L. G. (1982). Contribution of striate inputs to the visuospatial functions of parieto-preoccipital cortex in monkeys. *Behavioural Brain Research* 6: 57–77.

Mogenson, G. J. D., and Yim, C. (1980). From motivation to action—functional interface between the limbic system and the motor system. *Progress in Neurobiology* 14: 69–97.

Monchi, O., Petrides, M., Strafella, A. P., Worsley, K. J., and Doyon, J. (2006). Functional role of the basal ganglia in the planning and execution of actions. *Annals of Neurology* 59: 257–264.

Mullan, S., and Penfield, W. (1959). Illusions of comparative interpretation and emotion: Production of epileptic discharge and by electrical stimulation in the temporal cortex. *Archives of Neurology and Psychiatry (Chicago)* 881: 269–284.

Murphy, K. J., Racicot, C. I., and Goodale, M. A. (1996). The use of visuomotor cues as a strategy for making perceptual judgments in a patient with visual form agnosia. *Neuropsychology* 10: 396–401.

Noë, A. (2002). Is the visual world a grand illusion? *Journal of Consciousness Studies* 9: 1–12.

Noë, A. (2004). *Action in Perception*. Cambridge, Mass.: MIT Press.

Noë, A. (2005). What does change blindness teach us about consciousness? *Trends in Cognitive Sciences* 9: 218–218.

Noë, A. (2006a). Precis of *Action in Perception. Psyche: An Interdisciplinary Journal of Research on Consciousness* 12.

Noë, A. (2006b). Experience without the head. In T. S. Gendler and J. Hawthorne (Eds.), *Perceptual Experience*. New York: Oxford University Press, 411–433.

Noë, A., and Hurley, S. (2003). The deferential brain in action: Response to Jeffrey Gray. *Trends in Cognitive Sciences* 7: 195–196.

Noë, A., and O'Regan, J. K. (2000). Perception, attention and the grand illusion. *Psyche: An Interdisciplinary Journal of Research on Consciousness* 6.

Noë, A., and O'Regan, J. K. (2002). On the brain-basis of visual consciousness: A sensorimotor account. In A. Noë and E. Thompson (Eds.), *Vision and Mind: Selected Readings in the Philosophy of Perception*. Cambridge, Mass.: MIT Press, 567–598.

Noë, A., and Thompson, E. (2004). Are there neural correlates of consciousness? *Journal of Consciousness Studies* 11: 3–28.

O'Regan, J. K. (1992). Solving the "real" mysteries of visual perception: The world as an outside memory. *Canadian Journal of Psychology/Revue Canadienne de Psychologie* 46: 461–488.

O'Regan, J. K., and Noë, A. (2001). A sensorimotor account of vision and visual consciousness. *Behavioral and Brain Sciences* 24: 939–1031.

Oberauer, K. (2001). The explanatory gap is still there. *Behavioral and Brain Sciences* 24: 996–997.

Penfield, W. (1955a). The permanent record of the stream of consciousness. *Acta Psychologica* 11: 47–69.

Penfield, W. (1955b). The twenty-ninth Maudsley Lecture: The role of the temporal cortex in certain psychical phenomena. *Journal of Mental Science* 101: 451–465.

Penfield, W. (1959). The interpretive cortex. *Science* 129: 1719–1725.

Pessoa, L., Thompson, E., and Noë, A. (1998). Finding out about filling-in: A guide to perceptual completion for visual science and the philosophy of perception. *Behavioral and Brain Sciences* 21: 723–802.

Philipona, D. L., and O'Regan, J. K. (2006). Color naming, unique hues, and hue cancellation predicted from singularities in reflection properties. *Visual Neuroscience* 23: 331–339.

Philipona, D., O'Regan, J. K., and Nadal, J. P. (2003). Is there something out there? Inferring space from sensorimotor dependencies. *Neural Computation* 15: 2029–2049.

Prinz, J. (2006). Putting the brakes on enactive perception. *Psyche: An Interdisciplinary Journal of Research on Consciousness* 12.

Puce, A., Allison, T., and McCarthy, G. (1999). Electrophysiological studies of human face perception. III: Effects of top-down processing on face-specific potentials. *Cerebral Cortex* 9: 445–458.

Redding, G. M. (2007).

Redding, G. M., Rossetti, Y., and Wallace, B. (2005). Applications of prism adaptation: A tutorial in theory and method. *Neuroscience and Biobehavioral Reviews* 29: 431–444.

Redding, G. M., and Wallace, B. (2006a). Generalization of prism adaptation. *Journal of Experimental Psychology: Human Perception and Performance* 32: 1006–1022.

Redding, G. M., and Wallace, B. (2006b). Prism adaptation and unilateral neglect: Review and analysis. *Neuropsychologia* 44: 1–20.

Regan, D. (2000). *Human Perception of Objects.* Sunderland, N.Y.: Sinauer.

Regier, T., Kay, P. and Khetarpala, N. (2007). Color naming reflects optimal partitions of color space. *Proceedings of the National Academy of Sciences USA* 104: 1436–1441.

Regier, T., Kay, P., and Cook, R. S. (2005). Focal colors are universal after all. *Proceedings of the National Academy of Sciences USA* 102: 8386–8391.

Rensink, R. A. (2000). The dynamic representation of scenes. *Visual Cognition* 7: 1–42.

Rensink, R. A. (2002). Change detection. *Annual Review of Psychology* 53: 245.

Revonsuo, A. (2001). Dreaming and the place of consciousness in nature. *Behavioral and Brain Sciences* 24: 1000–1001.

Riesenhuber, M., and Poggio, T. (1999). Hierarchical models of object recognition in cortex. *Nature Neuroscience* 2: 1019–1025.

Rizzolatti, G. C. L. (2004). The mirror-neuron system. *Annual Review of Neuroscience* 27: 169–192.

Rizzolatti, G. L. G. (2001). The cortical motor system. *Neuron* 31: 889–901.

Rizzolatti, G., Fadiga, L., Gallese, V., and Fogassi, L. (1996). Premotor cortex and the recognition of motor actions. *Cognitive Brain Research* 32: 131–141.

Rizzolatti, G., Fogassi, L., and Gallese, V. (1997). Parietal cortex: From sight to action. *Current Opinion in Neurobiology* 7: 562–567.

Rizzolatti, G., Scandolara, C., Matelli, M., and Gentilucci, M. (1981a). Afferent properties of periarcuate neurons in macaque monkeys: I. Somatosensory responses. *Behavioural Brain Research* 2: 125–146.

Rizzolatti, G., Scandolara, C., Matelli, M., and Gentilucci, M. (1981b). Afferent properties of periarcuate neurons in macaque monkeys. II. Visual responses. *Behavioural Brain Research* 2: 147–163.

Robertson, A. R. (1997). Fluoxetine and involuntary recall of remote memories. *Australian and New Zealand Journal of Psychiatry* 31: 128–130.

Sacks, O. (1995). *An Anthropologist on Mars*. New York: Knopf.

Salzman, C. D., Britten, K. H., and Newsome, W. T. (1990). Cortical microstimulation influences perceptual judgements of motion direction. *Nature* 346: 174–177.

Schacter, D. (1989). On the relation between memory and consciousness: Dissociable interactions and conscious experience. In H. R. Craik (Ed.), *Varieties of Memory and Consciousness: Essays in Honor of Endel Tulving*. Hillsdale, N.J.: Erlbaum.

Schall, J. D. (2002). The neural selection and control of saccades by the frontal eye field. *Philosophical Transactions of the Royal Society London B Biological Sciences* 357: 1073–1082.

Schall, J. D. (2003). The neural selection and control of saccades by the frontal eye field. In A. Parker, A. Derrington, and C. Blakemore (Eds.), *The Physiology of Cognitive Processes*. New York: Oxford University Press, 173–189.

Schanz, F. A. (1923). New theory of vision. *American Journal of Physiological Optics* 4: 284–293.

Schneider, G. E. (1969). Two visual systems. *Science* 163: 895–902.

Serre, T., Kreiman, G., Kouh, M., Cadieu, C., Knoblich, U., and Poggio, T. (2007). A quantitative theory of immediate visual recognition. *Progress in Brain Research* 165: 33–36.Sesack, S. R., et al. (2004). In B. Moghaddam and M. E. Wolf (Eds.), *Glutamate and Disorders of Cognition and Motivation*. New York: New York Academy of Sciences, 36–52.

Simons, D. J., and Rensink, R. A. (2005a). Change blindness: Past, present, and future. *Trends in Cognitive Sciences* 9: 16–20.

Simons, D. J., and Rensink, R. A. (2005b) Change blindness, representations, and consciousness: reply to Noë. *Trends in Cognitive Sciences* 9: 219–219.

Singer, T. (2006). The neuronal basis and ontogeny of empathy and mind reading: Review of literature and implications for future research. *Neuroscience and Biobehavioral Reviews* 30: 855–863.

Singh, M., and Hoffman, D. (1998). Active vision and the basketball problem. *Behavioral and Brain Sciences* 21: 772–773.

Smeets, W., and Gonzalez, A. (2000). Evolution of the basal ganglia: New perspectives through a comparative approach. *Journal of Anatomy* 196: 501–517.

Smith, C. N., Clark, R. E., Manns, J. R., and Squire, L. R. (2005). Acquisition of differential delay eyeblink classical conditioning is independent of awareness. *Behavioral Neuroscience* 119: 78–86.

Smith, C., and Squire, L. R. (2005). Declarative memory, awareness, and transitive inference. *Journal of Neuroscience* 25: 10138–10146.

Sober, S. J., and Sabes, P. N. (2005). Flexible strategies for sensory integration during motor planning. *Nature Neuroscience* 8: 490–497.

Sprengelmeyer, R., Schroeder, U., Young, A.W., and Epplen, J. T. (2006). Disgust in pre-clinical Huntington's disease: A longitudinal study. *Neuropsychologia* 44: 518–533.

Squire, L. R. (2004). Memory systems of the brain: A brief history and current perspective. *Neurobiology of Learning and Memory* 82: 171–177.

Squire, L. R. (2007). Rapid consolidation. *Science* 316: 57–58.

Squire, L. R., Wixted, J. T., and Clark, R. E. (2007). Recognition memory and the medial temporal lobe: A new perspective. *Nature Reviews Neuroscience* 8: 872–883.

Stern, Y., and Langston, J. W. (1985). Intellectual changes in patients with MPTP-induced Parkinsonism. *Neurology* 35: 1506–1509.

Stich, S. (1983). *From Folk Psychology to Cognitive Science: The Case against Belief.* Cambridge, Mass.: MIT Press.

Stratton, G. M. (1897). Vision without inversion of the retinal image. *Psychological Review* 4: 463–481.

Taylor, J. G. (1962). *The Behavioral Basis of Perception.* New Haven, Conn.: Yale University Press.

Tulving, E. (1972). Episodic and semantic memory. In E. Tulving and W. Donaldson (Eds.), *Organization of Memory.* New York: Academic Press, 381–403.

Tulving, E. (1983). *Elements of Episodic Memory.* Oxford: Clarendon.

Tulving, E. (1985a). How many memory systems are there? *American Psychologist* 40: 385–398.

Tulving, E. (1985b). Memory and consciousness. *Canadian Psychology/Psychologie Canadienne* 26: 1–12.

Tulving, E. (2002a). Episodic memory: From mind to brain. *Annual Review of Psychology* 53: 1.

Tulving, E. (2002b). Chronesthesia: Conscious awareness of subjective time. In D. T. Stuss and R. T. Knight (Eds.), *Principles of Frontal Lobe Function.* New York: Oxford University Press, 311–325.

Tulving, E., and Schacter, D. (1990). Primary and human memory systems. *Science* 247: 310–306.

Tye, M. (1995). *Ten Problems of Consciousness.* Cambridge, Mass.: MIT Press.

Tye, M. (2000). *Consciousness, Color, and Content.* Cambridge, Mass.: MIT Press.

Umeno, M. M., and Goldberg, M. E. (2001). Spatial processing in the monkey frontal eye field. II. Memory responses. *Journal of Neurophysiology* 86: 2344–2343.

Ungerleider, L. G., and Pribram, K. H. (1977). Inferotemporal versus combined pulvinar-prestriate lesions in the rhesus monkey: Effects on color, object and pattern discrimination. *Neuropsychologia* 15: 481–498.

Velichkovsky, B.M., Joos, M., Helmert, J.R. & Pannasch, S. (2005). Two visual systems and their eye movements: Evidence from static and dynamic scene perception. In *Proceedings of the XXVII Conference of the Cognitive Science Society,* 2283–2288.

Walk, R. D., Shepherd, J. D., and Miller, D. R. (1988). Attention and the depth perception of kittens. *Bulletin of the Psychonomic Society* 26: 248–251.

Waller, A. D. (1909). Note on the latency of the photo-electrical response of the frog's retina before and after massage of the eyeball. *Quarterly Journal of Experimental Physiology* 2: 401–401.

Walls, G. L. (1928). The photo-mechanical changes in the retina of mammals. *Science* 67: 655–656.

Walls, G. L. (1934). Human rods and cones. the state of knowledge. *Archives of Ophthalmology (Chicago)* 12: 914–930.

Walls, G. L. (1942). *The Vertebrate Eye and its Adaptive Radiation.* Oxford: Cranbrook Institute of Science.

Walls, G. L. (1953). *The Lateral Geniculate Nucleus and Visual Histophysiology*. Berkeley: University of California Press.

Welchman, A. E., Deubelius, A., Conrad, V., Bülthoff, H. H., and Kourtzi, Z. (2005). 3-D shape perception from combined depth cues in human visual cortex. *Nature Neuroscience* 8: 820–827.

Wheeler, M. A., Stuss, D. T., and Tulving, E. (1997). Toward a theory of episodic memory: The frontal lobes and autonoetic consciousness. *Psychological Bulletin* 121: 331–354.

Witherington, D. C., Campos, J. J., Anderson, D. I., Lejeune, L., and Seah, E. (2005). Avoidance of heights on the visual cliff in newly walking infants. *Infancy* 7: 285–298.

Wolgin, D. L., Hein, A., and Teitelbaum, P. (1980). Recovery of forelimb placing after lateral hypothalamic lesions in the cat: Parallels and contrasts with development. *Journal of Comparative and Physiological Psychology* 94: 795–807.

Xing, J., and Andersen, R. A. (2000). Models of the posterior parietal cortex which perform multimodal integration and represent space in several coordinate frames. *Journal of Cognitive Neuroscience* 12: 601–614.

Yonas, A., and Granrud, C. E. (2006). Infants' perception of depth from cast shadows. *Perception and Psychophysics* 68: 154–160.

PART IV

NEUROCOMPUTATION AND NEUROANATOMY

CHAPTER 12

....

SPACE, TIME, AND OBJECTS

....

RICK GRUSH

1. INTRODUCTION

....

In this chapter, I outline a unified information processing framework whose goal is to explain how the nervous system represents space, time, and objects. In the remainder of this introductory section, I am more specific about the sort of spatial, temporal, and object representation at issue, and then I outline the structure of this chapter.

It is standard procedure to distinguish different kinds of spatial representation, and the most basic distinction is between *allocentric* (or *objective*) and egocentric spatial representation.[1]

The idea is that egocentric spatial representation is how an organism represents its environment for purposes of perception and action. The directions involved in egocentric spatial representation are *above, ahead, to the left*, and so forth. Allocentric or objective spatial representation lacks any explicit reference to the organism itself: When I grasp the thought that the Arc de Triomphe is between the Obelisk and the Grand Arche de la Défense, my spatial representation is in terms of objective spatial relations and perhaps objective units of magnitude as well. I am concerned exclusively with the egocentric variety of spatial representation, but to avoid baggage connected to that expression in the literature, I prefer the expression *behavioral space* to *egocentric space*.

A similar distinction can be made in the case of temporal representation. When I conceive of World War II as being after World War I, I am not thinking in terms of the temporal relation of those events to my current thought. The magnitudes and directions (so to speak) are independent of my current temporal location. By contrast, when I think that the traffic light is about to turn red, or that I went through the door just a moment ago, neither the units nor directions (past versus future) are independent of my current temporal location and capacities. I may have a very good idea of when the light will turn red, but a very poor capacity to specify this in objective units, such as milliseconds. I refer to the sort of time I am interested in as *behavioral time*: the time in whose terms the content of our current perception and action is given.

Finally, objects can be conceived of objectively, as things not tied to my current perception of or action on them. But it is also possible to grasp objects as entities in my behavioral field, as things on which I can perceive and act. I am likewise concerned with the representation of such *behavioral objects*.

Section 2 is a very brief introduction to the emulation theory of representation (more detail can be found in Grush, 2004). This theory holds that the nervous system constructs and uses models of the body and environment to represent them in perception, action, and imagery. It is important to note that the emulation theory itself is silent on *how* this internal model is implemented and also silent on what sorts of things can be represented. It is a general architecture that describes how an internal model, or emulator, can be comported within a larger system to play certain kinds of roles in perception, imagery, off-line planning, and so forth. I provide some details as to how the emulation theory can be applied to the specific cases of behavioral space, behavioral time, and behavioral objects, and the specific way this emulator is implemented neurally.

In section 3 I briefly describe an extension of the emulation framework for temporal representation (more detail can be found in Grush, 2005). This is an extension of the emulation theory from an internal model that, at any given point in time, represents the target domain as it is at a point in time, to an internal model that represents, at any given point in time, the behavior of the target domain over a temporal interval.

In section 4 I discuss spatial representation, in particular Alexandre Pouget's basis function model of spatial representation (see, e.g., Pouget, Deneve, and Duhamel, 2002). This is a specific proposal about the neural implementation of spatial representation, in particular of behavioral spatial representation.[2] In brief, the model has it that the locations of objects are represented as a set of basis function values of the sensory and postural signals involved in the perceptual episode.

In section 5 I describe how to combine the basis function model of spatial representation with the trajectory emulation model of temporal representation to yield an information processing framework that genuinely represents behavioral spatiotemporal trajectories of behavioral objects. Section 6 concludes.

2. EMULATION THEORY

In this section I introduce a theory of the information processing structure that the brain employs to construct and use representations of entities external to the brain, especially the body and the environment. This introduction is quite brief, and includes neither much of the supporting evidence to the effect that this is in fact the information processing structure that the brain uses nor many of the applications of the theory that supply tremendous explanatory leverage in the attempt to understand the brain's operation. Much of this omitted material can be found in Grush (2004). Readers familiar with the emulation theory can safely skip sections 2.1 and 2.3, though I still recommend section 2.2. If I am right, the brain has and uses many emulators, and I describe a number of them. There are emulators of the body that are used for various motor control purposes and to produce motor imagery; emulators of the visual scene that produce anticipations of what will be seen, and can be used to produce visual imagery; and amodal emulators of the environment that maintain representations of what is happening in the immediate vicinity. Many of these can be run in parallel, and in fact as we shall see, the operation of an emulator of the body and of the sensory modalities being run in parallel is arguably a big part of the explanation of our ability to represent egocentric space in an amodal way.

I should point out that in claiming that this is a way to understand representation, I am simultaneously trying to explain a phenomenon and define my use of terms. Other people may have some idea of what representations are that does not jibe with what I am about to say. That is fine. I am not interested in fighting over who gets to use the word *representation* but in understanding a certain kind of phenomenon—the capacity of a sophisticated system to construct and maintain "internal" states that track the behavior of other entities to assist it in its interactions with these other entities. It seems to me that the word *representation* and its cognates are a natural fit for this phenomenon, and if one wants to couch the issue in terms of providing an account of what representation is, or something like that, then what I am about to do, and the "representation" terminology I use in doing it, strikes me as reasonable and natural. But anyone who has their own ax to grind about the word *representation* is invited to provide their own terminology for what I am about to describe.

2.1. Control, Filtering, and Emulation Basics

The most basic division in control theory is between the thing doing the controlling, and the thing being controlled. I will typically call the first the *controller*, and the latter the *process*.[3] There are two basic kinds of classical control architectures that describe how the controller influences the process: open-loop (a.k.a. feedforward) and closed-loop (a.k.a. feedback) control. These are shown in figure 12.1.

The controller is provided with some goal state—the state that the process should be in. This goal is most often specified in terms of some measured state or states of the process. For example, a thermostat is given as its goal a temperature for the room or building, and this is measured by a sensor—a thermometer—that is sensitive to that state of the process. An autopilot controls an aircraft, and its goals are in terms of an altitude, heading, speed—all of which are measured by various instruments on the aircraft. There are, of course, many states of the room or aircraft

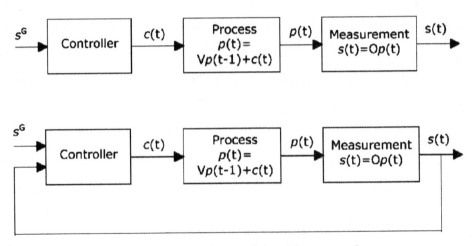

Figure 12.1. Open-loop and closed-loop control.

that are not measured, and some of these may be important for the operation of the process. The mass of the aircraft is not measured, nor is the force applied to the wing by the engine. *Measured* states will be called sensor signals, because they are typically produced by sensors that monitor or measure some state(s) of the process. The goal state then is a target sensor signal, which I call s^G.[4]

The controller's job is to produce a control signal, or sequence of control signals, that will, when issued to the process, cause the process to go into the goal state (as determined by the measured sensor signals). The controller can thus be described as a function that maps a specification of the sensory goal into control signals. The process is some system such that its state at any given time t is a function of (at least) two factors: its state at the previous time $t - 1$, and the current control signal $c(t)$. If we let V stand for the function that determines how the state of the process would evolve over time in absence of any external influence, we have: $p(t) = Vp(t - 1) + c(t)$.

The measurement is just some mechanism that measures one or more states of the process to produce a sensor signal. If we use the label $s(t)$ for the sensor signal that is produced at any given time t, we have: $s(t) = Op(t)$, where O is the measurement function. Notice that the sensory goal s^G does not change over time, like the sensory state $s(t)$ and process state $p(t)$ do.

An open-loop controller is one that determines the control signals without benefit of information about the state of the process as the control episode unfolds. A closed-loop controller has the benefit of a continual stream of feedback from the process (in the form of the sensor signal) to help determine the control signals. A thermostat is the standard example of a closed-loop controller. The process in this case is the room or building together with its heating system. The measurement is a measurement of one crucial state of the process, its temperature. The goal state is a goal temperature for the room or building, and this is often input to the controller by moving a lever along a calibrated set of marks. The controller compares the goal temperature with the actual temperature—which it has access to via a measurement of the process. In the simplest case, this measurement is implemented by the angle of a bimetallic strip. Based on this comparison, the controller either turns (or keeps) the heater on, or turns (or keeps) the heater off. The result of the controller's operation is that it produces a sequence of signals, typically in the form of electrical signals sent to the heating system, whose effect is to get the process to the goal state (as determined by the sensor signal).

An example of an open loop controller is an old-fashioned toaster. The process is the heating elements and bread. The controller is simply a timer that keeps the heating elements on for some period of time (this is as least one way toasters have been implemented, there are others). As with the thermostat, one sets the goal state by moving a lever along a calibrated scale, typically ranging from "light" to "dark." On the basis of this input, the controller produces a control sequence and issues it to the process, in the form of keeping a circuit that powers the heating elements closed for some period of time. Unlike the thermostat, the controller gets no feedback concerning how the process develops during the control episode. The control sequence is determined on the exclusive basis of the input of the desired goal state. If everything works well, when this control signal is acted on by the process, the effect is that the bread is toasted to the degree specified by the desired goal that was input.

My purpose in discussing control theory is not to discuss thermostats or toasters but to understand the operation of the brain. In the case of motor control (the most obvious application of control theory in the brain), much of the debate on this topic in the twentieth century was a debate between proponents of closed-loop and those of open-loop control as a model for human motor control. In the closed-loop camp (which was heavily influenced by the cyberneticists, themselves largely closed-loop control endorsers whether or not they used that terminology), the motor control centers know the current state of the body and the goal state, and issue commands that will reduce the distance between the two until the difference is zero. This is standard closed-loop thinking.

The open-loop proponents, driven by data that suggested that the initial stages of a given movement appear to be the same whether or not the feedback signal is tampered with, held that the initial stages of a movement are open-loop—a motor volley determined and executed without employing any feedback. One standard way to tamper with the feedback signal is tendon vibration. The two main mechanisms by which the nervous system gets information about the position of the body are stretch receptors, which are responsive to muscle length, and Golgi tendon organs, which are sensitive to tendon tension. Appropriate vibration at muscle–tendon interface can stimulate stretch receptors, fouling the feedback they provide. The finding is that this interference appears to make a difference to the motor control episode only toward the very end of the movement, earlier stages being largely unaffected. This led these researchers to suggest that motor control is closed-loop only at the very end of the movement (grasping and pointing are typical examples) when fine adjustments are needed. For more on this debate, see Desmurget and Grafton (2000).

Closed-loop and open-loop control, though the most well-known kinds of control scheme, do not exhaust the possibilities. In this subsection and the next I discuss a few additional schemes, all of which make use of a construct that has not yet been introduced, the *forward model* (which I also call an *emulator*). The simplest scheme to use a forward model is pseudo-closed loop control, which is shown in figure 12.2. In this scheme we have a controller and a process, as in the closed- and open-loop schemes. In addition there is an entity that implements the same (or close to the same) input-output mapping as the process. It is a model of the forward mapping.

In this scheme, the control signal $c(t)$ is split into two copies, one of which goes to the process as in closed- and open-loop schemes. The other copy is sent to the emulator (which here is a *model* of the process plus a model of the measurement). The process model models the states of the process and also models the way that those states evolve over time. While the real process has a state $p(t)$ at any given time, the model has an *estimate* of that state, $\bar{p}(t)$. Just as the real process evolves over time as a function of its previous state $p(t-1)$ and the control signal, so the process model's state evolves over time as a function of its previous state $\bar{p}(t-1)$ and the control signal. The process model is subjected to a measurement that produces a mock sensory signal $\bar{s}(t)$.

Because the emulator (process model + measurement) implements the same input-output mapping as the real process + measurement, and because it is being given the same input, it will produce the same output: that is, $\bar{s}(t)$ will be equal to $s(t)$. Because the output is the same, the emulator's feedback $\bar{s}(t)$ can be provided to the controller in lieu of the feedback produced by the measurement of the process. (These are ideal conditions, of course, and complexities such as noise and random disturbances will be introduced shortly.)

There are many uses for process models, including helping the controller deal with delayed feedback from the real process; running the emulator only, with the process completely idle, to test out counterfactuals, to see what the process would do if certain control signals were issued to it; running the emulator and process in

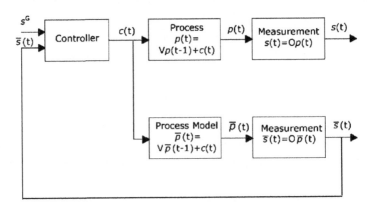

Figure 12.2. Pseudo-closed-loop control.

parallel and using the emulator's feedback to fill in or correct faulty or noisy sensor information from the measurement of the process. This last use requires some more sophisticated mechanisms, to which I turn.

The Kalman filter (Kalman, 1960; Kalman and Bucy, 1961; henceforth *KF*) per se is, as the name implies, a method of filtering noise from a signal. As such it is not necessarily involved in control structures. I first describe one standard version of the *KF* and then explain how it can be integrated into a control structure. For convenience I treat time as discrete, but extensions of *KF*s to continuous time are available, just more complicated. The top third of figure 12.3 exhibits the problem that the *KF* solves. A process evolves over time, in part as a function of its own inner dynamic, but possibly also under the influence of some external driving force and perhaps even random disturbances.

At each time t the process is measured to produce a signal $I(t)$. But this measurement process is not perfect, and the imperfection can be represented as the addition of noise $n(t)$ to $I(t)$. The *observed* (noisy) signal is $s(t) = I(t) + n(t)$. So we have made the process as described in the previous section more realistic by accommodating the possibility of unpredictable disturbances to the process's state, as well as noise in the measurement of the process.

The *KF*'s job is to determine what the real signal $I(t)$ is, or to put it another way, to filter the noise from the observed signal. (If the measurement function O is invertible, then this is equivalent to knowing the process's actual state.) The *KF* itself is diagrammed on the lower two-thirds of figure 12.3. The *KF* has knowledge of the function V that governs the evolution of the process, as well as the measurement function that produces signals based on the process's state. It also knows,

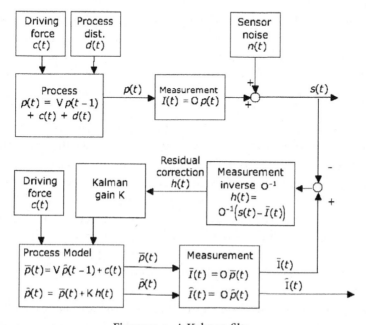

Figure 12.3. A Kalman filter.

at each time step, what the observed signal is and what the driving force (if any), is. What it does *not* know is the state of the process, the process noise, or the sensor noise.

This description may sound like it applies only to artificial situations, but in fact this is characteristic of many real-world situations, such as ship navigation. The navigation team knows the driving force if any (we can suppose that they simply listen in as the captain is giving orders), and they know the observed signals—the noisy measurements provided by the bearing takers, and so on. They have knowledge of how a ship's state evolves over time. For example, they know basic stuff, such as if a ship is at location X and is going at speed S and direction D, then at the next time it will be at Y. The team also knows how the measurement process works, in that they know how to translate from ship state to bearing measurements and vice versa (this is just basic trigonometry). They do not know how inaccurate the bearing measurements are (sensor noise), nor do they know the process disturbance—unknown winds and ocean currents, for example. The navigation team's job is to determine the ship's actual state, which, given the capacity to translate between process state and measurements, is equivalent to determining what perfectly accurate noise-free measurement would be.

There are many other situations that fit this general structure as well. A relevant example is the brain, which tries to keep an accurate estimate of the body's state. It has knowledge of motor commands that it has sent (it knows the driving force); it has a bunch of sensor information that is noisy and imperfect in various ways; it has, through experience, knowledge of how the body's state generally evolves over time; and on the basis of these sources of information it tries to determine what is really going on with the body.

Back to an explanation of the *KF*. The main trick of the *KF* is that it uses its various sources of information to maintain an optimal estimate of the state of the process. It then subjects this process state estimate to a measurement that is just like the real measurement of the real process that produces the real noise-free signal. The result is an optimal estimate of the real noise-free signal. So the question now is: How does the *KF* get and maintain an optimal estimate of the state of the process?

The *KF* begins each cycle with the state estimate it produced at the previous cycle. After I have explained the *KF*'s operation, I return to the question of how the *KF* first gets a workable estimate without any previous estimate. This turns out to be relatively trivial. For now, though, it is easiest to assume that it has a decent estimate from the *previous* cycle to begin with. The first thing the *KF* does is to produce an a priori estimate of what the current process state should be: $\bar{p}(t)$. This estimate is a priori in that it has not yet taken into account any of the information from the observed signal. The *KF* arrives at $\bar{p}(t)$ by taking its previous state estimate and the current driving force and applying its knowledge of how the process's state evolves over time, V. So for example, the navigation team can take its estimate of the ship's state at the previous fix cycle, together with the commands that have been issued by the captain concerning engine speed and rudder angle, to produce an a priori estimate as to what the ship's current state ought to be. This cycle of the *KF*'s operation is sometimes called the *time update*.

The second cycle, sometimes called the *measurement update*, of operation is where the *KF* adjusts its a priori estimate on the basis of the observed signal. The result of this adjustment is the a posteriori estimate, $\hat{p}(t)$, and this is the *KF*'s final estimate of the state of the process at that time. This cycle unfolds as follows. First, the a priori state estimate $\bar{p}(t)$ is measured to produce an a priori estimate of the real signal $\bar{I}(t)$. (I consistently use a straight bar over a variable to indicate an a priori estimate of that variable's value.[5]) This is what the *KF* expects the observed signal to be, given its a priori state estimate and current driving force. This is compared to the actual observed signal $s(t)$. The difference is the mismatch between what the *KF* expected to see, given its a priori estimate, and what it actually saw from the observed signal. By pushing this difference through an inverse of the measurement function,[6] the *KF* arrives at a measure of the difference between its own a priori estimate of the process's state and what the process's state would have to be if the observed signal were accurate. This is called the *sensory residual*.

The tricky part is that the sensor signal is not perfect. There is noise, and in the navigation example, this is a reflection of the fact that the people taking the bearings are not completely accurate. Because of this, one cannot assume that the existence of a nonzero sensory residual means that the a priori estimate was inaccurate. Even if the a priori estimate is entirely accurate, the existence of sensor noise will create a sensory residual.

Before explaining how the *KF* arrives at its a posteriori estimate, it is worth exploring the way that the a priori estimates $\bar{p}(t)$ and $\bar{I}(t)$ and the observed signal $s(t)$ differ with respect to how they handle the two kinds of unpredictability inherent in the process and measurement. These two sources of unpredictability are the process disturbance (unpredictable disturbances to the process's state during the last time step) and the sensor noise (imperfections in the signal produced). The a priori estimates are not affected by sensor noise for the simple reason that they do not make any use of the observed signal. The weakness of the a priori estimates is process disturbance. If there were no process disturbance, then the a priori estimates would be entirely accurate (given of course that the estimate available from the previous time was accurate). But because of unpredictable changes to the state of the process, the a priori estimates will not be entirely accurate even if the previous state estimate was. The sensor signal is exactly the opposite. It is unaffected by process disturbance for the simple reason that it is a measurement of the current actual state of the process. This measurement does not depend on how the process got to the state it is in.

These observations on the complementary strengths and weaknesses of the a priori estimate and the measured process state provide the rationale behind the way the *KF* produces its a posteriori estimate. If the magnitude of the process disturbance is large compared to the magnitude of the sensor noise, the *KF* will weight the observed signal more heavily than the a priori estimate when combining the two. In the navigation case, this would be a situation in which we know that there are strong unpredictable currents (we know we are in the middle of a storm, e.g.), but the people taking the bearing measurements are very accurate and reliable. In such a situation, if your prediction based on the last location of the ship was in significant conflict with what the people taking the bearings are telling you, you go with what the reliable bearing takers say and credit the disparity between what you predicted and what you observed to process disturbance that moved your ship off course. If, on the other hand, there is very little process disturbance (the seas and winds are calm), but the measurement process is very noisy—perhaps the bearing takers are drunk—then you will weight your prediction based on the last estimate more heavily and credit any major difference to noise in the observed signal.

The relative magnitude of the process disturbance and the sensor noise determines a factor, called the Kalman gain, that the *KF* uses when combining the a priori estimate and the measures process state. It is, roughly, a fraction that determines the relative weight given to each when they are combined to form the a posteriori estimate. Given the structure of the problem faced by the *KF* and the way this gain is determined, this estimate represents the optimal estimate in the sense that there is no better estimate that could be produced given the information that the *KF* has access to. The *KF* then subjects this a posteriori process state estimate $\hat{p}(t)$ to a measurement, and the result is the *KF*'s a posteriori estimate of what the real, noise-free signal is: $\hat{I}(t)$. The a posteriori estimate then forms the starting point for the a priori estimate of the next cycle, and the cycle repeats.

It is a trivial matter to integrate the *KF* into a control scheme. This is shown in figure 12.4.

The control architecture diagrammed in figure 12.4 has the various control structures discussed in the previous sections as special cases. An open-loop control scheme results if the mechanisms shown in the bottom two-thirds are ignored. A closed-loop system results if the Kalman gain is set so as to always use the entire residual correction. This is because if the entire residual correction is used, then the a posteriori estimate will always be equivalent to the observed signal, and hence the signal sent back to the controller will always be equivalent to the signal produced by the actual measurement of the process, just as in closed-loop control. Finally, if the Kalman gain is set to ignore the sensory residual altogether, the scheme becomes equivalent to pseudo–closed-loop control. If the sensory residual is ignored, then an a posteriori estimate is always equivalent to the a priori estimate, and in this case the process model simply evolves over time as a result of its own inner dynamic and the efference copies. Perhaps the most perspicuous way to understand the scheme is as a closed-loop control system that uses a *KF* to filter noise from the feedback signal.

I have used the *KF* as an example mostly because it is mathematically well defined, and by using an example that is so well defined, a number of distinctions can be made more efficiently than they could have been with a more qualitative example on hand. But the emulation theory is not identical to Kalman filtering. The *KF* is one example of the emulation framework, but not the only example. The emulation framework is an information processing strategy according to which a

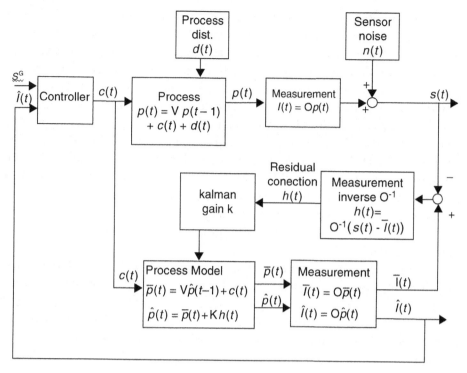

Figure 12.4. A control scheme that uses a Kalman filter.

system maintains a model of some other system and uses this model in various ways: It can operate on the model independently of the modeled system to get an idea of how the modeled system would behave in various circumstances; it can operate the model in parallel to the modeled system to overcome problems with sensory access to the modeled system, such as feedback delays, noisy sensors, and so on. The *KF* is relatively restricted: It does not run the model off-line, and when run in parallel with the process it does not use the model in such a way as to deal with feedback delays (the *KF* is set up to solve a problem other than feedback delays), and it combines the sensory information and the model's state in very specific ways. The emulation framework drops these restrictions. An emulator-employing system might use an emulator to help process sensor signals but not strictly determine anything like a Kalman gain to *optimally* combine then, but use some other method, perhaps including just giving each equal weight. It might use the emulator completely off-line to produce imagery or run thought experiments (more on this shortly).

2.2. Modal versus Amodal Emulation

In this subsection I very briefly introduce a distinction between two kinds of emulation, what I will call modal and amodal emulation. This will be a quick discussion, more detail on the difference between modal and amodal emulation can be found in Grush (2004). All of the emulators I have described so far have been models of the *process*. Additional components, specifically measurement functions, have been appended to the process and the process model to map states of the process or process model into signals in sensory format. These are all examples of what I will call amodal emulation. The emulator itself, the process model, is not tied to any sensory modality. Rather, the sensors are distinct mechanisms, and the modality would be the way the process (or process model) is measured. The following analogy should help make this clear. Your environment—the spatial vicinity around you and the objects in it—is not intrinsically visual or auditory or gustatory. The environment itself is amodal. Your body has various sensory modalities that can measure the environment in different ways. Visual sensors produce signals that give information about some of the states of the environment but are insensitive to others. Auditory sensors produce signals that pick up on features that vision is deaf to, but audition is itself blind to many features vision picks up on. And so forth for other modalities.

The situation is similar for emulators. A model of the process can be subjected to various measurements: measurements that produce estimates of what the visual signal will be, measurements that produce estimates of what the auditory signal will be, and so forth. (One might take a navigator's ship model and "measure" its location but not direction or speed; or one might measure its heading, but not location.) But another kind of emulator is possible—modality-specific emulators. This can be illustrated with an example, Bartlett Mel's Murphy (Mel, 1986, 1988). Murphy consists of a system that controls a robotic arm, its task being to move its arm around obstacles in a workspace and grasp targets. The arm's movement is confined to a plane. Murphy observes the workspace and its arm's motion via a video camera above the workspace. This camera drives a 64×64 grid of pixels that function as a low-resolution image, which is Murphy's sole access to what is happening in the workspace. As Murphy issues commands to its arm, in the form of changes to its shoulder, elbow, and wrist angles, it sees the results of its commands on the grid.

Murphy, however, implements a *modal* emulator of its environment. The units on the grid are actually connectionist units that learn to predict the results of given motor commands on the next workspace image. For example, if the pattern of activation on the grid is G_1, and Murphy issues motor command M_1, and this results in the pattern of activation on the grid changing to G_2, the units learn that in the future if the grid is displaying G_1, and M_1 is issued, the next image on the grid will be G_2. Once the grid has observed and learned from a sufficiently large sample of Murphy's overt operation, Murphy can take its arm and workspace off-line and operate only with the visual grid in emulation mode. Starting with an image of an initial arm and workspace configuration, Murphy issues motor commands that are suppressed from affecting the real arm (this is what it means to take the arm off-line) but are nevertheless processed by the visual grid such that the grid changes its state into an estimate of what the visual grid state would be if the arm were still online. Murphy is thus producing visual imagery by driving its visual grid with efference copies. Once Murphy has discovered a way to move its imagined arm around the

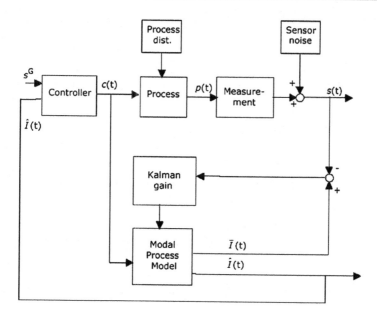

Figure 12.5. A modality-specific emulator.

imagined obstacles to grasp the imagined target, it puts its arm back online and implements the solution it found. The sort of emulation that Murphy implements can be diagrammed in figure 12.5.

Here, the emulator is not a model of the process per se but a modality-specific emulator of the system consisting of the process and a specific modality of measurement. Because of this, the emulator's output is not subjected to a measurement. Its output is already, by definition, in the format of the relevant sensory system. In Murphy's case, this was visual.

We can easily imagine systems that combine modal and amodal emulation. Such a system is shown in figure 12.6. Here, the same efference copies drive an amodal process model as well as a modality specific emulator. Both can be used to produce a priori estimates: one an estimate of what the state of the process will be, the other a modal estimate of what the sensory signal will be.

The system described in figure 12.6 employs two emulators: one an amodal process model, the other a modality specific emulator of the sensory systems. One copy of the command is provided to the amodal process model to produce an a priori estimate of the process's state; another copy is processed by the modal emulator to produce an a priori estimate of the next sensory state.

When the amodal process model's a priori state estimate is measured, another a priori estimate of the sensory state is produced. In figure 12.6 the a priori estimate produced by the modal emulator is called $\bar{I}^{M}$ (t), and the one produced by the measurement of the amodal process model is called $\bar{I}^{A}$ (t). A sensory residual is now determined by comparing the two a priori estimates with the observed signal.[7] This residual can then be used to produce a posteriori estimates of both the modal and amodal estimates.

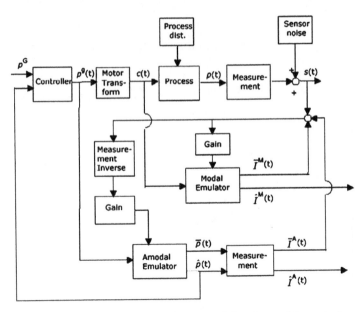

Figure 12. 6. A system that combines modal and amodal emulation.

Striking confirmation of the existence of a purely visual modality specific emulator comes from a phenomenon hypothesized by von Helmholtz (1910) and discussed and verified experimentally by Ernst Mach (1896). Subjects whose eyes are prevented from moving and who are presented with a stimulus that would normally trigger a saccade (such as a flash of light in the periphery of the visual field) report seeing the entire visual scene momentarily shift in the direction opposite of the stimulus. Such cases are very plausibly described as those in which the perceptual system is producing a prediction—an a priori estimate—of what the next *visual* scene will be on the basis of the current visual scene and the current motor command. Normally a motor command to move the eyes to the right will result in the image that is currently projected on the retina (and hence fed to downstream topographically organized visual areas of the brain) shifting to the left. Some region in the nervous system is apparently processing a copy of this driving force and producing an anticipation of such a shifted image—an anticipated image so strong that subjects actually report seeing it briefly. Normally such a prediction would provide to specific areas of the visual system a head start for processing incoming information by priming them for the likely locations of edges, surfaces, and so on. This a priori prediction would normally be largely confirmed and seamlessly absorbed into ongoing perception as part of the a posteriori estimates. You do not normally notice these images, but they are ubiquitous.

Nearly 100 years after Mach published his experimental result, Duhamel, Colby, and Goldberg (1992) published findings that seem to point to the neural basis of this effect. They found neurons in the parietal cortex of the monkey that remap their retinal receptive fields in such a way as to anticipate immanent stimulation as a function of saccade efference copies.

The situation is illustrated in figure 12.7. Box A represents a situation in which the visual scene is centered on a small disk. The receptive field of a given posterior parietal cortex (PPC) cell is shown in the empty circle in the upper left quadrant. The receptive field is always locked to a given region of the visual space, in this case above and just to the left of the center. Because nothing is in this cell's receptive field, it is inactive. The arrow is the direction of a planned saccade, which will move the eye so that the square will be in the center of the visual field. There is a stimulus, marked by an asterisk, in the upper right-hand quadrant. This stimulus is not currently in the receptive field of the PPC neuron in question, but it is located such that if the eye is moved so as to foveate the square, the stimulus *will* move into the cell's receptive field, as illustrated in Box B. The Duhamel et al. finding was that given a visual scene such as represented in Box A, if an eye movement that will result in a scene such as that in Box B is executed, the PPC neuron will begin firing shortly after the motor command to move the eye is issued, but before the eye has actually moved. The PPC neuron appears to be anticipating its future activity as a function of the current retinal projection and the just-issued motor command. The control condition is shown in Boxes C and D. In this case, the same eye movement to the square will not bring a stimulus into the receptive field of the neuron, and in this case the neuron does not engage in any anticipatory activity. (Or, more accurately, it *does* engage in anticipatory activity, and what it is anticipating, correctly, is that nothing will be in its receptive field.) The control condition effectively rules out the hypothesis that the PPC cell is firing merely as a result of the motor command itself. Only if the motor command will have a certain sensory effect does the PPC cell fire. This is a neural implementation of the construction of an a priori estimate.

A full set of these neurons, covering the entire visual field, would explain the Helmholtz phenomenon. They would also constitute a modality specific emulator of the visual scene.

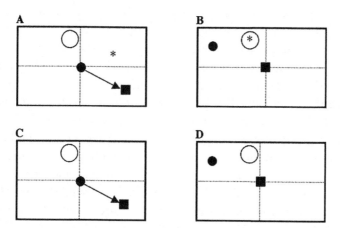

Figure 12.7. Anticipation of visual scene changes on eye movement. See text for details.

2.3. Application to Motor Control

2.3.1. *Motor Control*

One of the challenges in our understanding of motor control is the fact that the temporal length of the control loop—how long it takes for a signal to travel along biological axons from the motor areas of the brain to the body and for peripheral signals carrying information about the results of the execution of that command and be processed so that they can beneficially influence the ongoing motor commands—is not short. It is on the order of 250–400 ms (Dennier van der Gon, 1988; Ito, 1984). This by itself is interesting, for it seems as though motor control is relatively good during such short bursts, such delays notwithstanding. These twin facts have been one of the reasons that people have been drawn to models of motor control that are open-loop (a closed-loop control scheme with significantly delayed feedback would face significant problems) except for the very end of the movement, where feedback is presumed to be used to make refinements (see Desmurget and Grafton, 2000). Even more interesting, though, is the fact that it appears as though the motor centers make corrections to the motor plan as quickly as 70 ms or so after movement onset, corrections that appear to be made on the basis of peripheral information (van der Meulen et al., 1990). Thus it appears to be the case that the motor centers are getting and acting on peripheral feedback *before peripheral feedback should be available!*

In view of these facts and others, a growing number of motor control researchers are developing models of motor control that exploit forward models and (in some cases) Kalman filters (e.g., Blakemore, Goodbody, and Wolpert, 1998; Houk, Singh, Fischer, and Barto, 1990; Kawato, 1999; Krakauer, Ghilardi, and Ghez, 1999; Wolpert, Ghahramani, and Flanagan, 2001; for a very recent neurobiological vindication of forward models in motor control, see Mehta and Schaal, 2002). The main idea is that emulators of the body (specifically the musculoskeletal system and its dynamics) can process efferent copies and provide predictions of what the peripheral signal will be before the real peripheral signal is available (this was Ito's [1970, 1984] initial motivation for speculating on the existence of emulators in the cerebellum). A particularly clear example is Wolpert, Ghahramani, and Jordan (1995). These authors developed a model of the information processing structure of human motor performance with the aim of explaining the temporal patterns of errors and corrections in various movement conditions, one particular aspect being the potentially disruptive effects of feedback delays in fast real-time movement. The authors develop a model that is essentially of the form in figure 12.4, and show how patterns of movement errors under varying conditions can be explained on the assumption that during the initial phases of a movement, before proprioceptive feedback is available, the motor centers exploit feedback from an internal model of the musculoskeletal system (a priori predictions), while as time progresses, feedback from the periphery is incorporated into the estimate (a posteriori estimates).

2.3.2. *Motor Imagery/Motor Planning*

The previous subsection focused on the use of emulation during motor control—when the emulator is run in parallel with the real musculoskeletal system so that its timely feedback could stand in for the delayed feedback from the periphery. Now we turn to off-line uses. There has been a growing interest in the so-called simulation theory of motor imagery (Jeannerod, 2001; Johnson, 2000). According to this theory, motor imagery—the imagined proprioceptive feelings of movement and force—are the result of the off-line operation of the motor areas of the brain. This is entirely in line with the emulation theory, which holds that faux proprioception is the result of running the musculoskeletal emulator off-line, and the motor centers are what drive the emulator.[8]

The benefits of such off-line operations are many, but I mention only one here: *motor planning*. All movement tasks admit of an infinite number of solutions, some better than others. Depending on how your body is configured, and how your backpack is resting on the floor, and what you will be doing after you pick it up (opening it to look in it, grabbing it and walking away), taking an overhand or underhand grip on the strap might be better. We often choose the best grip quickly and without any conscious effort or awareness, but the motor systems are hard at work during the fractions of a second before the event. There is evidence (see Johnson, 2000, and references therein) to the effect that this motor planning involves covert motor imagery produced to determine which of a small number of options will work best.

3. TRAJECTORY EMULATION

3.1. Temporal Generalization of the Emulation Theory

The *KF* is temporally degenerate in two senses. First, it produces state estimates of only one time at a time. Second, these two times are always the same: for all times t_i, the state estimate that the *KF* produces at t_i is an estimate of the state of the process at t_i. This last claim might seem surprising at first, because doesn't the *KF* produce a *prediction* when it produces its a priori estimate? No. At least not in the relevant sense. At the beginning of each operational cycle, the *KF* produces an a priori estimate of the process's state. This estimate is a prediction in the sense that, once measured, it provides a prediction of what the observed signal is, and this "prediction" is compared with the observed signal to produce the sensory residual. But it is not a prediction in the sense that it is looking ahead in time. The a priori state estimate is an estimate of the state of the process as it *currently* is. It is a prediction in the sense that I might draw a card from a deck and ask you to predict what you will see when I turn it around. The card is already drawn when you produce your guess, so you aren't predicting what card I will draw. You are predicting what you will see when I turn the card around. It is only this sense in which the a priori estimate is a prediction.

The first generalization I undertake in this section takes us away from the *KF*'s ubiquitous focus on the co-temporaneous process state. The mechanisms already in place in the *KF* can easily produce a priori estimates of what are genuinely future states of the process. At time t, the *KF* can produce (as we have seen) an a priori estimate of the state of the process at t, by taking its previous a posteriori estimate together with any current driving force signal and updating it via the function V. Normally this estimate then gets measured and compared with the observed signal to produce the a posteriori estimate. But there are other options. The system might simply do another iteration of the time update. That is, it can take $\bar{p}(t)$, together with any driving force that *will* be executed at time $t + 1$, and use that as input to V again to produce an a priori estimate of the process's state at $t + 1$: $\bar{p}(t + 1)$. These iterations can continue indefinitely far into the future. The system can, at t, produce estimates of what the process's state will be at any arbitrary future time step by simply iterating the time update as many times as it takes.

There are obvious limitations. Depending on the magnitude of the process disturbance, these state predictions may fail to be reliably close to the real future state of the process beyond some number of iterations. Similar limitations arise if the driving force that is predicted to apply during future time steps is not perfectly predicted. But these limitations aside, the point is merely that such predictions can be produced by mechanisms already at hand. This production of estimates for genuinely future states of the process is *prediction*.

A similar but not entirely parallel process concerns the production of estimates of past states of the process. There are several ways that a system that has the tools of the *KF* could produce such past state estimates. First and easiest, it could simply *remember* the estimates that it actually produced at those previous times. Second, it could produce state estimates of previous states by taking its current state estimate and pushing it through an inverse of the time-update function. Just as one can produce a future estimate by employing the time update function V, as in $\bar{p}(t + 1) = V\bar{p}(t)$, one can produce a previous estimate from a current one, via $\bar{p}(t - 1) = V^{-1}\bar{p}(t)$. Of course, one would get a better estimate of the state at $t - 1$ if one used as input the a posteriori estimate at t: $\bar{p}(t - 1) = V^{-1}\hat{p}(t)$. This process can also be iterated to produce estimates of states arbitrarily far in the past (e.g., if the ship is now at location X, and its speed is S and heading is H, then it was probably at Y at the last fix cycle).

Though either of these will produce an estimate of the state of the process at some previous time, each has a shortcoming.[9] A third method, *smoothing*, effectively combines the two. At time t, a smoothed estimate of the state at time $t - 1$ is arrived at by combining the a posteriori estimate of the processes state at $t - 1$ that was actually produced at $t - 1$ (this is the first method discussed), with a state estimate arrived at by backtracking one time step from the a posteriori state estimate of the process at t that was produced at t (this is the second method discussed):

$$\hat{p}(t{-}1) = \hat{p}(t{-}1) + K_s(V^{-1}\,\hat{p}(t)). \tag{12.1}$$

Here, $\tilde{p}(t-1)$ is the smoothed estimate of the process's state at $t-1$; K_s is a factor analogous to the Kalman gain that determines the relative weight given to the a posteriori estimate from $t-1$ and the backtracked a posteriori estimate from t.

With the addition of smoothing and prediction we have generalized away from the *KF*'s myopic focus on the now, to a system capable of generating state estimates of the process as it was in the past or will be in the future. Next we must generalize from the focus on estimates of the process's *state* at a *single time* (whether past, present, or future) to estimates of the process's *trajectory* over a *temporal interval*. The basics of this are easy enough to do. We can describe a system that maintains estimates of the states of the process throughout an interval from $t-l$ to $t+k$. Of course, if $l=k=0$, then we have the degenerate case of an estimate of an interval that consists of only one time, t. I am interested in cases where l and k are both greater than 0:

$$(P_{t-l}, P_{t-l+1}, \ldots, P_t, \ldots P_{t+k-1}, P_{t+k}).\tag{12.2}$$

To make the notation a bit more elegant, I use $\tilde{p}_{[b,c]/a}$ to be the estimate of the trajectory of p over the interval from time b to time c, produced at time a. Hence the estimate in (12.2) would be $\tilde{p}_{[t-l,t+k]/t}$. I call a system that constructs and maintains estimates of the trajectory of the process over a temporal interval a *trajectory emulator*.

3.2. Psychological Phenomena

The overall idea that the brain employs a trajectory emulator that maintains a trajectory estimate over an interval can be illustrated with a number of phenomena. First consider apparent motion. Two successive flashing dots presented within some spatial distance and within some interstimulus interval will appear to be a single moving dot, moving from the location of the one that flashes first to the location of the one that flashes second (see figure 12.8). This can look to be merely a spatial illusion, in that it looks as though a dot has moved through spatial areas where no dot has been. For example, it appears as though the dot occupied and moved through location B as indicated on the right side of figure 12.8. To bring out the temporality of the phenomenon, consider that the subject will appear to see the dot first at the location A, then location B, and then finally at location C—the motion is actually perceived to be continuous, but I am just drawing attention to the temporal relations between three of the posits on the continuous path.

Notice, however, that if the second flashing dot were above, below, or to the left of the first, then the subject would have seen the dot as moving upward, leftward, or downward. Accordingly, the intermediate location B would be either above, to the left of, or below location A. But—and this is the crucial bit—until the second dot actually flashes, the subject cannot know in which of these four spatial regions the interpolated motion (the location of B) should occur. Yet the *subject sees the dot as being at the interpolated location before being at the terminal location where the second flash occurs*. It can seem as though the perceptual system is able to foretell where the second flash will be to appropriately begin filling in the intermediary phases of the apparent motion.

Figure 12.8. Apparent motion. The left-hand side represents actual stimuli, a flashing dot (1) followed by a second flashing dot (2). The right-hand side represents what is perceived: a single dot moving from location A (the location of the first dot's flash) through location B and to location C (the location of the second dot's flash).

The trajectory estimation model explains this without recourse to the supernatural. At the time of the first flash, the estimate is that there was a single flash at time t. If nothing else happens, then as time progresses this estimate will not change. At $t + 1$, and $t + 2$, and so on, the estimate will continue to be that there was a flash at t. Suppose, however, that at $t + 2$ a second flash occurs at location C. The visual system has models of what happens in the environment, and the relative likelihood of various events, according to which two discrete sensed flashes at A and C at times t and $t + 2$, respectively is, if the temporal and spatial magnitudes are small enough, more likely an imperfectly (noisily) sensed continuous stimulus traversing the path from A to C, than a perfectly sensed pair of distinct stimuli in close spatial and temporal proximity. So at $t + 2$, the trajectory estimate is revised to represent a stimulus as having been at location B at $t + 1$.

Another fascinating phenomenon that is potentially explained by the mechanisms introduced so far is *representational momentum*. The basic phenomenon is this: Subjects are shown a movie or sequence of images that shows some sort of movement, such as a rotating rectangle or moving ball. The scene stops, and subjects are probed to determine their assessment of the final state of the motion they saw. The result is that subjects judge that the motion or rotation continued farther than it in fact did. Not surprisingly, the phenomenon does require that the motion is predictable (Kerzel, 2002).

The trajectory emulation framework explains this phenomenon easily. Even though there is only a sensory signal corresponding to the motion up to time t, the prediction end of the trajectory emulator produces predictions of the future state of the process. These predictions will be possible because the emulator has knowledge of the way the process typically behaves. Senior, Ward, and David (2002) describe the situation this way:

> Representational momentum is thought to occur due to the encoding of specific contexts and semantics inherent within the stimuli (e.g., the encoding of the effects of gravity in a picture of a man jumping from a ledge). These contexts are encoded on the basis of prior knowledge of how complex objects behave in the real world.

When the subject is probed to determine the extent of their representation of the object's motion, this probe is picking up on representations that were constructed as predictions at the leading edge of the moving window.

4. SPATIAL INFORMATION PROCESSING AND BASIS FUNCTIONS

We switch gears now, from one kind of information processing structure to another—from time to space. The question of how the brain represents space is not as straightforward as one might have thought. Surprisingly, even though the brain makes use of a great many topographic maps—maps of the body surface and of the retinae, to name just two—it does not appear to represent egocentric space by means of anything like a map. The parietal cortex is certainly the most important cortical area for representing egocentric space. Lesions to this area result in characteristic spatial deficits, both perceptual and behavioral. But single cell recordings have failed to even hint at anything resembling such a map in the parietal lobes. What has been found are cells that are responsive to a number of sensory and postural signals. Understanding what these have to do with spatial representation requires the right theory, to which I turn.

Perhaps the major key to understanding the operation of PPC neurons and hence the PPC as a whole was a connectionist simulation by Zipser and Andersen (1988), a model that is also one of the most prominent triumphs of connectionist computational neuroscience. Zipser and Andersen constructed an idealized version of the problem confronted by the PPC. A system with a one rotatable eye was to determine the direction (in head-centered coordinates) of a stimulus projected onto its retina—in other words, determine the direction of an external stimulus given only information about stimulation on sensory receptors and postural information. The system in question was a connectionist network trained by back-propagation (see Zipser and Andersen, 1988, for details). During training the network was given an input vector that contained information about where on the retina a stimulus was projecting and how the eye was oriented. The output vector was a specification of the direction of the stimulus in head-centered coordinates. During training, the network was provided with training sets consisting of correct input-output pairs, and it was trained to learn to match them. Subsequent testing on novel inputs revealed that it could produce correct outputs.

Because this was an artificial network, it was possible to subject the units to any kind of analysis one might want, unlike real neurons, which are difficult to study. The key as always is the hidden units of the network—the processing elements that lie between the inputs and outputs, the details of whose operation is forged during the training period in such a way as to produce the correct output vector (in the output units) on receipt of an input vector (from the input units). The result of this analysis was that *each* of the hidden units was acting as a linear gain field combining both sensory and postural information, which in this case were the location of retinal projection and eye's orientation, respectively. In particular, each hidden unit's activity was the product of (1) a Gaussian function of the stimulus's distance on the retina from the unit's preferred retinal location, and (2) a linear gain determined by the unit's preferred eye orientation. The output units each performed a linear combination of the hidden units' activities.

It will help to walk through an example involving two hidden units, and restricting discussion to two dimensions (what I am about to describe are not actual hidden units in the model but fictitious exemplars of how the actual hidden units operate). Hidden unit h_1 would have a preferred location of retinal stimulation, and one factor in its response would be a Gaussian function of distance from that spot (see figure 12.9). If we number the retinal locations in order from 0 to 100 (we are simplifying to a two-dimensional realm, and so the retina will be one-dimensional), unit h_1 might have its preferred location at location 70, meaning that this factor in determining the unit's activity is strongest if the stimulus projects directly on retinal location 70, and decreases with distance from 70. It still is pretty strong at 68 or 72, but very weak at 10 or 98. The second factor influencing h_1's activity is a linear function of deviation from preferred eye orientation (see figure 12.10). This factor would be strongest if the eye was oriented either completely to the left or completely to the right (whichever the preferred direction is, let's say it is *right*), and would taper off linearly as the eye's orientation went to the other direction (left).

So for a given combination of retinal location of stimulation and eye orientation, h_1 would have its firing rate determined as a product of these two factors: a Gaussian of distance from preferred location and a linear function of eye orientation. If the eye is oriented completely to the right, and the stimulus falls directly at retinal location 70, h_1 will fire at its maximal rate (see figure 12.11). The actual location of the stimulus's projection on the retina together with the eye's orientation during the sensory episode will determine a firing rate. But of course the firing rate of h_1 by itself won't tell one where the stimulus is. Suppose that h_1 is firing at half its maximal rate. This might be a case where the eye orientation is all the way to the right, but the retinal stimulation is at location 80 or 60, and hence a bit distant from its preferred spot. Or the stimulus might project directly to retinal location 70, but the eye might be oriented halfway from its preferred direction. Many combinations

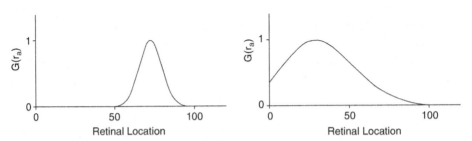

Figure 12.9. Gaussian functions. The graph shows the value of $G_1(r_a)$, the Gaussian used by unit h_1 (left), and $G_2(r_a)$, the Gaussian used by unit h_2 (right). The Gaussians differ both in terms of their preferred retinal location (peak response of $G_1(r_a)$ is at about 70; $G_2(r_a)$ is about 30), and their tuning ($G_1(r_a)$ is narrowly tuned, meaning it falls off quickly with distance from the preferred location; $G_2(r_a)$ is broadly tuned, meaning it falls off less quickly with distance from preferred location).

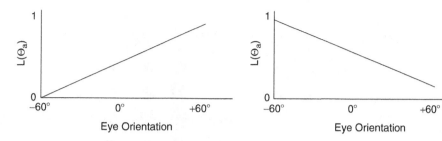

Figure 12.10. Linear functions. The graph shows the value of $L_1(\theta_a)$, a linear function used by unit h_1 (left), and $L_2(\theta_a)$, a linear function used by unit h_2 (right). The function is at its maximum when the eye is oriented either to the far left or far right, depending on the preferred orientation. The activity tapers off linearly as the eye's orientation differs from the preferred orientation.

would yield the same firing rate. In any case, each cell's activity is a function of these two factors:

$$h_1 = G_1(x_a)L_1(\Theta_a), \tag{12.3}$$

where h_1 is the activity (firing rate) of unit h_1; x_a is the actual location of retinal stimulation; G_1 is the Gaussian function used by unit h_1; Θ_a is the actual eye orientation; and L_1 is the linear function used by unit h_1.

The activity of unit h_2 will be determined similarly:

$$h_2 = G_2(x_a)L_2(\Theta_a). \tag{12.4}$$

The Gaussian function G_2 may be different from G_1 (see figure 12.9), in particular σ (a constant that determines how narrowly or broadly tuned the Gaussian curve is) may be larger or smaller; it may be centered at a different retinal location. The linear function L_2 may be different from L_1, that is, have a different slope. We can streamline our notation as follows:

$$h_1 = f_1(x_a, \Theta_a), \tag{12.5}$$
$$h_2 = f_2(x_a, \Theta_a). \tag{12.6}$$

The function associated with each unit (f_1, f_2, etc.) will be a linear gain field, a Gaussian multiplied by a linear gain. But because the exact form of the Gaussian (center and σ) and the slope of the linear gain might be different in each case, they are different functions. More generally, for each unit h_i, its activity can be expressed as

$$h_i = f_i(x_a, \Theta_a). \tag{12.7}$$

In Zipser and Andersen's model, as explained, the functions f_i are all linear gain fields. As is the case with such connectionist models, the output units' activities—where the answer gets produced—are simple linear combinations of the activities of the hidden units. That is, each output unit O_i is connected to each hidden unit with a scalar connection strength or *weight*, $w_{i,j}$, which is the strength of the connection from hidden unit i to output unit j. This output unit's output is the sum of all of these weighted connections:

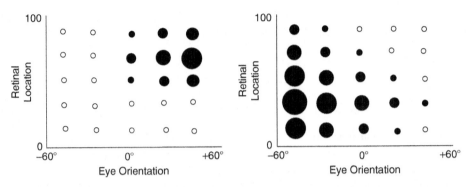

Figure 12.11. Graphical representations of the *product* of a Gaussian and linear gain. The figures show the activity of hidden unit h_1 (left) and h_2 (right) for 25 different combinations of retinal location and eye orientation. Empty circles represent no activity (a product at or very near 0), and filled circles' sizes are proportional to the unit's activity for that combination. As can be seen, the product of $L_1(\theta_a)$ and $G_1(r_a)$ is highest with a combination of retinal location around 70 and eye orientation fully to the right. The product of $L_2(\theta_a)$ and $G_2(r_a)$ is highest with a combination of retinal location around 30 and eye orientation fully to the left.

$$O_i = \sum_{j=1}^{n} w_{ij} h_j \tag{12.8}$$

That is, each output unit's activity O_i is the sum, for all j, of the product of the activity of hidden unit j and the weight from hidden unit j to output unit i. The set of these output unit's activities is the connectionist model's answer. It is a vector representation of the direction of the stimulus relative to the head:

$$S = (O_1, O_2, \ldots O_n). \tag{12.9}$$

The mathematical representation is helpful, but not essential. For those who have a distaste for math, the qualitative idea is this. There are two stages to the solution. In stage one, the set of hidden units has learned a particular way of combining the sensory and postural signal. This way, each unit has its activity determined as a slightly different function of both of these factors. This is what equation (12.7) expresses. The second stage involves decoding the activities of these hidden units in a certain sort of way. This is codified in equations (12.8) and (12.9).

Note that the fact that the model is limited to one sensory modality (vision), and one postural signal (eye orientation) is only for simplicity. The same mechanisms can easily generalize to more realistic cases where not only can the eyes move in the head, the head can move with respect to the torso, and so on. In such cases, additional signals are needed, such as signals coding the head's orientation with respect to the torso. Similarly, feeling something on the tip of my right index finger does not tell me where that object is located in egocentric space, unless I have postural information about how my index finger is angled with respect to my hand, how my wrist is comported with respect to my forearm, and my elbow and shoulder angles, and so forth. In this case, too, a sensory signal needs to be combined with postural signals to have enough information to narrow down the egocentric location of the stimulus.

Generalizing the notation to these more complicated cases is straightforward. In the special case described in (12.7), the value x_a is a sensory signal—information about what is happening on the sense receptor, where the sense organ is being stimulated. The value of Θ_a is a postural signal—information about how the sense organ is oriented with respect to other body parts. We can make the notation more general as in (12.10):

$$h_i = f_i(s_a, q_a). \tag{12.10}$$

Here, s_a and q_a are the sensory and postural signals associated with stimulus a, whatever form they may take.

What makes this model particularly interesting is that after it was determined that these artificial units had solved the problem by combining the sensory and postural signal in this particular way (linear gain fields as per equation [12.3]), this suggested that it was at least possible that this was what individual neurons in the PPC were doing. In fact, single cell recordings of neurons in the PPC during tasks that required spatial localizations of directions in head-centered coordinates revealed that many appeared to have their activity modulated in just this way (or close to it, see following discussion). That is, the activity of individual neurons in the PPC was found to vary with both eye orientation and location of retinal stimulation in the nonobvious way suggested by equation (12.3): close enough, anyway, to provide some plausibility to the claim that the way these artificial neurons were solving the problem might be a window into how the PPC neurons were solving it.

This leads to a more recent proposal by Alexandre Pouget. Pouget's Gauss-sigmoid model also can be discerned into two stages, both of which are similar to the corresponding stages of the Zipser and Andersen model, but with some significant differences. (Pouget describes his model as a "basis function" model, but for reasons I explain shortly, I want to reserve the name "basis function model"' for a generalization of Pouget's model, and so I use the specific kind of basis function encoding described by Pouget—Gauss-sigmoid—as the name for his model.) As in the Zipser and Andersen model, the first stage is an encoding stage, in which individual units or neurons combine the sensory and postural signals. The difference is that Pouget's model has each unit combining the signals not as a gain field (a Gaussian times a linear gain as with Zipser and Andersen's model) but by a nonlinear basis function consisting of the product of a Gaussian and a nonlinear sigmoid function (see figure 12.12). There are information-processing reasons and physiological reasons for preferring these basis functions to the linear gain fields of Zipser and Andersen. On the information processing side, it turns out that nonlinear basis functions have convenient computational and mathematical properties. I return to this shortly. The physiological reason is that on closer scrutiny, the PPC neurons look as though they may actually be implementing these Gauss-sigmoid functions rather than the linear gain fields. (The output of both of these is very similar over most of the dynamic range of neuron's response, and so it takes some subtle measurement

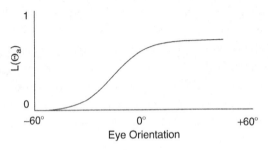

Figure 12.12. A sigmoid function.

to tell which is the better fit.) Generally, Gaussians and sigmoids are functions that real neurons are known to be able to compute.

The second stage is where the more interesting innovation is to be found. In Pouget's model, the basis functions are not just there to supply information to another set of units, the output units, that read out the correct answer, but are instead used to guide a motor response. This works as follows. Every possible *type* of behavior, such as "grasp with the right hand," involves a complex set of motor control signals, and the exact nature of this motor control sequence depends on where the stimulus is. Grasping the coffee cup in front of you with your right hand involves a different set of motor commands than grasping it when it is down near your left foot. What Pouget has shown is that given a nonlinear basis function representation of the sensory and postural information, the details of any behavior can be appropriately determined as a proprietary linear combination of the values of these functions.

Let's walk through this more carefully. A stimulus will be processed by the PPC as a set of basis functions of the form

$$B_i(s, q) \tag{12.11}$$

Here, each basis function $(B_1, B_2, \ldots)$ is an activity of a PPC neuron, its activity being a nonlinear function of the sensory and postural signal, a nonlinear version of the Zipser and Andersen model; that is, (12.3) is essentially a linear version of (12.11). The result of this stage is similar enough to the Zipser and Andersen model that the differences are not worth graphing: Except for the change from a line to a sigmoid and a corresponding slight difference in the exact form of graphs such as those in figure 12.11, a parallel set of figures corresponding to a Gauss-sigmoid field would look very similar. A given perception of a stimulus will involve a certain sensory signal and set of postural signals, the s and the q associated with the sensing of the stimulus, and the PPC applies a large number of basis functions of the form of (12.11) to these signals. The result is a lot of PPC neurons, each firing at a rate determined by its own version of (12.11).

A given kind of behavior, such as a grasp with the left hand or a foveating eye movement, is associated with a set of scalar coefficients (the mathematical version of neural connection strengths). For example a motor behavior, such as a left-hand grasp, would have a proprietary and constant set of numbers, $g_1, g_2, \ldots, g_n$, such that when those coefficients are used to produce a linear combination of the basis function values associated with stimulus a, the stimulus-a-targeted behavior is correctly executed:

$$m_j^{a,g} = \sum_{i=1}^{n} g_{i,j} B_i^a,$$

(12.12)

$$M^{a,g} = (m_1^{a,g}, m_2^{a,g}, \ldots, m_p^{a,g}).$$

(12.13)

What (12.13) says is that the neural motor commands that result in a left-hand grasp of stimulus a can be represented as a vector $M^{a,g}$, each component of which is $m_j^{a,g}$, and is arrived at by multiplying numbers associated with a left-hand grasp (the $g_{i,j}$ coefficients) and the basis functions associated with stimulus a (the B_i^a s) and adding them together, as per (12.12).

Of course a left-hand grasp directed at stimulus b will require a different motor command if b is located at a different spot in egocentric space. A left-hand grasp directed at b would be determined by:

$$m_j^{b,g} = \sum_{i=1}^{n} g_{i,j} B_i^b,$$

(12.14)

$$M^{b,g} = (m_1^{b,g}, m_2^{b,g}, \ldots, m_p^{b,g}).$$

(12.15)

Here, the different motor command $M^{b,g}$, the command that results in a left-hand grasp of stimulus b, is produced by taking *the same set of left-hand grasp coefficients*, the $g_{i,j}$s, and multiplying them with a different set of basis function values—the ones that the basis functions yield when applied to the sensory and postural signals produced during the sensing of stimulus b: B_i^b. A different kind of action, like an eye movement that foveates stimulus a or b, would be determined in an analogous way: by multiplying the eye movement coefficients ($e_{i,j}$) with the basis functions produced by the stimulus according to the following equations that should not need elaboration at this point:

$$m_j^{a,e} = \sum_{i=1}^{n} e_{i,j} B_i^a,$$

(12.16)

$$M^{a,e} = (m_1^{a,e}, m_2^{a,e}, \ldots, m_p^{a,e}),$$

(12.17)

$$m_j^{b,e} = \sum_{i=1}^{n} e_{i,j} B_i^b,$$

(12.18)

$$M^{b,e} = (m_1^{b,e}, m_2^{b,e}, \ldots, m_p^{b,e}).$$

(12.19)

5. EMULATION AND BASIS FUNCTIONS

The emulation theory and the basis function model are not in conflict. The emulation theory is a description of how a representation of some process can play a role in a larger information processing structure that underwrites various capacities, such as imagery, perceptual processing, the dulling of the detrimental effect of feedback delays, and the filtering of sensor noise. The emulation theory makes no requirements on *how* the emulator itself is implemented, with the exception of the requirement that however it is implemented, it must be able to play its role in the larger structure. The emulator might be implemented in a physical model, like in old-school ship navigation, or it might be implemented in a digital data structure. As long as it can be used to provide a priori estimates, be updated to form a posteriori estimates, be driven off-line to produce imagery, and so on, the details don't matter—at least not so far as the emulation theory itself is concerned.

I claimed that for higher organisms, including humans, normal perception of the environment involves the use of an amodal environment emulator. This emulator maintains representations of the spatial comportment of objects and surfaces in the environment, as well as their movement and force-dynamical interactions. One aspect of this is clearly the *spatial* aspect. The emulation theory does not specify how these spatial properties and relations are represented, so long as they are able to engage in the kinds of processes the emulation theory posits.

The basis function model is a theory of how the brain processes information to track the location of objects in the environment. This theory was presented (both by me in section 4, as well as by the original authors, though they did not put it in these terms) as a pure *measurement inverse*—one that goes from sensed signals (in this case, sensory and postural signals) to a construction of a representation of the spatial properties and relations of entities in the environment, which in this case is in terms of a set of basis function values that were determined by the relevant sensory and postural signals:

$$B_i(s, q). \tag{12.20}$$

The advantage of representing spatial locations as sets of basis function values is that in this format they can be used immediately (without further processing) by the motor centers to produce appropriate actions, as described in the previous section.

But note that the sensory and postural signals are *observed* signals—unfiltered signals going directly from the process (the body and its sense organs) to the PPC. These observed signals are then combined via basis functions and linearly combined with a set of coefficients appropriate to the target behavior. The result is a motor command that, if all works well, results in the target behavior being produced. To put it in other words, the basis function model as described by Pouget and collaborators, and as I have described it here, is an implementation of a closed-loop control scheme. It specifies one way to construct a closed-loop controller that will produce the right motor command when given feedback (the observed sensory and postural signals) from the process.

During the discussion of the control theoretic material, we never had a need for notation for a process state estimate that was nothing more than the observed signal pushed through a measurement inverse. I will now use an inverted hat for this purpose: $\check{p}(t) = O^{-1}s(t)$. Given this, the basis function values as discussed by Pouget and myself are:

$$\check{B}_i(\check{s},\check{q}). \tag{12.21}$$

Here, the sensory signal and the postural signal are completely unfiltered (hence the upside-down hats), and as a result the basis function values are an unfiltered measurement inverse.

Just like any other observed signal and associated process state estimate, the sensory and postural signals and the resulting basis function values might benefit from some filtering. What this requires in the present case is an emulator or emulators of the spatial features of objects in the environment. Such an emulator will simply be a mechanism that can take a representation of the spatial features at t, together with an efference copy, if any, and produce an estimate of the spatial features at $t + 1$. If we let $B_i(t)$ be the values of the basis functions produced at time t, then the spatial process model would be some mechanism that implemented the following:

$$\overline{B}_i(t{+}1)=V\hat{B}_i(t)+c(t). \tag{12.22}$$

That is, it produces an a priori estimate of what the next set of basis function values will be on the basis of the previous set (in this case, the previous a posteriori estimate) and any efference copies. There are two ways this might be implemented, and there is no reason to assume that only one of them is in play in the PPC.

First, because each set of basis function values is determined by sensory and postural signals, then any a priori estimate of the sensory and postural signals will be suitable to produce an a priori estimate of the basis functions:

$$\overline{B}_i(t{+}1)=B_i(\overline{S}(t{+}1), \overline{q}(t{+}1)), \tag{12.23}$$

$$\overline{S}(t{+}1)=V_s\hat{s}(t)+c(t); \overline{q}(t{+}1)=V_q\hat{q}(t)+c(t). \tag{12.24}$$

Here $\overline{S}(t)$ and $\overline{q}(t)$ are a priori estimates, at time t, of the sensory and postural signals. The functions V_s and V_q are functions that describe how the sensory states and postural states evolve over time (they are sensory and postural versions of the function V that was used by the *KF* to model the process's dynamics).

The attentive reader will have noted that all of this can be accomplished by mechanisms already discussed in previous sections: the a priori and a posteriori estimates of postural signals are just signals concerning the configuration of the body and are supplied by the musculoskeletal emulator, the same one used for motor imagery, motor planning, and so forth; the sensory signals are signals concerning the information incoming from the various sense organs and are supplied by modality-specific emulators of the various senses (e.g., the Duhamel et al., 1992, result that I analyzed as a visual image emulator in section 2.3). In other words, emulators already argued to be in play on independent grounds supply the information required to produce a priori estimates of the basis function values associated with a stimulus's spatial location.

A second method involves mechanisms that have not already been introduced. This would be a mechanism that simply evolves the basis function values themselves over time in accordance with information about how the spatial features of perceived objects typically evolve over time:

$$\bar{B}_i(t+1)=V_B\hat{B}_i(t)+c(t). \tag{12.25}$$

Here, V_B is a function that describes how the basis function values evolve over time, which maps the way that the spatial features of represented objects evolve over time.

At the same time an a priori estimate of the basis function values is produced as per (12.23) and/or (12.25) at time t, a purely bottom-up process—a measurement inverse—produces a set of basis function values that are what the sensors say about the spatial features of the environment at t. The two are combined in the way described in section 5.2 to produce an a posteriori estimate of the spatial features of the environment at t:

$$\hat{B}_i(t)=\bar{B}_i(t)+K[\bar{B}_i(t)-\check{B}_i(t)]). \tag{12.26}$$

This is exactly the procedure already discussed in section 2 as an amodal emulation of the spatial features of the environment. The current a posteriori estimate of the basis function values is the current a priori estimate plus a correction, which is the difference between the a priori estimate and the values based solely on the observed signal (the sensory residual) multiplied by a gain term K.

To this point, the synthesis of emulation theory and the basis function approach to spatial representation has been limited to temporally punctate the case of purely spatial representation. In this section I will expand this framework to explain the implementation of *spatiotemporal trajectory* representation. The generalization in the case of the emulation theory has already been discussed in section 3. What remains is to state the basis function model in such a way that it can be implemented in a trajectory emulation system.

A conceptually simple generalization is entirely straight-forward. The production of smoothed and predicted estimates of both the sensory and postural signals over the temporal interval $[t-l, t+k]$ can yield the set of basis function values subserving the representation of the spatial trajectory of the stimulus over that interval. If we let $\hat{B}_{i,a/[b]}$ be the estimate of the ith basis function value at time b, produced at time a, then this ordered set can be expressed as:

$$([\tilde{B}_{1,[t-l]/t},\dots,\tilde{B}_{n,[t-l]/t}],\dots,[\hat{B}_{1,[t]/t},\dots,\hat{B}_{n,[t]/t}],\dots,[\bar{B}_{1,[t+k]t},\dots,\bar{B}_{n,[t+k]/t}]). \tag{12.27}$$

This simple generalization posits, for each time step in the interval spanned by the trajectory estimation emulator, a separate set of basis function values, each based on the smoothed ($\tilde{B}_i$), filtered ($\hat{B}_i$), or predicted ($\bar{B}_i$) basis function value estimates corresponding to that time step. Although this generalization is conceptually simple, it is also conceptually inelegant. A slightly more sophisticated generalization is not only more aesthetically comely but interfaces with other elements of the basis function model better—and more realistically—than the simple generalization.

Given that there are estimates of the sensory and postural states throughout the interval available, it is not necessary to produce a separate set of basis function values for each time step. Rather, a single set of basis function values can be produced based on the entire interval estimates of the sensory and postural signals.

This requires the use of more complicated basis functions, but I won't explore the details of that here. If we let $\tilde{S}_{[t-l,\,t+k]/t}$ be the smoothed estimate, produced at time t, for the *trajectory* of sensory states over the interval $[t - l, t + k]$ (and use similar notation for postural estimates), then we can define a single vector of basis function values as:

$$(\tilde{B}_1(\tilde{s}_{[t-l,\,t+k]/t},\,\tilde{q}_{[t-l,t+k]/t}),\,\ldots,\,\tilde{B}n\,(\tilde{s}_{[t-l,t+k]/t},\,\tilde{q}_{[t-l,t+k]t})' \tag{12.28}$$

or more notationally conveniently as:

$$(\tilde{B}_{1,[t-l,t+k]t},\,\ldots,\,\tilde{B}_{n,[t-l,t+k]/t}). \tag{12.29}$$

This is not merely an exercise in notational parsimony. We must keep in mind the point of these basis functions, which is to guide motor behavior by combining with sets of coefficients appropriate for those behaviors. In the static case we had a motor behavior, such as a left-hand grasp of stimulus a, determined by something like (12.12) and (12.13), repeated here as (12.30) for convenience:

$$M^{a,g} = (m_1^{a,g}, m_2^{a,g}, \ldots, m_p^{a,g});\, m_j^{a,g} = \sum_{i=1}^{n} g_{i,j}\, B_i^a. \tag{12.30}$$

This was fine for a stationary object, for in such a case the fact that the motor behavior takes time can be ignored. The basis function values associated with the egocentric location of the object will not themselves change during the course of the motor behavior. But in the temporally nondegenerate case, this cannot be ignored. Grasping a moving object requires movement of the hand not to where the object *is now* but to where it *will be*. If there are different sets of basis function values for each time, then there will be different sets of basis function values associated with the object's location now and its location at the time of the grasp.

So why not just let each motor behavior be determined as in the static case, but with the right set of temporally punctate basis function values—the ones that correspond to the location of the object at the anticipated time of the grasp? If this could be done, then there would be no reason to prefer (12.29) over (12.27). The problem is that the time in the future appropriate for timing the grasp depends on the object's trajectory. If the object is moving very quickly then the grasp will have to be sooner than a case where the object is moving very slowly, even if the spatial location of the grasp is the same in both cases. If the trajectory is represented by an ordered set of sets of basis functions, then some other mechanism would have to have access to this set, and determine which of them is the appropriate time of a grasp interception, and then indicate to the motor system which set of basis functions it should use to combine with the behavior's coefficients.

Although this could work in principle, the approach cuts completely against the conceptual grain of the basis function model. The point of this model is to explain how combinations of sensory and postural signals combine so as to organically guide motor behavior without the need for intervening levels of representation or micromanagement. The simple generalization as expressed in (27), when we attempt to reintegrate it with the behavioral output part of the model, introduces exactly such intermediaries—a system that examines the set of basis functions, somehow picks one out as appropriate, and then feeds that one to the behavior-appropriate coefficients.

The more sophisticated generalization maintains the elegance of the static case. A motor behavior can still be associated with a set of proprietary coefficients that combine with a set of basis functions. A grasp will be produced by something like

$$M^{a,g} = (m_1^{a,g}, m_2^{a,g}, \ldots, m_p^{a,g}); \qquad (12.31)$$

$$m_j^{a,g} = \sum_{i=1}^{n} g_{i,j} B_{i,[t-1,t+k]/t}^{a}. \qquad (12.32)$$

Here (12.31) is just as before: The motor command $m^{a,g}$ to execute a left-hand grasp of moving stimulus a is a vector each of whose elements is described in (12.32). This is where the difference is. Each of these elements $m_j^{a,g}$ is a linear combination of basis function values coding the estimate for the target stimulus's trajectory over the window's interval, not simply its location at one time.

Because this single set of basis functions of the form $B_{i,[t-1,t=k]/t}^{a}$ contains all the relevant information about object a's trajectory over the represented interval (not just its location at the present time), the values these basis functions yield on any given occasion are capable in principle of combining with a set of behavior-specific coefficients to produce an appropriate motor output, even for moving stimuli.

6. Discussion

It will be noted that I advertised my goal as providing a unified neural information processing structure for the representation of behavioral space, behavioral time, and objects. Although I have had sections on space and time, objects seem to have not made an appearance. I close with a few words about objects.

Though it has been implicit, objects have been addressed all along. The behavioral-spatial representation, both in temporally punctate and temporally extended form, is built around behavioral objects as defined in section 1. The basis functions are functions of sensory and postural signals, and the sensory signals are, in the first instance, signals from some *stimulus*—such as a light that is detected on the retina. The basis functions' entire purpose is to support a linear decoding via a motor-behavior-specific set of coefficients to produce a bodily action that is directed on *that stimulus*—such as grasping or foveating the seen object. The stimulus, the entity that is the accusative of both perception and action, is the behavioral object that is represented by the basis function values.

Now of course this is not an object in the usual sense of *object* beloved of philosophers. The objects playing a role in my account could be rocks, bugs, or branches, but could just as well be shadows, luminance edges, or holes. There is little conceptual room at this stage of representation between a location in behavioral space and a behavioral object. They are objects in the sense of a potential focus of perception and action.

I believe that the capacity to represent behavioral-space, -time, and -objects is a very fundamental feature of cognition and mentality. Surely there are more basic functions of the nervous system, functions that predate those discussed here. There is regulation of internal processes, managing of reflexes, and central pattern generators. But my hunch is that if we are interested in those nervous system functions that are fundamental to cognition and mentality, then the capacity to represent an environment of actionable objects is about as fundamental as it gets.

ACKNOWLEDGMENTS

I thank Lisa Damm, Holly Andersen, and participants in seminars on temporal representation I taught at the University of Pittsburgh in 2004 and UC San Diego in 2005 for feedback on various parts of this project in various formats. I am grateful to the McDonnell Project in Philosophy and the Neurosciences, and the project's director, Kathleen Akins, for financial support during which this research was conducted.

NOTES

1. For more distinctions, see Grush (2000).

2. On my preferred use of the expression *representation*, the basis function model by itself is not a theory of representation at all but a theory of the information processing that extracts spatial information from various signals. It becomes representational, on my account, when operating within the superstructure of the emulation theory, as section 5 details.

3. *Controller* is fairly standard terminology for the thing issuing commands. The controlled system is often called the *plant* in the literature, but *process* is also used, especially in signal processing contexts.

4. In some cases my notation and terminology differ slightly from the standard notation and terminology used in control theory or signal processing. These divergences aren't too frequent, and when they occur the reason will typically be that slightly nonstandard terminology makes my overall goal of putting these tools to use in understanding neural information processing easier and more perspicuous. The vast bulk of my terminology and notation is entirely standard. Apologies to those readers who are surprised by the two or three deviations in notation, but such a reader should have no problem knowing what I am talking about: for example, that what I have called s^G is standardly called a *setpoint* or *reference signal*.

5. A straight bar was also used in the previous section in notation for the states of the process model in pseudo-closed-loop control. By the end of this section it should be clear

why this is appropriate: a pseudo-closed loop system does not provide for any influence from the real sensor signal to the process model, and so the process model is restricted to working with a priori estimates.

6. This is called a measurement inverse because it is the inverse of the measurement function. The measurement is a function that maps process states to sensor signals. For example, the people who take bearings on a ship are implementing a measurement. They produce signals, in this case bearings to known landmarks, on the basis of the process's state, in this case the location of the ship. The set of numbers produced by the bearing takers depends on the location of the ship. The inverse of this is a mapping from sensor signals to process states. When the navigation team is given a set of numbers from the bearing takers, they implement an inverse by determining where the ship would have to be if the sensor signals they have just received are accurate.

7. Generalizing the process of arriving at a sensory residual from a case of one a priori estimate and one observed signal to perhaps more than one of each is straightforward. In the case where one wants to maintain the optimal estimation capability of the *KF*, one would of course combine them as a function of their respective error covariation. Where optimality is not a desideratum, much simpler procedures would suffice, such as averaging the a priori estimates and then subtracting the observed signal.

8. In Grush (2004), I discuss the simulation theory in more detail, and point out differences between the simulation theory and the emulation theory, as well as considerations that favor the emulation theory.

9. I've decided to unburden the main text of an explanation of these shortcomings. But for those who are interested, the following remarks and reference should suffice. Neither of the two methods described makes use of all the available data. A previous remembered estimate does not take into account observations made after that estimate, and these observations may be crucial. Estimates of past states made by back-iterating a future estimate through an inverse of the time update tell us what the most likely past state is given only the current state. But the most likely past state given only the current state might differ from what is the most likely past state given both the current state and the past observations. Each of these methods ignores some chunk of the observed signal. See Bryson and Ho (1975).

REFERENCES

Blakemore, S. J., Goodbody, S. J., and Wolpert, D. M. (1998). Predicting the consequences of our own actions: The role of sensorimotor context estimation. *Journal of Neuroscience* 18: 7511–7518.

Bryson, A. E., and Yu-Chi, Ho. (1975). *Applied Optimal Control: Optimization, Estimation, and Control.* Washington, D.C.: Hemisphere.

Denier van der Gon, J. J. (1988). Motor control: Aspects of its organization, control signals and properties. In W. Wallinga, H. B. K. Boom and J. de Vries (Eds.), *Proceedings of the 7th Congress of the International Electrophysiological Society.* New York: Elsevier.

Desmurget, M., and Grafton, S. (2000). Forward modeling allows feedback control for fast reaching movements. *Trends in Cognitive Sciences* 4: 423–431.

Duhamel, J.-R., Colby, C., and Goldberg, M. E. (1992). The updating of the representation of visual space in parietal cortex by intended eye movements. *Science* 255: 90–92.

Grush, R. (2000). Self, world and space: The meaning and mechanisms of ego- and allocentric spatial representation. *Brain and Mind* 1: 59–92.

Grush, R. (2004). The emulation theory of representation: Motor control, imagery, and perception. *Behavioral and Brain Sciences* 27: 377–442.

Grush, R. (2005). Internal models and the construction of time: Generalizing from *state* estimation to *trajectory* estimation to address temporal features of perception, including temporal illusions. *Journal of Neural Engineering* 2: S209–S218.

Houk, J. C., Singh, S. P., Fischer, C., and Barto, A. (1990). An adaptive sensorimotor network inspired by the anatomy and physiology of the cerebellum. In W. T. Miller, R. S. Sutton, and P. J. Werbos (Eds.), *Neural Networks for Control*. Cambridge, Mass.: MIT Press.

Ito, M. (1970). Neurophysiological aspects of the cerebellar motor control system. *International Journal of Neurology* 7: 162–176.

Ito, M. (1984). *The Cerebellum and Neural Control*. New York: Raven Press.

Jeannerod, M. (2001). Neural simulation of action: A unifying mechanism for motor cognition. *Neuroimage* 14: S103–S109.

Johnson, S. H. (2000). Thinking ahead: The case for motor imagery in prospective judgements of prehension. *Cognition* 74: 33–70.

Kalman, R. E. (1960). A new approach to linear filtering and prediction problems. *Journal of Basic Engineering*, 82(d): 35–45.

Kalman, R., and Bucy, R. S. (1961). New results in linear filtering and prediction theory. *Journal of Basic Engineering* 83(d): 95–108.

Kawato, M. (1999). Internal models for motor control and trajectory planning. *Current Opinion in Neurobiology* 9: 718–727.

Kerzel, D. (2002). A matter of design: No representational momentum without predictability. *Visual Cognition* 9: 66–80.

Krakauer, J. W., Ghilardi, M.-F., and Ghez, C. (1999). Independent learning of internal models for kinematic and dynamic control of reaching. *Nature Neuroscience* 2: 1026–1031.

Mach, E. (1896). *Contributions to the Analysis of Sensations*. Open Court Publishing.

Mehta, B., and Schaal, S. (2002). Forward models in visuomotor control. *Journal of Neurophysiology* 88: 942–953.

Mel, B. W. (1986). A connectionist learning model for 3-d mental rotation, zoom, and pan. In *Proceedings of Eighth Annual Conference of the Cognitive Science Society*, 562–571.

Mel, B. W. (1988). MURPHY: A robot that learns by doing. In *Neural Information Processing Systems*. New York: American Institute of Physics, 544–553.

Pouget, A., Deneve, S., and Duhamel, J.-R. (2002). A computational perspective on the neural basis of multisensory spatial representations. *Nature Reviews: Neuroscience* 3: 741–747.

Senior, C., Ward, J., and David, A. S. (2002). Representational momentum and the brain: An investigation into the functional necessity of V5/MT. *Visual Cognition* 9: 81–92.

von Helmholtz, H. (1910). *Handbuch der Physiologischen Optik*, vol. 3, 3rd ed. A. Gullstrand, J. von Kries, and W. Nagel (Eds.). Leipzig: Voss.

Wolpert, D. M., Ghahramani, Z., and Flanagan, J. R. (2001). Perspectives and problems in motor learning. *Trends in Cognitive Sciences* 5: 487–494.

Wolpert, D. M., Ghahramani, Z., and Jordan, M. I. (1995). An internal model for sensorimotor integration. *Science* 269: 1880–1882.

Zipser, D., and Andersen, R. A. (1988). A back-propagation programmed network that simulates response properties of a subset of posterior parietal neurons. *Nature* 331 (6158): 679–684.

CHAPTER 13

NEUROCOMPUTATIONAL MODELS: THEORY, APPLICATION, PHILOSOPHICAL CONSEQUENCES

CHRIS ELIASMITH

1. INTRODUCTION

Theoretical (or computational) neuroscience has come to play a role in neuroscience akin to that played by theoretical physics in the physical sciences. However, unlike theoretical physics, theoretical neuroscience is not characterized by a few well-studied basic theories (e.g., string theory, loop quantum gravity, etc.). Instead, as can be seen by perusing the textbooks in the field, theoretical neuroscience is largely a collection of disparate methods, models, and mathematical techniques that relate to neurobiological systems (see, e.g., Dayan and Abbott, 2001; Koch, 1998). For any given neural system of interest, some subset of these methods is chosen (or new ones developed), and they are applied in the analysis or simulation of that system. In short, although theoretical neuroscience has helped provide a quantified understanding of neural systems, it has done so in a largely unsystematic manner.

As a result of this diversity of techniques, and the accompanying variety of assumptions, it is difficult to discern what philosophically interesting conclusions can be drawn about neural systems *in general*. As a result, rather than focusing on the entire range of techniques used by theoretical neuroscientists, in this chapter I describe a systematic approach to studying neural systems that has collected and extended a set of consistent methods that are highly general. These methods have come to be called the neural engineering framework (NEF), and can be summarized by three basic principles, which I describe next. These principles have been extended in more recent work (Tripp and Eliasmith, 2007), and here I present their original formulation (Eliasmith and Anderson, 2003), which is simpler and does not detract from subsequent discussion. An indication of the generality of these three principles is the wide variety of neural systems they have been used to characterize. These include the barn owl auditory system (Fischer, 2005), the rodent navigation system (Conklin and Eliasmith, 2005), escape and swimming control in zebrafish (Kuo and Eliasmith, 2005), the translational vestibular ocular reflex in monkeys (Eliasmith, Westover, and Anderson, 2002), working memory systems (Singh and Eliasmith, 2006), and language-based deductive inference (Eliasmith, 2004). These models span sensory, motor, and cognitive systems across the phylogenetic tree. This broad range of applicability, which is a consequence of the generality of the NEF, makes subsequent philosophical consequences of greater interest (see section 4).

2. The NEF

2.1. Introduction

The NEF draws heavily on past work in theoretical neuroscience, integrating work on neural coding, population representation, and neural dynamics to enable the construction of large-scale biologically plausible neural simulations. The three principles that form the basis of the framework are:

1. *Representation:* Neural representations are defined by a combination of nonlinear encoding and optimal linear decoding.
2. *Transformation:* Transformations of neural representations are functions of the variables that are represented by a population.
3. *Dynamics:* Neural dynamics are characterized by considering neural representations as control theoretic state variables.

These principles are quantitatively defined by Eliasmith and Anderson (2003) to (a) apply to a wide variety of single cell dynamics; (b) incorporate linear and nonlinear transformations; (c) permit linear, nonlinear, and time-varying dynamics; and (d) support the representation of scalars, vectors, functions, or any combinations of these. In addition, the principles are formulated to preserve our current understanding of the biophysical limitations of neural systems (e.g., the presence of significant noise, the intrinsic dynamics of neurons, largely linear somatic interactions of dendritic currents, etc.). In the next four subsections, I describe each principle in more detail and discuss how they provide a unified view of the function of neural systems for the behavioral sciences.

2.2. Representation

The notion of representation is broadly employed in neuroscience.[1] In general, if a neuron fires relatively rapidly when an animal is presented with a certain set of stimuli, the neuron is said to represent the property that the set of stimuli share (see, e.g., Felleman and van Essen, 1991). This kind of experiment has been performed on mammals since Hubel and Wiesel's (1962) classic research in which they identified cortical cells selective to the orientation and size of a bar in a cat's visual field. The slightly earlier bug detector experiments of Lettvin, Maturana, McCulloch, and Pitts (1959/1988), perhaps better known to philosophers, take a similar approach. In these experiments, retinal ganglion cells were found that respond to small, black, fly-sized dots in a frog's visual field. These were referred to as "bug detectors" because they fired rapidly when such dots were present and fired less rapidly when they were not. More recently, this method has been used to find face-selective cells (i.e., cells that respond strongly to faces in particular orientations) in monkey visual cortex (Desimone, 1991). In all of these cases, what is deemed important for representation is how actively a neuron responds to some known stimuli.

The two central difficulties with this use of the term *representation* are that it assumes (1) *single* neurons are the basic carriers of content, and (2) content can be determined by what has been called the naive causal theory—the view that a brain state represents whatever causes it to be active—which is well known to be highly problematic (Dretske, 1988). Little thought has been given in neuroscience to trying to establish a principled means of determining what appropriate representational vehicles are or how they might be related to the stimuli they are taken to represent. Why, for instance, should we assume that cells that selectively fire in the presence of faces actually represent faces? If the system is unable to use the information carried by such a cell to detect faces, or if the neuron is only partly informative of the presence of a face, or if as yet untested nonface stimuli can cause the cell to be active, such content claims will be misleading.

Work in theoretical neuroscience has been more careful regarding such claims. In particular, researchers examining neural coding are often careful not to assume that the stimuli presented to an animal are automatically or fully represented despite observed correlations (Rieke, Warland, de Ruyter van Steveninick, and Bialek, 1997). As a result, one of the most significant conceptual contributions of theoretical neuroscience to a neuroscientific understanding of representation is an emphasis on *decoding*. As mentioned, characterizing the responses of neurons to stimuli in the environment has been the mainstay of neuroscience. This, however, describes only an *encoding* process. That is, the process of responding to some physical environmental variable through the generation of neural action potentials, or spike trains. By adopting an information theoretic view of representation, theoretical neuroscience holds that to truly understand what information is preserved through the encoding process, we must be able to demonstrate that we (or the system) can (at least in principle) decode the spike train to give the originally encoded signal. As a result, to fully define representations, we must characterize both encoding and decoding.

In addition, theoretical neuroscientists have distinguished two aspects of representation: temporal representation and population representation. The former deals with how neurons represent time-varying signals. The latter deals with issues of distributed representation. That is, how a single cell's response contributes to a complex representation over a large group of neurons (i.e., allowing content claims to encompass more than single cells). In the next two subsections, I describe the theoretical characterization of encoding and decoding over time and neural populations employed by the NEF.

Temporal representation. Perhaps the best understood aspect of how neural systems represent time-varying signals is the encoding process. In some ways, this should not be too surprising because the focus of neuroscience in general has been on encoding. This is probably because the encoding process can be largely characterized by focusing on single cells. So the highly successful work on quantifying the dynamics of action potential generation in single cells—including mathematical descriptions of voltage-sensitive ion channels of various kinds (Hodgkin and Huxley, 1952), the use of cable equations to describe dendritic and axonal morphology (Rall, 1957, 1962), and the introduction of canonical models of a large class of neurons (Hoppensteadt and Izhikevich, 2003)—supports a highly mechanistic understanding of encoding. However, fully describing the encoding process also necessitates the identification of the particular, perhaps external parameters to which a neuron may be sensitive (partially in virtue of its relation to other neurons in the brain). These more holistic considerations are implicitly captured by the ubiquitously reported neuron "tuning curves." Improving our understanding of the encoding process is largely an empirical undertaking, one that has a long, successful history in both experimental and theoretical neuroscience. However, this is not true of temporal decoding.

There are two main kinds of theory of temporal decoding in neuroscience. These are referred to as the "rate code" view and the "timing code" view. Generally speaking, rate code theories are those that assume that information about temporal changes in the stimulus is carried by the average rate of firing of the neuron responding to that stimulus. In contrast, timing code theories assume that information about the stimulus is carried by the approximate distance between neighboring spikes in the spike train generated by the neuron responding to the stimulus.

Despite a wide-ranging debate over which code is used by neural systems, when carefully considering rate codes and timing codes, it becomes evident that they are variations on the same theme. Both codes assume that we choose some time window and count how many spikes fall in that window. In the case of rate codes, the time window is usually about 100 ms, and in the case of timing codes, the size of the window varies depending on the distance between spikes. It should not be too surprising, then, that methods have been developed for understanding temporal decoding that vary smoothly between rate codes and timing codes (Rieke et al., 1997). In the end, the distinction between rate codes and timing codes is not significant for understanding temporal representation.

These methods are surprisingly simple because they are linear (i.e., rely only on weighted sums). Suppose we are trying to understand the representational role of two neurons. To do so, we present this population with a signal and then record the spikes it produces in response to the signal. These spikes are the result of some (well-characterized) highly nonlinear encoding process. As discussed earlier, to properly characterize the representational properties of this neuron, we should be able to use those spikes to reconstruct the original signal. However, to do this we need to identify a decoder that takes those spikes as input and produces an estimate of the original signal. We can begin by assuming that the particular position of a given spike in the spike train does not change the meaning of that spike; that is, the decoder should be the same for all spikes. Essentially, every time a spike occurs, we place a copy of the decoder at the occurrence time of the spike. We can then sum all of the decoders to get our estimate of the original input signal (see figure 13.1). There are well-tested techniques for finding optimal decoders of this sort. As a testament to the effectiveness of these assumptions, it has been shown that this kind of decoding captures nearly all of the information that *could* be available in the spike trains of real neurons (Rieke et al., 1997, pp. 170–176).

A limitation of this understanding of temporal representation is that it is not clear how *our* ability to decode the information in a spike train relates to how that spike train is actually *used* by the organism. The NEF addresses this issue by

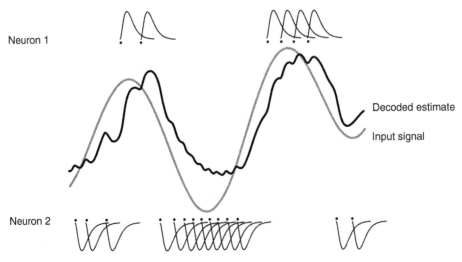

Figure 13.1. Temporal decoding. This diagram depicts linear decoding of a neural spike train (dots) using stereotypical decoders (skewed bell-shaped curves) on an input signal (gray line). The result of the decoding from two neurons (black line) is a reasonable estimate of the input signal. This estimate can be indefinitely improved with more neurons. Adapted from Eliasmith and Anderson (2003).

identifying the postsynaptic currents (PSCs) observable in the dendrites of receiving neurons with these temporal decoders (Eliasmith and Anderson, 2003, chapter 4). Although these decoders are no longer optimal, they are biologically plausible (unlike the noncausal optimal decoders found with past methods). Increasing the number of neurons in the representation can make up for any loss in fidelity of the represented signal. An example of this kind of decoding for two neurons is shown in figure 13.2a. That figure demonstrates how a rapidly fluctuating signal can be decoded from a neural spike train by a receiving neuron using a timing code (it is a timing code because significant jitter in the position of the spikes would greatly change the estimate). An example of decoding a much slower signal, which is encoded using something more like a rate code, is shown in figure 13.2b.

Together, these diagrams show that linear temporal decoding with PSCs is biologically plausible and can capture both rate and timing codes, depending on the demands of the situation. As a result, the NEF incorporates a method of characterizing temporal coding in neurons that is unique in its combination of biological plausibility and applicability to understanding the representation of signals at a variety of time scales.

The examples discussed to this point are only time-varying scalar values. To support representations of sufficient complexity to handle the vast variety of behaviors exhibited by neurobiological systems, it is essential to understand how large groups of neurons can cooperate to effectively encode complex, real-world objects.

Population representation. In a well-known series of experiments, Georgopoulos and colleagues explored the idea that the representation of physical variables in the cortex could be understood as a weighted sum of the individual neuron responses (Georgopoulos, Lurito, Petrides, Schwartz, and Massey, 1989; Georgopoulos, Schwartz, and Kettner, 1986). By recording from a population of neurons in the motor cortex, they demonstrated that a good prediction of a monkey's arm movement could be made by multiplying neuron firing rates by their preferred direction of movement and summing the result over the population. Essentially, Georgopoulos discovered a decoding method for extracting information carried by the neural firing rates that captured how this information was used by the motor system.

It is generally agreed that Georgopoulos provided a demonstration of how to decode a scalar variable (arm angle) encoded by a population of neurons. This kind of decoding, we should notice, is identical to that described in the temporal case. It is a simple linear decoding where the temporal decoder is replaced by a population one (i.e., preferred direction). However, the particular decoding chosen by Georgopoulos is far from optimal. Nevertheless, it is a simple matter to determine the optimal linear decoder (Salinas and Abbott, 1994). Furthermore, it is easy to generalize this kind of understanding of neural representation to more complex mathematical objects than scalars (Eliasmith and Anderson, 2003). For instance, instead of understanding neurons in motor cortex as encoding a one-dimensional scalar (i.e., direction), we can take them to be encoding a two-dimensional vector (i.e., direction and distance of arm movements). Indeed, there is evidence that the

a)

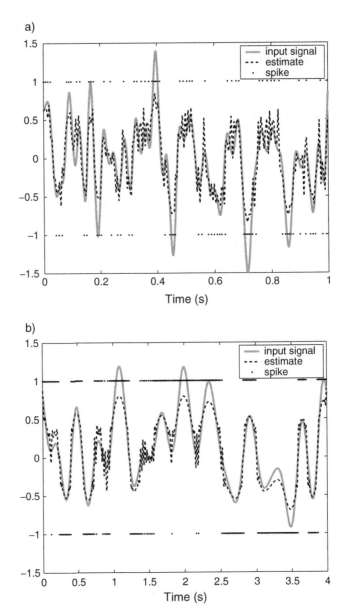

Figure 13.2. Biologically plausible timing and rate coding. (a) A high-frequency signal effectively decoded using postsynaptic currents (PSCs) as the decoders. This demonstrates a timing code. (b) A low-frequency signal (note the difference in time scale) similarly decoded. This demonstrates a typical rate code. Adapted from Eliasmith and Anderson (2003).

neurons Georgopoulos originally recorded from carry information about both of these dimensions (Moran and Schwartz, 1999; Schwartz, 1994; Todorov, 2000).

However, the discussion so far does not make it evident how to capture the wide variety of neural responses observed by experimental neuroscientists. For instance, one of the most common kinds of tuning curves observed in cortex is a Gaussian-shaped bump (sometimes called cosine tuning) around some preferred stimulus. For example, in lateral intraparietal cortex (LIP), neurons have these bump-like responses centered around positions of objects in the visual field (Andersen, Essick, and Siegel, 1985; Platt and Glimcher, 1998). On first glance, it may be natural to see them as encoding a scalar value that indicates the current estimate of the position of an object in the visual field. However, there is evidence to suggest that these representations are more sophisticated. For instance, the representation in this area can encode multiple object positions simultaneously and can have differing heights of bumps at those positions (Platt and Glimcher, 1997; Sereno and Maunsell, 1998). As a result, a more natural characterization of the representation in this area is as a *function*. That is, the activity of the neurons encodes a function whose height at a location is determined by the presence of various features at that location, such as brightness, shape, and so on.

Conveniently, function representation can be understood analogously to scalar and vector representation. Rather than a preferred direction vector in some parameter space, we can take neurons to have preferred functions. This would (approximately) be the function that best matched the neuron's tuning curve over the parameter space (e.g., object position and shape). It is then possible to find the optimal linear functional decoder for estimating some set of functions that the neural population can represent (Eliasmith and Anderson, 2003). With the introduction of function representation, the NEF shows how essentially any definable mathematical object can be represented over a population of neurons.

To this point, I have described both population representation and temporal representation independently. However, since both descriptions are cases of nonlinear encoding and linear decoding, it is a simple matter to combine these two kinds of representation. That is, rather than having a separate temporal decoder and a separate population decoder, we can define a single population-temporal decoder which can be used to decode a spiking, population-wide encoding of some mathematical object that captures the properties to be represented. This, then, completes a computational neuroscientific description of the representational vehicles employed by neurobiological systems.

In sum, this discussion demonstrates the wide variety of kinds of mathematical objects that can be represented in a neurobiologically plausible way with the NEF. This degree of generality suggests that the representational assumptions embodied in Principle 1 (section 2) are very broadly applicable to neurobiological systems. And, because this characterization of neural representation is simply variations on a common theme (i.e., nonlinear encoding and linear decoding), the NEF serves to unify our understanding of representation in neurobiological systems.

2.3. Computation

Conveniently, the NEF characterizes neural computation in the same way as neural representation. That is, in terms of a nonlinear encoding and a linear decoding. The difference is that representation consists of estimating the identity function, whereas computation, more broadly, consists of estimating arbitrary linear or nonlinear functions of the encoded variable. That is, when representing a variable, the system is concerned with decoding the value of that variable as it is encoded into neural spikes trains. The NEF labels decoders for this purpose "representational decoders." However, it is possible to identify decoders for computing any function of the encoded input; the NEF labels these "transformational decoders."

For example, if we define the representation in the LIP to be a representation of the position of an object, we can find representational decoders that estimate the actual position given the neural firing rates. However, we can also use exactly the same encoded information to estimate where the object would be if it was translated 5° to the right. For this, we could identify a transformational decoder. This particular example is merely linear transformation of the encoded information, and so is not especially interesting. However, the same methods can be used to find the transformational decoders for estimating nonlinear computations as well (e.g., perhaps the system needs to compute the square of the position of the object).

This account of computation is successful largely because of the nonlinearities in the neural encoding of the available information. When decoding, we can either attempt to eliminate these nonlinearities by appropriately weighting the responses of the population (as with representational decoding) or emphasize the nonlinearities necessary to compute the function we need (as with transformational decoding). In either case, we can get a good estimate of the appropriate function, and we can improve that estimate by including more neurons in the population encoding the information.

2.4. Dynamics

Given the previous characterizations of representation and computation, it is possible to build neurally realistic circuits that take time-varying signals as input and compute arbitrary functions of those signals. However, these techniques, as they stand, apply only to feedforward computations. As is well known, recurrence or backward projection is ubiquitous in neural systems. This kind of complex interconnectivity suggests that feedforward computation is not sufficient for understanding neurobiological function. As a result, theoretical neuroscientists need a means of characterizing the sophisticated, possibly recurrent, internal dynamics of the representations they take to be present in neural populations.

The third principle of the NEF incorporates the suggestion that neural dynamics can best be understood by taking neural representations to be control theoretic state variables. Control theory is a set of mathematical techniques developed in the 1960s to analyze and synthesize complex analog physical systems (Kalman, 1960a, 1960b). For linear, time-invariant systems, control theory provides a canonical way of expressing, optimizing, and analyzing the set of possible behaviors of the system. More complex dynamics, such as nonlinear and time-varying dynamics, can also be expressed using control theory, although analysis of the systems is no longer guaranteed to be analytically tractable.

The standard state-space form for control theoretic descriptions of physical systems is a set of differential equations defined over variables called the "state variables" (figure 13.3a). For any system so described, the current value of the state variables and the set of differential equations governing their dynamics completely determine the future behavior of the system. In neural systems, the set of differential equations can be taken to describe how the representation in a neural population changes over time. The value of the variables at any particular time is determined by the (spiking) neural representation at that time, and the governing equations are determined by the connection weights between that population and any others providing input to it (possibly including that population itself).

Notably, the standard control system depicted in figure 13.3a assumes that the dynamics of the physical system being described can be characterized as integration (hence the transfer function being an integral). However, neurons have their dynamics determined by intrinsic properties (e.g., ion channel speed, membrane capacitance, etc.) and do not naturally support integration. As a result, it is necessary to translate the standard control theoretic equations into a form appropriate for neural systems (figure 13.3b). Fortunately, this translation can be done in the general case (Eliasmith and Anderson, 2003, chapter 8). Such a translation allows any standard control theoretic description of a system to be written in an equivalent neural control theoretic form. The ability to effect such a translation can prove a great benefit to theorists. In particular, it allows mobilizing the vast theoretical

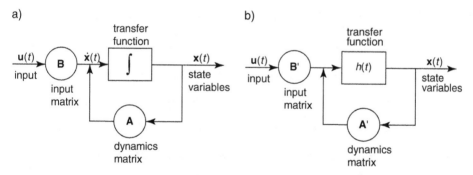

Figure 13.3. A diagram of the dynamics equation for LTI control theoretic descriptions of (a) a standard physical system, $\dot{x}(t) = \mathbf{A}x(t) + \mathbf{B}u(t)$ and (b) a neural system, $x(t) = h(t)*$ $(\mathbf{A}'x(t) + \mathbf{B}'u(t))$. The input signal, $u(t)$, can be modified by the parameters in the input matrix, B, before being added to any recurrent signal that is modified by the parameters in the dynamics matrix, A. The result is then passed through the transfer function, which defines the dynamics of the state variable, $x(t)$. In (a), the canonical form, the transfer function is integration. In (b), the neural form, the transfer function is determined by intrinsic neural dynamics. Fortunately, given the canonical form and the transfer function, $h(t)$, A' and B' can be determined for any A and B, for any linear, nonlinear, or time-varying system.

resources of control theory when hypothesizing about some observed biological function: a function that may already be well characterized by control theory.

2.5. Synthesis

The previous sections have defined the three principles of the NEF for characterizing neurobiological systems. However, it may not yet be clear how these principles interact, and, more importantly, how they are intended to map onto the observable properties of real neural systems.

Figure 13.4 depicts how these principles can be integrated to characterize the functioning of neurobiological systems at various levels of description. Specifically, figure 13.4 shows the components of a generic neural subsystem, including temporal decoders, population decoders, control matrices, encoders, and the spiking neural nonlinearity. A series of such subsystems can be connected to describe larger neural systems, because both the inputs and outputs of the subsystems are neural spikes.

Additionally, figure 13.4 depicts what it means to suggest that neural representations are control theoretic state variables. The state variables are defined by the temporal and population decoders and encoders, the dynamics of the control system are defined by the control matrices, and any functions that must be computed to

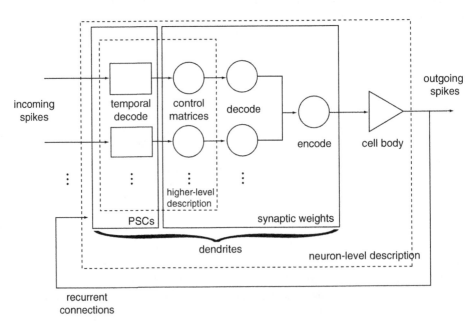

Figure 13.4. A generic neural subsystem. The outer dotted line encompasses elements of the neuron-level description, including PSCs, synaptic weights, and the neural nonlinearity in the soma. The inner dotted line encompasses elements of the control theoretic descriptions at the higher level. The gray boxes identify experimentally measurable elements of neural systems. The elements inside those boxes denote the theoretically relevant components of the description. See text for details. Adapted from Eliasmith (2003b).

implement the control system can be estimated by replacing the appropriate representational decoders with transformational decoders.

This figure also captures how the theoretical elements of this description map onto real neural systems. In particular, the control matrices, decoders, and encoders can be used to analytically compute the connection weights necessary to implement the desired control system in the neural population. The temporal decoders, as noted earlier, are mapped onto the PSCs produced in dendrites as a result of incoming neural spikes. Finally, the weighted dendritic currents arriving at the soma (cell body) of the neuron determine the output of the neural nonlinearity, that is, the timing of neural spikes produced by neurons in this population.[2]

Notably, the theoretical elements in this description are not identical to physically measurable properties of neural systems. As a result, there is a sense in which neural systems themselves never internally decode the representations they employ. This is because decoding, encoding, and the dynamics determined by the control matrices are all included in the synaptic weights, so their individual effects are not measurable. Nevertheless, if our assumptions regarding representation or dynamics of the system are incorrect, the model that embodies these assumptions will make incorrect predictions regarding the responses of individual neurons. So, although we cannot directly measure decoders, we can justify their inclusion in a description of neural systems insofar as the description is a successful one at predicting the properties we can measure (e.g., spike patterns and tuning curves). This, of course, is a typical means of justifying the introduction of theoretical entities in science. Encouragingly, this approach has been successfully applied to simulating and predicting the behavior of a large number of neurobiological systems, including sensory, cognitive, and motor systems, as previously enumerated at the end of section 1.

3. Rat Navigation

To better ground the subsequent philosophical claims regarding the NEF, and to show an application of these principles, I describe a detailed model of part of the rat navigation system first presented in Conklin and Eliasmith (2005).

The behavior of interest for this model is called path integration. It has been observed that rats are able to return directly to a starting location in an environment after having searched the environment in a somewhat random path (Alyan and McNaughton, 1999; Tolman, 1948; see figure 13.5a). Notably, in these experiments, the only available cues for the rat are self-motion (i.e., only idothetic cues). As a result, it has been hypothesized that the rat constantly updates an internal representation of its location in an environment relative to its starting point. Based on numerous neurophysiological investigations, it has been demonstrated that the representation can be thought of as a bump of activity that is centered on the rat's current estimate of its location (see figure 13.5b).

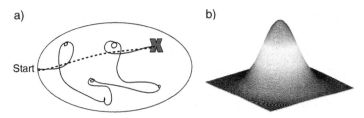

Figure 13.5. (a) Path integration in the rat. This is a schematic illustration of the rat's behavior while searching for a target ("X"). Not knowing the target location, it searches the environment (solid line) somewhat haphazardly. However, on locating the target, it is able to plot a course (dashed line) directly back to its starting position. (b) Internal representation of location in the rat. This is an idealization of the internal neural representation in a rat if it were located in the middle of the environment. This type of plot is generated by topographically arranging the receptive fields of cells in the relevant areas (subiculum, parasubiculum, and superficial layers of the entorhinal cortex). The bump indicates the firing rates of neurons in a population so arranged, and the center of the bump indicates the current estimate of the rat's location.

The challenge from a modeling point of view is to take the known physiological and anatomical properties of neurons in these areas and suggest an arrangement of such neurons that could implement a path integration mechanism that reproduces this observed behavior. Adopting the NEF, Conklin and I addressed this challenge with a detailed neural model that captures a variety of behavioral and neural observations and provides novel predictions.

In our publication, we begin by characterizing this bump of activity as a two-dimensional bell-shaped function representation. The nonlinear encoding is determined by the response properties of neurons observed in these brain areas (Sharp, 1997), and the neural model we employ (a leaky integrate-and-fire neuron).

Next, we suggest a high-level mechanism for performing path integration using only self-motion velocity commands available from the vestibular system. The details of the mechanism are not essential. However, it is notable that this suggestion is in the form of a dynamical/control system whose state variables are used to represent the two-dimensional bump. In short, we define a stable function attractor that will hold a bump at any location without input (i.e., when the rat is not moving), and then slide the bump to a topographically appropriate position given self-motion information. This specification is done independently of neural implementation.

We then embed the representation into the suggested control system as suggested by principle 3. The necessary representational transformations to implement the system in neurons are accomplished by drawing on the second, computational principle of the NEF. In short, we calculate the feedforward and feedback connections between the relevant populations of neurons by incorporating the appropriate dynamics, decoding and encoding matrices into the neural weights. Interestingly, we find that the resulting weight matrices have a center-surround organization, consistent with observed connectivity patterns in these parts of cortex.

Most significant, we provide a number of simulations of the resulting model (see figure 13.6). These simulations are the result of the activity of 4,000 spiking neurons. Notably, there is small drift error (11 percent) in completing a circular path (figure 13.6a). This demonstrates that the model has no biases in any particular direction while updating the representation. This also compares very favorably to the best past model of path integration, which had an error of approximately 100 percent using a network of 300,000 neurons to traverse a circular path (Samson-ovich and McNaughton, 1997).

A number of other results of the model are of particular interest for subsequent discussion.

- *Phase precession.* When a theta rhythm[3] is introduced into the model as global excitation, two phasic phenomena observed in rats are also observed in the model: phase precession (acceleration and deceleration of the representation in phase with theta) and phasic bump width changes.
- *Types of tuning curves.* The model shows the variety of tuning curves observed in vivo, including directionally selective cells in opposing directions, and nonselective cells.
- *Tuning curve resemblance.* When tuning curves are generated from model data using the same methods as for real cells (i.e., random foraging paths), details of the curves are very similar.
- *Sensory input for calibration.* The model shows the same effects as observed in the rat for weak (smooth, accelerating updating of the represented location) and strong (a jump in the location of the population activity) sensory input.

In addition to these replications of available data, the model makes three main predictions. First, it predicts that all cells will be velocity (as well as position) sensitive, if they are probed correctly. Second, cells in the path integrator (unlike typical

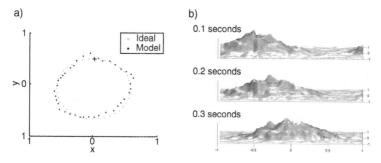

Figure 13.6. (a) The performance of the path model on a circular path (i.e., heading in every direction). The black dots indicate the center of the bump moving clockwise at samples taken every 50 ms. (b) Three points in time of the bump moving in a linear path from left to right. The bump is a result of counting spikes in a sliding window to determine firing rate. It is smoothed with a 5-point moving average for legibility. Adapted from Conklin and Eliasmith (2005).

place cells) will have the same relative location in different environments. Third, path integration should work regardless of the head direction of the rat (e.g., if the rat's head is pointing in a direction other than its direction of motion, this will not affect path integration). This last prediction is in contradiction with past models, and so is of particular interest.

4. PHILOSOPHICAL CONSEQUENCES

There is much to be said about the consequences of the NEF for our understanding of neural systems: That aspect of the framework has been extensively discussed in neuroscientific journals. In contrast, much less has been written about the philosophical consequences of this means of characterizing neural systems (although see Eliasmith, 2003a). In this section I briefly comment on several philosophical issues to which the NEF is relevant. These include the unity of science (i.e., theory reduction), theory construction in the behavioral sciences, and mental representation.

4.1. Theories, Models, and Levels

On occasion, cognitive scientists have expressed hostility toward the idea that our understanding of cognitive processes can be improved by a better understanding of how the brain functions (Fodor, 1999; Jackendoff, 2002; Lycan, 1984). They have suggested that knowing where things happen in the brain or how they are implemented is not relevant for answering the more important question of what the cognitive architecture is. These kinds of arguments have driven some to a view of brain sciences that draws sharp distinctions between cognitive and biological approaches to understanding neural function (Davies, 2000). More generally, this has been taken to suggest that science, in general, is not unified (Fodor, 1974). Often, the reduction of psychology to biology motivates these concerns precisely because the gap between these two modes of characterizing neural systems strikes many as insurmountable.

Despite the adoption of fMRI, PET, event-related potentials, and similar research methods by psychologists, there are no well-established techniques for integrating such temporally or spatially broad views of neural function with work in the electrophysiology or biochemistry of neurons. Similarly, models that incorporate biologically realistic single neurons tend to focus on low-level perception (e.g., receptive fields, motion, contour sensitivity), motor control (saccade generation, vestibular ocular reflex, invertebrate locomotion, digestion, etc.), and single-cell learning (e.g., retinal wave effects, receptive field learning, cortical column organization).

Given the principles and applications of the NEF, it seems plausible to suggest that this theoretical approach to neural systems stands to bridge this gap. That is, the NEF integrates single cell models (via nonlinear encoding) with cognitive mechanisms (via control theoretic descriptions). This integration is highly precise (i.e., each principle is quantitative); relates directly to underlying, measurable physical processes; and scales as computational power permits. The rat model presented earlier provides a somewhat uncognitive example of this sort of integration. However, Eliasmith and colleagues (Stewart and Eliasmith, in press; Eliasmith, 2004) present a similarly derived (though much larger) model of language-based deductive inference which effectively characterizes the well-known Wason selection task (Wason, 1966), and exhibits cognitive behavior found only in human reasoners. Models of these sorts make the brain sciences look much less disunified than has been argued in the past.

In fact, I propose that application of the NEF can suggest a particular kind of scientific unification. In particular, we can see from the rat model that the application of the general NEF principles boils down to the continually more precise specification of sets of boundary conditions. Some of these conditions are in the form of a hypothesis regarding the dynamics (e.g., integration), some are in the form of a control mechanism (e.g., the particular matrices defining the path integrator), and others are in the form of empirically measured neuron tuning curves (e.g., the distribution of tuning curves of cells in subiculum). In general, as we progress from general theory (NEF) to specific model (rat path integration) we have followed a route of increasing specificity. Were we to continue on that route—that is, were we to match each model neuron with a specific neuron in a specific rat (rather than matching neuron property distributions across rats)—we would end up with a highly detailed (perhaps too much so) model that would be able to make specific predictions regarding the behavior of a particular rat. Of course, the model as originally presented is not interested in such questions, so the level specificity stopped much earlier. Nevertheless, this notion that increasingly detailed boundary conditions can serve to traverse a model-to-theory hierarchy seems a potentially useful description of how the brain sciences may be unified. The unification stems from the fact that at each step in the specification, the basic principles do not change.

Unlike past models, those derived from the NEF can be placed in such a unification hierarchy. This allows for general principles of neural function that might not otherwise be evident to become obvious. For instance, the close relation between rat path integration, mechanisms of horizontal eye control by the nucleus prepositus hypoglossi, the head direction system, and working memory (all of which can be characterized as vector integrators) might have gone unnoticed without this principled underpinning (see Eliasmith, 2005, for details of these and related generalizations).

Although much remains to be said about the potential unification or disunification of brain sciences, the NEF provides a first plausible and detailed story about how such a unification might be worked out. As a result, it is in a unique position to support replies to the notion that "the description of mental processes at the cognitive level can be divorced from the description of their physical realization" (Fodor and Pylyshyn, 1988, p. 54).

4.2. Theory Construction in the Behavioral Sciences

I have argued elsewhere that current approaches to cognitive science have their theoretical foundations grounded in metaphor (Eliasmith, 2003a). I suggest that the NEF is unique in its avoidance of metaphor for theoretical insight (though not for explanation). An important consequence of this reliance on metaphor by past approaches that I have not emphasized in past discussions is the adverse effect it has on theory construction in the behavioral sciences. In short, if the theoretical import of a metaphor is not explicitly grounded, that is, directly related to independently observable quantities, then it will be difficult to construct empirically testable theories. I take notions like "empirical testability" and "directly related" to be matters of degree. However, in both cases, the more the better.

I suggest that the NEF is unique among approaches to the behavioral sciences in that the elements of the theory are (very) directly relatable to observables, and hence the models stemming from the NEF are highly testable. For instance, the elements in the path integration model can be mapped directly onto elements in the brain (or, more precisely, the distribution of element properties can be so mapped). That is, model neurons produce spike rates, tuning curves, spike patterns, somatic currents, and so on that can be compared directly to spike rates, tuning curves, spike patterns, somatic currents, and so on in real rat neurons. In contrast, when classical cognitive science assumes the mind is like a computer, and imports notions of data structure, symbolic representation, and so on into behavioral models based on such a metaphor, we are left wondering how such theoretical entities relate to the physical system that they are supposed to be describing. This is largely because we do not know how to measure (independent of this theory) such entities in a real behaving system. In short, the ability of NEF-generated models to be mapped in detail onto independently measurable physical properties makes them more convincing (because more empirically testable), than those generated by classical models. But what of other approaches in the behavioral sciences? I briefly consider two other paradigms, dynamicism, and connectionism.

The dynamicist view in cognitive science emphasizes dynamical descriptions for behavioral systems (Port and van Gelder, 1995). However, there is an extremely important difference between these dynamical descriptions and those generated by the NEF. For dynamicists, the variables over which the differential equations are defined are not explicitly related to the physical system itself (Eliasmith, 1997, 2003a). For example, the "motivation" variable in motivational oscillatory theory, which is intended to characterize some high-level property of the animal, is never related to any specific physical property of the system (Busemeyer and Townsend, 1993)—and it is entirely unclear how it could be. In contrast, the NEF is explicit on the relation between higher level neural representations and the activations of single cells. It is precisely these representations that serve as the variables over which the dynamics are defined. Again as in the classical case, the explicitness of the mapping, and hence empirical import, of models generated by the NEF is far more impressive.

What about connectionism? The difficulty with connectionism is precisely that while endorsing brain-like models, it is far too abstracted from neurobiological constraints. That is, because only the barest features of neural architectures are preserved in connectionist models, it is difficult to relate the resulting models back to real brains. Earlier I expressed concern with Fodor and Pylyshyn's distancing of cognitive from neural approaches to the behavioral sciences, they clearly understand the importance of exploiting any available constraints:

> Understanding both psychological principles and the way that they are neurophysiologically implemented is much better (and, indeed, more empirically secure) than only understanding one or the other. That is not at issue. The question is whether there is anything to be gained by designing "brain style" models that are uncommitted about how the models map onto brains. (Fodor and Pylyshyn, 1988, p. 62)

Although Fodor and Pylyshyn suspect that there is no interesting interplay between these levels of description, they do realize the import of both. I suggest that the NEF helps integrate high-level and low-level approaches, thus providing more empirically secure models that can draw directly from various levels of description in the behavioral sciences. The path integration model is able to make the specific, empirical predictions it does precisely because of the detailed mapping between the model and the neurobiological system it simulates. Notably, these predictions are both behavioral (relating head direction to integration bias), and neural (predicting specific relations between neural tuning curves and the rat's environment). The ability of a single model to successfully address multiple levels of description make it reasonable to think that Fodor and Pylyshyn's dismissal of intertheoretic unity is premature.

In conclusion, the lesson to be learned is that the more explicit and independently testable the mappings of your theories or models, the more success you will have in constructing interesting theories. In the behavioral sciences, the NEF uniquely provides such mappings across traditionally distinct levels of description.

4.3. Mental Representation and Semantics

One useful distinction that has arisen out of the philosophical discussion of representation is that between the contents (semantics) and the vehicles (syntax) of representations (Cummins, 1989; Fodor, 1981). In general, contents are thought to be determined by the object in the world that the representation picks out, the relation of that representation to other representations, or a combination of both. The vehicles of representations are the physical realization of objects that play the role of representations (i.e., carrying a content) in a system. Theoretical neuroscience can contribute to improving our understanding of both representational vehicles and their contents.

The characterization of representation in section 2.2 is most clearly about vehicles. The NEF (and previous work on which it draws) tells us how to characterize structures in the brain as able to carry contents as values of scalars, vectors, functions, and so on. I suspect this characterization is sufficient for understanding the complete set of vehicles available to neural systems. However, let me emphasize one particular class that is generally overlooked by the philosophical community. As far as I am aware, there are no discussions in the philosophical literature of representational systems that include the uncertainty of the representations in the representations themselves. Because the NEF can describe how neural systems represent functions, it can describe how neural systems represent probability distributions over possible states of the world—just such a representation of uncertainty. In fact, the rat's bump of activity can be interpreted as just such a representation. Rather than supposing that the center of the bump represents the rat's location, we can more interestingly suppose that the bump represents a distribution of the possible locations of the rat with varying certainties. Thus, a wider bump would indicate more uncertainty (variance) in the representation, and a narrower bump less uncertainty. In either case, the best estimate of the rat's actual location will be the mean, but understanding the bump in this way increases the amount of information that such a representation carries and allows the representation to support sophisticated reasoning strategies that employ statistical inference (Eliasmith and Anderson, 2003).

This is not merely idle speculation. There is increasing evidence that precisely this kind of representation is used to encode information about the uncertainty of the estimate of the stimulus being encoded and that this information is used by the nervous system for (nearly optimal) statistical inference (Britten and Newsome, 1998; Knill and Pouget, 2004; Kording and Wolpert, 2004; Stocker and Simoncelli, 2006). It seems essential, given the noisy, complex, and uncertain environment in which neurobiological systems reside, for such systems to be able to make decisions with partial, incomplete, or noisy data. So it is only to be expected that the representations in neural systems can support statistical inference. In sum, an important class of vehicles for understanding minds, those that carry a content and its uncertainty, has been overlooked in philosophical discussions.

Let me now turn to a brief consideration of semantics (see Eliasmith, 2006, for a more detailed discussion of a semantic theory consistent with the NEF). There are three broad classes of semantic theories: causal, conceptual role, and two-factor theories. Causal theories of meaning have as their main thesis that mental representations are about, and thereby mean, what causes them (Dretske, 1981, 1995; Fodor, 1990, 1998). In the context of the previous discussion this means that the encoding process alone determines meaning. Conceptual role theories hold that the meaning of a term is determined by its overall role in a conceptual scheme (Harman, 1982; Loar, 1981). Under such theories, the meaning of a term is determined by the inferences it causes, the inferences it is the result of, or both. Here, the focus is on the decoding of whatever information happens to be in some neural state.

One theoretical move, to avoid the difficult problems that arise when adopting either a causal theory or a conceptual role theory, is to combine them into a two-factor theory (Block, 1986; Field, 1977). On two-factor theories, causal relations and conceptual role are equally important, independent elements of the meaning of a term: "The two-factor approach can be regarded as making a conjunctive claim for each sentence" (Block, 1986, p. 627). So only two-factor theories explicitly acknowledge both encoding and decoding.

Given the NEF characterization of representational vehicles, a representation is only defined once both the encoding and decoding processes are identified. This means that contrary to both causal and conceptual role theories of content, both how the information in neural spikes is used (decoding) as well as how it is related to previous goings-on (encoding) are relevant for determining content. In the rat example, the bump indicates the rat's location precisely because it is caused by (or correlated with) the rat's actual location in the world and because it is used by the rat to determine how to move (e.g., making a beeline back to the starting location once the goal has been achieved). So given the characterization of vehicles we have seen, two-factor theories of content seem most plausible.

However, as just noted, it is assumed by past two-factor theories that the factors are *independent*. This property raises a grave difficulty for such theories. In criticizing Block's theory, Fodor and Lepore remark, "We now have to face the nasty question: *What keeps the two factors stuck together?* For example, what prevents there being an expression that has the inferential role appropriate to the content *4 is a prime number* but the truth conditions appropriate to the content *water is wet?*" (1992, p. 170). If, in other words, there is no relation between the two factors (i.e., they are simply a conjunction), it is quite possible that massive misalignments between causal relations and conceptual roles can occur.

However, in the NEF, characterization of representation there is a tight relation between the encoding and decoding processes—they are not independent. Broadly speaking, the population-temporal decoders are found to estimate some function of the encoded parameter. For simple representation this function is identity, but it need not be in the case of transformational decoding. That is, all of the inferences derivable from some particular neural encoding depend on the information carried by that encoding. As a result, if there is no relation between the "wetness of water" and "4 being a prime number," it would it be impossible for the latter to be part of the conceptual role of the encoding of the former given the NEF characterization. Such considerations suggest that this characterization can avoid the main weakness of past two-factor theories, though more work must be done to propose a full-fledged theory of representation.

5. CONCLUSION

Admittedly, each of these discussions of the philosophical consequences of the NEF deserves much more careful, full-length treatment. Nevertheless, these suggestions hopefully demonstrate the utility of looking beyond traditional philosophical or psychological approaches to the behavioral sciences for addressing a variety of philosophical problems.

It is also worth emphasizing that there is much subtlety to the NEF itself that has not been addressed here. The framework has been designed to account for the ubiquitous effects of noise, allow novel methods for the analysis of learning rules, and incorporate the wide variety of single cell dynamics (e.g., adaptation, bursting) seen across neurobiological systems. Each of these developments may also serve to highlight new approaches to related philosophical problems.

ACKNOWLEDGMENTS

Parts of sections 2 and 4 of this article are based on Eliasmith (2007).

NOTES

1. A search of PubMed indexed neuroscience journals (53 journals) over the past 5 years for the term *represent* returns over 2,300 hits.
2. This nonlinearity can be captured by a set of differential equations that describes the dynamics of the channel conductances that control the flow of ions through the cell membrane resulting in action potentials, or it could be a simpler reduced model of neural spiking (like the common leaky integrate-and-fire model).
3. In much of the hippocampal complex, there is a globally observable voltage oscillation at 7–10 Hz. This is called the theta rhythm.

REFERENCES

Alyan, S. H., and McNaughton, G. L. (1999). Hippocampectomized rats are capable of homing by path integration. *Behavioral Neuroscience* 113: 19–31.

Andersen, R. A., Essick, G. K., and Siegel, R. M. (1985). The encoding of spatial location by posterior parietal neurons. *Science* 230: 456–458.

Block, N. (1986). Advertisement for a semantics for psychology. In P. French, T. Uehling, and H. Wettstein (Eds.), *Midwest Studies in Philosophy*. Minneapolis: University of Minnesota Press, 615–678.

Britten, K. H., and Newsome, W. T. (1998). Tuning bandwidths for near-threshold stimuli in area MT. *Journal of Neurophysiology* 80: 762–770.

Busemeyer, J. R., and Townsend, J. T. (1993). Decision field theory: A dynamic-cognitive approach to decision making in an uncertain environment. *Psychological Review* 100: 432–459.

Conklin, J., and Eliasmith, C. (2005). An attractor network model of path integration in the rat. *Journal of Computational Neuroscience* 18: 183–203.

Cummins, R. (1989). *Meaning and Mental Representation*. Cambridge, Mass.: MIT Press.

Davies, M. (2000). Interaction without reduction: The relationship between personal and sub-personal levels of description. *Mind and Society* 1: 87.

Dayan, P., and Abbott, L. H. (2001). *Theoretical neuroscience: Computational and mathematical modeling of neural systems*. Cambridge, Mass.: MIT Press.

Desimone, R. (1991). Face-selective cells in the temporal cortex of monkeys. *Journal of Cognitive Neuroscience* 3: 1–8.

Dretske, F. (1981). *Knowledge and the Flow of Information*. Cambridge, Mass.: MIT Press.

Dretske, F. (1988). *Explaining Behavior*. Cambridge, Mass.: MIT Press.

Dretske, F. (1995). *Naturalizing the Mind*. Cambridge, Mass.: MIT Press.

Eliasmith, C. (1997). Computation and dynamical models of mind. *Minds and Machines* 7: 531–541.

Eliasmith, C. (2003a). Moving beyond metaphors: Understanding the mind for what it is. *Journal of Philosophy* 100: 493–520.

Eliasmith, C. (2003b). Neural engineering: Unraveling the complexities of neural systems. *IEEE Canadian Review* 43: 13–15.

Eliasmith, C. (2004). Learning context sensitive logical inference in a neurobiological simulation. In S. Levy and R. Gayler (Eds.), *AAAI Fall Symposium: Compositional Connectionism in Cognitive Science*. AAAI Press, 17–20.

Eliasmith, C. (2005). A unified approach to building and controlling spiking attractor networks. *Neural Computation* 17: 1276–1314.

Eliasmith, C. (2006). Neurosemantics and categories. In C. Lefebvre and H. Cohen (Eds.), *Handbook of Categorization in Cognitive Science*. Amsterdam: Elsevier.

Eliasmith, C. (2007). Computational neuroscience. In P. Thagard (Ed.), *Philosophy of Psychology and Cognitive Science*. Amsterdam: Elsevier.

Eliasmith, C., and Anderson, C. H. (2003). *Neural Engineering: Computation, Representation and Dynamics in Neurobiological Systems*. Cambridge, Mass.: MIT Press.

Eliasmith, C., Westover, M. B., and Anderson, C. H. (2002). A general framework for neurobiological modeling: An application to the vestibular system. *Neurocomputing* 46: 1071–1076.

Felleman, D. J., and van Essen, D. C. (1991). Distributed hierarchical processing in primate visual cortex. *Cerebral Cortex* 1: 1–47.

Field, H. (1977). Logic, meaning, and conceptual role. *Journal of Philosophy* 74: 379–409.

Fischer, B. (2005). *A Model of the Computations Leading to a Representation of Auditory Space in the Midbrain of the Barn Owl*. PhD dissertation, Washington University in St. Louis).

Fodor, J. (1974). Special sciences (or: The disunity of science as a working hypothesis). *Synthese* 28: 97.

Fodor, J. (1981). *Representations*. Cambridge, Mass.: MIT Press.

Fodor, J. (1990). *A Theory of Content and Other Essays*. Cambridge, Mass.: MIT Press.

Fodor, J. (1998). *Concepts: Where Cognitive Science Went Wrong*. New York: Oxford University Press.

Fodor, J. (1999). Let your brain alone. *London Review of Books* 21.

Fodor, J., and Lepore, E. (1992). *Holism: A Shopper's Guide*. Oxford: Basil Blackwell.

Fodor, J., and Pylyshyn, Z. (1988). Connectionism and cognitive architecture: A critical analysis. *Cognition* 28: 3–71.

Georgopoulos, A. P., Lurito, J. T., Petrides, M., Schwartz, A., and Massey, J. (1989). Mental rotation of the neuronal population vector. *Science* 243: 234–236.

Georgopoulos, A. P., Schwartz, A. B., and Kettner, R. E. (1986). Neuronal population coding of movement direction. *Science* 243: 1416–1419.

Harman, G. (1982). Conceptual role semantics. *Notre Dame Journal of Formal Logic* 23: 242–256.

Hodgkin, A. L., and Huxley, A. F. (1952). A quantitative description of membrane current and its application to conduction and excitation in nerve. *Journal of Physiology* 117: 500–544.

Hoppensteadt, F., and Izhikevich, E. (2003). Canonical neural models. In M. Arbib (Ed.), *The Handbook of Brain Theory and Neural Networks*. Cambridge, Mass.: MIT Press.

Hubel, D., and Wiesel, T. (1962). Receptive fields, binocular interaction and functional architecture in the cat's visual cortex. *Journal of Physiology (London)* 160: 106–154.

Jackendoff, R. (2002). *Foundations of Language: Brain, Meaning, Grammar, Evolution*. New York: Oxford University Press.

Kalman, R. E. (1960a). Contributions to the theory of optimal control. *Boletin de la Sociedada Matematica Mexicana* 5: 102–119.

Kalman, R. E. (1960b). A new approach to linear filtering and prediction problems. *ASME Journal of Basic Engineering* 82: 35–45.

Knill, D. C., and Pouget, A. (2004). The Bayesian brain: The role of uncertainty in neural coding and computation. *Trends in Neurosciences* 27: 712–719.

Koch, C. (1998). *Biophysics of Computation: Information Processing in Single Neurons*. Oxford: Oxford University Press.

Kording, K. P., and Wolpert, D. M. (2004). Bayesian integration in sensorimotor learning. *Nature* 427: 244–247.

Kuo, D., and Eliasmith, C. (2005). Integrating behavioral and neural data in a model of zebrafish network interaction. *Biological Cybernetics* 93: 178–187.

Lettvin, J., Maturana, H., McCulloch, W., and Pitts, W. (1959/1988). What the frog's eye tells the frog's brain. In W. McCulloch (Ed.), *Embodiments of Mind*. Cambridge, Mass.: MIT Press.

Loar, B. (1981). *Mind and Meaning*. London: Cambridge University Press.

Lycan, W. (1984). *Logical Form in Natural Language*. Cambridge, Mass.: MIT Press.

Moran, D. W., and Schwartz, A. B. (1999). Motor cortical representation of speed and direction during reaching. *Journal of Neurophysiology* 82: 2676–2692.

Platt, M. L., and Glimcher, G. W. (1997). Responses of intraparietal neurons to saccadic targets and visual distractors. *Journal of Neurophysiology* 78: 1574–1589.

Platt, M. L., and Glimcher, G. W. (1998). Response fields of intraparietal neurons quantified with multiple saccadic targets. *Experimental Brain Research* 121: 65–75.

Port, R., and van Gelder, T. (1995). *Mind as Motion: Explorations in the Dynamics of Cognition*. Cambridge, Mass.: MIT Press.

Rall, W. (1957). Membrane time constant of motoneurons. *Science* 126: 454.

Rall, W. (1962). Theory of physiological properties of dendrites. *Annual New York Academy of Science* 96: 1071–1092.

Rieke, F., Warland, D., de Ruyter van Steveninick, R., and Bialek, W. (1997). *Spikes: Exploring the Neural Code*. Cambridge, Mass.: MIT Press.

Salinas, E., and Abbott, L. (1994). Vector reconstruction from firing rates. *Journal of Computational Neuroscience* 1: 89–107.

Samsonovich, A., and McNaughton, B. L. (1997). Path integration and cognitive mapping in a continuous attractor model. *Journal of Neuroscience* 17: 5900–5920.

Schwartz, A. B. (1994). Direct cortical representation of drawing. *Science* 265: 540–542.

Sereno, A. B., and Maunsell, J. H. R. (1998). Shape selectivity in primate lateral intraparietal cortex. *Nature* 395: 500–503.

Sharp, P. E. (1997) Subicular cells generate similar spatial firing patterns in two geometrically and visually distinctive environments: Comparison with hippocampal place cells. *Behavioural and Brain Research* 85: 71–92.

Singh, R., and Eliasmith, C. (2006). Higher-dimensional neurons explain the tuning and dynamics of working memory cells. *Journal of Neuroscience* 26: 3667–3678.

Stewart, T., and C. Eliasmith. (In press) Compositionality and biologically plausible models. In W. Hinzen, E. Machery, and M. Werning (Eds.), *Oxford Handbook of Compositionality*. Oxford University Press.

Stocker, A. A., and Simoncelli, E. P. (2006). Noise characteristics and prior expectations in human visual speed perception. *Nature Neuroscience* 9: 578–585.

Todorov, E. (2000). Direct cortical control of muscle activation in voluntary arm movements: A model. *Nature Neuroscience* 3: 391–398.

Tolman, E. C. (1948). Cognitive maps in rats and men. *Psychological Review* 55: 189–208.

Tripp, B., and Eliasmith, C. (2007). Neural populations can induce reliable postsynaptic currents without observable spike rate changes or precise spike timing. *Cerebral Cortex*. 17:1830–1840.

Wason, P. C. (1966). Reasoning. In B. M. Foss (Ed.), *New Horizons in Psychology*. Harmondsworth: Penguin, 135–151.

CHAPTER 14

NEUROANATOMY AND COSMOLOGY

CHRISTOPHER CHERNIAK

A bounded-resource paradigm is by now familiar in mind–brain science. The discussion here focuses not on the levels of psychology or physiology but on brain wiring, in particular, on an apparent paradox: Available connectivity in, say, the cerebrum, is stringently limited, yet deployment of interconnections shows fine-grained optimization, sometimes without detectable limits. Virtually perfect network optimization, rather than just network satisficing, sometimes applies well to neuroconnectivity architecture. Such layout cost-minimization problems are a major hurdle of microcircuit design and are known to be NP-complete (explained shortly). How does biology effectively solve such problems? Briefly, some odd wrinkles of the computational realm seem to be exploited. This line of thought suggests extensions to the anthropic principle of cosmology—that is, further possible constraints on models of a universe in which our intelligence can arise. This in turn may narrow the conventional hardware-independence thesis of computational psychology.

1. Brain Wiring Minimization and Optimization Landscapes

The tension discussed here is a picture sometimes emerging in our work: seemingly almost limitless refinement in use of clearly limited connection resources (e.g., Cherniak, 1994a, 1994b; Cherniak, Mokhtarzada, and Nodelman, 2002). Prima facie, this embodies an antagonism. The bounded-resource perspective (e.g., Cherniak, 1986) is that the mind–brain has moderate-scale resources—not zero, not perfect. The natural expectation regarding their use that harmonizes with this resource model would be that available resources are satisficed, that is, employed *moderately* well. On the one hand, they cannot be used with profligate inefficiency because they are limited. Of course, optimal use of connections in effect would maximize available connection resources. However, on the other hand, the wiring would not be anticipated to be (nearly) perfectly deployed, because that refinement itself in turn typically has its own cosmically high costs.

Network optimization theory characterizes the minimized use of limited connection resources (e.g., wirelength) in a system. A main feature of the optimization landscape is that many of the problems are nondeterministic polynomial–time complete (NP-complete) or NP-hard; that is, such problems are conjectured to require computation time typically on the order of a brute-force search of all possible solutions and are often therefore intractable.

Over the past decade or so, our laboratory has uncovered a pattern of very efficient connection use in the nervous systems of various animals (e.g., roundworm, rat, cat, primate), at different levels (from positioning of whole brain, through layout of ganglia and cortex, down to subneuronal structures like somata and arbors), and for different types of network optimization (e.g., Steiner tree, component placement optimization) (Cherniak et al., 2002). We are also beginning to find connection-minimization patterns in genomic systems. Generally, the verdict of history is that Nature just solves tractable special cases of hard optimization problems. However, we have found some odd twists. The interrelation between the neuroanatomy and cosmology in the title of this chapter is that brain structure optimization seems to mesh finely with some convenient coincidences of the computational order of the universe. These instances of biology exploiting anomalies of the computational universe operate against the background of a "nongenomic nativism" (Cherniak, 2005): We have found some complex biological structure originating directly from simple physical processes, without need of DNA involvement.

For example, we described neuron arbor approximations of Steiner tree optimization (Cherniak, Changizi, and Kang, 1999; see Chklovskii and Stepanyants, 2003). A Steiner tree is a minimum-cost arbor connecting a set of terminal loci, for example, root to synapse sites as "leaves." The exact solution of the problem has two parts: (1) Brute force search of an exponentially exploding set of alternative tree topologies or connection patterns (the NP-hard part of the problem); (2) then embedding each topology (adjusting branch lengths for the various weights of the arbor branches, because trunks cost more than their branches), achievable via simple vector-mechanical processes. (This type of post hoc analysis applies despite the "intrinsically" driven character of typical dendrites, where leaf node loci are in fact not targets fixed in advance.) Perhaps we acquire a romantic picture from graph theory: The heart of the matter is searching the topologies (each is like a different universe, inaccessible from any other), whereas the embedding is trivial, just classical continuous mathematics.

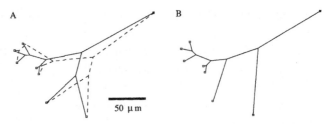

Figure 14.1. Mouse thalamus axon subarbor (wireframe representation). (A) Actual multijunction tree in broken lines; optimal embedding of actual topology (with respect to volume minimization) in solid lines. Volume error of actual tree is 2.2 percent. (B) "Best of all possible topologies" (with respect to volume); volume error is 2.5 percent. Only 10 of the 10,395 alternative topologies here have lower total volume costs, when optimally embedded, than the actual topology. Topology search yields little improvement compared with embedding. Embedding can be accomplished by a simple fluid mechanical process; topology cannot.

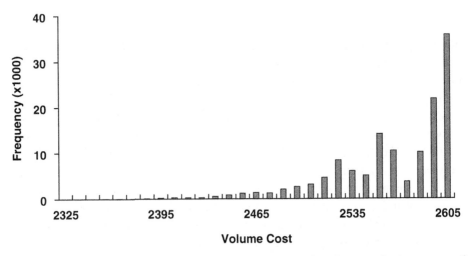

Figure 14.2. Nine-terminal arbor of mouse thalamus axon: distribution of volume costs of all 135,135 possible topologies, each optimally embedded. The histogram shows the usual pattern for natural arbors, living and nonliving—more costly topologies are more common, cheapest ones are rarest. The most costly optimally embedded "pessimal" layouts have only about 12 percent greater volume than cheapest one. Hence, for optimization, "topology does not matter."

However, the unintuitive story we found is that roughly, "Topology does not matter." Figures 14.1 and 14.2 illustrate that in fact relatively little tree cost-minimization seems to be at stake in selecting a topology; much more can be gained in just refining the embedding. (So also for classical uniform-cost Steiner trees, with all branch junctions at 120°.) Thus, Nature seems to "solve" the Steiner tree problem via a lucky if counterintuitive factoid of computational geometry, that embedding dominates over topology; topology can in effect be ignored at comparatively little cost. (This strategy may also be worth exploring for rectilinear Steiner tree design in microchip engineering.) Neuron arbors solve their minimization problem to within a few percent of optimality, about as well as nonliving arbors, such as river drainage networks; the neurons seem to attain their volume minimization via the same basic fluid dynamic processes as do water networks.

Another exploitation of special cases emerges in mechanisms for optimization of layout of ganglia in the nematode nervous system. This is a component placement optimization problem, involving positioning of a system of interconnected components to minimize total connection costs. Again, the general quadratic assignment problem (QAP) here is NP-hard. Yet the worm's actual layout is the unique cheapest one in total wirecost (Cherniak, 1994a). As we have reported, a very simple genetic algorithm, with total wirelength of nervous system as fitness measure, will robustly and reliably find that optimal layout (Cherniak et al., 2002). Yet so will a force-directed placement algorithm (FDP) or vector-mechanical "mesh of springs." See figures 14.3 and 14.4 (see also Chklovskii, 2004).

Such energy-minimization approaches have not proven very successful for microchip layout because of trapping in local minima. Why do they work for worm brain layout? One strange feature we found is that the FDP algorithm has a knife-edge sensitivity to the worm connectivity matrix: We found some changes of adding or cutting a *single* worm brain connection that can paralyze the algorithm in local minima. So the moral seems to be that the worm brain may indeed constitute a

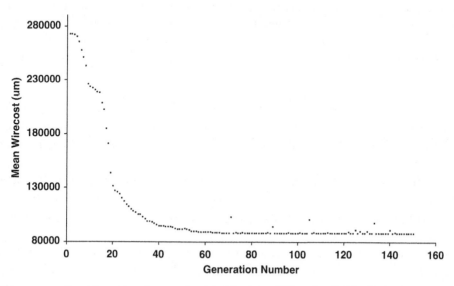

Figure 14.3. GenAlg, a simple genetic algorithm, rapidly and reliably finds the optimal (minimum wirelength) layout of *C. elegans* ganglia among 11! alternatives. The initial population of this run was only 10 individuals, all with reverse of actual ordering of ganglia. (For another GenAlg run with the same initial population, see Cherniak et al., 2002, figure 5.)

```
                                                    Input: rid.add


                  T E N S A R A M A

Head                                          Tail
0    0    1    1    2    2    3    3    4    4    5
0    5    0    5    0    5    0    5    0    5    0    Tetrons

   PH    (152.000000)
     AN    (352.000000)
      RNG   (492.000000)
DO   (26.000000)
          LA    (616.000000)
         VN    (796.000000)
        RV    (1000.000000)
              VCa   (1908.000000)
                              VCp   (3908.000000)
                                    PA    (4778.000000)
                                    DR    (4862.000000)
                                    LU    (4936.000000)


Final layout popped out after:   150,000 iterations
Tension Constant:   0.0100
Total Wirecost:   90,743.7500   um
```

Figure 14.4. Tensarama, a force-directed placement (FDP) algorithm that optimizes layout of *C. elegans* ganglia. This "tug of war" vector-mechanical energy-minimization simulation represents each of the worm's approximately 1,000 connections acting on the movable ganglia PH, AN, and so on. The key feature of Tensarama performance for the actual worm connectivity matrix is its low susceptibility to local minima traps—unlike Tensarama performance for small modifications of the actual connectivity matrix (a "butterfly effect"), and unlike FDP algorithms in general for circuit design. Here Tensarama is locked in a nonoptimal layout by a "killer" connectivity matrix that differs from the actual matrix by only one added connection. See also Cherniak et al. (2002, figure 6) and Cherniak (2005, figure 5.2).

special tractable case of QAP; but the picture may be that the abstract connectivity matrix itself (the "mind") co-evolves with its wirecost-minimized physical layout. Instead of the top-down design methodology familiar in computer engineering, this is a cart-before-horse (cart-beside-horse?), tail-wags-dog picture.

Finally, we have found a peculiar fine-tuning of a quick-and-dirty heuristic for connection cost minimization of layouts of worm ganglia (also perhaps of mammalian cerebral cortex). The adjacency rule wiring heuristic is: If two components are connected, then place them next to each other. It can be used for laying out a system and also as an easily applicable wirecost measure for such layouts (instead of measuring actual wirelengths, which is often unfeasible). We have described a calibration of performance of this heuristic for worm ganglia (Cherniak et al., 2004; see figures 14.5 and 14.6). In general, the adjacency heuristic does not yield especially low-wirecost ganglion layouts. However, again, a very narrow range of special cases behaves quite well, namely, layouts that conform best to the adjacency rule do have the cheapest wirecosts. The

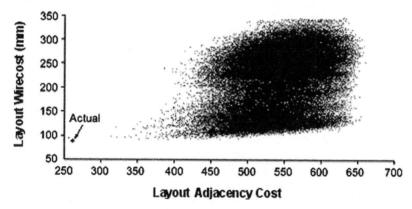

Figure 14.5. Adjacency rule conformance, versus total wirecost, of a sample of 100,000 *C. elegans* ganglion layouts. (Adjacency rule: "If components *a* and *b* are connected, then *a* and *b* are adjacent.") Generally, the adjacency rule is not an effective heuristic for good wirecost. However, the small set of layouts best fitting the adjacency rule (points at far left) behave markedly differently: They correlate well with the *best* wirecost layouts.

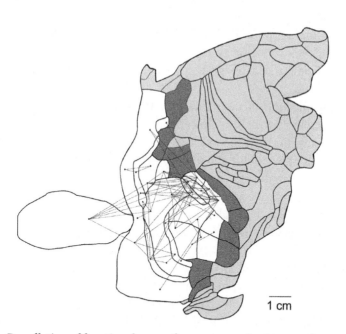

Figure 14.6. Parcellation of functional areas of macaque cerebral cortex. Component placement optimization analysis of layout of 17 core areas (white) of visual cortex, along with immediately contiguous edge areas (dark gray). Lighter straight lines indicate reported interconnections among core areas. Rostral (forward) is to right. In a connection cost analysis (with respect to the adjacency rule), this actual layout of the core visual system ranks in the top one-millionth of all alternative layouts (Cherniak et al., 2004). For 39 areas of cat cortex, actual layout may rank in top 100 billionth of all possible layouts. "Best of all possible brains?"

computational order is such that for arbor optimization, topology does not matter; yet for component placement optimization, it suffices. So once more, the leitmotif seems to be exploitation of happy accidents of the fine scale microtopography of the optimization landscape.

What these cases convey is the need to develop means of systematically mapping such "chaotic" problem terrains—concepts beyond simple sampling.

2. Brain Wiring Optimization and the Anthropic Principle

The simplest relation of the brain to the universe, stemming from the LaPlacean picture of the cosmos as a vast clock, comes from a tradition of calculating the maximum total computational capacity of the cosmos. A recent estimate, based on an entropic theory of information, and taking account of quantum phenomena, is 10^{50} operations/second (Lloyd, 2002). With the familiar speculation (e.g., Donofrio, 2001) that one human brain is capable of around 10^{16} flops (10 petaflops, or 10 quadrillion floating-point arithmetic operations/second), the universe then has the computing capacity of 10^{34} human brains. Or, with ~10^9 human brains presently alive on Earth, the universe-as-computer is equivalent to 10^{25} Earth human brain-populations.

Another connection of neuroanatomy to cosmology would proceed via the anthropic principle (Barrow and Tipler, 1986). A weak form of the anthropic principle asserts that any model of the universe must meet the adequacy condition that it permits the development of life and intelligence—as has in fact occurred. (Although the idea is much older, the phrase "anthropic principle" is credited to Carter, 1974.) In particular, the physical constants—the number of dimensions, energy states of the electron, strength of the weak nuclear force, and so on—must be fine-tuned to permit carbon-based life, and human intelligence, to arise.

For instance, in the search for extrasolar planets capable of supporting life, the focus is on ones in the habitability range, not too hot or cold. Similarly, on the largest scale for the universe: Its physics must not yield just Big Bang conditions with too high temperatures for stable structure, nor only heat death conditions with too little energy exchange for information-processing—neither bang nor whimper.

In the previous section, we reported brain-wiring optimization in a number of nervous systems, at a number of levels. If such extreme neural network optimization is not just gratuitous, but in fact somehow is a prerequisite for brain functioning (Cherniak et al., 2002), we can now contemplate a possible further set of brain-enabling conditions of the universe.

1. For the generation of approximations of optimal Steiner trees, search of topologies does not have a significant downside risk, compared to embedding. This is a lucky accident of computational geometry, because exhaustive topology search in fact is intractable, whereas embedding is straightforward.

2. There are connectivity matrices for the "mind" of the nematode, and of other creatures (that implement required brain functions) for which energy-minimization placement processes are not trapped in local minima—as FDPs often are, and as very small variations from the actual worm brain matrix are.

3. Regarding worm nervous system layouts, in the vast majority of cases, adjacency heuristic conformance does not correlate with cheap wirecost. However, the few cases of *best* adjacency rule performance do correspond to the cheapest wirecost cases. Worm ganglia, and rat, cat, and macaque cortex areas in fact do optimize well with respect to the adjacency heuristic, with a Size Law included (Cherniak et al., 2004).

In concluding, we refrain from intelligent design speculations about such fortunate harmony of universe and brain. There are traditions of haruspicating messages in natural patterns, for example, from extraterrestrials in bacteriophage DNA (Yokoo and Oshima, 1979), and from Someone in the cosmic microwave background radiation (Hsu and Zee, 2006). As a caveat, we cite a universal nonde-nominational prayer that social commentator Emo Phillips proposed, in another context: Approximately, "Please arrange the universe for my convenience." Reality is the ultimate Rorschach.

A modest moral concerns modeling mind: Some of the landscape of philosophy of mind begins to shift. Namely, seeing neuroanatomy so intimately meshed with the computational order of the universe prompts reconsideration of constraints on the computationalist thesis of hardware-independence of mind. To the extent that wiring optimization seems both requisite, and a hostage to brain-friendly compu-tational anomalies of the universe, practical latitude for alternative realizations of mind narrows.

Acknowledgment

A version of this chapter was presented as an invited contribution to a symposium on Computational Complexity Analyses of Cognitive Models at the Society for Mathematical Psychology annual meeting, July 2006, Vancouver.

REFERENCES

Barrow, J., and Tipler, F. (1986). *The Anthropic Cosmological Principle*. Oxford: Oxford University Press.

Carter, B. (1974). Large number coincidences and the anthropic principle in cosmology. *International Astronomical Union Symposium* 63: 291.

Cherniak, C. (1986). *Minimal Rationality*. Cambridge, Mass.: MIT Press.

Cherniak, C. (1994a). Component placement optimization in the brain. *Journal of Neuroscience* 14: 2418–2427.

Cherniak, C. (1994b). Philosophy and computational neuroanatomy. *Philosophical Studies* 73: 89–107.

Cherniak, C. (2005). Innateness and brain-wiring optimization: Non-genomic nativism. In A. Zilhao (Ed.), *Evolution, Rationality and Cognition*. London: Routledge, 103–112.

Cherniak, C., Changizi, M., and Kang, D. (1999). Large-scale optimization of neuron arbors. *Physical Review E* 59: 6001–6009.

Cherniak, C., Mokhtarzada, Z., and Nodelman, U. (2002). Optimal-wiring models of neuroanatomy. In G. Ascoli (Ed.), *Computational Neuroanatomy: Principles and Methods*. New York: Humana: 71–82

Cherniak, C., Mokhtarzada, Z., Rodriguez-Esteban, R., and Changizi, B. (2004). Global optimization of cerebral cortex layout. *Proceedings of the National Academy of Sciences USA* 101: 1081–1086.

Chklovskii, D. (2004). Exact solution for the optimal neuronal layout problem. *Neural Computation* 16: 2067–2078.

Chklovskii, D., and Stepanyants, A. (2003). Power-law for axon diameters at branch point. *BMC Neuroscience* 4: 18.

Donofrio, N. (2001). Turing Memorial Lecture. *Computer Journal* 44: 67–74.

Hsu, S., and Zee, A. (2006). Message in the sky. *Modern Physics Letters A* 21: 1495–1500.

Lloyd, S. (2002). Computational capacity of the universe. *Physical Review Letters* 88: 1–4.

Yokoo, H., and Oshima, T. (1979). Is bacteriophage ϕX174 DNA a message from an extraterrestrial intelligence? *Icarus* 38: 148–153.

PART V

NEUROSCIENCE OF MOTIVATION, DECISION MAKING, AND NEUROETHICS

CHAPTER 15

THE EMERGING THEORY OF MOTIVATION

ANTHONY LANDRETH

1. INTRODUCTION

Some people are highly motivated, whereas others are not. Some people are motivated to run, others are motivated to fight. When we describe the patterns of motivation we see in ourselves and others, we talk about what we want, in terms of outcomes and actions, and we talk about what we intend to do and how we intend to do it. A desire we intend to satisfy supplies us with a goal or an end. By virtue of a desire's incorporation into an intention, the desire drives us in a direction we believe will bring about the relevant end. Motivated behavior is intentional behavior, and what we intend to do, we want to do.[1] Thus, the theory of desire and intention are parts of the theory of motivation.

As part of our commonsense psychology, we know that motivation has many aspects. We know that motivation both directs behavior and invigorates it (Dickinson and Balleine, 2002). Aside from what we see in behavior itself, we know that motivation comes and goes, and various motivational states compete within us for control of our actions. We also know that motivation directs our practical reasoning capacities, turning them toward the formation of plans for action.

In this chapter, I relate aspects of our commonsense understanding of motivation to an emerging, mechanistic account of motivation in neuroscience. According to the emerging theory, motivational states depend on specific control systems in the brain. These systems supply us with goals for thought and action, as well as the drive to act on behalf of those goals.

The discussion canvasses various points in neural processes where motivational control will have an opportunity to play a role. These points of influence, I argue, occur (1) in the early stages of planning a course of action by sequencing a set of subgoals, (2) at the stage of action selection when the type of instrumental action to be performed is chosen, and (3) at the stage of online action correction when adjustments are made in the midst of performance.

The work of many neuroscientists and philosophers guides our discussion. In relating feedback control to the explanation of motivation's directional capacity, I open with a theory of goal-directed systems, based on the work of Fred Adams (1979). According to Adams, goal-directed systems implement feedback control. If he is correct, motivation mechanisms should be a species of feedback control system. To flesh out this insight, I draw on the neurocomputational work of Randy O'Reilly and Michael Frank, the work of James Houk, and results from Richard Andersen's lab. To account for motivation's drive capacity, I turn to the work of Yael Niv, Nathaniel Daw, and Daphna Joel. Then, to relate theory from neuroscience to our commonsense understanding of motivation, I draw on the work of Timothy Schroeder, Alfred Mele, and Elisabeth Pacherie.

2. THE DIRECTIONAL CAPACITY

A motivational state provides an agent with at least one goal. Typically, the way we individuate motivational states suggests that each provides what we might call a basic goal. The basic goal of hunger is to be fed. The basic goal of lust is to have sex.

The basic goal of a motivational state can serve as a foundation for the subgoals that are instrumental in the satisfaction of the basic goal. Thus, having the basic goal of being fed, one might be led to form the subgoal of opening a refrigerator door. That subgoal, in turn, might lead to a subgoal for reaching out to grasp the refrigerator door handle.

Notably, the word *goal* has a certain kind of ambiguity. For example, sometimes the word refers to a mental state—an unsatisfied want held by the goal's bearer. Other times, the word is used to refer to an object of desire. For the sake of clarity, let's call the psychological state underlying a goal for action *desire*. We can then let *goal* refer to a state that satisfies a desire. Thus, we can distinguish between intrinsic desires and instrumental desires (i.e., psychological states) and basic goals and subgoals (i.e., objects of desire). Like basic goals, intrinsic desires are held for their own sake. Instrumental desires, like subgoals, are held for the sake of satisfying intrinsic desires.

Motivational states are psychological states, so it seems intuitive to say that they consist of desires. In consisting of desires, motivational states supply their bearers with goals and thus a purpose or target at which to aim thought and movement. Thus, one of the first steps in developing a theory of motivation is to specify the role goals should play in the explanation of thought and behavior.

Preferably, a state of affairs being a goal will be an objective matter, independent of our opinion. That is to say, a thing being a goal should depend not on people adopting an anthropomorphic attitude toward that thing but on the way that the thing is otherwise situated in the world. Let us call systems that are goal-directed in this objective sense *intrinsically goal-directed systems*.

In a paper published in 1979, Adams argued that intrinsically goal-directed systems qualify as such because they realize feedback control processes. For a process to be goal-directed, it must be under feedback control. Feedback control systems provide an intuitive model for understanding the nature of goal-directedness, because the manner in which these systems work and rest is contingent on a specific match between a sensed environmental condition—our model for a goal state—and a specific internal parameter—our model for desire.

The most familiar cases of feedback control are driven by negative feedback. Others are driven by positive feedback. In engineering contexts, negative feedback control is implemented in air conditioning systems, missile guidance, and the cruise control systems in cars. In the abstract, each of these systems has a common set of components causally organized into negative feedback loops (see figure 15.1a). For example, each such system has a component sensitized to a state variable that needs to be controlled, that is, a "sensor," like the speedometer in your car. There is a controller that affects the parameter to be controlled in the environment, for example, that adjusts the gas flow to the engine. There is also a component that supplies an input to the controller that determines the equilibrium state of the control system, called the "setpoint." In cruise control, the setpoint is what you adjust through your console to set the speed. Negative feedback control systems also have a comparator, such as a device that tracks the difference between the setting and the actual speed, and a controller that adjusts the gas flow to the engine, based on the comparator's output. We say that the system involves a feedback loop because the effect the controller has on the car's speed in turn

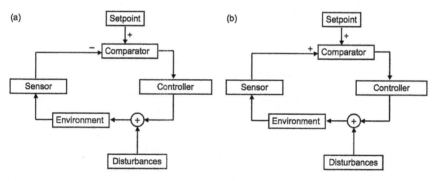

Figure 15.1. Feedback control systems. (a) Negative feedback control system. Disturbances include any unforeseen influences on the controller's output, once the output is sent to the environment. The comparator's output is based on the difference between the sensor's input and the setpoint (goal). The process controlled by the controller is taken to be in the environment external to the other systems components. (b) Positive feedback control system. The comparator's output is based on the sum of the setpoint and the feedback signal.

affects (or feeds back into) the controller through the comparator. Negative feedback control systems have a tendency to neutralize the effects of the setpoint on the controller via the feedback signal. Thus, the feedback tends to be negative.

Positive feedback control works somewhat differently (figure 15.1b). In contrast with a negative feedback controller, which tends to produce feedback that minimizes the controller's rate of output, a positive feedback controller tends to produce positive feedback that increases work output. Whereas a negative feedback loop subtracts the return value from the setpoint value, a positive feedback loop adds the values. In some cases, a positive feedback loop has a deactivation condition that cuts off output at a particular sensor measurement, a kill switch that serves as a deactivation condition for the controller.

The parallels between feedback control and motivational states are familiar. When motivated to eat, we seek to reduce the discomfort that hunger brings, and when the hunger is gone, the motivation to eat may be set to rest. Motivation to eat has an intuitive negative feedback structure. The more we eat, the less we want to eat.

Yet, some aspects of hunger appear to follow a certain kind of positive feedback pattern, evinced in the salted peanut effect. Sitting on a plane, not feeling particularly hungry but a bit bored, you might find yourself opening a complimentary packet of peanuts. (It's something to do after all.) Taking the first peanut, you might notice that the saltiness tastes quite good. So you eat more and, up to a point, you eat more quickly.

The salted peanut effect refers to the kind of increase in response vigor that occurs at the beginning of a consummatory episode. Eating peanuts makes you want to eat more peanuts, until you reach a cut-off point—satiety for salt appetite, which may not mean satiety for other flavors. Thus motivation appears to have both negative and positive feedback facets.

Relating feedback control to our understanding of goals and desires, we might want to identify the specific goals of motivational states with the setpoints that guide the controllers of our actions. In analogy to the equilibrium conditions determined by setpoints, we might say that goals are those sensed conditions that bring the controller to rest.

But the analogy is a bit simplistic. Unlike the paradigm cases of feedback control, our control systems are multipurpose. For example, we can use our bodies and motor control systems to reach for a flower or reach for a weapon, to woo a mate or cheer on an athlete. We can pursue categorically distinct goals at different times, and we need not come to rest just because one of our goals has been met. Thermostats only regulate temperature, but motivation regulates all kinds of variables. Thus, if we are to use feedback control as a model for understanding motivational states, we will have to upgrade the kind of system that will constitute our model.

To capture the multifunctionality of motivation, let us build into our control system a mechanism I call a *feeder*. The function of a feeder is to supply the comparator with setpoints. When the system's goal state obtains, the feeder swaps out the old setpoint and plugs in a new one. Thus, the operations of the feeder will parallel our understanding of the manner in which different desires command our behavior at different times. For example, when the satisfaction of an intrinsic desire requires the satisfaction of a sequence of instrumental desires, the feeder can supply the comparator with each setpoint in serial order as the prior setpoint is met. Then, when the intrinsic desire is satisfied, the feeder can shift to another intrinsic desire and start feeding a different series of setpoints into the comparator. Different motivational states specify categorically distinct basic goals for action and specify subgoals instrumental to the attainment of a basic goal.

Because an agent can satisfy one goal and move on to the next without coming to rest, we probably shouldn't think of reaching a setpoint as a matter of our internal motor control systems turning off. It would make much more sense, instead, if when the sensor signal came to match the setpoint, this would cause the setpoint to come unplugged from the comparator, thereby allowing a new one to take its place. Thus, the "rest" condition that occurs in simpler feedback control systems could be highly transitory in a motivational feedback system, amounting to a goal-switching condition. A sequence of subgoals could then be pursued in serial order until a basic goal obtains.

The capacity of a motivational state to match subgoals to basic goals links motivation to learning and thus adds another layer of complexity to our feedback conception of motivation. Environments change, as well as one's capacities to navigate those environments. The learned subgoals and associated actions sufficient to obtain basic goals yesterday may no longer be sufficient today. Motivation must be able to adapt action to environmental change. Thus, a motivational feedback system must have built into it a capacity to update its action biases as well.

There are three locations where we will need to build in an update function for learning in feedback control. One location, as my comments suggest, is at the mechanism for storing sequences of instrumental desires—the memory bank from which the feeder draws when it plugs setpoints into the comparator. Another location is at the point where the kind of action to satisfy each desire's subgoal is chosen. A third location is in the process of action execution itself, where motor commands may need to be corrected to account for unexpected environmental contingencies.

Concerning the update function in the first instance, sometimes it will be necessary to alter a bank of instrumental desires when a new set of initial conditions is necessary to bring about a goal state. For example, suppose that recent road construction has blocked your usual driving route to the grocery store. If you have a basic goal of acquiring food, many of the normal subgoals associated with driving the route from home to the store are no longer going to work for you. New subgoals for arriving at a different set of intersections will have to replace the old. Obviously we are capable of adopting and abandoning subgoals when it has a bearing on desired outcomes. So the control systems model should have the capacity to modify its bank of instrumental desires.

Our control system should also have the capacity to modify the motor control signals it uses to bring about goal states. The adoption of a new subgoal will require the adoption of a new motor control policy for bringing about the subgoal. For example, knowing that you have to take a new route to the store, you might adopt the instrumental desire of doing so. But having the instrumental desire does not ensure that you have the knowledge of the new route. Thus, there should also be a capacity for instrumental learning.

The adoption of subgoals involves prediction (regarding what will get us what we want), based on learning (sometimes from experience), in the service of planning (which in execution expresses an operative form of motivation). Insofar as the predictive, learning, and planning capacities involve operations on mental representations, we should expect motivation to operate on mental representations. It follows that our model of motivation should help us understand how basic goals interface with representations. There is a class of feedback control system that combines many of these features. These systems have internal models that enable the system to represent action-outcome contingencies and adjust behavioral tendencies based on real and simulated feedback. Using the same, feedback-based learning signal, these systems can also adjust their subgoals. Furthermore, these systems appear to actually be realized in our brains. Following precedent, I call these systems model-driven reinforcement learning systems (Sutton and Barto, 1998). In subsequent sections, I refer to the application of reinforcement learning concepts to the explanation of motivation mechanisms as the reinforcement learning framework. Let's look at how the framework operates.

3. THE ADOPTION OF INSTRUMENTAL DESIRES

Distinct motivational states fix in mind at least one intrinsic desire and one set of instrumental desires. Let us refer to this pair as a desire system. In the previous section, I suggested that model-driven reinforcement learning might provide a good model for understanding motivation. If that's the case, then the model should help us understand the nature of desire systems.

In the first application of the reinforcement learning framework, I would like to consider the acquisition of instrumental desires. To that end, I focus on a specific computational model developed by Randy O'Reilly and Michael Frank (2006). In my discussion of the model, I introduce the foundational concepts of reinforcement learning theory. For the sake of clarity, I first present the conceptual details of the model (without the neuroscience) and then relate those details to the neural system whose processes the model is supposed to capture. (In section 4, I relate the present discussion to desire selection.)

O'Reilly and Frank call the framework for their model PVLV. Like other reinforcement learning systems, PVLV relies on a prediction error signal to drive the learning process. In this framework, the goal quantities are called *rewards*. Expectations of reward combine with reward returns to generate the prediction error signal, which in its simplest form can be defined thus:

$$\delta = r - r'. \tag{15.1}$$

In the formula, r is the magnitude of a perceived reward return, r' is the magnitude of an expected reward return, and δ is the difference between them. Thus, r is the output of a function, called the "reward function," which takes a specific

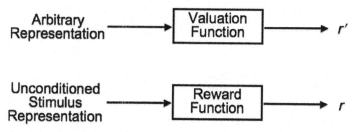

Figure 15.2. Determinants of δ. The valuation function takes an arbitrary representation and assigns a scalar value ($0 \leq n < \infty$). The reward function takes an unconditioned stimulus and assigns a scalar as well. When r exceeds r', δ is positive.

category of representation as input (e.g., food) and has as its output a scalar value. The r' term corresponds to the output of a "valuation function," which takes any arbitrary representation as input and assigns a scalar as output (see figure 15.2). When a representation is fed into the valuation function and a positive number comes out, the valuation function treats the representation's referent as a predictor of reward. However, if the valuation function assigns a zero to an input representation, then that representation is not associated with reward and is neutral.

When the difference between r and r' is positive, the reward expectations are increased and the action tendency active at the time is strengthened. When the difference is 0, *ideally* behavioral and cognitive dispositions remain the same. When the difference is less than 0, reward expectations decrease and the active action tendency at the time weakens.

PVLV is an instance of a reinforcement learning system that uses an Actor-Critic architecture (see figure 15.3). A Critic is a mechanism that simultaneously updates the reward predictions in the valuation function and alters the input-output profile of the Actor, which is a kind of controller. The Critic interacts with the Actor by sending it a δ-signal. The Actor's action tendencies are then biased or altered by receiving the δ-signal.

Like other kinds of Actor-Critic systems, PVLV is capable of forming what Read Montague (2006) calls "value proxies," The formation of a value proxy amounts to a transference of reward function from an unconditioned stimulus to a conditioned stimulus. The reader may recall from Pavlov's famous experiments on dogs the transference of an unconditioned response (salivation) from the sight of an unconditioned stimulus (e.g., food) to a conditioned stimulus (e.g., a ringing bell that predicts the presentation of food). The transference indicates that the dogs learned to expect food when the bell rang. The formation of a value proxy is a neural counterpart to this kind of learning process.

A value proxy, in Montague's terms, is a stimulus predictive of reward that is treated by the brain as though it were the reward itself. Thus, a value proxy is something that the Critic can learn to treat as a reward but on first encounter would not have been treated as such. For example, the sight of fresh salmon might not be rewarding until one has come to associate salmon with a pleasant flavor and various

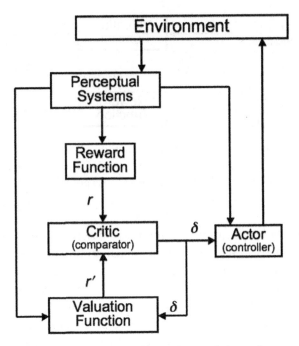

Figure 15.3. Simple Actor-Critic architecture. The *r* and *r′* signals converge on the Critic to generate a negative feedback signal, δ. In the figure, δ acts as both a biasing and training signal, working on both the valuation function and the Actor.

health benefits. Once the association is learned, the sight of salmon, and not just eating it, will be treated by the Critic as a reward. The PVLV framework accounts for the formation of value proxies by defining two distinct pairs of reward and valuation functions. One set of functions corresponds to the operations in what the authors call a Primary Value system (PV for short). The other set of functions corresponds to the operations of what they call a Learned Value system (LV). Each of these systems can independently drive the Critic to produce the δ-signal (figure 15.4).

Because the two kinds of value systems generate the δ-signal by means of distinct reward and valuation functions, PVLV distinguishes two kinds of δ-signal:

$$PV_\delta = r_{PV} - r'_{PV},$$ (15.2)

and

$$LV_\delta = r_{LV} - r'_{LV}.$$ (15.3)

The LV system's reward function is defined on the representations that have been assigned positive scalar values in the PV system's valuation function. So what the LV system treats as rewards depends on what the PV system treats as *predictors* of reward. As the PV system gets better at predicting reward returns, PV_δ will approach 0. But the minimization of PV_δ will not in turn minimize LV_δ. The LV system must learn how to predict signs of impending reward to minimize its error, and though the LV system will rely on the Critic's signal to perform this function, the LV system's update is a distinct process.

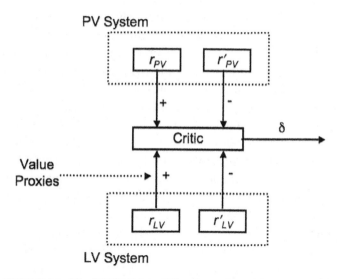

Figure 15.4. PVLV Critic. The PVLV Critic differs from the Critic in a simpler Actor-Critic architecture. As in the simpler architecture, the δ-signal affects the Actor and updates valuation functions. However, in PVLV, there are two distinct valuation functions (r'_{PV} and r'_{LV}) whose predictive outputs can be used to cancel out the effects of the reward functions (r_{PV} and r_{LV}) on the Critic.

The minimization of LV_δ will lag behind the minimization of PV_δ. This is significant, because (as I mentioned a moment ago) both PV and LV systems rely on the same comparator, that is, the same Critic, to compare reward predictions to reward returns, and produce the basic δ-signal. The manner in which the LV system treats a predictor of reward as a proxy for reward is by failing to accurately predict returns of r_{LV}. Thus, when the PVLV system has learned that a stimulus's occurrence predicts primary reward return (i.e., a basic goal quantity), the basic δ-signal migrates away from the reward event back to the event that predicts reward. In other words, the PVLV system will treat a predictor of reward as though it were the reward itself, that is, as a value proxy.

The only reason the LV system treats a predictor of reward as a value proxy is that the predictor is reliable. If the predictor stops being reliable, then the LV system will stop treating it as a value proxy. Similarly, if the satisfaction of an instrumental desire ceases to be conducive to the satisfaction of an intrinsic desire, we can expect the instrumental desire to be abandoned. Thus, we can see a parallel between the ways an intrinsic desire relates to an instrumental desire and a PV system's reward function relates to an LV system's reward function. Now let's consider how PVLV maps onto neural systems.

First, let us consider the δ-signal itself, which is taken to model the behavior of phasic dopamine in particular neural pathways. In the phrase "phasic dopamine," the word *phasic* refers to a burst of spikes in the cells that release dopamine from vesicles at these cells' axon terminals. Cells releasing dopamine are called "dopaminergic cells." *Phasic* stands in contrast to *tonic*. A tonic dopamine response is a baseline spiking response, which contrasts with a pause, which is a moment when a cell simply does not spike. Dopamine cells have a baseline spike rate, exhibited in the tonic response, and they have a bursting rate, exhibited in the phasic response.

Dopaminergic cells are located in the hypothalamus, substantia nigra pars compacta (SNc), and the ventral tegmental area (VTA) (figure 15.5). Reinforcement learning models focus on dopaminergic cells in the SNc and the VTA to the exclusion of hypothalamic dopamine production. The reason for this is that dopaminergic cells in these structures appear to meet the functional profile of the δ-signal and because dopamine released from these cells is known to be critical for a variety of important functions. For example, reductions in levels of dopamine from the SNc are regarded as the mechanism of Parkinson disease, which causes impairments in voluntary movement, working memory, and learning.

Dopamine itself is regarded as a relatively slow-working agent that binds to receptors on target cells in portions of the basal ganglia, and cells in neocortex and the cerebellum. But dopaminergic cells, when they release dopamine, do not release dopamine alone. Some of these cells also release fast-acting neurotransmitters, such as glutamate.

Wolfram Schultz and colleagues performed the classic experiments associating phasic dopamine with error in predicted reward. In these experiments, Schultz,

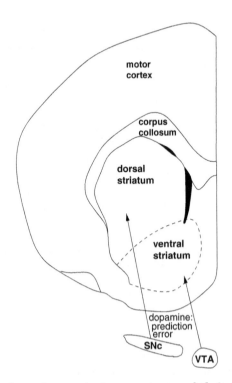

Figure 15.5. Midbrain dopamine-producing structures and their targets. VTA = ventral tegmental area; SNc = substantia nigra pars compacta. Modified from Daw, Niv, and Dayan (2005).

Apicella, and Ljungberg (1993) found that when a monkey encountered an unpredicted reward, midbrain dopamine cells would evince the phasic response—a burst of firing when the monkey was given a squirt of juice. When an expected reward was omitted, dopamine cells would pause in their firing, momentarily ceasing to exhibit even a tonic response. Over a series of trials in Pavlovian and instrumental conditioning tasks, a monkey would learn to predict reward on the basis of a cue (see Schultz, Dayan, and Montague, 1997; Schultz and Dickinson, 2000). Once the monkey learned to predict the amount of impending reward, something unexpected occurred. The phasic dopamine response shifted to the presentation of the predictor of reward, and the same dopaminergic cells remained silent when the reward was received. The dopaminergic cells came to treat predictors of reward like substitutes for actual rewards. But if a stimulus that was previously a reliable predictor of reward ceased to serve that role, that stimulus would no longer elicit the phasic response. Thus, the predictor of reward can come to serve as a value proxy on these cells.

Based on the likeness of the phasic dopamine response to the δ-signal, Schultz and colleagues (1997) hypothesized that phasic dopamine was simultaneously an agent of reinforcement and the training signal for reward expectations. If the hypothesis was correct, then cells should be found encoding a prediction of reward and reward return, and these cells should synapse onto dopaminergic cells that could then generate a phasic response on the basis of the difference between these two signals. Finding evidence of a Critic, we should therefore expect to find evidence of reward functions and valuation functions. And that is what we find. Electrophysiology and functional neuroimaging confirm the existence of reward prediction in orbitofrontal cortex and the ventral striatum (a component of the basal ganglia).

The orbitofrontal cortex projects directly into the VTA, which in turn releases dopamine into the nucleus accumbens (a portion of the ventral striatum) and most areas of cortex. Of course, for the VTA to serve as a Critic, mechanisms implementing reward functions must project into the VTA as well, so that the difference between r and r' can be calculated there. One possibility is that separate projections from orbitofrontal cortex send the r signal, at least when we are talking about r proxy signals. Cells in the medial orbitofrontal cortex have been found to respond preferentially to reward stimuli and reliable predictors of reward.[2] The response magnitude of these cells scales to the amount of reward received and the satiety of the animal. For example, a cell that responds to a stimulus predicting a food reward will fire in response to that predictor until the animal is full.

A wide variety of reward and punishment types are tracked by orbitofrontal cells, including erotica, food, drinks, brand names, monetary gains, pleasant touch, pleasant music, attractive faces, and orgasm (see Holstege et al., 2003; Rolls, 2005; Zald and Rauch, 2006). From the looks of things, the orbitofrontal cortex would be a natural place to find desire systems. But the orbitofrontal cortex is not the only place to look. Evidence suggests that at least two distinct networks underlie the formation of reward expectations, the other being the ventral striatum. These two systems are believed to serve different functions.

The orbitofrontal cortex has often been regarded as a fast learning system for predictors of reward, because the electrophysiological response profiles of orbitofrontal cells can change fairly quickly. By contrast, the ventral striatum has been regarded as a slow reward learning system, likely involving it in the formation and selection of habitual responses (Daw et al., 2006). Where the orbitofrontal system has the VTA as its Critic, the ventral striatum has the SNc (Frank and Claus, 2006; O'Reilly and Frank, 2006).

Habitual responses are considered to be only weakly under motivational control and more strongly under the control of external stimuli. But habitual responding is not totally free of motivation's influence. For example, a habitual response can be performed more or less quickly, depending on recent returns of a desired quantity, regardless of whether the habitual response is related to the desired returns (see Niv, Joel, and Dayan, 2005).

Generally speaking, systems-level models of dopamine treat the relationship between the performance of habits and dopamine's effect on the ventral striatum as quasi-independent. The dopamine δ-signal is needed to acquire habits and can be used to bias for or against the performance of habitual responses, but the δ-signal is not taken to be necessary for an Actor to do its job. Of course, that is not to say that tonic dopamine is not necessary for action selection (see section 8). But it is important to recognize that dopamine *biases* the selection of activation patterns at its targets. Dopamine is not a complete action selection mechanism.

How are the ventral striatum and orbitofrontal systems supposed to interact? Roughly, the idea is that the orbitofrontal cortex can inhibit the ventral striatum's actions on the dorsal striatum, thereby overriding a habitual response in favor of an alternative response. The ventral striatum, being part of a habit system, is believed to rely strictly on the agent's total reinforcement history to bias habitual responses. In contrast, the orbitofrontal system is believed to rely on recent reinforcement information and forward-looking planning capacities to form its action preferences. Planning intersects with motivation in the selection and sequencing of instrumental desires. Let us now consider how PVLV might explain this kind of sequencing process.

4. SEQUENCES OF GOALS

In the next application of the reinforcement learning framework, I want to consider how instrumental desires could be sequenced so that a feeder will be able to serially route them to a comparator for motor correction. In this section, we consider how phasic dopamine could affect active maintenance (i.e., working memory) by acting on midbrain dopamine targets. Motivation continuously affects behavior through desires. Thus, one would expect there to be an active maintenance mechanism to sustain desires.

Generally speaking, "active maintenance" refers to the capacity to hold online a piece of information. The capacity is fairly mundane. For example, when I wave to you from across the street and a bus passes between us, I don't wonder where you went. I actively maintain a representation of your location based on the immediately preceding perceptual experience. When the bus passes and I see you on the other side, things are as I expect them to be because I didn't forget you were over there. Our brains can actively maintain what our senses take in.

In an application of the PVLV framework, O'Reilly and Frank (2006) built a neural network whose output layers fed back into their input layers—what is known as a recurrent network. Thus, when a signal was sent to the network by an external system, the signal could be maintained by the network resending the signal to itself. In the model, recurrent networks were strung together in series to create a system capable of maintaining a sequence of signals. Gating functions were then built into the recurrent networks. These functions enabled each network either to admit a new signal for active maintenance or to be shielded from potentially distracting signals.

The challenge for the model designers was to create a system capable of learning the right time to open and close the gates to approximate human performance in sequential working memory tasks. The testbed for the model was a task called the 1-2-AX task. In the 1-2-AX task, symbols are presented one after another. As the symbols are presented, the subject's goal is to identify target sequences and ignore distracters.

In the task, there are two target sequences, one of them being 1-A-X, the other 2-B-Y. The onset of a "1" signals the beginning of a new trial for the 1-A-X string, "2" for the 2-B-Y string. The strings can be intermingled, for example, 1-A-2-B-X-Y, in which case the subject should signal (with a button press) 1-A-X at the presentation of X and 2-B-Y at the presentation of Y. The challenge for the task subject is to ignore intervening stimuli while keeping track of the beginning and end of a sequence. For example, one might encounter a sequence like 1-A-C-4-X, in which 1-A-X should be signaled at the presentation of the X.

In the task, the order of stimuli matters. If you don't pay attention to the order of the stimuli, you'll fail. If you do, you might succeed. Thus, success in the model is treated as a reward signal and failure is treated as an omission of reward.

When training simulations begin, the PVLV system is not "informed" of the task directions. The gating operation works randomly, until the PVLV system discovers the rules by trial and error. Thus, the system must learn when to open and close working memory buffers to know when to signal that a target sequence has been presented.

The model has two button-press responses: one button to signal detection of a complete target sequence, another to signal that a target sequence has not been completed. The signal that opens the buffer is called a Go signal; the signal that keeps the buffer shut is called a NoGo signal.

The model decomposes into an Actor-Critic architecture, the Actor being the network that sends the Go and NoGo signals, and the Critic being a structure that biases and reinforces Actor responses. The valuation mechanism learns to associate buffer contents and a button press with a quantity of reward return, using the PVLV formulae for producing the δ-signal.

In the model, there are separate recurrent networks for each moment in the task. One can think of these moments as instants at which a stimulus can be captured by working memory and held in active maintenance. Because there is a limit to how many stimuli one can hold in working memory, there is nothing particularly artificial about limiting the number of these networks.

A sequence of stimuli will be captured by the model in a series of simultaneously active recurrent networks. Thus, once the model has learned to maintain the sequence 1-A-X, the three component signals in the sequence will be simultaneously maintained in three adjacent recurrent networks. Of course, if the system is to learn to maintain the correct signal sequences and block the distractors, it must be designed to maintain stimulus signals in general for some duration. Initially all stimulus signals will receive limited maintenance with relatively rapid decay rates. So a C might be maintained briefly, though it is not part of any target sequence. However, when an X is gated into the correct recurrent network and when the correct button press is performed, a positive δ-signal might be received before that signal decays. When this occurs, a bias begins to form in favor of active maintenance for that signal in that network. Because the δ-signal tracks unpredicted predictors of reward, and the complete sequence predicts reward, the Critic will learn that not just X and a particular button press predict reward but that A-X and a correct button press predicts reward, and so on.

The upshot is that the system can use value proxies (stimulus sequences) to regiment its policy for gating signals into the buffer. So eventually, when a 1 comes in, its receipt by the valuation function will release a δ-signal biasing a Go response in the Actor, opening the buffer to 1. If the 1 is followed by a C, there will be no δ-signal, because the valuation function will not have assigned a positive reward value to that representation. However, if the C is followed by an A, the A will evoke a δ-signal because the sequence 1-A is associated with reward, and so on for the sequence 1-A-X. The result is that the system can learn which mnemonic actions are conducive to reward return and reward omission, which is the essence of planning. Now, let's take a look at the interpretation of the model with respect to neural mechanisms.

First, the δ-signal in the model is taken to represent phasic dopamine sent from the SNc to dorsal and ventral components of the striatum. The dorsal striatum corresponds to the Actor; the ventral striatum corresponds to the valuation function. The source of reward signals is taken to be the hypothalamus.

When the SNc sends phasic dopamine to the dorsal striatum, dopamine molecules then bind with D1 and D2 receptors. The action of dopamine at D1 receptors facilitates Go signaling, and on D2 receptors suppresses NoGo signaling via the direct and indirect pathways of the basal ganglia (see figure 15.6).

In their discussion of the dopamine signal, O'Reilly and Frank propose a localization of the components of the PV and LV systems. Recall that both systems have

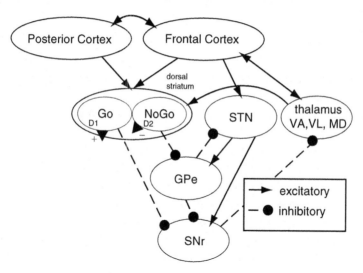

Figure 15.6. The direct and indirect pathways in working memory. The dorsal striatum composes the Actor, which receives signals from the Critic (not shown) at D1 and D2 dopamine receptors. The NoGo pool of cells feeds into the indirect pathway, and the Go pool feeds into the direct pathway. The working memory buffers on which O'Reilly and Frank focus are located in the frontal cortex. Sensor signals come in through the posterior cortex. STN = subthalamic nucleus; GPe = external globus pallidus; SNr = substantia nigra pars reticulata; in the thalamus: VA = ventral anterior, VL = ventrolateral, MD = mediodorsal. Compliments of O'Reilly and Frank (2006).

a reward function and a valuation function. The reward function in the PV system is assigned to the lateral hypothalamus, and the corresponding valuation function is assigned to the ventral striatum. The reward function in the LV system is assigned to the central nucleus of the amygdala, and the corresponding valuation function is again found in the ventral striatum. Thus, the system that O'Reilly and Frank describe does not include the orbitofrontal cortex (see Frank and Claus, 2006, for more on orbitofrontal cortex). However, there is no reason we cannot speculate that in the case of sequencing items in working memory that the orbitofrontal cortex and the ventral striatum might compete with each other for control of the Critic, just as they are believed to compete in the selection of planned and habitual actions.

Based on physiological evidence, O'Reilly and Frank estimate that prefrontal cortex holds approximately 4,000 buffers of the sort depicted in their model. They call the systems containing these buffers *stripes* and note that evidence supports the existence of stripes in posterior cortex as well. In the model, each cortical stripe involved in a working memory task gets a corresponding stripe in the dorsal striatum. The stripes in the dorsal striatum consist of networks of Go and NoGo cells. As information comes in, instrumental to selecting an action conducive to reward, each stripe can be either updated or shielded from distracters by the gating mechanism (i.e., the Go/NoGo stripes). Once the complete signal sequence is in place, the instrumental response can then be taken.

To support the case that the kind of mechanism O'Reilly and Frank describe might also underlie the adoption of sequences of instrumental desires, it would help if we could narrow down the location of the relevant stripes in prefrontal cortex. Perhaps the most promising locus is dorsolateral prefrontal cortex. In functional neuroimaging experiments, this region of prefrontal cortex is preferentially activated in tasks that require subjects to prepare sequential movements (Pochon et al., 2001). In cell recording experiments, it has been found that cell activity in this region correlates with sequences of target stimuli in delayed match-to-sample tasks (Funahashi, Inoue, and Kubota, 1997). Most important, it has also been shown that cells in dorsolateral prefrontal cortex will encode the expected reward value of reaching to represented targets (Wallis, 2007).

O'Reilly and Frank's model shows how the phasic dopamine signal could function in a mechanism that causes us to hold in mind sequences of stimuli and might thereby provide a starting place for thinking about how phasic dopamine could enable us to arrange instrumental desires in planning. If an Actor-Critic system could learn to base a one-step action (button press) on a sequence of representations held online, then perhaps the same sort of system could learn to base a multi-step action on each representation in the sequence, once the total sequence has become associated with reward. Each representation in the sequence could then be passed on to a motor planning system and fit into a motor plan.

Taking these ideas seriously raises an important question: How do we relate the operations of a feeder, plugging setpoints into a comparator, to sequences of desires affecting motor planning? There are at least two ways suggested in the literature. One of them is through the disinhibition of prepotent motor plans (see Schroeder, 2004). If a motor plan is already primed and ready to go, then in the same manner the Critic disinhibits a gating mechanism to open a working memory buffer, the Critic might be able to unleash the relevant primed motor program. The other way we can relate the two operations is through the online correction of behavior. If the learned instrumental desires are fed to a distinct motor control comparator (not the Critic) that improves the accuracy of the specific movements performed in the execution of a motor plan. In the next two sections, we consider these operations in detail.

5. Routing Instrumental Desires

Dopamine is important for sequencing representations in working memory, but it is also important for engaging in sequential actions. In this next application of the reinforcement learning framework, we consider how a sequence of instrumental desires, held in active maintenance, could be fed to motor control mechanisms. Toward that end, I review the work of James Houk and colleagues (2007), which suggests that the principles of sequential action selection are importantly similar to those of sequential working memory. To support the notion that prefrontal cortex sends value proxies to action planning mechanisms, I review work from Richard Andersen's lab.

To study sequential action selection, Houk et al. used fMRI to image subjects performing the Replicate task. In this task, subjects are presented with a sequence of targets on a grid. Subjects must remember the sequence for a delay period, and then use a joystick to move a cursor to each target location in sequence. Like the 1-2-AX task, subjects must encode and maintain perceptual information. Unlike the 1-2-AX task, there are no distracters, and the response to the sequence is itself sequential.

A control task, called Chase, was used to extract the activation related to the Replicate task from fMR images. In Chase, subjects are presented with a sequence of targets but are directed to track each target with the joystick as the target appears. In Chase, it is assumed that subjects will maintain the target signals, thereby eliminating the working memory component. More fine-grained contrasts were created to tease out the motor execution phase of the task and the decoding phase of the task (see Houk et al., 2007, for details).

Because it is widely believed that action selection occurs in the striatum, special attention was given to imaging striatal components. As mentioned in section 4, the striatum can be divided into dorsal and ventral components. These components further subdivide. For example, dorsal striatum components can be separated into medial nuclei (caudate) and lateral components (putamen). During the execution phase, a significant increase in activation was found in the putamen, and during the decoding phase, a significant decrease in activity was found in the caudate nucleus.

Cellular studies reveal that caudate neurons have inhibitory connections with one another. Houk and colleagues interpreted the deactivation results to mean that substantial presynaptic inhibitory activity had occurred in the caudate. This local inhibition results in only select neurons in the caudate being able to influence caudate target cells. The caudate nucleus is part of a synaptic loop running through M1, the cortical gateway to the spinal cord, and back into the basal ganglia. Thus, the deactivation results suggest that during the task, caudate cells competed to influence Go signaling in M1.

The putamen is part of a synaptic loop that runs through the working memory networks of prefrontal cortex. Putamen output is believed to drive the disinhibition signal (i.e., the Go signal) described by O'Reilly and Frank. So naturally, increased activation in the putamen during the execution phase would suggest that active maintenance gates are being opened in working memory buffers. Opening the gate to a working memory buffer not only lets a new representation into the buffer, it also lets a maintained representation out. Thus, we should expect that during the execution phase, subgoal representations held in working memory then feed into a target network that can influence M1.

Here is the basic picture of action selection up to this point: (1) The putamen controls a gate on working memory buffers in prefrontal cortex; (2) the working memory buffers hold sequences of desire representations in active maintenance; (3) when the feeder acts on a maintained sequence, desires can be fed to a motor control network; (4) the motor control network associates each desire with a set of motor commands—a motor plan; and (5) the caudate disinhibits one of these motor plans at M1. As in the O'Reilly and Frank model, dopamine biases disinhibition of reward-associated representations and motor plans. But where, one might wonder, is the association between desire representations and motor plans made? Evidence from Andersen's lab suggests that components of that network are in the posterior parietal cortex.

The posterior parietal cortex is known to be important for visuomotor planning and performance. This region of the brain is sometimes called the "where" or "how" pathway, because it encodes visual information in egocentric frames of reference specifically for action. Researchers believe this region to be involved in motor planning, because its components encode, for example, in reaching with one's arm, both the target of the reach and the initial position of the hand before the reach begins (Andersen and Buneo, 2002). This region is known to be important for performance, because damage restricted to portions of it can selectively disrupt adaptive interaction with objects.[3]

Posterior parietal cortex both sends and receives projections from prefrontal cortex (Chafee and Goldman-Rakic, 2000; Fuster, 2001). Thus, the posterior parietal cortex can receive the representations held in active maintenance in sequence as a series of performance targets. Predicting from a representation of the target the motor commands that, for example, will bring the hand to touch the target, the posterior parietal cortex and prefrontal cortex can collaborate in the formation of motor plans. One piece of evidence to suggest that learned value systems are involved in this process comes out of research directed at the development of brain–machine interfaces (BMIs). Functioning BMIs—communication channels between brain cells and prosthetic devices—can be found on at least four campuses in the United States. Some BMIs decode motor control signals for arm movements from activity in motor and premotor areas to drive a computer display cursor in a pointing task (Taylor, Tillery, and Schwartz, 2002). Others extract a variety of motor parameters (i.e., hand position, velocity, gripping force, and the electromyograms of multiple arm muscles) from the electrical activity of frontoparietal neuronal ensembles and use these to drive a robot arm (Carmena et al., 2003). BMI research tends to focus on motor commands, leaving closed the black box of cognitive states that often cause such commands. Recently, an effort has been made to uncover goal-related signals.

To determine the goal of a monkey's reaching actions, Musallam, Corneil, Greger, Scherberger, and Andersen (2004) took recordings from part of the posterior parietal cortex they call the parietal reaching region (PRR). The PRR includes Brodmann area 7a, medial intraparietal cortex (MIP), and the dorsal portion of the parieto-occipital (PO) area (Andersen and Buneo, 2002, pp. 189–220). Though it is well established that all three of these areas are reach-related, area 7a is a predominantly visual area, and evidence speaks to MIP and PO supporting visual representations as well (Klam and Graf, 2003; Musallum et al., 2004). The experimental set-up was as follows.

Three monkeys were trained on a memory task that required them to interact with a touch-sensitive video screen. A green icon would appear at the center of the screen. The monkeys would touch this icon and look at a red fixation point also on the screen. Then, 500 ms later, a peripheral target would flash for 300 ms. A memory period then ensued, lasting between 1,200 and 1,800 ms. At the end of the memory period, the green icon would disappear. This served as a "go" cue for the monkeys to touch the location where the target had been. The monkeys were rewarded only if they touched the target area at the end of the memory period, and if their gaze did not stray from within an angular threshold of the red fixation point. If they touched the target area before the go signal, they received no reward.

Once activity from the PRR could be used to predict where on the screen monkeys would reach (the reach control task), the monkeys were trained in a new task (the brain control task). The brain control task differed from the reach control task in the action the monkeys were to perform. During the memory period, activity in the PRR was decoded to predict where the monkey would move its arm. Monkeys were no longer rewarded for reaching after the memory period. Instead, 200 ms after the target was extinguished, PRR activity was decoded. The decoding process took no more than 900 ms, and then a cursor was placed at the decoder's predicted location. If hand movement occurred or if the monkey's eyes strayed too far from the red fixation point, the trial stopped. If the decoder predicted the wrong location on the screen, the green icon was extinguished, cuing the monkeys to reach for the area where the target had been.

An important result of the experiment was that PRR activity could be dissociated from motor activity. During brain control, the characteristic motor bursts in recorded cells were absent in successfully decoded cells. The goal-related signal was present when the monkeys withheld movement and present when the monkeys could not see their hands.

It would appear that Musallum and colleagues uncovered sensory representations of desired reach goals. But they also demonstrated that spike trains in the PRR carry preference information. Musallum et al. (2004) ran a variant of the memory task in a different series of experiments, where the size of the go cue was varied to indicate the amount, probability, or type of reward that monkeys would receive on successfully completing a trial (p. 260). The task described in the previous section used juice rewards to motivate performance. In the variant task, rewards could vary between orange juice and water. Sometimes monkeys would be rewarded and sometimes not. The quantity of reward varied as well. But only one of these three aspects (type, probability, and amount of reward) was varied in a session. Reach control and brain control were used as before.

When the go cue indicated that the monkey would receive its preferred reward, PRR responses became more precise—they increased their tuning or mean rate of firing in response to their preferred spatial location. When the probability of receiving a reward was high, or when the amount of reward was large, tuning also increased. This change resulted in an overall improvement in successful decoding of 12.2 percent during the brain control segment.

The upshot is that expected reward value is encoded in the same neurons that encode the visual representation of the spatial location for reach. The strength of the response in PRR neurons varies with the predicted reward value of the reach-destination. Like value proxies, the goal representations described by Musallum et al. vary in magnitude, contingent on expected rewards, and can be dissociated from activity in motor areas. The representations in the PRR can be sustained without triggering action, thus they can be held online to serve as setpoints for a model-driven control system.

6. Online Correction

The reinforcement learning framework can be applied to the problem of explaining how the brain uses goals to select subgoals and actions. Dopamine can drive the selection of instrumental desires by updating valuation functions in working memory networks. Dopamine can facilitate action selection by disinhibiting Actor networks. But these are not the only ways the reinforcement learning framework can be applied to understanding a motivational state's directional capacity. Another way is in terms of online action correction.

By "action correction," I mean the processes leading to an adjustment of one's intended movements while movement is under way. For example, suppose that you are boxing an opponent who is slipping your strikes. You know what your goal is: to hit your opponent in the head. You also know how you're going to do it: You're going to time his head movements and throw a left cross when he comes up. But your opponent is not stationary. You throw the punch and find that your opponent's head is slightly lower than you expected. In the midst of your punch, you adjust your angle and connect.

During action correction, the goal for the movement is known. The ballpark form of the movement plan is decided. The movement is under way, but in the midst of executing the plan, revisions may occur. Adjustments, called corrective submovements, will be made (Houk et al., 2007). These corrective submovements will require motor commands to diverge from the initial motor plan. Our capacity to engage in corrective submovements suggests that the value proxies fed to the posterior parietal cortex can serve as setpoints for correcting motor plans.

To study the neural basis of corrective submovements, Fishbach, Roy, Bastianen, Miller, and Houk (2007) took electrophysiological measurements from monkeys performing a step-tracking task. To perform the task, a monkey is trained to use a rotating handle to move a cursor horizontally across a computer screen. The handle was equipped with sensors that tracked the position and angular velocity of the handle. At the beginning of a trial, a box-shaped target occurred randomly at one of three possible target locations (left, center, right). The monkey would rotate the handle to place the cursor on the target, and then the target would extinguish and another would appear at one of the two remaining locations. The monkey had unlimited time to move the cursor to the location of the new target.

On two-thirds of the trials, the second target was perturbed. Perturbation of the target amounted to an abrupt shift of the target once the monkey had started rotating the handle. The handle was low-friction, so a quick corrective submovement could ensure that the cursor lined up with the target.

To study neural mechanisms of corrective submovements, electrodes were inserted into cells in M1 and the internal globus pallidus (GPi) that project to M1. The globus pallidus is part of a pathway from the basal ganglia that inhibits motor neurons in M1 (i.e., the indirect pathway). So pauses in GPi cell activity should be correlated with spikes in M1 cell activity if the GPi is part of the action selection mechanism for corrective submovements. That is what Fishbach and colleagues found.

The electrophysiological recordings support the idea that the selection of corrective submovements relies on the kind of disinhibition mechanism operative in the other functions discussed. But these recordings do not locate the correction process itself. To relate the activity in the GPi and M1 to a correction process, we need to find a causal pathway to a good candidate corrective mechanism.

For a number of reasons, the most promising candidate for such a mechanism can be found in the cerebellum. Lesion experiments suggest that the cerebellum is involved in predictive feedback control of movements. For example, damage to the cerebellum preserves the capacity to make goal-directed (though shaky) reaching movements in the presence of visual feedback (Ito, 2006). But if the eyes are closed, patients lose the capacity to make such movements accurately (e.g., one will have difficulty touching one's nose with one's eyes closed). Electrophysiological recordings demonstrate that cells in the cerebellum encode visual, auditory, vestibular, and somatosensory information. In particular, somatosensory information is encoded in a fractured somatotopy, where patches of the cerebellum code for neighboring patches of the subjects body (Ito, 2006). Presently, it is believed that the cerebellum contains internal models of sensory feedback whose predictions can be evoked by motor commands. Roughly, when motor cortex generates a motor command, it is believed that a copy of that signal (an efference copy) is sent to the cerebellum. Internal models in the cerebellum use the efference copy to predict the sensory feedback that should follow that motor command and enable the motor cortex to correct its next output if the predicted outcome diverges from the target (i.e., the setpoint).

Looking at the action selection and correction mechanism's components in total, we can see that the system is highly distributed. Desire representations are sent from the prefrontal cortex to the posterior parietal cortex. M1 receives projections from posterior parietal targets, the cerebellum, and the subcortical loops in which these sites are embedded. Thus, when the posterior parietal cortex receives value proxies and is thereby enabled to identify action targets, signals can be sent to the motor cortex and the cerebellum to program a sequence of motor commands. Dopamine, acting on dorsal striatum targets, can then disinhibit one of these motor programs.

Returning to the boxing example, if your opponent's head moves, then your setpoint has moved.[4] Because you're in the midst of throwing a punch, somehow you are going to have to adjust the movement in progress to match the new setpoint. The basic idea here is that the cerebellum will predict what additional motor command signals will be needed to redirect your hand trajectory, and then tells the motor cortex to use the new signals. The predicted result of following the cerebellum's suggestion can be checked against the value proxy to make sure that the prefrontal and posterior cortical systems are in agreement. If they are, then the corrective submovement's motor commands will be approved and the basal ganglia will disinhibit them.

To sum up, we can see predictive feedback control at work in at least three locations in motivated behavior: (1) in the selection of instrumental desires, (2) in the selection of motor plans, and (3) in the correction of selected motor plans. This concludes the discussion of motivation's directional capacity and leaves us to attend to motivation's drive capacity. To get the discussion of drive under way, it will help to consider the conditions that account for a motivation mechanism's activation and strength. We begin with a discussion of the activation and deactivation of a motivation mechanism. In section 8, we turn to a discussion of the means by which an activated motivation mechanism shows its strength when it summons the energetic resources that account for vigorous action.

7. Turning It On and Off

Desires turn on and turn off. They compete with each other and when they win, they control our focus and direct our actions. How might we understand these processes in causal terms? It will help to introduce a bit of vocabulary.

Let us call the conditions that activate, strengthen and weaken desire the volume control, or the d-volume for short. Think of the control dial on a stereo that when turned clockwise both activates the stereo and increases the volume. The d-volume is what is responsible for a desire becoming occurrent. In a negative feedback system, a difference between setpoint and feedback will turn on the system and simultaneously turn up the volume. Behavior will be directed at turning the volume down and off. In a positive feedback system, imagine the volume having a slightly different design.[5] Thus, the satiety conditions on desires, those conditions that both satisfy and deactivate a desire, are specified by the desire's d-volume. The representations determining the off positions in d-volumes therefore constitute the conditions that unplug desires from motor planning systems. What is it that's turned on and off by d-volumes?

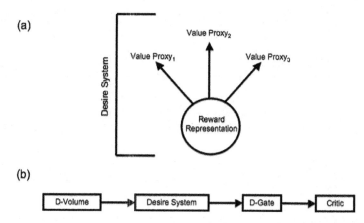

Figure 15.7. A desire system. (a) A desire system consists of a primary reward system, which defines the reward function, and value proxies, which can substitute as rewards when fed into the reward function. A set of primary reward representations forms the core of an intrinsic desire mechanism, and value proxy representations form the core of an instrumental desire mechanism. (b) The d-volume controls activation in the desire system. The d-gate accounts for the desire system's relative influence on the Critic—the structure through which the desire system influences cognitive and motor systems.

I think a good first guess is that a d-volume will operate on the components of a desire system, comprised of reward representations and associated value proxies. Turning up the d-volume or turning it off should then result in the activation and deactivation of representations that feed into PVLV systems. Thus, a d-volume simultaneously affects mechanisms of intrinsic and instrumental desire (see figure 15.7a).

Common sense tells us that some desires are intensified by deprivation of the desired stimulus, whereas others are intensified by the imposition of an aversive stimulus. When my stomach empties, I become hungry (in perhaps overly simple terms). The hunger increases as I continue to go unfed. So we should expect that some d-volumes will be turned up by a specific deprivation condition and turned down or off with stimulation of the same category.

Other d-volumes will be turned on as the result of an imposition and turned down or off with the imposition's removal. For example, the load of a bully planting his knee on my chest will motivate me to escape. In this case, it is not the absence of a stimulus (such as food) driving me to action. Rather, something directly pushing on me intensifies my motivation. Thus, in the way desires sort into appetites and aversions, motivation correspondingly divides into the appetitive (stimulated by deprivation) and the aversive (stimulated by imposition).

Notably, many of the paradigmatic motivational states are recurrent, which is not surprising given our various routines. Hunger recurs. The need for social interaction recurs. Sex drive recurs. These motivational states have a rhythm that to a large extent seems to depend on the rhythms within us, some of which are hormonal. Others, such as the motivation to avoid a harsh light, appear to be driven by environmental circumstances. Some motivational states have a rhythm set by the environment. Still other motivational states will occur only once (e.g., in my case, the motivation to skydive).

The basis of hunger's rhythm is not too difficult to follow. When the stomach empties, it contracts, and the stores of fat and sugar it held are broken down and transported elsewhere. Through stretch receptors and fat receptors, and hormonal receptors in other places, food deprivation can be sensed. The structure of the stomach and associated receptor systems helps us understand how going without food can turn on a hunger mechanism. Time elapses, the stomach drains, and you feel that something is missing. You eat again, and the rhythm is set.

Like hunger, social needs can be activated by deprivation. For example, when someone who is not lonely is placed in an empty cell, changing none of the contents of the cell, it will only take time for him or her to become lonely. It is not some occurrence going on outside that renders the confined person lonely. Rather, it is something *not* going on outside—a persistent absence—that turns up the d-volume. How does one perceive the absence?

Social needs obviously have no stomach, so what we need is a functionally comparable detection mechanism. We need something to clock the time one spends alone in the way that digestion (and the decline of blood glucose and hormones) clocks the time since the last feeding. What we need is an internal timer, connected to the social need's d-volume, so that when the timer approaches some temporal threshold, the volume will turn up.

We should allow this kind of timer to be reset in the manner that hunger's rhythm can be reset when we break with our routines (e.g., by eating snacks when you're not supposed to). Being reset, the timer will in turn reduce (or turn off) the respective d-volume, thereby deactivating the desire system. For an example of what I have in mind, imagine that you unexpectedly have to deal with people all day at work. Though you weren't seeking company at the time, you found lots of it. At the end of the day, unlike other days, you may have no desire for conversation. You've been talking all day and now would like some solitude. "Sorry, honey," you say to your spouse. "I just need to be alone." (Then your spouse forces you to sleep on the couch for that night.)

Now imagine that the number of people you must deal with varies from day to day, and at various times of day, you find yourself engaged in more or less interaction. In such an environment, we would expect the timer on your social need to be haphazardly reset. Thus, if the social environment is haphazard and lacking in periodicity, the environment will obscure the periodicity of the corresponding form of motivation. But if the agent is capable of imposing periodicity on its habitat, the clocks within will be able to guide that sort of environmental engineering.

Some desire systems are on internal timers. But for motivation to be adaptive, desire systems must take turns. Turning a desire system on may put it in a position to here-and-now affect thought and behavior. But turning on a desire system does not by itself place that system in command of cognition and motor control. Since I know of no name for that which enables a desire to influence thought and behavior, let us call that thing the desire's d-gate (see figure 15.7b). To the extent that a desire has an effect on other capacities, we can say that it is more or less "gated." In terms of the Actor-Critic architecture, the d-gate will stand between a particular desire system and the Critic.

Because desires compete, we should expect desire systems to compete. Thus we should expect the opening and closing of one d-gate to depend on that of the others, which in turn depend on the volume settings of the various desire systems. It seems readily apparent that we can pursue more than one desire at a time. For example, I can simultaneously satisfy my desire to find a good place to work, have a good cup of coffee, and be close to a kickboxing gym by going to CyberJava in Hollywood. I can simultaneously satisfy my desire to have a quiet walk, find a trashcan, and get to campus by going through the park. However, I cannot simultaneously satisfy my desire to hike in the Rockies and throw neck kicks in Hollywood. The competition among my desires is one in which there can be more than one winner, but not one in which all can win at the same time. Thus there is a limited form of mutual inhibition among desire systems. In terms familiar to theoretical neuroscientists, we might say that the competition is a *k*-Winners-Take-All process, where what is *taken* is what lies on the other side of the d-gates for the *k* number of *winners*—that is, access to the Critic, which in turn facilitates control of planning and motor control capacities.

So desire systems get turned on and turned off. Their volume gets turned up and down. I have called the conditions responsible for these functions a desire system's d-volume. When one desire overpowers the others, or when a coalition of desires forms, the d-volume is turned up and a d-gate opens. Thus a desire system (perhaps in orbitofrontal cortex) can then influence a Critic (e.g., the VTA). What is the d-volume and how does d-gating happen? I only offer a brief gesture toward an answer.

Just to start, we might make the observation that many nervous systems, including human nervous systems, contain intrinsically bursting cells. The textbook pyramidal neuron is a cell that emits a spike train only when its membrane potential has crossed a voltage threshold. The cells I am speaking of are quite different. Intrinsically bursting cells are neurons that emit brief high-frequency spike trains periodically, when the surrounding extracellular environment is held constant. What is interesting about these cells is that they *drive themselves* across the voltage threshold (hence, they are *intrinsically* bursting).

Other kinds of cells exhibit a conditional form of rhythmicity. For example, in a portion of the hypothalamus called the arcuate nucleus, cells have been found that oscillate when bound with orexin, an agent associated with hunger (van den Top, Lee, K., Whyment, Blanks, and Spanswick, 2004). One exposure to orexin is sufficient to induce periodic bursting potentials in these cells on the order of 30 minutes. When exposed to leptin, a hormone associated with satiation, these conditional pacemaker cells cease activity. Orexin application can then be used to restore periodic behavior. Thus, we have an example what looks like an internal timer, regulating the hunger system.

Though we focus on hunger in this example, I think there is a suggestion of what resources might be available to handle the nonhunger cases. Slow oscillation occurs in VTA cells. But this oscillation appears to depend on forebrain input (Shi, 2005). Knowing that the VTA receives substantial inputs from orbitofrontal cortex, we should expect to find either intrinsic or conditionally rhythmic cells indigenous to that region.

Of course, for rhythmic cells to work as timers on desire systems, there must be something that can accumulate their output. Applied to the control of d-volumes, if a team of intrinsically bursting and conditionally rhythmic cells can come to fire in-phase with each other, they might be sufficient as a group to turn on a desire system and increase its volume until their entrainment is broken. Thus, if the deactivation condition is what disrupts entrainment in these teams, then perhaps we can explain the activation and deactivation of appetitive desire systems. Absence of reward will relieve the group of oscillating cells from disruption as they become increasingly entrained. Provision of reward will break the rhythm.

Perhaps impositions have a similar rhythmic mechanism, but rather than punishments reducing entrainment, we should expect them to facilitate it. Thus, perceiving an imposition (and stimuli predictive of an imposition) would increase excitation in an aversion system. Removal of punishment would then follow the removal of the imposition, with a successful anticipative response rendering an aversion inactive sooner. Of course, it is less obvious that recurrent aversive motivation is based on internal timers. But the hypothesis is worth exploring.

8. VIGOR AND GRADIENTS OF REWARD

Motivated runners run lots of laps. Motivated mice run in their wheels for many revolutions. Speed and repetition—these are signs of drive.

It is well established that dopamine depletion leads to sluggishness, whereas raising dopamine levels reestablishes vigorous action. On the basis of these observations and against the backdrop of the reinforcement learning framework, Niv, Joel, and Dayan (2005) proposed that tonic dopamine is responsible for energizing action. To draw the connection between tonic dopamine and motivation's energizing function, the authors looked for a reinforcement learning explanation of response rates.

In their account, the phasic dopamine response facilitates action selection, signaling error in predicted reward in the way we have discussed. But the phasic response is functionally quite different from the tonic response, which they believe signals the current average rate of net reward. Thus, the bursting dopamine signal biases the choice of action plans, and the sparse signal controls the rate of action performance.

The average rate of reward is calculated by averaging the phasic dopamine signal. Over time, the average error in predicted reward should equal the average reward rate, because the predictive error signal (LV_δ) should come to approximate rewards received, and the feedback error signal (PV_δ) should correct for inaccuracies in the predictive error signal. A net average rate of reward can then be calculated by subtracting costs, per unit of time, from the average rate of reward.

Once the net average rate of reward is known, this knowledge can be factored into a decision concerning which action to take and how fast to perform it. This decision is based on the opportunity cost of inactivity, which is a function of the net average rate of reward multiplied by the inverse of response latency for an action under consideration. Multiplying these two numbers allows you to compare how much reward you would expect to get from performing action a at latency l to how much reward you would expect to get from performing a at l'. If the average net rate of reward is high and you move slowly, you might end up forfeiting rewards that you would have gotten had you moved quicker. If the average net rate is low, then moving slower won't cost you as many opportunities for reward. According to the model, we should expect an optimal reinforcement learning system to choose latencies with the highest expected rate of reward returns. Thus, the mechanism of response rate selection (i.e., latency) will follow a gradient of rewards, working like a positive feedback control system.

Based on our discussion of dopamine's involvement in the striatum, we can relate Niv's model of drive to Go and NoGo signaling, allowing the availability of free-floating tonic dopamine to set a baseline for the facilitation of Go responses. Low tonic levels of dopamine should make it difficult to update working memory buffers, disinhibit motor plans, and learn new action-outcome contingencies. Phasic dopamine bursts should have a weaker effect on target cells without having the elevated tonic level to ride on (see figure 15.8). Thus, when representations make it into active maintenance, they will not be easy to get out, because NoGo responses (which keep the buffer gates closed) will be difficult to suppress.

Niv's model fits with recent speculation that the reason Parkinson sufferers have difficulty moving is because a trick has been played on their reward-learning systems. It is well known that Parkinson disease results from damage to dopaminergic structures. Aside from difficulty moving, symptoms of Parkinson include working memory deficits, which agrees with the model of working memory proposed by O'Reilly and Frank. But as we know from the discussion of the habit system,

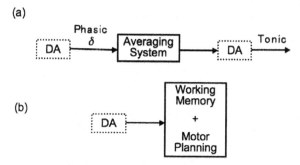

Figure 15.8. (a) Phasic dopamine updates the averaging system and thereby alters the rate of tonic release. (b) The combined dopamine responses (phasic and tonic) modulate working memory and motor planning.

working memory may not be needed to select actions. The habit system does not need dopamine to select actions, only to learn new actions. Thus, it might make sense to consider that dopamine depletion might indicate to the brain's reinforcement learning systems that moving is simply not worth it.

Or as Montague (2006) puts it, reduced dopamine levels might teach valuation functions that moving is only slightly more conducive to reward than stillness.

If this idea is correct, the reduced motivation suffered by Parkinson patients might be on the drive end, rather than the desire end of motivation mechanisms. Parkinson sufferers might have their motivation mechanisms activated, but those mechanisms may not be able to exert control over cognitive and motor systems. Wanting might be high, while drive is low. Is there any evidence for this hypothesis?

According to one psychiatric study, sufferers of Parkinson, without treatment, tend to report higher levels of hunger than those with treatment (Rosenberg, Herishanu, and Beilin, 1977). The study is small, so we cannot treat it as very weighty evidence, but dopamine-depleted animals showing reduced drive (in terms of response rates) also show increased appetite (Cousins, Wei, and Salamone, 1994). This suggests that a goal state can be represented in the brain without dopamine, but the goal's capacity to regulate and drive behavior requires dopamine. The upshot is that the story we tell about the activation of motivational states will likely require more than appeal to various causal roles played by dopamine (see Landreth, 2007).

Returning to the feedback conception of motivation with which this chapter began, we can see that Niv's model of tonic dopamine describes a positive feedback control system. The more you encounter signs that your desires will be satisfied, and the more often you experience pleasant surprises, the more driven you should be, according to the model. To some extent, this seems intuitive. Of course, we could imagine motionless people who are endlessly rewarded, and hardworking folk who never get anything they want. Do they exist? I don't know. I doubt it, but I may be in the grip of a theory.

Attending to more serious challenges for Niv's model, we must admit that there are also aversive sources of drive, such as fear. The terror felt by someone knowing that they have become quarry can generate extraordinary motivation to flee. It cannot be the promise of reward that generates this form of drive. Rather, it must be the promise of punishment's omission and the experience of relief that follows from successful escape. Punishments figure into response rate selection, too.[6]

9. NEURAL MECHANISMS AND THE PROATTITUDES

There has been a lot of discussion of desire in this chapter, and one might wonder how much of the meaning of the term as I've used it is merely stipulative and how much overlaps with our commonsense understanding of desire. One might also wonder what bearing the discussion of motivation I've offered has on more tradi-tional philosophical discussions, which focus on intentional action. In this section, I address some of these questions, focusing first on the theory of desire and then on the theory of intentional action.

In his book, *Three Face of Desire* (2004), Timothy Schroeder argues that our commonsense understanding of desire attributes to it three core capacities: (1) reward, (2) motivation, and (3) pleasure (see Landreth, 2006, for a more detailed review). Schroeder associates desire with reward, because knowledge of what people want can be used to instill habits in them. For example, if you know that a child wants a particular toy, you might promise to buy the toy if the child brushes her teeth twice a day for the next 3 weeks. The hope is that using the toy as leverage will make oral hygiene a habit.

Motivation is associated with desire for obvious reasons. If one wants Q and believes that doing A will provide Q, then unless other wants intervene, one will do A for the sake of Q. Desire, combined with means-end belief, motivates action.

Pleasures arise in us, by and large, when we get what we want—displeasure when we don't, or when something happens that we wanted *not* to happen. If I want to please you, then I should figure out what you want and give it to you. If I really want to please you, I should give you something better than what you expected.

In Schroeder's view, reward is the essence of desire, and by this he means that the mechanisms of motivation and pleasure asymmetrically depend on the mecha-nism of reward. Schroeder takes the mechanism of reward to be the neural systems I have described in this chapter. Thinking of desire in Schroeder's terms, as the mechanism of reward, enables us to account for the nature of intrinsic desire as the determinant of the instrumental desires we will form, relying on PV and LV systems.[7] If reward is the essence of desire, then the perception of stimuli as rewards should be essential to motivation and pleasure. I have argued at length here that reward processing is fundamental to motivation. Pleasure is another matter, but it is worth mentioning that substantial evidence suggests the involvement of orbitof-rontal cortex in pleasant and unpleasant experience (see Rolls, 2005). Thus, it would seem that Schroeder's account of desire is on track (though see Landreth, 2007, for a critique of the details of Schroeder's account of pleasure).

It should not be too difficult to understand how one might relate desire as I have used to the term to our commonsense understanding of desire. What about intention?

Typically we think of motivated behavior as intentional behavior. If you were motivated to do A, then it is likely that you did A on purpose. Of late, it has become popular to regard an intention as a plan that one is settled on carrying to fruition. In Alfred Mele's (1992, 2002) terms, an intention is an executive attitude toward a plan. When one intends to A, one has decided to do A—hence, one has taken an execu-tive attitude toward A. If one is to do A intentionally, then the doing of A must be guided by one's reasons. One of these reasons is the goal for which the performance of A is instrumental. For example, I might intend to make a sandwich so as to eat the sandwich. Other reasons can be found in the plan for accomplishing the goal, for example, the plan for making a sandwich, which can be part of a plan for eating a sandwich. Thus, intention is an executive attitude toward a plan.

In taking intention to be an executive attitude toward a plan, Mele and others do not mean to suggest that intentions all involve well-formed plans (see Bratman, 1987). For example, I might intend to visit the Great Wall of China someday without having any step-by-step, worked-out plan for satisfying that intention. But failing to have a worked-out plan is not failing to have any plan at all. When I intend to visit the Great Wall, I at least plan on achieving the goal of visiting it. Forming the intention, I have decided that I have a goal and am settled on pursuing it. My plan has a basic goal. Later, through a planning process, it may come to include many subgoals.

Based on the discussion in section 1, we should expect the goals of intentional actions to be set by setpoints in motivational mechanisms. Once a decision to pursue the goal has occurred, retrieval and planning mechanisms can be governed by that setpoint until a subjectively suitable means for achieving the setpoint has been uncovered. Thus the feedback control conception of motivation intersects with Mele's conception of intentions in the formation and execution of plans.

The feedback control conception of motivation is not foreign to philosophical discussions of intention and intentional action. Harry Frankfurt (1978), under the influence of Ernest Nagel (1977), was one of the earliest advocates of this sort of view, arguing that intentional actions must be amenable to corrective guidance when they depart from their intended course.[8] Later work by John Searle (1983) proposed a distinct kind of intention, called intention-in-action, to capture the sense that intentional actions are under guidance on a moment-to-moment basis. In more recent work, Marc Jeannerod (1997) formulated a theory of motor intentions meant to account for the goal-directedness of the specific movements instrumental to the attainment of more fundamental goals.

Not all intentions are of the sort to guide action on a moment-to-moment basis. An intention can be formed in the present to perform an action well in the future. As Bratman (1987) notes, this kind of future-directed intention is capable of initiating and directing planning processes, as well as determining when a planning process should be terminated. Having settled on the goal of planning a trip to the Amazon, I might then search widely through tourist guides and discuss with travel agents all that I want to see and do on my trip. The intention to go on the trip initiates this planning process and incorporates into itself the results of the process. As I plan the trip, my basic goal becomes progressively more distinct. I make reservations for transportation, shelter, and food, and as I make the arrangements it becomes clear to me that I want more leisure than adventure from this experience. With the resulting higher resolution goal, I can then determine when I have accumulated enough subplans that I may stop the planning process.

If I can expect my plan to work, then I can call planning to a stop until it is time to execute the plan. When finished, my trip is planned, guided by intention. But this intention is not directed at a goal for present action; rather, it is directed at a goal for future action—for traveling perhaps several months from now. For several months,

I may intend to go to the Amazon without doing anything Amazon-related. I have a plan of action that I will be ready to execute at a later time.

Taking the various distinctions among intention-types mentioned, Elizabeth Pacherie (2006) has proposed a dynamic theory of intentions involving interactions among future-directed intentions (F-Intentions), present-directed intentions (P-Intentions), and motor intentions (M-Intentions) (see figure 15.9). An F-Intention involves a decision to pursue a goal in the future, which may induce a process of planning as described. The plan can then be stored and later retrieved for execution. A P-Intention involves a decision to presently execute an F-Intention's plan or to formulate and execute a new plan presently. In either case, a P-Intention will adapt instrumental knowledge to the unforeseen demands of the current context. An M-Intention receives the various subgoals set by the P-Intention, transforms them into goals for specific bodily movements, and then selects the motor plans best suited to achieve those movement goals. Thus, in some cases, forming an F-Intention leads later to forming a P-Intention, which then leads to forming M-Intentions. But P-Intentions can be formed without the need of F-Intentions.

Each of the kinds of intention described by Pacherie is a negative feedback process, whose products are plans and actions. Each process is initiated by a decision to pursue a particular goal or subgoal. Each goal or subgoal chosen then provides a setpoint for the formation and execution of plans. Once the distance between the goal state and the perceived or predicted state of the controlled system is minimized, the process is terminated. Thus, in forming and elaborating my F-Intention,

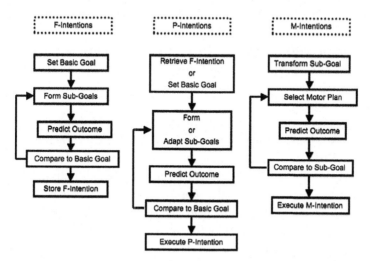

Figure 15.9. Three kinds of intention (my portrayal). The process of forming each kind of intention first involves the selection of a basic goal or a subgoal to be pursued. Planning takes place in the F- and P-stages when subgoals are formed. Planning takes place in the M-stage by taking the various subgoals and sequencing the motor commands that could achieve those subgoals. Each kind of intention involves a planning process based on feedback control.

I revise and elaborate a plan. In the process of revision and elaboration, I attempt to minimize the distance between the predicted result of following my plan and the desired result. When I find a result that satisfices, I can then stop planning for the trip. In forming and elaborating my P-Intention for the trip, I work to minimize the distance between the present state of the trip and my goals and subgoals for that stage of the trip. In my M-Intentions, systems within me work to minimize the distance between target movements and the actual movement that I take, such as hiking without stumbling, casting a fishing rod without losing my grip, or following a pink Amazonian river dolphin with my gaze.

Pacherie's dynamic theory of intentions is helpful for understanding each segment of a motivational process consisting of the various types of intention. In many cases, a P-Intention will be formed without reference to an F-Intention.[9] For example, I might presently, at 5:30 P.M., form the intention of casting my fishing line without having in the past (e.g., 2:30 P.M.) planned on taking that action. Having formed this P-Intention, the content of the intention can now interact with motor planning systems to satisfy the P-Intention's basic goal, such as catching a piranha.

In the interaction between P-Intentions and M-Intentions, the content of the intentions will change. For example, now P-Intending to catch a piranha, I might intend to cast left, and thereby form and hold in inhibition a motor plan for casting left. But if I see someone else catch a piranha to my right, I might shift to the subgoal of casting in that direction. As these subgoals change in my P-Intention's plan, a new goal for my muscles will have to be formed—a different motor plan will have to be selected. The instrumental content of the intentions will change, but the basic goal remains the same. Thus, we should expect P-Intentions and M-Intentions to participate in interacting feedback loops. The feedback loops underlying simple instrumental actions (M-Intentions) will be embedded in a larger feedback mechanism (a P-Intention). The setpoints sent in sequence to motor planning mechanisms will be transformations on the basic goal and subgoals found in the P-Intention. Thus, one goal (e.g., to catch a piranha) will regulate the variety of movements performed to satisfy that goal.

In her discussion of planning, Pacherie suggests that internal models might form the doxastic basis for planning activity. As mentioned earlier, internal models mimic the effects that various stimuli (or stimulus contexts) have on the nervous system. Thus, a controller can interface with internal models and thereby anticipate feedback that will come through the senses, when a given course of action is followed. In the execution of a motor plan, internal models can help motor control systems overcome feedback delays. In the formation of a motor plan, internal models can be used in the simulation of actions and outcomes (see figure 15.10).

Internal models come in two varieties: forward models and inverse models. Forward models make predictions that roughly go forward in the temporal order of events. Inverse models make predictions that go backward. So if you want to know what will happen next if you find yourself doing A, consult a forward model. If you want to know what most likely happened immediately preceding A, consult an inverse model. The value of an inverse model is that although you may have a solid

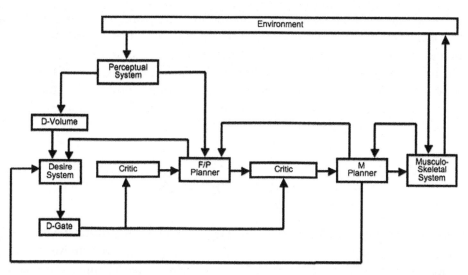

Figure 15.10. Hierarchical structure of a motivational control system. The perceptual system may affect the setpoint (determined by the "off" position in the d-volume). The setpoint is the basic goal of the motivational state. The d-gate determines whether the comparator controlling the F/P-Planner will receive this particular basic goal. The F/P-Planner constructs the plans founds in F-Intentions and P-Intentions and passes setpoints (subgoals) to a comparator that regulates the output of the M-Planner. The M-Planner and F/P-Planner will likely mutually interact with each other via efference copies. The predicted consequence of following a plan can then be compared to the basic goal for the plan. The M-Planner forms the motor plans found in M-Intentions.

sense of the goal you would like to pursue, you may be unaware of the means to achieving that goal. If you are looking for means, you are looking for what will cause the goal state to obtain. So you want to work backward from the goal to a course of action. If you are engaged in executing a course of action, and the outcome differs from what you expected, you want to be able to work forward and see if the course of action is still conducive to your goal. Thus, forward and inverse models can work together in correcting plans for action.

As Pacherie observes, planning for the future and planning for the present likely involve different forms of representation from those involved in motor planning. Correspondingly, the format of the internal models should differ. Motor planning requires representations in an egocentric frame of reference so that motor plans are based on the current location of one's limbs and one's current orientation to environmental stimuli. The planning processes involved in F- and P-Intentions are probably more abstract than this. For example, I can form a future- or present-directed plan to fly to Tampa without knowing where the airport is located with respect to my current location. But I cannot form a motor plan to get on a plane without knowing where I am with respect to the plane. Thus we should expect there to be a mechanism for M-Planning distinct from the mechanism for F- and P-Planning.

If we are willing to countenance the notion that planning can be based on the operations of internal models, then we should expect that reward and valuation functions could be active in the planning process, and we can thereby relate our understanding of intentional action to the circuits discussed in this chapter. Although a full understanding of planning mechanisms remains to be attained, a fruitful start could be made by applying the reinforcement learning framework.

10. CONCLUSION

I have argued that we can advance our understanding of motivational states by modeling them on reinforcement learning principles. Basic goals are constitutive of motivational states and likely exert their control over behavior by determining the set of subgoals to be followed in pursuit of the basic goal. Thus, we should think of the kind of feedback control system underlying motivation in terms of a system capable of adopting new subgoals, by forming instrumental desires, plugging those instrumental desires into motor planning and correction mechanisms, and unplugging them when sensory feedback matches the content of the corresponding instrumental desire.

What should a mechanism of motivation look like in the brain? According to the account pieced together in this chapter, motivational mechanisms should look like pulsating synaptic cascades across vast breadths of neural tissue. From a seed of rhythmic activity, perhaps in orbitofrontal cortex and the hypothalamus, motivation would reach through planning mechanisms in prefrontal cortex, posterior parietal, and motor cortex and all of the loops connecting these areas through the basal ganglia and thalamus.[10] Basically, a motivation mechanism should extend through most of the brain. But not every part in the mechanism would do the same thing. Thus, we must posit desire systems, d-volumes and d-gates, forward and inverse models, and so on.

There is a lot of work to be done in the theory of motivation, not addressed in this chapter (see Landreth, 2008). For example, it has yet to be explained what mechanisms account for the prioritization of our desires, for example, whether there is a principle creating in us a hierarchy of needs as Maslow (1943) suggested. Is there a common scale that the brain uses to rank desires? That question remains unanswered.

It also must be determined where aversive motivation fits into the reinforcement learning framework. Are there systems that track punishments in the same way that reward systems track rewards? If so, what is the carrier of the punishment-error signal? Recent research suggests that the periaqueductal gray are importantly involved in punishment prediction, but the evidence is far sparser for this hypothesis than the dopamine reward-error hypothesis (Cole and McNally, 2007).

Ultimately, the neuroscience of motivation should lead to a taxonomy of primary motives based on distinct desire systems. The history of motivation theory is plagued by debates over ad hoc lists of needs (see Chulef, Read, and Walsh, 2001). How many desire systems do we have? How many more can we add? If an appetitive desire system runs on dopamine, what does an aversive desire system run on?

One would also like to know whether there is a causal structure in the brain that answers to the distinction between higher and lower order desires. For example, I might desire to smoke a cigarette. I also might desire not to desire to smoke a cigarette. The latter is a higher order desire with respect to the former. How do we distinguish among these kinds of desires in terms of mechanisms? Why do we more closely identify ourselves with some of these desires and not others? Why do we feel more responsible for the actions driven by some of these desires instead of others? How is it that we come to feel responsible—feel the sense of agency—about our wants and actions at all? Where does the will fit into this picture?[11]

There is also work relevant to motivation which I have neglected to discuss, because it is already quite prominent. I'm thinking mainly of work on the emotions. How do motivational states *qua* reinforcement learning systems interface with mechanisms of emotion (see Landreth, 2008; Rolls, 2005)? When our desires are satisfied and frustrated, we display distinct facial expressions, parasympathetic responses, and feelings. These responses no doubt feed back into motivational processes. There is a massive amount of data and theory that could be used to build bridges between the theory of motivation and the theory of emotion.

In closing, I must stress the importance of uncovering motivation's mechanisms. Motivation is not simply the problem of turning underachievers into Tony Robbins. It is a problem for moral conduct and the pursuit of a satisfying life. Considering the enormous budget devoted to the war on drugs, the success rates of current treatments, and the toll addiction takes on people's private lives, any advance on understanding motivation mechanisms is attractive. Perhaps one day a precise delivery system could be developed to work on the specific desire mechanisms underlying an addictive condition. Taking the notion a step further, one could imagine a future where people are given direct control over any number of their desires, enabled to turn down the volume on self-defeating forms of motivation, and turn up the volume on nobler motives. Imagine a future where substances more powerful than religious sermons, pep rallies, and motivational lectures, more precise than antidepressants and caffeine, could be self-administered by people interested in getting control over their lives. We will never know this future unless sustained and concerted effort is devoted to articulating the mechanisms of motivation.

NOTES

1. We may not always intend what we *most* want to do, but that doesn't negate the fact that what we intend to do we want to do.

2. Cells in the lateral orbitofrontal cortex respond to predictors of punishment.

3. For example, the calibration of an appropriate grip for picking up an object can be disrupted, though a subject is still capable of describing the relevant visual attributes of the object (Goodale and Humphrey, 1998).

4. Assuming that the value proxy was only used to pick the goal object represented in posterior parietal cortex, there should be no need to formulate a new value proxy to guide the action process.

5. Turning the volume clockwise will turn on the desire and continuing to turn up the desire's strength until it clicks again, turning the desire off. The on and off switches are in the same direction for a positive feedback system, such as we see in the salted peanut effect.

6. In the rabbit VTA, putative dopaminergic cells have been found that respond to aversive shock to the ear as well as predictors of aversive shock to the ear (Guarraci and Kapp, 1999). However, Ungless et al. (2004) demonstrated that VTA cells that respond to aversive stimuli do not release dopamine (nor are they likely GABA cells). It would seem that an aversive motivation system is at least partially colocalized at the VTA.

7. Here, I am not, strictly speaking, reviewing Schroeder's account but fitting it with O'Reilly and Frank's (2006) ideas.

8. Frankfurt writes: "Behavior is purposive when its course is subject to adjustments which compensate for the effects of forces which would otherwise interfere with the course of the behaviour, and when the occurrence of these adjustments is not explainable by what explains the state of affairs that elicits them. The behaviour is in that case under the guidance of an independent causal mechanism, whose readiness to bring about compensatory adjustments tends to ensure that the behaviour is accomplished" (1979/1997, p. 48).

9. It makes sense not to require the involvement of F-Intentions for an act to be intentional. To keep the theory of intentional behavior sufficiently general to encompass beings with less developed planning capacities and to simply account for decisions to act made on the fly, it should be sufficient that action be guided by P- and M-Intentions. Furthermore, it should be allowed that such intentions could be very simple, involving no more than one outcome goal and one action-oriented subgoal.

10. One should expect the mechanism of motivation to affect the cerebellum as well.

11. See papers from Andersen's lab on cognitive neuroprosthetics for an interesting starting place on this issue.

REFERENCES

Adams, F. (1979). A goal-state theory of function attributions. *Canadian Journal of Philosophy* 9: 493–518.

Andersen, R. A., and Buneo, C. A. (2002). Intentional maps in posterior parietal cortex. *Annual Review of Neuroscience* 25: 189–220.

Bratman, M. (1987). *Intention, Plans, and Practical Reason*. Cambridge, Mass.: Harvard University Press.

Carmena, J. M., Lebedev, M. A., Crist, R. E., O'Doherty, J. E., Santucci, D. M., Dimitrov, D. F., et al. (2003). Learning to control a brain-machine interface for reaching and grasping by primates. *PLoS Biology* 1: E42.

Chafee, M. V., and Goldman-Rakic, P. S. (2000). Inactivation of parietal and prefrontal cortex reveals interdependence of neural activity during memory-guided saccades. *Journal of Neurophysiology* 83: 1550–1566.

Chulef, A. S., Read, S. J., and Walsh, D. A. (2001). A hierarchical taxonomy of human goals. *Motivation and Emotion* 25: 191–232.

Cole, S., and McNally, G. P. (2007). Temporal-difference prediction errors and Pavlovian fear conditioning: Role of NMDA and opioid receptors. *Behavioral Neuroscience* 121: 1043–1052.

Cousins, M. S., Wei, W., and Salamone, J. D. (1994). Pharmacological characterization of performance on a concurrent lever pressing/feeding choice procedure: Effects of dopamine antagonist, cholinomimetic, sedative and stimulant drugs. *Psychopharmacology* 116: 529–537.

Daw, N., Niv, Y., and Dayan, P. (2006). Actions, policies, values and the basal ganglia. In E. Bezard (Ed.), *Recent Breakthroughs in Basal Ganglia Research*. New York: Nova Biomedical, 91–106.

Dickinson, A., and Balleine, B. (2002) The role of learning in the operation of motivational systems. In C. R. Gallistel (Ed.), *Learning, Motivation and Emotion*, vol. 3. New York: Wiley, 497–533.

Fishbach, A., Roy, S. A., Bastianen, C., Miller, L. E., and Houk, J. C. (2007). Deciding when and how to correct a movement: Discrete submovements as a decision making process. *Experimental Brain Research* 177: 45–63.

Frank, M. J., and Claus, E. (2006). Anatomy of a decision: striato-orbitofrontal interaction in reinforcement learning, decision making, and reversal. *Psychological Review* 113: 300–326.

Frankfurt, H. (1978) The problem of action. *American Philosophical Quarterly* 15: 157–62. Reprinted in A. Mele (Ed.), *The Philosophy of Action*. Oxford: Oxford University Press, 1997.

Funahashi, S., Inoue, M., and Kubota, K. (1997). Delay-period activity in the primate prefrontal cortex encoding multiple spatial positions and their order of presentation. *Behavioral Brain Research* 4: 203–223.

Fuster, J. M. (2001). The prefrontal cortex—an update: Time is of the essence. *Neuron* 30: 319–333.

Goodale, M., and Humphrey, K. (1998). The objects of action and perception. *Cognition* 67: 181–207.

Guarraci, F. A., and Kapp, B. S. (1999). An electrophysiological characterization of ventral tegmental area dopaminergic neurons during differential Pavlovian fear conditioning in the awake rabbit. *Behavioural Brain Research* 99: 169–179.

Holstege, G., Georgiadis, J. R., Paans, A. M., Meiners, L. C., van der Graaf, F. H., and Reinders, A. A. (2003). Brain activation during human male ejaculation. *Journal of Neuroscience* 23: 9185–9193.

Houk, J. C., Bastianen, C., Fansler, D., Fishbach, A., Fraser, D., Reber, P. J., et al. (2007). Action selection and refinement in subcortical loops through basal ganglia and cerebellum. *Philosophical Transactions of the Royal Society of London, B: Biological Sciences* 362: 1573–1583.

Ito, M. (2006). Cerebellar circuitry as a neuronal machine. *Progress in Neurobiology* 78: 272–330.

Jeannerod, M. (1997). *The Cognitive Neuroscience of Action*. Oxford: Blackwell.

Klam, F., and Graf, W. (2003). Vestibular signals of posterior parietal cortex neurons during active and passive head movements in macaque monkeys. *Annual New York Academy of Sciences* 1004: 271–282.

Landreth, A. (2006). Review: *Three Faces of Desire* by Timothy Schroeder. *Philosophical Psychology* 19: 562–566.

Landreth, A. (2007). *Far Beyond Driven: On the Neural Mechanisms of Motivation*. Doctoral dissertation, University of Cincinnati.

Landreth, A. (2008). The neural substrate of moral judgment. In P. Zachar and L. Charland (Eds.), *Fact and Value in Emotion*. Amsterdam: John Benjamins.

Maslow, A. H. (1943). A theory of human motivation. *Psychological Review* 50: 370–396.

Mele, A. (1992). *The Springs of Action*. New York: Oxford University Press.

Mele, A. (2002). *Motivation and Agency*. New York: Oxford University Press.

Montague, R. (2006). *Why Choose This Book? How We Make Decisions*. New York: Dutton.

Musallam, S., Corneil, B. D., Greger, B., Scherberger, H., and Andersen, R. A. (2004). Cognitive control signals for neural prosthetics. *Science* 305: 258–262.

Nagel, E. (1977). Teleology revisited: Goal-directed processes in biology. *Journal of Philosophy* 74: 261–301.

Niv, Y., Joel, D., and Dayan, P. (2005). A normative perspective on motivation. *Trends in Cognitive Sciences* 10: 375–381.

O'Reilly, R. C., and Frank, M. J. (2006). Making working memory work: A computational model of learning in the prefrontal cortex and basal ganglia. *Neural Computation* 18: 283–328.

Pacherie, E. (2006). Towards a dynamic theory of intentions. In S. Pockett, W. P. Banks, and S. Gallagher (Eds.), *Does Consciousness Cause Behavior? An Investigation of the Nature of Volition*. Cambridge, Mass.: MIT Press.

Pochon, J. B., Levy, R., Poline, J. B., Crozier, S., Lehericy, S., Pillon, B., et al. (2001). The role of dorsolateral prefrontal cortex in the preparation of forthcoming actions: An fMRI study. *Cerebral Cortex* 11: 260–266.

Rolls, E. T. (2005). *Emotion Explained*. New York: Oxford University Press.

Rosenberg, P., Herishanu, Y., and Beilin, B. (1977). Increased appetite (bulimia) in Parkinson's disease. *Journal of American Geriatric Society* 25: 277–278.

Schroeder, T. (2004). *Three Faces of Desire*. New York: Oxford University Press.

Schultz, W., Apicella, P., and Ljungberg, T. (1993). Responses of monkey dopamine neurons to reward and conditioned stimuli during successive steps of learning a delayed response task. *Journal of Neuroscience* 13: 900–913.

Schultz, W., Dayan, P., and Montague, P. R. (1997). A neural substrate of prediction and reward. *Science* 275: 1593–1599.

Schultz, W., and Dickinson, A. (2000). Neuronal coding of prediction errors. *Annual Review of Neuroscience* 23: 473–500.

Searle, J. (1983). *Intentionality*. Cambridge: Cambridge University Press.

Shi, W. X. (2005). Slow oscillatory firing: A major firing pattern of dopamine neurons in the ventral tegmental area. *Journal of Neurophysiology* 94: 3516–3522.

Sutton, R. S., and Barto, A. G. (1998). *Reinforcement Learning: An Introduction*. Cambridge, Mass.: MIT Press.

Taylor, D. M., Tillery, S. I., and Schwartz, A. B. (2002). Direct cortical control of 3D neuroprosthetic devices. *Science* 5574: 1829–1832.

Ungless, M. A., Magill, P. J., and Bolam, J. P. (2004). Uniform inhibition of dopamine neurons in the ventral tegmental area by aversive stimuli. *Science* 303: 2040–2042.

van den Top, M., Lee, K., Whyment, A. D., Blanks, A. M., and Spanswick, D. (2004) Orexigen-sensitive NPY/AgRP pacemaker neurons in the hypothalamic arcuate nucleus. *Nature Neuroscience* 7: 493–494.

Wallis, J. D. (2007). Neuronal mechanisms in prefrontal cortex underlying adaptive choice behavior. *Annals of the New York Academy of Sciences* 1121:447–460.

Zald, D. H., and Rauch, S. L. (Eds.). (2006). *The Orbitofrontal Cortex*. New York: Oxford University Press.

CHAPTER 16

INFERENCE TO THE BEST DECISION

PATRICIA SMITH CHURCHLAND

Anyone who is tempted to explore the possibility of neuroethics—the idea that what is and is not valuable is rooted in basic biology—can expect to be scolded with dictum: "You cannot derive an *ought* from an *is*."[1] For those of us who recognize evolutionary biology as the essential backdrop for inquiries into human nature and human behavior, the old dictum seems based on a narrow idea of how values and facts are related. Morality is not the product of a mythical pure reason divorced from natural selection and the neural wiring that motivates the animal to sociability. It emerges from the human brain and its responses to real human needs, desires, and social experience; it depends on innate emotional responses, on reward circuitry that allows pleasure or fear to be associated with certain conditions, and on cortical networks, hormones, and neuropeptides. Its cognitive underpinnings owe more to case-based reasoning than to conformity to rules.

That we are social animals with social dispositions is a central fact owed to our evolutionary history (Darwin, [1871] 1981; Allman, 1999; Dunbar, 1998). Sociability has been selected for in humans, as well as in baboons, wolves, ravens, jays, dolphins, chimpanzees, and many other species. Oxytocin, known to play a role in parturition and parent–offspring interactions, also plays a role in affiliative behaviors, such as sex and grooming.[2] Vasopressin also plays a crucial role, especially in males. As always in biology, there are individual differences within a species, and certainly one can observe individual differences among humans with respect to social dispositions and the capacity to learn what is expected in our own social group; for example, in the case of monoaminoxidase-A genetic variants.[3] There are also individual differences in temperamental features, such as risk aversion, sensitivity to disapproval, impulsivity and capacities for self-control.

At a neurobiological level, we are beginning to understand how sociability is supported in the brain and the role of experience in learning group standards of behavior. We are also beginning to understand the relationship between gene expression and epigenetic factors, and their impact on socially appropriate behavior in maturity (Weaver et al., 2004). For example, research shows that infant cuddling (licking in rats) initiates a cascade of neurochemical events that eventually alters gene expression that modifies the circuitry mediating social capacities. At a more general level, biologically constrained models demonstrate how traits of cooperation and social orderliness can spread through a population; how the virtues can be a benefit, cheating a cost, and punishment of the socially dangerous a necessity.[4] All this is consistent with natural selection and in no way implies group selection. In short, owing to developments over the past three decades, a tension has developed between the sanctity of the "ought/is" dogma and what is known about the neurobiology of social behavior. As I argue, the cognitive process that we loosely call *inference to the best decision* is a solution to this tension. First, I consider the epistemological background.

The idea of "inference to the best *explanation*," often referred to by philosophers as "abduction," is also known in experimental psychology as "case-based reasoning."[5] Essentially, case-based reasoning yields a solution to a problem (what is this, how does this work, why did this happen) by using memory for relevantly similar cases and applying past knowledge to present circumstances. The point I emphasize shortly is that case-based reasoning, whether used for addressing scientific or moral questions, does not rely on universal propositions—neither laws, in the domain of science, nor maxims nor moral theories nor moral rules, in the domain of social behavior (Churchland, 1998). What it does rely on are prototypes, similarity metrics, and analogies (Johnson, 1998; Lakoff, 1996). Moreover, neural network models demonstrate that networks easily learn from examples and the response patterns of the inner units display a similarity metric. The parameter spaces the inner units represent during training, even unsupervised training, are in fact similarity spaces.

In philosophy, abduction has been embraced as a solution to a problem in epistemology. The problem was this: According to one plausible theory—the deductive-nomological (D-N) theory of explanation—acceptable explanations of a phenomenon are deductive arguments that must contain nomological statements (natural laws) of the form, "All X's are Y's." An illustration of where the theory works is the following: Why did that copper expand? Because (Premise 1) copper expands when heated (nomological statement) and (Premise 2) that piece of copper was heated. Therefore, (3) that piece of copper expanded.

The trouble was, in actual scientific practice, as well as in the day-to-day business of life, people routinely generate good, powerful, and highly predictive explanations without relying on natural laws or other generalizations in their explanations. The D-N theory of explanation, though apparently plausible, turned out to be deeply problematic for many exemplary scientific explanations. For example, consider the explanation of how information is coded in DNA; the explanation of the origin of the Earth, the origin of species, the function of the heart and lungs, how the pancreas works, why the dinosaurs became extinct, the cause of aurora borealis, the tides, and cervical cancer. Moreover, many routine, commonplace explanations likewise fail to conform to the requirement that a universal statement be included in the premises. They are good explanations in the sense that they launch powerful predictions that turn out to be correct and inspire manipulations that turn out to be successful. But they do not depend on universal propositions, and they do not involve derivation in any straightforward logical sense.

How do these nomically impoverished explanations nonetheless succeed in explaining? As Peirce argued, and as we all know now, empirical understanding is mainly acquired by recognizing an event as relevantly similar to a familiar class and inferring that the event has a cluster of properties similar to that of the class. Abduction relies on the capacities to generalize usefully from observed cases and draw suitable analogies from the familiar to the unfamiliar (Bogaerts and Leake, 2005; Leake, 2002). Thus abductive—case-based—explanations address mechanism, origins, causal organization, and so forth.[6] Much of the cognitive business of abduction, like the cognitive business of perception and behavioral control, is probably nonconscious and largely inarticulable. In some instances, case-based reasoning may reach for rather abstract analogies between the familiar and the puzzling; other instances may be fairly humdrum. As Peirce noted, abduction sometimes amounts to sophisticated perceptual pattern recognition, as when the neurologist instantly recognizes a tremor as a sign of Parkinson's disease, or an astronomer recognizes a fuzzy spiral in the night sky as a distant galaxy (Churchland, 1998). Sometimes they involve quite abstract analogies, as when Newton realized that the revolution of the moon was, at bottom, like falling toward a large gravitational mass (Churchland, 1995), and when Darwin realized that the natural origin of new species was essentially like breeding dogs but without the breeder.

Why does it hurt, screams the child, and the mother, given her background understanding (it is summer and wasps are about) and her observation of the growing red welt, along with her own similar experience in similar conditions, infers that the child has been stung by a wasp. Inference to the best explanation. She need not invoke, implicitly or otherwise, a nomic statement about red welts in general. To simplify, she recognizes this red welt as relevantly like others she has seen—welts that were caused by wasp stings. In short, *pattern recognition* rather than *discursive argument* is the essential cognitive platform.

The space shuttle *Challenger* explodes, the scientific committee investigates. Many possible explanations are ruled out. Feynman puts sample O-rings (gaskets) in ice water and observes the onset of brittleness. Probably the cold temperature of the O-rings was the critical factor that precipitated the catastrophe. Inference to the best explanation of the explosion. Watson and Crick, using background knowledge in chemistry and physics, and mulling over the X-ray photograph of the DNA crystal, build a model of how the DNA molecule might be structured. They realize that the four base-pair organization of the inner ladder is like a code, and the double helix can split and reform to replicate itself. Inference to the best (albeit, incomplete) explanation of a mechanism whereby copying of information from parent to offspring is achieved. Empirical science being what it is, the inferred explanations are only probable and may be revised in the light of new understanding, but case-based explanation is often the best one can do, relative to the conceptual and evidential resources available in the time available. In addition, because scientific data are always partial and understanding may vary when conceptual frameworks vary, there may well be disagreements that cannot be resolved, at least in the short run. It is also significant that no one argues for the need for a background rule for prudential *oughts*. So if we can infer what prudentially we ought to do, without aid of a prudential background rule, why can't we do this in the moral domain?

Drawing on evolutionary biology, experimental psychology, and neurobiology, we can approach case-based reasoning as a brain phenomenon. Nervous systems were selected for because they allow an organism to move, rather than passively take what comes (Llinas, 2001). The fundamental functions of nervous systems are to move, survive, and make predictions that inform movement, thereby enhancing the organism's chances of surviving long enough to reproduce. Other things being equal, an organism that can predict events—where good food and shelter are, whether it is best to run or hide, whether another is a good mate—will gain in the competition to survive and reproduce. Behaviorally useful categorizations of relevantly similar events, and the retrieval capacity swiftly to access a category for use when needed, are fundamental to prediction and hence to survival.

Case-based reasoning, whatever exactly the neural mechanisms involved, is rooted in neurobiological dispositions to categorize "me-relevant" stimuli for the purposes of prediction that will guide behavior, either in the short or the long run. Some of this understanding may be nonconscious, much of it is undoubtedly organized in prototype mode rather than in propositional mode, especially for animals with no language. What experimental psychologists have discovered is that by and large our work-a-day categories have fuzzy boundaries, and a graded internal structure such that some members are more prototypical than others. Membership is not determined by necessary and sufficient conditions, and categories have a radial structure involving degrees of similarity to the most central members. Moreover these kinds of categories form the fundamental platform for reasoning (Johnson, 1998). This sort of empirical understanding is more akin to exercising a skill than to constructing an argument in discursive form.

Now for inference to the best decision. Notwithstanding Hume's injunction against deriving an *ought* from an *is*, sensible people often do make wise and good decisions about what ought to be done in a social context—what their children or their nation ought to do or they themselves ought to do. They do so without invoking normative premises, maxims, rules, or what have you (Johnson, 1998). They judge the situation on the basis of their recognition that one social situation is relevantly similar, perhaps in quite abstract ways, to other social situations whose sequelae are remembered and evaluated. They are using case-based reasoning, not deduction. Case-based reasoning does not require generalizations, normative or otherwise. As Paul Churchland (1998) has argued, it probably does depend on fuzzy, radially organized categories whose members occupy positions or trajectories in similarity spaces (see figure 16.1).

The person recognizes a situation as relevantly similar to the cases where courage or kindness or acquiescence or biding one's time was the best strategy. This is cased-based reasoning in decision making and is very like case-based reasoning in explanation, except that it targets the social domain, rather than the domain of non-social phenomena. Sometimes inference to the best decision calls for action in the very short run, sometimes it calls only for a judgment without immediate action, as when one decides that the United States ought (*morally* ought) to pursue an energy policy that aims for independence on foreign oil. For our purposes, however, the

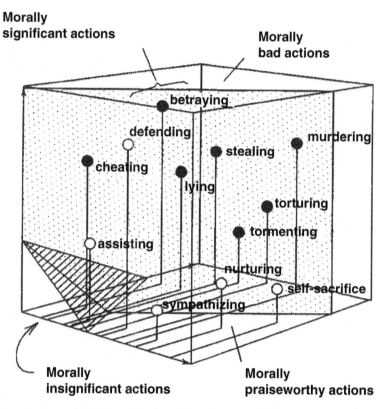

Figure 16.1. A schematic diagram characterizing the parameter space for that subset of social categories with ethical relevance. The aim of the diagram is purely conceptual; namely, to augment the text by showing what is meant by a parameter space, how categories cluster, and how similarity can be understood in terms of distance in a parameter space. It relies on principles of the parameter-space approach to representation in sensory systems, such as taste, vision, and audition, or to representation of more complex categories, such as faces and furniture. In sensory systems, there is a lot of evidence from neurophysiology supporting the hypothesis of parameter-space representation. The morally blameworthy categories are black and cluster on the far side of the main divide, and the morally praiseworthy actions cluster on the near side of the divide. Adapted from Churchland (1998, p. 87).

salient point is that these judgments can be understood as inferences to the best decision (as instances of case-based reasoning). As such, they typically make no reference to moral rules or normative generalizations.

What should I do when Adam kicks me? What do I do when I know my close friend is cheating on exams? What do I do if I know my brother murdered someone? These are the questions children ask, and parents, drawing on their own understanding and assessing the complex social situation as best they can, infer to a good decision.

In 1945, President Harry S. Truman decided that the United States would drop atomic bombs on Japan. Did he *deduce* that the bomb ought to be dropped from facts about the state of affairs? No. Did he use a normative rule plus initial conditions from which the decision followed? No. But he did draw an inference to what he took to be the best decision. The decision was about what ought to be done, given his beliefs about the stubbornness of the emperor and the widespread Japanese conviction that "better death than dishonor," his judgment about American casualties in a greatly prolonged war, the likely impact of the bomb's detonation on Japanese determination, and so forth. On the basis of the same data, others might have come to a different decision, and some would have made the same decision. As with empirical understanding, there are bound to be differences between people regarding the best decision that are not easily resolved. When a collective decision is required despite differing opinions, differences might be safely negotiated (Churchland, 1998). Thus, many women who would themselves not wish to have an abortion under any circumstances nevertheless agree that women who feel differently should be allowed to the opportunity to abort. Of course, sometimes a decision will be negotiated, but once the consequences of the legislation are weighed, the decision may require renegotiation. But many decisions are wise and, by serving the group well, serve the interests of the individual and its capacity to reproduce.[7]

Does not "best" make this approach circular? No more than it does in "inference to the best explanation." Does it not require too much of us—that our decisions be not only good, but the *best*? No more than in inference to the best explanation. "Best" in this context is just relative to the creature's understanding of the situation, including the social understanding, rooted in neurobiology, of the importance of group flourishing, the creature's needs, and the desire to avoid suffering. Use the label "case-based reasoning," and the problem disappears anyhow.

An additional point should be made regarding case-based reasoning. Some philosophical discussion of morals seems "academic," in the pejorative sense of the word, because examples presented often lack substantive detail. The lack of detail prevents case-based reasoning from getting traction; too many or too few prototypes are available to guide our reasoning. For example, we are asked to consult our "moral intuitions" and render a decision even though the circumstances are grotesquely underdescribed ("when the end of the world is nigh, ought one to punish the guilty anyway?"), or the imagined circumstances are so outlandish that no useful analogies to known experience can be drawn; for example, suppose you are in a lifeboat and you have to sacrifice Kant or your mother, which should you sacrifice?[8]

The nature of decision making, in humans and other animals, is beginning to be understood at both the psychological and the neurobiological levels. The emergence of a social decision depends on background conditions including emotions, motivational factors, and social understanding, some of which may be nonconscious and inarticulable (Hsu et al., 2005; Vohs, Meade, and Goode, 2006). It is anchored by social dispositions that are tuned by the reward system as a result of prior experiences. Given a normal reward system, the young of social species internalize what counts as acceptable behavior; they begin routinely to exhibit it, and they come to expect it from others in the group.[9] We see this in social animals generally—wolves, baboons, vampire bats, Steller's jays, and humans. For example, the developing baboon comes to recognize the requirements of reciprocity in grooming, after having been slapped for failure to reciprocate, just as the child recognizes the paradigmatic requirements of truth-telling after having been punished for lying.

As Aristotle realized, making wise decisions is probably a kind of skill for navigating the social world and is quite unlike learning the rules of chess or the Ten Commandments. Early moral learning is organized around prototypes and relies on the reward system to make us feel emotional pain in the face of some events (e.g., stealing), and emotional joy in the face of others (e.g., rescuing) (see Hare, 1981). The child comes to recognize the prototype of being fair, being rude, sharing, and cooperating. His understanding is also shaped by the stories of Chicken Little, the Ant and the Grasshopper, and the Little Red Hen. Some understanding may be discursive and rules of thumb may be a provisional guide, in both natural and moral domains: You can't push on a rope; cheaters never prosper. But these are not exceptionless rules, and knowing about exceptions is not learning the order in which rules get trumped. Sometimes you can push on a rope (it was wet and is now deeply frozen) and sometimes cheaters do prosper, though the social cost can be huge. Consequently, much reorganization of understanding occurs as the child matures, just as in the case of his understanding of the natural world. Reflection, mediated by the emulation circuitry (Grush, 2004), may occasion significant changes, and some change may occur as part of general, ongoing neuronal consolidation of learning and memory.[10] In any case, as Andy Clark (2000) wisely argues, case-based reasoning and rule-based (linguaform) reasoning are, at least in modern times and in linguistically competent humans, complementary. My point is that case-based reasoning is more fundamental in the cognitive economy.

The role of the brain's reward system in social learning normally engenders respect or even reverence for whatever local social institutions happen to exist. Change in those institutions, therefore, may be neither fast nor linear, and may be vigorously resisted even by those who stand to benefit from the change; for example, women who opposed the vote for women; the poor who oppose taxation of the very rich. Despite the power of social inertia, modifications, and sometimes revolutions, do occur, and some of these changes can reasonably be reckoned as moral progress (Churchland, 1998).

A complaint will be that the decisions herein discussed are not genuinely moral but merely pragmatic. The genuinely moral choice must be made for moral reasons alone. Loftily, the moral purist may insist that one must do the right thing simply and only because it is the right thing, whatever our biology. But real morality is not independent of its relevant domain—namely, getting on in life.

As remarked earlier, our social motivation and our urge to belong are rooted in our evolutionary past (Darwin, [1871] 1981). Great benefits accrue to organisms living in a social group; individuals share food and other resources, share knowledge of how to hunt and find the essentials of life, and share defense of the group against predators and invaders. We understand reasonably well the conditions permitting social traits to spread throughout a population, and they include the capacity to detect and remember who are the socially dangerous individuals, and the willingness to punish them and punish those who will not share the burden of punishment (Ridley, 1996).

Darwin had the basic story right, when he remarked in *The Descent of Man* ([1871] 1981): "A tribe including many members who, from possessing in high degree the spirit of patriotism, obedience, courage and sympathy, were always ready to aid one another and to sacrifice themselves for the common good would be victorious over most other tribes; and this would be natural selection" (p. 162). The very purest of the moral purists have missed the day-to-day nature of real, flesh-and-blood morality. They have certainly missed the significance of the selective advantage generally accruing to individuals who exhibit social behavior, including moral behavior. I think they have missed the opportunity to understand how morally exemplary behavior can be displayed in, for example, Inuit communities, which lack rule codification but rely on categories of virtue and case-based reasoning.

Monogamous pair bonding is typical in certain species, such as humans, Canada geese, and prairie voles. The behavior exists not because pure reason sees its universal propriety but because the species evolved so that most individuals have high concentration of receptors for the peptides oxytocin and vasopressin in limbic structures of the brain (Young, Gingrich, Lim, and Insel, 2001). The limbic pathways connect to the dopamine-mediated reward system (mainly the ventral tegmental area and the nucleus accumbens).

Fundamentally, punishment of cheaters (in the broadest sense) is justified because social traits such as cooperation and sharing cannot spread through a population unless cheaters are punished. Dispositions to punish are likely also to be regulated by neural modulators, such as dopamine in the reward system, serotonin in frontal structures, and vasopressin in limbic structures. The precise nature of the punishment—shunning, beating, biting, or whatever—may, in some species such as humans be a matter for negotiation and cultural standards. Like the importance of punishment in social groups, the higher priority typically given to the welfare of kith and kin over distant strangers, wired up by normal brain development, is unlikely to be significantly changed by any categorical imperative repudiating the morality of such priorities.

A caveat is now in order. Certain social practices may allow the tribe to thrive in one condition, but not another. Lethal outgroup hostility, seen in chimpanzees and humans, for example, may be a case in point. According to one model, extinction of competitor out-groups along with high level of in-group sharing, especially of the spoils, gave rise to the distinctive form of altruism seen in human societies (Bowles, 2006). As resource availability changes, as the costs of hostile exchanges escalate, as common goals emerge, cooperation may turn out to be a more productive option. Under such conditions, hostile skirmishes acquire moral condemnation and "the melting pot" acquires moral approval. We crack down on urban gangs and hold out incentives for diversity. Assuming our savanna ape ancestors as well our own human ancestors engaged in outgroup raids, as chimps and several South American tribes still do, can we be confident in moral condemnation of *their* behavior? I see no basis in reality for such a judgment. If, as Bowles argues, the altruism typical of modern humans plausibly coevolved with lethal out-group competition, such a judgment will be problematic.

Concluding Remarks

Ultimately, one wants a deeper account of the neurobiological mechanisms of both inference to the best explanation, and inference to the best decision—of case-based reasoning in its many manifestations. My own expectation is that psychology and neuroscience will eventually uncover at least the general principles concerning how neural networks perform these functions and that the two domains (explaining and deciding) will have much in common. My guess (though of course it could be wrong and anyhow is rather vaguely stated here) is that the account will involve neural networks settling into a local minimum in ways that are now quite familiar and well understood. I conclude with this point not because it neatly sews things up but because I want to emphasize how very much remains to be understood. My main point in this context, however, is that naturalism in ethics should no longer be hobbled by the dictum that you cannot infer an ought from an is. Fine—you cannot deduce an ought from an is. What you *can* do, however, is come to a decision about what you ought to do without relying on any normative rules or maxims. That is what humans, and undoubtedly other animals, in fact do. From this perspective, many new questions in ethics arise. These questions present philosophers with a unique opportunity to collaborate with scientists on matters of great social importance.

Acknowledgment

The basic idea for this chapter comes from Casebeer (2001), who observed that many judgments about what ought to be done are abductive, and from Churchland (1998), who showed how parameter-space representation yields prototypes and a similarity metric. I also got sensible advice from Anne Churchland, Mark Churchland, Dan Dennett, David Brink, John Jacobson, and Michael Stack.

NOTES

1. For a recent and uncompromising defense of Hume's claim, see Kitcher (2006). See also Wilson (2000).

2. For a comprehensive review article, see Insel and Fernald (2004). See also Champagne and Curley (2005) and Carter et al. (2008).

3. The MAOA gene is carried on the X chromosome, and some individuals carry a variant that results in decreased expression of the gene. MAOA is an enzyme that metabolizes serotonin and norepinephrine. If the individual carrying the MAOA is male, then the probability that he will display irrational and self-destructive violent behavior is very high if, as a child, he is abused. See Caspi et al. (2002).

4. For an accessible overview of the literature, see Ridley (1996).

5. See Leake (1998). There does exist an extensive research program into the nature of case-based reasoning.

6. For a discussion of how children acquire causal understanding, see Glymour et al. (2004). See also Craver (2005).

7. As the virtue ethicists have pointed out, there is no evidence that as a matter of fact, Kantians, for example, are more morally upstanding than the general population. In fact, lot of very ordinary, non-Kantian people act in morally superlative ways without knowing a thing about the categorical imperative or reflective equilibrium. See Annas (2004).

8. The so-called trolley cases are examples in this vein.

9. Here is the connection I see to Searle's (1964) paper. Once the reward system of the young baboon has been tuned up to the prevailing standard for grooming reciprocity, then the baboon normally acts in accord with the standard. He recognizes a situation wherein another baboon expects grooming for past services, and case-based reasoning takes him to the decision the he ought to reciprocate.

10. Some of the consolidation and reorganization likely occurs during sleep. See Borbely, Hayaishi, Sejnowski, and Altman (1996).

REFERENCES

Allman, J. M. (1999). *Evolving Brains.* New York: Scientific American Library.

Annas, J. (2004). Being virtuous and doing the right thing. Presidential Address to the Pacific Division of the APA. *Proceedings and Addresses of the American Philosophical Association* 78: 61–75.

Bogaerts, S., and Leake, D. B. (2005). A Framework for Rapid and Modular Case-Based Reasoning System Development. Technical Report TR 617. Bloomington, Ind.: Computer Science Department, Indiana University.

Borbely, A. A., Hayaishi, O., Sejnowski, T. J., and Altman, J. S. (Eds.). (1996). *The Regulation of Sleep*. Strasbourg: Human Frontiers Science Program.

Bowles, S. (2006). Group competition, reproductive leveling, and the evolution of human altruism. *Science* 314: 1569–1572.

Carter, C. S., Grippo, A. J., Pournajafi-Nazarloo, H., Ruscio, M. G., and Porges S. W. (2008) Oxytocin, vasopressin and sociality. *Progress in Brain Research* 170: 331–336.

Casebeer, W. (2001). *Natural Ethical Facts*. Cambridge, Mass.: MIT Press.

Caspi, A., McClay, J., Moffitt, T., Mill, J., Martin, J., Craig, I., et al. (2002). Role of genotype in the cycle of violence in maltreated children. *Science* 297: 851–854.

Champagne, F. P., and Curley, J. P. (2005). How social experiences influence the brain. *Current Opinion in Neurobiology* 15: 704–709.

Churchland, P. M. (1995). *The Engine of Reason, The Seat of the Soul*. Cambridge, Mass.: MIT Press.

Churchland, P. M. (1998). Toward a cognitive neurobiology of the moral virtues. *Topoi* 17: 83–96.

Clark, A. (2000). Word and action: Reconciling rules and know-how in moral cognition. *Canadian Journal of Philosophy* 26 (supplement): 267–289.

Craver, C. (2005). Beyond reduction: Mechanisms, multifield integration, and the unity of science. *Studies in History and Philosophy of Biological and Biomedical Sciences* 36: 373–395.

Darwin, C. ([1871] 1981). *The Descent of Man, and Selection in Relation to Sex*. J. T. Bonner and R. M. May (Eds.). Princeton, N.J.: Princeton University Press.

Dunbar, R. I. M. (1998). The social brain hypothesis. *Evolutionary Anthropology* 6: 178–190.

Grush, R. (2004). The emulation theory of representation: Motor control, imagery, and perception. *Behavioral and Brain Sciences* 27: 377–442.

Glymour, C., Gopnik, A., Sobel, D. M., Schultz, L. E., Kushnir, T., and Danks, D. (2004). A theory of causal learning in children: Causal maps and Bayes nets. *Psychological Review* 111: 1–31.

Hare, R. M. (1981). *Moral Thinking*. Oxford: Oxford University Press.

Hsu, M., Bhatt, M., Adolphs, R., Tranel, D., and Camerer, C. F. (2005). Neural systems responding to degrees of uncertainty in human decision-making. *Science* 310: 1680–1683.

Insel, T. R., and Fernald, R. D. (2004). How the brain processes social information: Searching for the social brain. *Annual Review of Neuroscience* 27: 697–722.

Johnson, M. L. (1998). Ethics. In W. Bechtel and G. Graham (Eds.), *A Companion to Cognitive Science*. Oxford: Blackwell, 691–701.

Kitcher, P. (2006). Biology and ethics. In D. Copp (Ed.), *The Oxford Handbook of Ethics*. Oxford: Oxford University Press, 163–185.

Lakoff, G. (1996). *Moral Politics*. Chicago: University of Chicago Press.

Leake, D. B. (1998). Case-based reasoning. In W. Bechtel and G. Graham (Ed.), *A Companion to Cognitive Science*. Oxford: Blackwell, 465–476.

Leake, D. B. (Ed.). (2002). *Case-Based Reasoning: Experiences, Lessons, and Future Directions*. Cambridge, Mass.: AAAI Press/MIT Press.

Llinas, R. (2001). *I of the Vortex: From Neurons to Self*. Cambridge, Mass.: MIT Press.

Ridley, M. (1996). *The Origins of Virtue: Human Instinct and the Evolution of Cooperation*. New York: Viking.

Searle, J. (1964). How to derive "ought" from "is." *Philosophical Review* 73: 18–26.

Vohs, K. D., Meade, M. L., and Goode, M. R. (2006). The psychological consequences of money. *Science* 314: 1154–1165.

Weaver, I., Cervoni, N., Champagne, F., D'Allesio, A., Sharma, S., Seckl, J., et al. (2004). Epigenetic programming by maternal behavior. *Nature Neuroscience* 7: 847–854.

Wilson, C. (2000). The biological basis and ideational superstructure of ethics. *Canadian Journal of Philosophy* 26 (supplement): 211–244.

Young, L. J., Gingrich, B., Lim, M. M., and Insel, T. R. (2001). Cellular mechanisms of social attachment. *Hormonal Behavior* 40: 133–139.

CHAPTER 17

EMERGENTISM AT THE CROSSROADS OF PHILOSOPHY, NEUROTECHNOLOGY, AND THE ENHANCEMENT DEBATE

ERIC RACINE AND JUDY ILLES

1. Introduction

The continuous stream of advances in biomedical engineering and neuroscience have led to a spectacular array of functional interfaces between living neurons and electronic signals. Though strong efforts at the intersection of biology and engineering have animated research and theoretical speculation since the 1970s, contemporary research has been narrowing the gap between neurons and electrodes. Deep brain stimulation is now used to treat Parkinson's disease, for example, and represents a source of hope for improved quality of life for these patients. Other brain-machine technologies are leading the way to clinical benefits, including unprecedented possibilities for restoring motor function in paralyzed patients. However, even if therapy is the stated final aim for these efforts, some investigators also envision nontherapeutic applications. In fact, the possibility of using neurotechnology for enhancing human function that falls outside parameters defined by pathology (Racine, 2002) is believed to be increasingly plausible, if not inescapable given current neuroscience advances (Farah et al., 2004; Sahakian and Morein-Zamir, 2007).

Ethical debate on the possibility of neurotechnological enhancement has focused on pharmacology (Chatterjee, 2004; Dees, 2004; Hauser, 2004; Rose, 2002; Whitehouse, Juengst, Mehlman, and Murray, 1997; Wolpe, 2002). With the aim of contributing to and elaborating on this debate, we review capabilities for enhancing brain function with brain–machine interfaces (BMIs). Given the invasive nature of BMIs, their potential use for enhancement provides a basis for illustrating how different philosophies of neuroscience lead to diverging ethical frameworks for evaluating their scientific, ethical, regulatory, and cultural implications. If the mind is a property per se that is independent of the brain (holism), or if the mind is a concept eliminated by advances in neuroscience (reductionism),[1] then the question of how these technologies have the potential to modify the way we conceive of ourselves as human beings cannot be part of the ethical analysis. In the case of holism, the cultural challenges of enhancement and reflection on its philosophical implications are unclearly framed because of related strong dualist beliefs between mind and brain properties obscure the possibility that brain intervention can have an impact on the workings of the mind. In the case of reductionism, scientific challenges are emphasized, but other issues are left unattended. More problematic, however, is that reductionism might actually threaten normative principles such as respect for person and autonomy and eschew relevant cultural issues. In this chapter, we discuss these approaches in philosophy of neuroscience—reductionism, holism, and emergentism—for framing the ethics discussion. We argue that the emergentist approach, for which reduction is necessary but insufficient to understand the higher level properties of the self, provides the strongest option for guiding the present ethical debate. Emergentism leads to a more complete ethical analysis that includes scientific, normative, and cultural considerations. The implications of this analysis are considerable, we believe, for investigators, physicians, health care providers, and neuroethicists insofar as it reveals the interdependence of philosophical and ethical frameworks as well as the more concrete implications of such fundamental approaches.

2. BMIs

The dream of developing a symbiosis between neurons and electrodes has been pursued for a number of decades (Nicolelis, 2001), and new advances in neuroscience linking engineering and computer science are bringing this to reality. Currently, major efforts are focused on finding appropriate theoretical and practical methods to (1) record neural signals, (2) extract these signals with the help of software and mathematical processing, and (3) use the extracted signal to guide either computer displays (such as cursors) or robots (such as artificial arms) (Schwartz,

2004, p. 490). Current experimental designs deal extensively with the transformation of motor cortex signals. Accordingly, restoration of motor skills is a major target that makes disease such as amyotrophic lateral sclerosis (ALS) and paralysis due to trauma likely candidates for clinical implantation (Birch, Bozorgzadeh, and Mason, 2002; Chapin, 2000; Millan Jdel, Renkens, Mourino, and Gerstner, 2004; Musallam, Corneil, Greger, Scherberger, and Andersen, 2004; Mussa-Ivaldi and Miller, 2003; Nicolelis, 2003; Prochazka, Mushahwar, and McCreery, 2001; Sanchez et al., 2004).

A single name is yet to be recognized for this technology, and it therefore remains variously referred to as brain–computer interfaces (BCIs) (Schwartz, 2004; Wickelgren, 2003), BMIs (Donoghue, 2002; Nicolelis, 2003) or hybrid BMIs (Nicolelis, 2001).[2] Two families of BMIs, indirect and direct BMIs, are generally described in the literature (Donoghue, 2002; Nicolelis, 2001, 2003; Schwartz, 2004; Wickelgren, 2003).

It is not within the scope of this chapter to present exhaustive details of these technologies, but in brief, direct and indirect BMIs both attempt to transduce neural signals into meaningful movement codes that can be used to guide computer displays or motor devices (Donoghue, 2002; Mussa-Ivaldi and Miller, 2003; Nicolelis, 2003; Schwartz, 2004). Indirect BMIs record signals on the scalp with EEG electrodes. Some EEG variants include the implantation of electrodes under the dura or on the surface of the cortex itself. The signals are then collected and treated using computers as decoding instruments. Such paradigms have allowed paralyzed humans to move cursors on computer screens, for example, and indicate choices. Historically, a team led by Birbaumer has provided the basis for a "spelling device for the paralyzed" (Birbaumer et al., 1999). Limitations of indirect BMIs include the practical challenges of fastening them to tissue. Others concern the low-precision level of EEGs as indicators of movement. These have led some researchers to explore possibilities of using direct neuronal signals rather than EEGs.

Direct BMIs are inserted intracortically to capture the discharge activity of neurons. This activity represents very low-voltage electric signals, and miniature microelectrodes are used to detect and encode the electrical activity of numerous neurons. Following the insight of Canadian psychologist Donald Hebb, we know that neuron populations work in small networks. The motor cortex in particular has proven to be a fertile ground for promoting neural network principles. In a now classic neurophysiology study, Georgopoulos, Schwartz, and Kettner (1986) demonstrated that motor cortex neuron populations can code for arm movement. According to neural networks approaches, vectorial algebra, and other mathematical tools, neural signals are thus encoded into meaningful limb-related patterns. Once this is realized, an actuator transforms the converted computer signal into a representation, such as an animated computer display or a robot movement. Newer technologies use microwires, assemblies of tiny wires that have proven reliable to record signals for up to hundreds of neurons. Safety issues are presently a principal concern because BMIs need to work reliably for years (Donoghue, 2002).

Whereas indirect EEG-based BMIs aim principally at restoring communication capabilities, direct BMIs aim to restore sensorimotor function as well. BMIs have primarily focused on motor and sensory areas. Neuroanatomy studies have revealed principles of spatial representation of the body in the brain that exist in the cochlear (tonotopy), the primary visual cortex (retinotopy), and the motor and sensory primary areas of the brain (somatotopy). Regarding the latter, Wilder Penfield's homunculus constitutes a visual representation. Although the orientation of the face on the homunculus has been debated (Servos, Engel, Gati, and Menon, 1999), the mapped representation of the body in the brain is a guiding principle for current BMI research and applications. The intimate relationship with neural tissue, the invasive nature of direct BMIs, and also their potential restorative power make them a more compelling model than indirect BMIs to discuss enhancement tissues (table 17.1). Hereafter, we use the term BMI to represent direct BMIs.

Though obstacles must be tackled before BMIs are implanted into patients, many significant technological advances are paving the way toward this goal. For example, tens of thousand of patients have benefited from cochlear implants, the original BMI (Mussa-Ivaldi and Miller, 2003 Nicolelis, 2001). Neural prostheses that use electrical stimulation of neurons in visual pathways are being explored intensively. Preliminary human trials of retinal prosthesis have been approved by the U.S. Food and Drug Administration, though many significant challenges exist (Hetling and Baig-Silva, 2004).

Deep brain stimulation[3] is an example of electric signal transfer to central nervous system (CNS) structures. Neurostimulation devices targeting basal ganglia activity have been used successfully to alleviate tremor, rigidity, and bradykinesia

Table 17.1. Direct and indirect BMIs

	Direct BMIs	Indirect BMIs
Description	Invasively and directly record neural signals with microelectrodes. Intracortical implantation.	Noninvasively record neuroelectrical signals using methods such as EEG. Neural signals are recorded indirectly. Extracortical implantation.
Successes	Potential recovery of motor function.	Important communication channels for patients with severely limited communication abilities.
Limitations	Many technical challenges given sophisticated signal processing and algorithms. Grafting procedures require the placement of stable electrodes that decode neuronal population activity.	Cumbersome and slow compared to natural behavior given the indirect nature of signals. A substitute for recording directly neural activity.

Source: Adapted from Donoghue (2002).

in patients suffering from Parkinson's disease (Blank, 1999, pp. 107–108; Donoghue, 2002).[4] Kennedy and colleagues developed a cerebral implant enabling a paralyzed ALS patient to express himself verbally (Emory University, 1998; Kennedy and Bakay, 1998). A glass-encapsulated neurotrophic cone electrode was inserted in the motor cortex of the patient and neurotrophic factors inside the electrode facilitated the growth of coupling motor cortex neurites. The electrode converts neuronal discharges in a computer-usable signal. The latter is received by a computer and serves to move a cursor on the screen.

Using a very small number of neurons in the primary motor cortex, Serruya and colleagues have observed that monkeys can successfully use the activity of their motor cortex to guide a cursor in any position hands-free. This result represents an important achievement since previous attempts were based on extensive subject training or were based on a limited movement repertoire (Serruya, Hatsopoulos, Paninski, Fellows, and Donoghue, 2002). Overall, use of the neural signal instead of hand motions was only slightly slower to reach targets. Previously, Chapin and colleagues had demonstrated that rats could trigger with brain signals a robot arm to obtain water (Chapin et al., 1999), albeit using larger neuron populations. Wessberg and colleagues demonstrated the same phenomenon in monkeys (Wessberg et al., 2000).

From what may have seemed to be a mere dream 30 or 40 years ago, BMIs have emerged as therapeutic hope for some neurological diseases. Patients suffer from cognitive, mnesic, motor, visual, auditory, thermo-algesic, and language symptoms as well as dementia. Interest for new treatments and therapies is clear given the gravity of symptoms and related costs. Accordingly, significant funding is now backing BMI research efforts. For example, the National Institutes of Health (NIH) has invested $3.3 million in 2002 for software testing of several BMIs (Wickelgren, 2003). The National Institute for Neurological Disorders and Strokes (NINDS) of the NIH has a designated neural prostheses program. Other NINDS-funded researchers are also grouped under the Deep Brain Stimulation Consortium. Treatment is the prime goal of these BMIs efforts. With Defense Advanced Research Projects Agency (DARPA) investments of a staggering $26 million in the early 2000s, the improvement of direct BMI techniques has been intensively pursued for several years (Wickelgren, 2003).

3. Framing BMI Enhancement and Philosophy of Neuroscience in Neuroethics

3.1. Neuroethics of BMI Enhancement

Neuroethical discussion of BMI has focused on what we identify as four classes of interdependent issues—scientific and medical, ethical and legal, policy and

Table 17.2. Sets of interdependent BMI-related issues

Issues	Description	Examples
Scientific and medical issues	Technological readiness of BMI implantation.	Safety, risks, and side effects. Efficacy of BMI implantation. Medical appropriateness.
Ethical and legal issues	Respect for person and patient preferences.	Respect for autonomy. Protection of confidentiality. Respect for privacy. Distributive justice.
Policy and regulatory issues	Regulatory framework and approval mechanisms for uses of BMIs.	Regulation for commercialization and marketing of BMI technology. Public input into policy making.
Cultural and social issues	Impact of BMIs on our view of ourselves and our identity in a multicultural context.	Considerations of our self-definition as human beings in the analysis of the potential impact of BMI enhancement on personhood. Health coverage and public health impact of BMI enhancement.

regulatory, and cultural and social (table 17.2). They are distinguished and artificially separated for the purpose of further clarifying the impact of different philosophies on the ethical analysis of BMI use, especially on enhancement, which is our prime focus. Some would consider scientific and medical issues to be the most important, given the state of current research. For example, when Maguire and McGee (1999) urged for a discussion on implantable brain chips in the *Hastings Center Report*, these considerations were dismissed as alarmist, speculative, or even ridiculous because recent technical advances remain far from enhancement interventions. At best, the most current interventions aim to restore lower level functions that may appear to have little to do with higher functions typically associated with personhood such as cognition and emotion. This was the reaction of White to Maguire and McGee's paper: "At present then, there is no bioethical issue surrounding the placement of 'chips' in the human brain, for there is no evidence that it can be accomplished" (White, 1999). Still, others would contend that ethical and legal issues, such as respect for autonomy, are key in dealing with the ethics of enhancement. For example, Caplan (2003) argues from a libertarian point of view that individuals can pursue enhancement as long as they freely choose to do so. There are of course social pressures that may shape the impetus for enhancement, but a separate discussion would be needed to fully assess this proposal. However, our goal here is more modest. We identify sets of issues without arguing for the priority of one.

Underlying this strategy is a minimal commitment that we should open the debate to all types of related concerns to warrant fuller ethical analysis of BMIs.

The technical readiness of BMIs for clinical uses raises an inescapable set of scientific issues. As noted, many neuroengineering challenges need to be surmounted before clinical uses are warranted. Brain tissues can get infected, and microelectrodes can move and become inefficient neuronal sensors. These are especially acute concerns for patients who may be desperately ill and turning to BMIs as a last resort.

3.2. Ethical and Legal Issues

If we imagine a scenario of safe, effective, and reliable implantation, ethical and legal issues related to, for example, the assessment of patient preferences or to the respect for person and autonomy surface. Individuals or their proxies would need to consent to make their preferences known to the physician and the health care team. More imaginative issues of BMIs raise additional concerns for privacy and justice. For example, employee monitoring or storage of information through BMIs will have ethical consequences. How would such applications and the information to which they give access be regulated (Moreno, 2003)? Will they lead to social injustice (Farah et al., 2004)?

3.3. Regulatory and Policy Issues

Safety of BMIs and respect for autonomy can only be fulfilled if appropriate mechanisms are in place to regulate the production of BMIs and monitor the quality of information available to individuals through public marketing of BMI technology. Public input in the policy-making process may also be crucial for BMIs given the wide range of existing public opinions.

3.4. Cultural and Social Issues

A fourth set of issues—cultural and social issues,[5] such as the impact of BMIs on cognition and personhood—has also been discussed.[6] For example, chairing the third meeting of the International Bioethics Committee of UNESCO, which explored ethical issues of neuroscience, French neurobiologist Jean-Didier Vincent (1996) suggested that implantation of microelectrodes "might be envisaged to replace or supplement higher cognitive functions." In 2001, preeminent BMI researcher Nicolelis suggested BMI technologies could "trigger a revolution in the way future generations interact with computers, virtual objects and remote environments, by allowing never-before-experienced augmentation of perceptual, motor and cognitive capabilities" (Nicolelis, 2001). Donoghue expressed this possibility while invoking the necessity of ethical discussion:

> If direct neuromuscular BMIs are successful, they will provide extraordinary
> options for those who have lost major neural pathways. Future BMIs may
> further complement biological solutions to repair damaged nervous system,

approaches such as gene or stem cell therapy. One can further envision more imaginative uses of BMIs. For example, they could be used to augment human capabilities by providing novel information input-output channels or added memory capacity. However, the neural augmentation prospects of BMIs resurrect important ethical and social issues that have been raised in the past. Discussion on these topics should resume. (2002)

Once intervening on the nervous system in ways that could change personality is technically and safely feasible, individuals could choose to do so based on personal values and beliefs. However, a set of issues bearing on the wider cultural meaning of enhancement would still remain. Are we changing what it means to be human? Is the use of enhancement—like in sport competition—an illegitimate way of self-achievement? Are we replacing what was the realm of culture—searching for the meaning of one's personal life and achieving self-realization by personal effort—by the realm of technological means and the instrumental rationality it follows? This set of questions may present the most daunting challenge of BMIs.

BMI research with animals has also further fueled the debate. One controversial study used stimulation of the somatosensory cortex (right and left whisker representation) and the medial forebrain bundle to produce a remote-controlled rat. Rats were backpacked with a microprocessor that rendered possible the delivery of neurostimuli in the implanted brain sites. The animals were trained to interpret remote brain stimulation as instructions for directing their trajectory of locomotion, and stimulation of the whisker-representing areas of somatosensory cortex served as a virtual touch, whereas forebrain stimulation served as the reward, even as a trigger message. The authors suggested that "the ability to receive brain sensory activity remotely and interpret it accurately could allow a guided rat to function as both a mobile robot and a biological sensor" (Talwar et al., 2002). This experiment was rapidly seen as opening the possibility of reconfiguring human behavior using BMIs. Moving away from the traditional territory of BMIs—the primary motor cortex—to higher order cortex neurons, Musallam and colleagues (2004) used cells of the parietal reach region of monkeys to guide cursors. This cognitive-based approach is not restricted to the higher order motor area and opens up new neuroengineering possibilities by suggesting that many kinds of cognitive signals may be decoded from a patient (Musallam et al., 2004). These efforts are still remote from enhancement, but they illustrate how rapidly basic insights could lead the way to neurotechnology that modifies normal function.

Some investigators have already begun stretching the frontiers of neuroengineering closer to enhancement. English researcher, Kevin Warwick, underwent surgery in August 1998 to implant a microprocessor underneath the skin of his arm (Warwick, 2000). According to Warwick, this microprocessor could replace Social Security numbers and save information such as blood type and bank information. For Warwick, his personal experiments all point in the direction of progress and a natural coevolution of man and computer. Warwick's rhetoric on BMI enhancement seems far-fetched to many, but it nonetheless forces us to accept that some may actually want to pursue enhancement efforts. Military interest in BMIs is also indisputable (Blank, 1999). DARPA stated that its intentions are to eventually use such technologies to improve the performance of military personnel, allowing, for example, information to be relayed directly to the brains of the personnel (Hoag, 2003). One is also left wondering what the biomedical goals stated at the beginning of BMI articles mean: actual goals or therapeutic disguised pretexts?[7] Perhaps enhancement is still a remote possibility given the state of BMI research, but impressive developments constitute steps in this direction. Enhancement could be pursued for individual and robot ethics ideals as Warwick's endeavors illustrate or for military concerns as DARPA exemplifies. These developments show that we need to address all relevant issues, including cultural and social issues, such as the impact of technology on personhood and enhancement. To this end, we wish to illustrate how different philosophies highlight the various challenges of BMIs.

4. Philosophy of Neuroscience and Ethical Analysis of BMIs

Given the intimate relationship between direct BMIs and brain tissue, we now argue that implicitly or explicitly held philosophical approaches and related views on the nature of neuroscientific explanations of mind and body inform ethical perspectives on BMIs. As Blank (1999) hinted and Illes and Racine (2005) argued, research on the brain brings into play mind–brain relationship topics that impact views on ethical issues. As a theoretical and practical endeavor, bioethics has been especially attentive to the sorting of facts, especially in comparison to other forms of ethics (Toulmin, 1982). This is clearly illustrated when we consider the emergence and the focus of clinical ethics, or the use of casuistry in case analysis (Jonsen, Siegler, and Winslade, 1998). However, addressing neuroethical issues such as BMI enhancement will be complicated because establishing facts also means wrestling with interpretation of neuroscientific findings—a task with considerable philosophical ramifications. For example, analysis of the implications of neurotechnology on free will, and legal or moral responsibility introduce the need for conceptual analysis and philosophical reflection (Moreno, 2003). Scrutiny of mind–body reductionism is another traditional philosophical forte and is also necessary to assess in depth the impact of neuroscience on culture and self-conception. For example, will neuroscience eliminate folk psychology, our ordinary view of ourselves, since the ultimate ontology is the scientific one (reductive monism) like Churchland (1989) contends? Or is neuroscience completely irrelevant to understanding the mind because it is an independent substance (substance dualism) or another type of reality description (semantic or property dualism) like many philosophers such as Ricoeur maintain (Changeux and Ricoeur, 2000)? As these different questions suggest, neuroethics

Table 17.3. Philosophy of neuroscience and BMIs

Philosophy	Blitz (1992) Part–Whole: Ontology	Part–Whole: Epistemology	Racine (2002) Mind-Body Thesis	Ethical Scope of Neurotechnologies	Racine, Illes, and Bar-Ilan (this chapter) Neurotechnology
Reductionism	Properties of the whole are always found among the properties of their parts—all properties are resultants.[a]	Knowledge of the part is both necessary and sufficient to understand the whole.	Reductive monism and eliminativism: The mind does not exist because it does not reduce to its components, the activity of the nervous system. Mind concepts must be eliminated.	Neurotechnological interventions do not cause particular problems because mind-related issues are based on false folk psychology concepts. Traditional ethics language is or will be reshaped by scientific ontology. Ethics could be evacuated.	**Reductionism focuses on scientific and medical issues.** BMIs operate within a positivistic framework in which ethics concepts are replaced or eliminated by neuroscience. Reductionism leads us to consider whether BMIs are efficient and safe, but those concerns do not include specific analysis of ethical or cultural issues. For example, reductionism allows (even facilitates) physicians, health care providers, and neuroethicists to uncritically reproduce a problematic view of the role of science in the clinical setting.
Holism	The basic unit is that of the whole—wholes are independent of parts.	Knowledge of the parts is neither necessary nor sufficient to understand the whole.	Dualism: Mind is a whole and cannot be explained or understood from its components, the activity of the nervous system.	Neurotechnological interventions do not cause particular problems because the mind is independent of the body. Respect for traditional ethical norms is fostered.	**Holism does not highlight cultural and social issues.** Some religious and philosophical traditions based on dualism have proven to be important critical resources for the assessment of bioethical issues. However, cultural and social issues such as BMI enhancement are difficult to frame within a dualist philosophy. If the mind is completely independent from the brain, how is enhancement even possible? Worries about enhancement and defense of strict dualism seem incompatible.

Emergentism	Some properties of wholes are not the properties of any of their parts.	Knowledge of the parts is necessary but not sufficient to understand the whole.	Emergentist monism: Understanding the activity of the components of brain systems is necessary but insufficient to understand higher level properties of the brain.	Neurotechnological intervention could affect working of the mind. New ethical questions are raised given that the components of the brain give rise to mind-level phenomena.	**Emergentism highlights cultural and social issues.** Emergentism allows for the evaluation of both the possibility and ethics of BMI enhancement. It illuminates new ethical issues bearing on the concept we have of ourselves and urges open dialogue about the cultural and narrative dimensions of BMI enhancement.

[a] A resultant property is a property that both a system and its components have, whereas an emergent property is a property that a system has but is not found in any of its components (Mahner and Bunge, 1997).

Source: Extended from Racine (2002) and Blitz (1992).

must address philosophy of mind and philosophy of neuroscience issues to fully analyze the impact and the risks of neurotechnology. To get a clearer picture of the ethical implications of neurotechnology such as BMIs, we need to bring these philosophical discussions into the realm of bioethics. With the goal of exploring such a contribution, we now introduce three philosophical theories[8]—reductionism, holism, and emergentism—and discuss how they highlight different sets of ethical concerns for BMIs (table 17.3).

4.1. Reductionism

Reductionism is a philosophy stating that properties of the whole are always found among the properties of their parts and knowledge of the part is both necessary and sufficient to understand the whole (Blitz, 1992). Concerning the mind–body problem, this approach supports complete reduction of higher order functions to the properties of the nervous system. It is, for example, Crick's astonishing hypothesis that "You, your joys and your sorrows, your memories and your ambitions, your sense of personal identity and free will, are in fact no more than the behavior of a vast assembly of nerve cells and their associated molecules" (Crick, 1995). In the eliminativist variant of reductionism, ordinary-language descriptions of psychological phenomena called folk psychology or propositional attitude psychology could be replaced by neuroscientific explanations. They are in fact bound to disappear to the profit of a scientific ontology (P.M. Churchland, 1981, 1989, 1995; P.S. Churchland, 1986; Rorty, 1965).

From an ethical point of view, the implications of a strong reductionist stance are problematic. If the self is the "detailed behavior of a set of nerve cells" (Crick, 1995), then the framing of ethical problems becomes difficult. What happens to ethical concepts and principles that deal with person and autonomy if these are reduced to neuronal activity? What becomes of the social and normative dimensions of the concept of person and the consideration of others as persons? Can this ethical concept really translate into neurobiological concepts? The prospect of eliminating propositional attitude psychology and seeing ourselves and others only as complex neuronal organisms threatens the scope and relevance of ethical concepts. Sensitivity to ethical issues raised by neurotechnologies could be jeopardized by the replacement of ordinary worldview of phenomena such as thought processes and emotions by neurobiological explanations. Proponents of reductionism may argue that this is not the case, and the elimination of folk psychology will only bring more precise ethical concepts in our cultural landscape. For example, contenders argue that replacing our lay understanding of conceptualization and reasoning with more scientifically warranted neural network views, might dismiss some possibly erroneous ethical perspectives (Churchland, 1989, 1995). However, precedent in the history of medicine and neuroscience suggests that the power of biomedical language is great and can have unintended consequences. The case of lobotomy, for example, illustrates both its disastrous consequences and the related overenthusiastic and uncritical public portrayal of the procedure (Diefenbach et al., 1999). Engelhardt's analysis of biomedical language as descriptive and etiological and, at the same time, social and evaluative (Engelhardt, 1996) further supports this argument. Replacing ordinary views with neurobiological ones could lead to hasty attempts to discredit some moral perspectives as being erroneous based on preliminary scientific data or by not taking into account the value-laden character of scientific and medical language, especially when the public appropriates it. Hence, one can only be skeptical of explanations that depict mind–body reductionism as a neutral and harmless process.

When we look precisely at BMIs, our analysis further supports that reductionism is unsuitable for voicing ethical and legal or cultural and social concerns over enhancement. In the reductionist stance, neuroscientific materialism constitutes the epistemological authority and consequently the final judge of our ontology. If ethical principles or concepts such as respect for persons or autonomy are not understandable in neuroscientific terms, that is, if they do not reduce to neuroscientific concepts, they will be eliminated. Revision of our ontology has proven to be an important scientific accomplishment of modernity. For example, we no longer believe that phlogiston explains chemical interactions between molecules, nor does modern science warrant radical creationism. However, we must be prudent in stating that neuroscience will change the way we see ourselves, in particular the ethical dimension of human beings. By overemphasizing neuroscientific revision of folk psychology, we may lose our ordinary insights into the ethics of neuroscientific advances. In an early discussion of ethical implications of mind–brain philosophies, Gunther Stent provided a relevant comment on Patricia Chuchland's *Neurophilosophy* emphasizing how reductionist statements are ethically problematic (Stent, 1990). At best, reductionism will force us to question if BMIs work, are effective, and are safe—an important set of concerns—but it falls short of accommodating a more in-depth analysis of social and cultural issues, such as enhancement. If we reduce ethical concepts to neurobiological explanations, we may in fact lose the ability to take some distance and look more critically at BMIs. Ethical discourse is also very complex, and reduction of ethical language may not carry this complexity forward, leaving aside the variety of moral views. In this respect, reductionism could even threaten to eschew other sets of concerns. Could globally rejecting the relevance of neuroscience to our understanding of the self, as Stent suggests, be the path to follow?

4.2. Holism/Dualism

Holism is a philosophy that espouses the whole as the basic unit of analysis because wholes are independent of their parts (Blitz, 1992). Therefore, according to holism, knowledge of the parts is neither necessary nor sufficient to understand the whole (Blitz, 1992). As with reductionism, advocates of this approach can be found in both biological sciences as well as social sciences. In cognitive science, some argue that the mind can be studied independently of the brain, whereas in sociology some defend that social facts can always be understood without studying individual psychology (Bunge, 1996, 1998).

In philosophy of mind, holism translates into dualism given that the mind—a whole—can be considered independent of the brain. Apart from Descartes's thesis, many contemporary philosophers have argued for a form of dualism. For example, in a classic essay Nagel (1974) has sustained that qualitative properties are not amenable to scientific inquiry. Similarly, Ricoeur argued in his dialogue with neurobiologist Changeux for semantic dualism because language used to describe oneself phenomenologically is betrayed by scientific investigation of the same language or concept (Changeux and Ricoeur, 2000; Nagel, 1974). Though it is not within the scope of this chapter to review differences between the various forms of dualism, when we focus more narrowly on the ethical implications of holism and its dualism counterpart, we find that if dualism is maintained, BMI enhancement could prove unproblematic. If mind is completely independent from brain, how is enhancement even possible (Moreno, 2003, p. 150)? Hence, worries for enhancement and defense of strict dualism seem incompatible. However, and unlike reductionism, this does not mean dualism cannot attend to ethical scrutiny of BMIs. Some religious and philosophical traditions based on dualism have proven to be important critical resources for the evaluation of ethical and legal issues in abortion or establishing brain death criteria. However, cultural and social issues, such as the possibility of enhancement, are framed only with difficulty within a dualist framework because enhancement recognizes the impact of brain intervention on the mind. Discussing enhancement in the context of pharmacology, Cole-Turner (1998) reports this implication of dualism:

> Some, of course, will argue that psychopharmacology or genetic alteration may affect the body or the brain but not the person as person, not the soul or the mind, not the self as a psychological dimension of being.... This view is based on some form of dualism of brain and mind or body and soul and is probably very widespread, even if its religious or philosophical antecedents have disappeared.

We come to the conclusion that such opposing positions as reductionism and holism converge on their inability to fully attend to the challenges of BMIs. Either they emphasize technical issues and threaten the value of personhood with eliminativism, or they highlight ethical issues while rejecting the possibility of a relationship between mind and brain. Thus they make BMI enhancement unintelligible and hardly amenable to analysis, if at all. Reductionism is conducive to the belief that folk psychology is false and will eventually be eliminated. Dualism does not sufficiently emphasize the specifics of brain intervention. Both are too restrictive in scope and perspective for framing cultural issues of BMIs.

4.3. Emergentism

Emergentism can be conceived as a middle ground between reductionism and holism. Emergentism states that some properties of wholes are not the properties of any of their parts and therefore knowledge of the parts is necessary but not sufficient to understand the whole (Blitz, 1992). A qualitative novelty is possible with increasing complexity of biological organization, but these novel emergent properties of the whole are not independent of their components.

This form of scientific emergentism has been defended in philosophy of biology (Blitz, 1992; Mahner and Bunge, 1997; Mayr, 1985, 1988), philosophy of mind (Bunge, 1977a, 1977b, 1980), and more implicitly by some neuroscientists (Changeux and Dehaene, 1989; Dehaene and Changeux, 1993). For example, biological life is an emergent property of cell activity, but none of the cell's organelles are living things as such (Mahner and Bunge, 1997). In the same manner, mind properties emerge from the interaction of nervous system components, but these properties do not all reduce to their components. This is in accordance with the neuroscientific hypothesis that consciousness is an integrative process stemming from the synchronization of activity of various brain regions. It is also consistent with the discovery of neural networking principles that indicate emergent properties of local brain activity. As we have seen, the success of some BMIs is in fact grounded in the existence of emergent properties of neuron population because these code for the higher order property of movement.

Accordingly, emergentism contrasts with the radical stance of holism for which mind properties are not amenable to scientific investigation. Emergentism is more in line with the commitment of reductionism to current research that shows that studying the brain is a fruitful strategy to understand the mind and its dysfunctions. However, it also provides for an understanding that certain higher level mind properties are part of our ontology and will not necessarily simply be eliminated by lower order explanation. Consequently, some content of ordinary language may be lost if we follow strong reductionist commitments. Within emergentism, BMI enhancement not only becomes intelligible, but its implications are also apparent.

Changing the brain could change us as human beings, and this challenges who we think we are. Modern neuroscience provides overwhelming evidence to support this claim. Neuropsychological observations indicate that specific functions can be impaired by brain lesions, leading to loss of inhibitory behavior, anosognosia, and even dyscalculia. Neurological and psychiatric diseases can also interfere with brain functions that lead to dramatic personality changes. Creutzfeldt-Jakob disease stems from microdamage to the brain associated with infected prion proteins. Neurodegenerative diseases like Alzheimer's disease are accompanied by profound changes in memory, language, and ultimately executive function. Some diseases are more primarily disorders of neurotransmission than neurodegeneration. For example, a common hypothesis is that schizophrenia is related to excessive dopamine neuronal activity (Cooper, Bloom, and Roth, 2003). Given the effect of pathological brain changes on the mind, the prospect of intervening on the brain with pharmacological agents or computerized devices thus brings potentially heavy consequences on personality, memory, emotional processing, or thinking, all fundamental aspects of personhood. These consequences are brought to the foreground by emergentism because it recognizes the relationship between mind and brain, and the potential impact of brain intervention on the self as a higher order property that has some ontological standing. Consequently, in this perspective, ethical discussion must be anchored in the depth of interactions between mind-level reality descriptions and brain processes. Neither dualism nor reductionism provides the grounds for analyzing this impact of BMI enhancement on humans. In this respect, emergentism is the most constructive and insightful theoretical and interpretive framework to grasp cultural and social issues of BMIs such as enhancement.

5. Two Implications of Emergentism

The emergentist framework implies an important call to attend to cultural and social issues, such as enhancement, because is sustains that higher biological levels of analysis could be changed by lower level interventions. We therefore need to extend the scope of ethical reflection by including not only scientific, ethical, and regulatory but also cultural issues.

The first implication of our emergentist analysis is to bring attention to enhancement with BMIs as a reality that we may face soon, and in which philosophical frameworks can have a significant impact on the ethical discussion. Reductionist beliefs are strong within the medical curriculum and reinforce a tendency to dismiss the importance of narratives and patient history in clinical medicine. In parallel, media accounts of neuroscience research in popular culture sometime suggest that we are our brains, that the brain is our essence, and that social practices should be informed by neuroscientific advances (Racine, Illes, and Bar-Ilan, 2005). With respect to BMIs, both this latter ambient or lay reductionism, and the former biomedical reductionism join market-driven pushes for enhancement products, possibly leading to uncritical acceptance of eventual social pressures for nontherapeutic enhancement. If we reduce individuals strictly to their brains and accordingly reject normative and cultural concerns that cannot comply with the epistemological authority of neuroscience, we will miss much in our ethical analysis of enhancement. Indeed, there is more to the ethics of cognitive enhancement than considerations of safety or efficiency. Hence, we need to move away from reductionism even if it may constitute the implicit dominant paradigm of contemporary science. In fact, part of the goal of bioethics is to overcome reductionism (Callahan, 1976). Only emergentism emphasizes the cultural consequences of BMIs and brings clear attention to their impact on issues related to personhood.

In addition to the philosophical approach of emergentism, the sheer reality of emerging neurotechnologies supports increased attention to enhancement. One study documenting the recreational use of methylphenidate (trade name Ritalin) in college students, reports that out of 283 respondents, 17 percent had taken methylphenidate for fun, and a majority of students (53 percent) knew others who had done so (Babcock and Byrne, 2000). The same study indicates that the medication is sometimes used as an aid to enhance normal function. Currently, research is ongoing on molecules that have enhancement potential (Lynch, 2002; Rose, 2002). A currently available acetylcholinesterase-inhibiting drug, donepezil (trade name Aricept), used in the treatment of Alzheimer's disease, has been reported to improve the performance of commercial aircraft pilots during flight simulation (Chatterjee, 2004). Increased understanding of the neurobiology of memory is also yielding insights into molecules that could enhance memory formation (Hall, 2003). This neurotechnological possibility of being better than well is bound to bring different philosophical and cultural perspectives to the discussion (Wolpe, 2002). Again, an emergentist outlook brings attention to the cultural consequences of BMIs or other neurotechnology and highlights these significant and pressing challenges that join a host of scientific and normative issues.

The second implication of the emergentist framework is the needed focus on the cultural and social implications of BMI enhancement. Discussions of ethical and legal issues (such as patient preferences in health care intervention) are of utmost importance. Scientific standards must also be respected for obvious reasons. Regulatory issues must clearly be addressed. However, to this we may want to add a set of cultural and social issues that include beliefs of patients and health care providers on the mind–body relationship that may be challenged by the nature of BMIs and, more specifically, by enhancement uses. Some new questions follow logically: How would BMI enhancement interact with broader cultural beliefs held by patients on self-achievement? Will cultural diversity impact our views of non-therapeutic enhancement of the brain? What are the concomitant risks and benefits? Clinical practice could bring situations along these lines where fundamental religious and cultural beliefs on the mind and the brain collide. In this respect, clarification of belief systems and basic philosophical stances may contribute to a more complete ethical analysis of neurotechnology. However, this would extend bioethical reflection, which has heavily focused on ethical and legal issues and partly left aside thicker and more reflexive cultural considerations.

Concerning the transformative powers of biotechnology on human nature, Jonas stated that our answers to such challenges will be based on our concept of what it is to be human (Jonas, 1983), clearly emphasizing the cultural dimension of such a possibility. However, another field of neuroscience, neuroimaging, illustrates the complex cultural impact of neurotechnology and offers us a glimpse at the social context in which we will make choices concerning BMIs. As a contributor to the New York Times, Stephen Hall self-reported his neuroprofiling experience to explore his own personality with functional imaging. Of interest to gain insight into the cultural impact of neuroscience here are the repeated comparisons between his personal narratives to aspects of his brain's physiology as revealed by fMRI. He concludes:

> In our age-old struggle to understand the mind, we have always been
> empowered—yet oddly constrained—by the vocabulary of the moment, be it
> the voices of the gods in ancient myth, buried conflicts in the idiom of Freudian
> analysis or associative memories in Proustian terms. But as psychology and

neuroscience begin to converge, brain imaging may provide a new, visual vocabulary with which to rethink, and perhaps reconcile, some of these older ideas on mind. (Hall, 1999)

Science certainly does not warrant all the interpretations Hall put forward. But such personal brain narratives illustrate how neuroscience interacts with wider cultural presuppositions and concerns, namely, the interaction of brain findings with cultural beliefs and our capacity for self-interpretation. Media accounts of patients undergoing experimental treatments with BMIs are readily depicted as cyborgs (Duncan, 2004), while self-experimenter of the technology Kevin Warwick has provided a literary account of his own cyborg experience (Warwick, 2004). Media portrayal of neuroimaging suggests that the brain is our essence and that pictures of the brain depict our reality, thereby reinforcing the hunger for neurotechnological innovation (Racine et al., 2005). Such accounts also suggest that cultural assumptions such as free will or individual responsibility could be challenged aggressively by neuroscience. However, some content could be left out prematurely or lost if the persuasive power of biomedical science triumphs over other belief systems (Stent, 1990). This suggests that the neuroethics of BMIs will benefit from further exploration of philosophical commitments and their relationship to ethical analysis of neurotechnology to further clarify the choices we could have to make.

6. Conclusion

BMIs can constitute groundbreaking therapeutic interventions as applications in Parkinson's disease and epilepsy illustrate. Enhancement for nonmedical uses is also a possibility, and related concerns are not unwarranted. Accordingly, we have argued that unlike reductionism and dualism, emergentism enables consideration of how neurotechnologies can change human nature. In this respect, Parens's fundamental question, "Is better always good?" (Parens, 1998), is more profound than ever. It challenges scientists, health care providers, and neuroethicists to tackle the enhancement issue from not only a scientific or normative but also a cultural point of view.

Acknowledgments

This research was supported by the Greenwall Foundation and NIH/NINDS R01 NS045831 (J.I.), and the SSHRC and FQRSC (E.R.). Thanks to Agnieszka Jaworska and Marisa Gallo for helpful comments.

NOTES

1. Our discussion is based on a strong—eliminativist—version of reductionism as proposed by Patricia and Paul Churchland. Emergentism as we define it could also be called moderate or revisionary reductionism (Bickle, 1992) but we use the terminology proposed by Bunge (1980) and Blitz (1992) for reasons that will become apparent as well as to bring to the forefront a form of multilevel scientific emergentism that has not been extensively discussed in the philosophy of mind literature.

2. BCIs, neurostimulators, and also recording electrodes (mostly used for research purposes) are grouped under the name of "cortical neural prostheses" (Schwartz, 2004).

3. Neurostimulation is sometimes distinguished from BMIs and considered an indirect BMI (Nicolelis, 2001) or variously as part of a larger class of neural prostheses (Schwartz, 2004).

4. Neurostimulation is also used outside the CNS; for example, certain forms of epilepsy are now treated by neurostimulation of the vagus nerve (Fisher and Handforth, 1999; Henry, 1998; Morris and Mueller, 1999). Some impressive advances have been in the successful implantation of motor BMIs.

5. As mostly featured in continental philosophy under the name of philosophical anthropology.

6. Lively discussions of enhancement uses of psychopharmaceuticals are also ongoing (e.g., Butcher, 2003; Farah et al., 2004; Rose, 2002; Whitehouse et al., 1997; Wolpe, 2002). For our purposes, enhancement is considered a cultural and social issue, and this explains our lengthy treatment of this set of issues.

7. There is now an international journal, *Augmented Cognition*, dedicated to research area "that has the potential to enhance human cognitive capacity and capability under complex, stressful conditions." Foreseeable applications are wide-ranging, and involvement of DARPA is extensive. For example, within the Small Business Innovation Research Program, one business is trying to develop a noninvasive recognition system. Because emotions affect the performance of individuals, the detection and classification of emotions could help eliminate mistakes they provoke. Another funded initiative aims to create high-resolution processes to identify thermal signals caused by neuronal activity associated with dishonesty (AugCog, 2004). Although these do not all constitute BMIs per se, they are in the range of human–computer interface and illustrate how the appeal of enhancement can be strong in the real-world setting.

8. We use three of David Blitz's description of five philosophies of biology (reductionism, mechanism, emergentism, organicism, and holism) (Blitz, 1992). We judge reductionism, holism, and emergentism to be the three most relevant for the purpose of this neuroethics discussion because they have been most extensively argued and can relate to our discussion.

REFERENCES

AugCog. (2004). New phase one small business innovative research. *AugCog International Quarterly* 2: 6–7.

Babcock, Q., and Byrne, T. (2000). Student perceptions of methylphenidate abuse at a public liberal arts college. *Journal of American College Health* 49: 143–145.

Bickle, J. (1992). Revisionary physicalism. *Biology and Philosophy* 7: 411–430.

Birbaumer, N., Ghanayim, N., Hinterberger, T., Iversen, I., Kotchoubey, B., Kubler, A., et al. (1999). A spelling device for the paralysed. *Nature* 398: 297–298.

Birch, G. E., Bozorgzadeh, Z., and Mason, G. S. (2002). Initial on-line evaluations of the LF-ASD brain-computer interface with able-bodied and spinal-cord subjects using imagined voluntary motor potentials. *IEEE Transactions on Neural Systems and Rehabilitation Engineering* 10: 219–224.

Blank, R. H. (1999). *Brain Policy: How the New Neuroscience Will Change Our Lives and Our Politics*. Washington, D.C.: Georgetown University Press.

Blitz, D. (1992). *Emergent Evolution: Qualitative Novelty and the Levels of Reality*. Boston: Kluwer Academic Press.

Bunge, M. (1977a). Emergence and the mind. *Neuroscience* 2: 501–509.

Bunge, M. (1977b). Levels and reduction. *American Journal of Physiology* 233: R75–R82.

Bunge, M. (1980). *The Mind-Body Problem: A Psychobiological Approach*. Oxford: Pergamon Press.

Bunge, M. (1996). *Finding Philosophy in Social Science*. New Haven, Conn.: Yale University Press.

Bunge, M. (1998). *Social Science under Debate: A Philosophical Perspective*. Toronto/Buffalo: University of Toronto Press.

Butcher, J. (2003). Cognitive enhancement raises ethical concerns. *Lancet* 362: 132–133.

Callahan, D. (1976). Bioethics as a discipline. In J. Humber and R. F. Almeder (Eds.), *Biomedical Ethics and the Law*. New York: Plenum Press, 1–11.

Caplan, A. L. (2003). Is better best? *Scientific American*, September, 104–105.

Changeux, J.-P., and Dehaene, S. (1989). Neuronal models of cognitive functions. *Cognition* 33: 63–109.

Changeux, J.-P., and Ricoeur, P. (2000). *Ce qui nous fait penser: La nature et la règle*. Paris: Odile Jacob.

Chapin, J. K. (2000). Neural prosthetic devices for quadriplegia. *Current Opinion in Neurology* 13: 671–675.

Chapin, J. K., Moxon, K. A., Markowitz, R. S. and Nicolelis, M. A. (1999). Real-time control of a robot arm using simultaneously recorded neurons in the motor cortex. *Nature Neuroscience* 2: 664–670.

Chatterjee, A. (2004). Cosmetic neurology: The controversy over enhancing movement, mentation, and mood. *Neurology* 63: 968–974.

Churchland, P. M. (1981). Eliminative materialism and the propositional attitudes. *Journal of Philosophy* 77: 67–90.

Churchland, P. M. (1989). *A Neurocomputational Perspective: The Nature of Mind and the Structure of Science*. Cambridge, Mass.: Bradford Books/MIT Press.

Churchland, P. M. (1995). *The Engine of Reason, the Seat of the Soul: A Philosophical Journey into the Brain*. Cambridge, Mass.: Bradford Books/MIT Press.

Churchland, P. S. (1986). *Neurophilosophy: Toward a Unified Science of the Mind-Brain*. Cambridge, Mass.: Bradford Books/MIT Press.

Cole-Turner, R. (1998). Do means matter? In E. Parens (Ed.), *Enhancing Human Traits: Ethical and Social Implications*. Washington, D.C.: Georgetown University Press, 151–160.

Cooper, J. R., Bloom, F. E., and Roth, R. H. (2003). *The Biochemical Basis of Neuropharmacology*. Oxford: Oxford University Press.

Crick, F. (1995). *The Astonishing Hypothesis: The Scientific Search for the Soul*. London: Simon and Schuster.

Dees, R. H. (2004). Slippery slopes, wonder drugs, and cosmetic neurology: The neuroethics of enhancement. *Neurology* 63: 951–952.

Dehaene, S., and Changeux, J.-P. (1993). Pensée logico-mathématique et modèles neuronaux des fonctions cognitives. L'exemple des capacités numériques. In Q. Houdé and D. Miéville (Eds.), *Pensée logico-mathématique: Nouveaux objets interdisciplinaires.* Paris: PUF, 123–146.

Diefenbach, G. J., Diefenbach, D., Baumeister, A., and West, M. (1999). Portrayal of lobotomy in the popular press: 1935–1960. *Journal of the History of the Neurosciences* 8: 60–69.

Donoghue, J. P. (2002). Connecting cortex to machines: Recent advances in brain interfaces. *Nature Neuroscience* 5: 1085–1088.

Duncan, D. E. (2004). Paraplegic fitted with brain sensor ushers in cybernetic age. *San Francisco Chronicle*, December 5, B1 and B6.

Emory University. (1998). Emory neuroscientists use computer chip to help speech-impaired patients communicate. Available at: whsc.emory.edu/_releases/1998october/101398bakay.html.

Engelhardt, H. T. (1996). *The Foundations of Bioethics.* New York: Oxford University Press.

Farah, M. J., Illes, J., Cook-Deegan, R., Gardner, H., Kandel, E., King, P., et al. (2004). Neurocognitive enhancement: What can we do and what should we do? *Nature Reviews Neuroscience* 5: 421–425.

Fisher, R. S., and Handforth, A. (1999). Reassessment: Vagus nerve stimulation for epilepsy. *Neurology* 53: 666–669.

Georgopoulos, A. P., Schwartz, A. B., and Kettner, R. E. (1986). Neuronal population coding of movement direction. *Science* 233: 1416–1419.

Hall, S. S. (1999). Journey to the center of my mind. *New York Times*, June 6, 122.

Hall, S. S. (2003). The quest for a smart pill. *Scientific American* 289: 54–65.

Hauser, S. L. (2004). The shape of things to come. *Neurology* 63: 948–950.

Henry, T. R. (1998). Most commonly asked questions about vagus nerve stimulation for epilepsy. *Neurologist* 4: 284–289.

Hetling, J. R., and Baig-Silva, M. S. (2004). Neural prostheses for vision: Designing a functional interface with retinal neurons. *Neurological Research* 26: 21–34.

Hoag, H. (2003). Neuroengineering: Remote control. *Nature* 423: 796–798.

Illes, J., and Racine, E. (2005). Imaging or imagining? A neuroethics challenge informed by genetics. *American Journal of Bioethics* 5: 5–18.

Jonas, H. (1983). *The Imperative of Responsibility: In Search of an Ethics for the Technological Age.* Chicago: University of Chicago Press.

Jonsen, A. R., Siegler, M., and Winslade, W. T. (1998). *Clinical Ethics: A Practical Approach to Ethical Decision in Clinical Medicine.* New York: McGraw-Hill.

Kennedy, P. R., and Bakay, R. A. (1998). Restoration of neural output from a paralyzed patient by a direct brain connection. *Neuroreport* 9: 1707–1711.

Lynch, G. (2002). Memory enhancement: The search for mechanism-based drugs. *Nature Neuroscience* 5 (supplement): 1035–1038.

Maguire, G. Q., and McGee, E. M. (1999). Implantable brain chips? Time for debate. *Hastings Center Report* 29: 7–13.

Mahner, M., and Bunge, M. (1997). *Foundations of Biophilosophy.* New York: Springer.

Mayr, E. (1985). How biology differs from the physical sciences? In D. J. Dephew and B. H. Weber (Eds.), *Evolution at the Crossroads: The New Biology and the New Philosophy of Science.* Cambridge, Mass.: MIT Press, 43–63.

Mayr, E. (1988). *Toward a New Philosophy of Biology.* Cambridge, Mass.: Harvard University Press.

Millan Jdel, R., Renkens, F., Mourino, J., and Gerstner, W. (2004). Noninvasive brain-actuated control of a mobile robot by human EEG. *IEEE Transactions on Biomedical Engineering* 51: 1026–1033.

Moreno, J. D. (2003). Neuroethics: An agenda for neuroscience and society. *Nature Reviews Neuroscience* 4: 149–153.

Morris, G. L., and Mueller, W. M. (1999). Long-term treatment with vagus nerve stimulation in patients with refractory epilepsy. *Neurology* 53: 1731–1755.

Musallam, S., Corneil, B. D., Greger, B., Scherberger, H., and Andersen, R. A. (2004). Cognitive control signals for neural prosthetics. *Science* 305: 258–262.

Mussa-Ivaldi, F. A., and Miller, L. E. (2003). Brain-machine interfaces: computational demands and clinical needs meet basic neuroscience. *Trends in Neuroscience* 26: 329–334.

Nagel, T. (1974). What is it like to be a bat? *Philosophical Review* 83: 435–450.

Nicolelis, M. A. (2001). Actions from thoughts. *Nature* 409: 403–407.

Nicolelis, M. A. (2003). Brain-machine interfaces to restore motor function and probe neural circuits. *Nature Reviews Neuroscience* 4: 417–422.

Parens, E. (1998). Is better always good? In E. Parens (Ed.), *Enhancing Human Traits: Ethical and Social Implications.* Washington, D.C.: Georgetown University Press, 1–28.

Prochazka, A., Mushahwar, V. K., and McCreery, D. B. (2001). Neural prostheses. *Journal of Physiology* 533: 99–109.

Racine, E. (2002). Thérapie ou amélioration? Philosophie des neurosciences et éthique des neurotechnologies. *Ethica* 14: 70–100.

Racine, E., Illes, J., and Bar-Ilan, O. (2005). fMRI in the public eye. *Nature Reviews Neuroscience* 6: 159–164.

Rorty, R. (1965). Mind-body identity, privacy, and categories. *Review of Metaphysics* 19: 24–54.

Rose, S. P. (2002). "Smart drugs": Do they work? Are they ethical? Will they be legal? *Nature Reviews Neuroscience* 3: 975–979.

Sahakian, B., and Morein-Zamir, S. (2007). Professor's little helper. *Nature* 450(7): 1157–1159.

Sanchez, J. C., Carmena, J. M., Lebedev, M. A., Nicolelis, M. A., Harris, J. G., and Principe, J. C. (2004). Ascertaining the importance of neurons to develop better brain-machine interfaces. *IEEE Transactions on Biomedical Engineering* 51: 943–953.

Schwartz, A. B. (2004). Cortical neural prosthetics. *Annual Review of Neuroscience* 27: 487–507.

Serruya, M. D., Hatsopoulos, N. G., Paninski, L., Fellows, M. R., and Donoghue, J. P. (2002). Instant neural control of a movement signal. *Nature* 416: 141–142.

Servos, P., Engel, S. A., Gati, J., and Menon, R. (1999). fMRI evidence for an inverted face representation in human somatosensory cortex. *Neuroreport* 10: 1393–1395.

Stent, G. S. (1990). The poverty of neurophilosophy. *Journal of Medicine and Philosophy* 15: 539–557.

Talwar, S. K., Xu, S., Hawley, E. S., Weiss, S. A., Moxon, K. A., and Chapin, J. K. (2002). Rat navigation guided by remote control. *Nature* 417: 37–38.

Toulmin, S. (1982). How medicine saved the life of ethics. *Perspectives in Biology and Medicine* 25: 736–750.

Vincent, J.-D. (1996). Ethics and neuroscience. In International Bioethics Committee of UNESCO (Eds.), *Proceedings: Third Session*, 1–8.

Warwick, K. (2000). Becoming one with your computer. Available online at www.wired.com/wired/archive/8.02/warwick_pr.html.

Warwick, K. (2004). *I, Cyborg.* Chicago: University of Illinois Press.

Wessberg, J., Stambaugh, C. R., Kralik, J. D., Beck, P. D., Laubach, M., Chapin, J. K., et al. (2000). Real-time prediction of hand trajectory by ensembles of cortical neurons in primates. *Nature* 408: 361–365.

White, R. J. (1999). Brain chips: postpone the debate. *Hastings Center Report* 29: 4.

Whitehouse, P. J., Juengst, E., Mehlman, M., and Murray, T. H. (1997). Enhancing cognition in the intellectually intact. *Hastings Center Report* 27: 14–22.

Wickelgren, I. (2003). Neuroscience: Tapping the mind. *Science* 299: 496–499.

Wolpe, P. R. (2002). Treatment, enhancement, and the ethics of neurotherapeutics. *Brain and Cognition* 50: 387–395.

CHAPTER 18

WHAT'S "NEU"
IN NEUROETHICS?

ADINA L. ROSKIES

THERE has been considerable skepticism among bioethicists regarding whether neuroethics ought to be recognized as a subfield of the discipline. Presumably, the main issue is whether neuroscience raises new ethical questions, or presents them in a novel enough light, to justify distinguishing neuroethics from bioethics more generally. In other words, do the questions raised by neuroethics differ substantially from those raised by other fields in bioethics? Genetics may be the best example we have of a science that has raised novel philosophical issues in virtue of scientific insights and powerful new technologies. The ethics of genetics is reified by the name *genethics*. Does the ethics of neuroscience deserve the same? Some may contend that any philosophical terra nova that can conceivably be staked out by biological disciplines has already been staked out by genethics, thus obviating the need for a new bioethical discipline. This is not so. Elsewhere I argue that neuroethics comprises not only the ethics of neuroscience but also the neuroscience of ethics (Roskies, 2002), which makes it unique among bioethical fields. This essay highlights some of the more exciting ethical issues raised by neuroscience, illustrating the way some philosophical issues are new or newly framed by neuroethics. My hope is that this brief survey will justify treating neuroethics as at least a distinctive subdiscipline of bioethics.

I begin with a few caveats. My argument is not intended to deny or downplay the obvious truth that the territory of neuroethics largely overlaps with that of genethics. Moreover, I wholeheartedly endorse the claim that neuroethics can and should look to previous work on shared questions for guidance and insight. It would be a mistake for neuroethicists to ignore or discount a rich body of relevant ethical thought merely because it treats of genes rather than brains. Examples of questions that are common to genethics and neuroethics are the ethics of access, including issues of consent, who can obtain information about a person's genome or brain, and what information they can have access to; the social implications of the misuses of that information; questions of distributive justice; questions about how to handle probabilistic or statistical information about future health; and the vexing question of how to conceptualize and identify pathology and normality. These issues have all been addressed by genethics as well as other areas of applied bioethics (Illes and Racine, 2005). Although addressing these same issues in the context of neuroscience may prompt us to think about them somewhat differently, the resulting analysis will likely be rather consistent with previous thought. However, in what follows I focus on questions that I think are unique to neuroethics.[1] I begin with a brief discussion about our understanding of the role of the brain that motivates the intuition that neuroscience raises novel ethical issues.

1. WE ARE OUR BRAINS

In the early days of the genetic revolution, the relation between genetic sequence and phenotype was thought to be relatively straightforward, and the idea that "we are our genes" seemed to reflect a simple truth. This idea has persisted in some form even to the present. For instance, Burley and Harris, in *The Companion to Genethics* write, "Because so much about us is determined or influenced by genes, they have come to have a special role in our understanding of, and indeed our feelings about, ourselves and our sense of own uniqueness. In this role genes have replaced the previous contenders for this special place, the heart, and more recently, the brain" (2002, p. 3). The sentiments expressed in this quotation illustrate the commonly held idea that what makes us who we are is our genetic makeup. However, I believe Burley and Harris overstate the role played by genes in our sense of ourselves and err in thinking that genes are more central to our self-conception than is the brain.

Call the view that we would be different people if we had different genes "genetic essentialism." It is debatable, but not clearly false that no one could be quite the person they are without the genetic sequence they have: In that sense, genes may be an important element of our identity. However, genetic essentialism should be distinguished from a related view, also implicit in the quote: the view that our genes *determine* the person we are. This idea, genetic determinism, is deeply mistaken. Our genes do not determine who or what we are, we now know, for the complex interactions between genes, regulatory mechanisms, and environment in determining phenotype defy any straightforward mapping from genetic makeup to outcome. It may be more accurate to think of genes as defining a space of potentialities for an organism: the range of phenotypes that could result under different environments and different background conditions. That range may be broad indeed, for widely different phenotypes can result from the very same genotype. For example, research on polymorphisms in the serotonin transporter nicely illustrates the dependence of phenotype on both genes and environment. In one study (Barr et al., 2003), macaque monkeys heterozygous for the short form of the serotonin transporter allele and those with two copies of the long form were either raised normally or deprived of maternal care as infants. The study found that heterozygous and homozygous animals raised by their mothers showed no differences in levels of aggression. In contrast, heterozygous animals with maternal deprivation displayed much higher levels of aggression, whereas similarly raised animals homozygous for the long allele did not. Abundant evidence about gene–environment interactions such as these confirms the falsity of genetic determinism. (Indeed, because of its persistence in the face of its falsity it is often referred to as "the myth of genetic determinism.") To the extent that the idea that we are our genes is rooted in the idea of genetic determinism, it is also mistaken.

We may not be our genes, but are we our brains? The brain seems to have supplanted the gene as the new candidate for that which determines who we are, and indeed, the connection between our brains and our selves appears to be more robust. In a rather direct way, our mental lives and behavior are a result of the functioning of our brains. In addition, there is a widely shared intuition that our personal identity depends in some essential way on psychological characteristics (such as temperament, memories, etc.; see, e.g., Locke, [1694] 1975; Parfit, 1986). Our psychological characteristics are rooted in the way our nervous system functions, and this provides additional reason to think that we are our brains. Neuroscience is devoted to exploring how the brain works, and cognitive neuroscience the biological basis of the mental. It is no longer incredible to think we might come to understand the physiological basis of many aspects of ourselves most closely associated with who we are. If so, these sciences are bound to raise novel philosophical issues.

Because neuroscience and genetics have so many parallels in terms of the ethical issues each raise, it is fair to ask how far the parallels go. Recent work in genetics tells us that genetic determinism is false. Will learning about the brain show us that the idea that we are our brains is likewise mistaken? Will the myth of genetic determinism be paralleled by a myth of neural determinism? Although it is difficult to predict what the future will hold, it is harder to see a parallel development here. In most cases, our genes alone do not ensure the presence of certain diseases or mandate the exact phenotypic trait we manifest. The genetic sequence is usually causally far removed from the phenotypic outcome. Not so with the brain. In general, brain events cause other brain events and behaviors, and the operations of the nervous system are causally proximate to the behavior, with few intervening processes. Granted, we may come to understand the dispositional capacities of the brain on behavior as well as the occurrent ones, and realize that in addition to direct causal control of our behaviors, brains also have indirect effects. Even so, it does seem that if one traces a causal path from genes through to behavior, the brain events are much more proximal to behaviors than are details of the genetic code. It is unlikely that science will overthrow the view that it has heretofore upheld—that the brain is the organ that controls behavior and mental life. Moreover, insofar as we believe that personal identity (both in the senses of numerical identity and what we psychologically and emotionally identify with) depends on psychological aspects of the person, we have support for the idea that we are our brains. Even a straightforward body criterion of personal identity seems to admit a close connection between the brain and the person, for the brain is one of the major bodily organs.

These remarks are meant to make plausible the intuition that we are our brains, or very nearly so. One open question involves spelling out in more scientific and philosophical detail what this means. But this chapter is more focused on exploring some of the consequences of this view. In the rest of the chapter, I combat the claim that neuroethics raises no new issues for bioethics mainly by suggestive counterexample. I briefly discuss four topics that I think raise interesting and novel ethical problems: consciousness; the self and personhood; decision making, control, and free will; and understanding moral cognition. My goal is not to defend any particular views but to illustrate areas in which I expect future work to prompt novel neuroethical thought.

2. Consciousness

Consciousness is perhaps the greatest mystery in science: How is it that a 3-pound mass of tissue can give rise to the thing we call consciousness, awareness, or a subject of experience? How can a collection of relatively simple (albeit highly organized) physical components make it possible to experience pain or have an experience of that particular shade of red or the ephemeral smell of a fine burgundy? So far, both science and philosophy have been stymied by this problem, and it would be folly for me to suggest that neuroscience is on the verge of answering it. But to understand this mystery remains an aspiration of many neuroscientists, and it does seem that if any scientific enterprise is to shed light on the question of consciousness, it will be the brain sciences.

Our inability to conceptualize how such a thing as consciousness can arise from brain activity has been offered as an argument against materialism (Chalmers, 1996), but other philosophers instead suggest that such reasoning is mistaken, and the inability to conceive of how consciousness could arise from mere matter merely reflects the poverty of our current understanding of brain function (Stoljar, 2006). The question of consciousness has primarily been and remains a philosophical question, but it is now inescapably also a scientific one. Neuroscience is increasingly in a position to address the questions "What is consciousness?" and "How is consciousness possible?" When we find organisms we think possess consciousness, we can now investigate the physical basis for being in such a state. Nevertheless, specifying what the hallmarks of consciousness are, when we are entitled to attribute it to other beings, and what sorts of rights or considerations having it entails remain philosophical endeavors. Therefore, determining what consciousness is and what has the property of being conscious should be thought of as a joint project between philosophy and neuroscience. Among the questions raised by this joint enterprise are ethical questions. The demystification of consciousness, if it occurs, will almost certainly affect how we think of ourselves, may impact on religious beliefs, and will likely have ramifications for how we understand our place in the natural world and the place of other organisms.

Realistically speaking, such a scenario is far in the future, if it is in the future at all. We must not thereby conclude that the issue of consciousness has no bearing on ethics in the short to medium term. Long before the problem of consciousness is solved there will be related questions that arise in ethics associated with various degrees of understanding consciousness. For instance, for the time being, neuroscientists have been working to find the neural correlates of consciousness (Crick, 1995; Dehaene, 2001; Koch, 2004). Significant advances have been made in that area, but we should not forget that this scientific project is always hostage to our philosophical commitments.

Let us consider one case in which our views on consciousness have immediate ethical implications. Severe brain trauma can leave a person in impaired states of consciousness, such as the minimally conscious state (MCS) or the persistent vegetative state (PVS). It is estimated that there are 112,000–280,000 MCS patients and 14,000–35,000 PVS patients in the United States alone (Steinberg, 2005). Though these patients groups differ subtly in degree of damage, both groups are characterized by a lack of awareness of self and environment, as assessed by their ability to respond to a variety of stimuli. In PVS, though basic functions like sleep–wake cycles and respiration remain intact, higher cognitive functions are not in evidence. The financial and emotional costs of preserving the life of someone in a vegetative state are considerable, and there are excellent arguments for terminating life support if these people are not conscious and will never again regain consciousness. If they are aware, commonsense morality speaks against removing life support, but if they are unaware, what to do remains tendentious. Views on these matters are deeply held and often accompanied by a quasi-religious zeal, as the public furor over the Terri Schiavo case illustrated. In past cases, such as Schiavo's, decisions were made based on opinion and wishful thinking, not fact. With a growing neuroscientific understanding of consciousness, future decisions may be far more informed. What can neuroscience tell us about the conscious state of brain-damaged individuals who are verbally and physically unresponsive?

Some inroads have recently been made in determining these patients' states of consciousness, but not without generating controversy and public misconception. Schiff et al. (2005) used functional magnetic resonance imaging (fMRI) to scan two patients in MCS while reading them personalized narratives and the same speech streams presented in a time-reversed fashion. The two MCS patients demonstrated increased activity to personal narratives in brain areas comparable to those of a normal control group (in response to emotionally neutral speech, not these personalized narratives), despite their decreased resting brain metabolic level. However, they showed reduced response to the time-reversed, meaningless stimuli compared to controls. Schiff et al. (2005) concluded that these patients had preserved functional networks for processing speech and meaning, and speculated that these could be involved in awareness.

The Schiff et al. (2005) publication received a lot of press, in part due to its appearance at the height of the Terri Schiavo controversy. Some heralded it as evidence that Schiavo was in fact conscious and should have been saved (despite the fact that she was in a PVS, not MCS, and despite the fact that these were single case studies, from which generalizations to an entire population would be unwarranted). Those who lobbied for Schiavo's continued maintenance regarded this study as vindication for their views. However, the implications of the Schiff et al. paper are far from clear, and the results were misunderstood and misused, in part for political gain and in part because of a lack of public understanding of what the relevant factors are for such a study.

One can conclude from the study that in these two MCS patients, widely distributed areas of neural tissue remained viable and connected to their normal input faculties, and were capable of similar gross patterns of processing as in normal brains. These findings were not surprising when one considers that these patients demonstrated occasional awareness of environment and the ability to respond to verbal stimulation. However, demonstrating the integrity of some regions of neural tissue is a far cry from demonstrating the integrity of a neural system capable of sustaining complex cognitive functions. Furthermore, a number of factors make the experimental results difficult to interpret functionally. For example, MCS patients displayed differentially reduced responses to reversed speech compared to normals. More important, the implication that response of brain areas to verbal stimuli indicates comprehension or consciousness is misleading. We know that quite a bit of neural processing goes on in the processing of verbal stimuli in the absence of awareness, in many of the same brain areas that are employed during conscious processing of verbal stimuli. For example, priming studies use presentation of stimuli of which the subject is unaware, but many higher order processes can be affected by the prime nonetheless (Dehaene et al., 2001; Dehaene et al., 1998; Naccache and Dehaene, 2001).

Because priming is paradigmatically unconscious, yet priming stimuli activate many of the same areas as stimuli of which a subject is aware, it is evident that merely documenting neural activity in the same brain areas as a control group provided with similar stimuli fails to indicate anything in particular about the cognitive status of the agent. All we can conclude from studies like this one is that some MCS patients retain enough viable neural tissue in distributed networks to show activation on an fMRI scan, with sufficient preserved connectivity to result in more or less normal-looking activation patterns at the macroscopic level. Importantly, these methods provide no particular information about the health or normalcy of the local networks in those regions.

One might be tempted to conclude from this story that the contributions neuroscience can make to this issue are so limited as to be uninteresting, but this would be too hasty an inference. With appropriate creativity and care, headway can be made on this difficult problem. Several studies indicate that frontal and parietal activations are reliably correlated with conscious perception (see, e.g., Dehaene, Changeaux, Naccache, Sackur, and Sergent, 2006). Additionally, in a recent short paper, Adrian Owen and colleagues provided much clearer evidence for awareness in a severely brain-damaged patient (Owen et al., 2006). Like Schiff et al. (2005), Owen and colleagues used functional neuroimaging on a patient that had been in a PVS for 5 months. They reported that the patient showed activity in the normal range in a network of brain areas in response to verbal stimulation, despite the fact that the patient was entirely unresponsive to verbal commands. However, Owen et al. recognized the illegitimacy of drawing conclusions about the patient's conscious state from this data, noting the extensive neural processing that can take place in response to verbal stimuli in the absence of awareness (Dehaene et al., 2001; Kotz, Cappa, von Cramon, and Friederici, 2002; Portas, 2000; Rissman, Eliassen, and Blumstein, 2003). They thus conducted a second experiment in which the patient was given verbal instructions to imagine herself playing tennis or imagine herself navigating through her house. Rather unexpectedly, the patient showed sustained activation of brain areas involved in motor imagery when asked to imagine playing tennis and in other regions involved in navigation when asked to imagine walking through her house. The regions activated overlapped with those activated during the same two tasks in a group of control subjects.

The beauty of this experiment is that it helps deconfound the factors of neural activity and awareness. By asking the patient to do two different cognitively demanding tasks, neither of which require a motor response and each of which has a neural signature distinct from the other, Owen and colleagues provided the best evidence we have yet that a physically unresponsive patient can still comprehend verbal instructions and act differentially in response to them. The fact that the activations were prolonged suggested that they were not stimulus-bound automatic processes. This study suggests that the patient was indeed conscious and retained a power of volition or intention. In this case, the inference that the patient was aware of the meaning of the commands and could respond appropriately seems warranted.

The implications of this study are staggering, not merely for the prospects for understanding what is and is not relevant to consciousness but also for future decisions regarding the treatment of brain-damaged patients. In this case, imaging provides the potential of a window into the state of consciousness of a patient unable to outwardly respond. It is easy to imagine how one might extend these studies not only to determine which patients have some awareness of their environment but also to communicate with people who retain some awareness and volition but cannot express themselves verbally or with bodily movements. For example, if indeed this patient in a vegetative state is mentally aware and able to comprehend and cognize, we can prompt her to associate different types of imagery with "yes" and "no" responses, and we can use neuroimaging to monitor the different patterns of brain activity in response to questions to understand her desires. Doing this will enable us to significantly improve the quality of these patients' lives and, perhaps most important, respect their autonomy by endowing them with the ability to choose if and when to end theirs.

3. Personhood and the Self

One standard philosophical move is to argue that what decisions to make about how to treat other beings (e.g., MCS and PVS patients) may depend in part on their status as persons. What is a person? Over the years, philosophers have given varied and conflicting accounts of what a person is, what (if any) are its essential characteristics, what makes a person the same person over time. Recently, some neuroscientists have considered whether there is any coherent concept of person at all. Farah and Heberlein (2007) argue that the philosophical problems involved in determining what a person is suggest that "person" is not a natural kind at all. They consider the option of trying to naturalize the concept by looking at what sorts of neural processes go into recognizing things as persons, with the reasoning that perhaps by understanding how we determine which things are persons and which aren't, we can understand what persons are. Although they ultimately conclude that the goal of naturalizing personhood is misconceived, the findings they report and their conclusions are interesting.

On the basis of evidence compiled from a large number of studies, Farah and Heberlein (2007) argue that there are two different, largely separate systems of brain regions involved in identifying people. One system responds to superficial stimuli like eyes and faces, seemingly goal-directed or self-induced actions, and the like. This system is innate, automatic, and yields binary (yes/no) judgments about whether something is a person. A separate nonspecialized system (or systems), presumably for recognizing objects in general, also recognizes people, in part by recognizing many of the more abstract qualities we take persons to have. Many of those qualities come in degrees: Things can be more or less person-like. This system can yield graded judgments of personhood, just as it can yield graded judgments about furniture, vehicles, and so on. In our evolutionary past, Farah and Heberlein (2007) conjecture, things that were person-like had qualities that would lead to congruent judgments in both systems, but in today's world there are cases that are more ambiguous: There are machines that evince goal-directed behavior, and people who are biologically alive but lack the ability to respond flexibly to stimuli, such as the brain-damaged people already discussed. They surmise that it is the incongruent responses of these two systems that leads to the conflicting intuitions in hard cases of personhood, and that also underlies the difficulties we find with conceptual clarity regarding personhood.

It is too soon to say whether this picture of the neural basis of person-recognition is correct. But what if it is? Farah and Heberlein (2007) draw strong conclusions from their study: They argue that the difficulties in spelling out the concept of personhood and the conflicts between our systems for identifying persons argue for an abandonment of the concept in our theoretical approaches to ethics, but they accede that we cannot escape the workings of our biological endowment that are called on in everyday interactions with others. They urge us to jettison the concept for ethics and instead to pursue a utilitarian ethics, one not predicated on "personhood" at all, while accepting our judgments for the purposes of ordinary life. I don't think this is feasible or advisable. First, any ethical theory we have has to have some domain, and in the past we have used persons to delineate the proper domain of our theories. Whether utilitarian or deontological, we have to determine the boundaries of our ethical theories, and some rather ill-defined concept, whether persons or something else, will need to be invoked. I do not think the concept is expendable. Second, recognizing the nature of the two systems for person recognition might give us some insight into how we view person-judgments, and alter the importance we put on them, but not in the ways they suggest.

According to Farah and Heberlein (2007), the first system, evolutionarily older, operates on superficial characteristics and yields quick binary responses; the second is more recently evolved, involves deliberation and complex cognitive processing, and yields graded responses. Their suggestion, therefore, amounts to accepting the operation of the first system but rejecting the dictates of the second. However, I think it can be argued that ideally a concept like personhood is rather abstract and sophisticated, and so our considered judgments and not our primitive reactions should prevail in determining what is and is not a person (Roskies, 2007, and other commentaries in the same volume). Thus, if anything, we should welcome a nuanced concept of personhood in ethics and pay more attention to the deliverances of the graded system; at the same time, we should be more skeptical of the outputs of the binary system. Thus, rather than excising the concept from our moral deliberations but keeping them for everyday purposes, we ought to be less prone to rely on our judgments in everyday, knee-jerk types of situations and more likely to question them. Furthermore, I suggest that a more refined abstract notion of personhood will only improve our ethical thought, not hopelessly mire it in confusion.

There are connections to be drawn between personhood and consciousness. Some think that persons are conscious (or potentially conscious) beings; others think that in addition to consciousness, persons must be self-conscious. Certainly normal humans are endowed with is a sense of self: We represent ourselves as distinct, continuant beings with persisting beliefs, desires, life hopes, projects, and so on. But what is the self? This is a traditional philosophical question. Is the self a substance, a process, an illusion? Neuroscience can approach questions about the self a little more obliquely, but perhaps quite fruitfully. It is likely that self-representation is one aspect of self-consciousness. Neuroscientists have begun to investigate the nature of self-representation: What is our conception of self (or, less abstractly, of ourselves), and how does it play a role in cognition? How do we represent the bodily self, or the mental self? How are various aspects of self-representation integrated? What happens when they fail to be properly integrated or are deficient, as occurs in some delusions? What differences are involved in representation of self and representations of others? The hope is that inquiry in this area combined with techniques used to investigate the basis of awareness will help elucidate the relation between consciousness and personhood.

Other beings share certain aspects of self-representation, but there is debate as to whether they are self-conscious. Although neuroscience has yet to reveal deep truths about these matters, the sort of understanding of self-representation and self-consciousness that neuroscience may eventually provide will likely impact both our view of personhood, as well as various other ethical views. For instance, it may cause us to reconsider the role the concept of the self does or should play in free choice, deliberations about moral status, determining ethical priorities, and so on. Even if it doesn't, if we think moral consideration should be afforded to beings that are self-conscious and self-concerned, and we find evidence that some other animals have the properties that we think underlie self-consciousness, we may modify our views about how they ought to be treated. It is also probable that our concept of self is connected in interesting ways to concepts such as free will, which is the next topic.

4. DECISION MAKING, CONTROL, AND FREE WILL

Although the issues of free will and determinism have been visited in genethics, genetics has raised the issue of freedom in the face of a certain kind of determinism: genetic determinism. But two factors make the challenge to free will from genetics a lame one. First, genetic determinism is a deeply mistaken view, and second, our genes are causally far removed from our behaviors. Thus, beyond raising the question, genethics has not contributed much insight to discussions about free will.

The brain, on the other hand, poses a more potent challenge to freedom of the will, because unlike genetics, the relation of brain to behavior is, on the face of it, subject to neither of the two mitigating factors. The brain is the proximate cause of our bodily movements, intentional actions, feelings, reactions, and the like. In some very tangible sense, we act as we do because of how our brain works, and there are few intervening variables between neural activity and our behaviors. Although it may be philosophically confused to ask for *the* cause of a person's behavior, brain activity meets the standard philosophical tests for a cause of our behaviors, and one of the most direct ones at that.

When we think of free will we typically think of the ability to freely make decisions. Recent work on the neurobiology of decision making (in monkeys) has shown that neural activity during decision making in perceptual tasks can be interpreted as reflecting the accumulation of evidence by neuronal populations representing alternative hypotheses. These neural data can be mathematically modeled, and the outcomes of the decision process predicted on that basis (Kim and Shadlen, 1999;

Leon and Shadlen, 1999; Mazurek, Roitman, Ditterich, and Shadlen, 2003). This research is consistent with the view that decision making obeys purely mechanistic rules for determining outcome, further strengthening the view that brains are just complicated biological machines. There is no reason to think human brains work differently. That strengthens the worry: If the brain is just mechanism, can we have free will?

Because of its causal proximity to behavior, what our brains do does determine, to a large extent, what our bodies do. Neural firing, coupled with facts about our bodies, for example, determines how we swing the bat, with what force, and what timing. (However, it does not determine whether we hit the ball—that depends on how our movements interact with the world: what trajectory the ball takes, how heavy the bat is, and so on. So we must be careful when we talk about how brains "determine" behavior.) It seems that if we know enough about how the brain works and know its input and current state, in principle we could predict its output. Most neuroscientists, and scientists in general, assume that all the relevant elements for understanding the operation of a biological system are those ordained by physics: There is no spooky stuff. If the brain is purely a physical mechanism, if there is no spooky stuff, and if the brain causes our behavior, then we are left with the uncomfortable conclusion that all our actions, choices, and decisions are due to the purely mechanistic functioning of the brain: Like a complicated 3-pound machine, it makes us do what the laws of physics and the structure of the mechanism determine we will do. There is no room in this picture for volition, let alone freedom.

One obvious response to this scenario is that there is room for volition, just as there is room for the self or subject of experience in a materialistic world. Volition is some (still not understood) function of brain structure and activity, due (let's speculate and oversimplify) to the operation of some subset of neurons in frontal areas interacting with representations of how the world is and how we want the world to be. If so, the will can coexist with the brain. But what of freedom? Here things get tricky, for we have to be clear about what we mean by freedom. It may be tempting to argue that "I can't be free, because if my will is caused by my brain then it is not caused by me: My brain is controlling me." However, this seems confused because in some sense (perhaps one to be specified by further research on the nature of the self) I am my brain, so if my brain is governing the behavior of my body then I am doing so. However, this will appease few people worried about freedom, for then I am the mechanism, and thus I am not free: Given the truths about my brain and the laws of physics I could not have done other than I do. I am not free.

These musings may indicate that the challenge to free will from neuroscience is more pressing than it is from genetics. However, though the problem of freedom is difficult, I have argued elsewhere that despite appearances, it is not neuroscience that gives rise to the problem (Roskies, 2006). Indeed, any physicalist or materialist view of the world gives rise to a paradox about freedom: Either the world is deterministic, in which case all events are due to natural law and the facts about the world at some prior time, so there is no freedom, or the world is indeterministic, so some events are not determined. But if this is so, they are random, and thus cannot be attributed to a subject's volition. Either way, we are not free. The only thing that can rescue free will from this dilemma is the admission of some extraphysical force of will, but this metaphysical view goes against prevailing physical doctrine. Moreover, I have argued that neuroscience cannot address the question of physicalism, nor can it adjudicate between the (seemingly both problematic) possibilities of determinism and indeterminism (Roskies, 2006).

Despite neuroscience's irrelevance in generating the problem of free will, it will likely cause people to doubt the existence of freedom as it continues to discover the neural mechanisms that have predictive value for behavior. It is the rhetorical force of the neuroscientific understanding, rather than what it can actually reveal, that causes potential ethical issues to arise. One might reasonably worry that skepticism about freedom will affect people's behavior and their ethical views. For example, because freedom is often thought to be essential for moral responsibility, some worry that if the folk abandon their commitment to the belief in freedom, they may conclude that moral responsibility is likewise an illusion, and nihilism may result (Smilansky, 2000). Others concur that neuroscience will undermine our common-sense notion of morality, and we will be forced to rethink our conception of justice. Greene and Cohen (2004), for instance, argue that our retributivist notions will be indefensible if our commonsensical conception of free will is jettisoned, and we will consequently mete out punishment purely due to utilitarian calculations. Though Greene and Cohen champion such an outcome, surely such a considerable change in our conception of justice and corresponding alterations in our legal system will force us to rethink many of our current moral views.

Not all visions of the future are so reversionary. Neuroscience could also be the salve for the wound, not just the salt. In a recent paper (Roskies, 2006), I argue that despite the possibility that people will come to believe they are not free, it is unlikely that their moral judgments will be altered. Evidence from this comes from experiments on the nature of folk intuitions (Roskies and Nichols, 2008) and from understanding the neural basis of moral cognition (the topic of the next section).

Finally, a deeper understanding of the brain may help us revise our conception of freedom and what it requires, thereby circumventing the standard paradox of freedom for physicalism. Recognition of the incoherence of our commonsense conception of freedom in a universe such as the one we think we inhabit may encourage us to develop a robust notion of freedom anchored in a scientifically informed view of the brain and how it operates in the world. I believe we must look for a compatibilist notion of freedom, perhaps one that opposes freedom to coercion, as Ayer (1954) suggested, but more substantially fleshed out. If I may sketch a rough idea in brief, we may come to realize that the type of freedom required for moral responsibility is one grounded in a picture of the proper functioning of an organism in a complex social network of others, together with an understanding of the sorts of mechanisms underlying that proper functioning. In particular, a neuroscientifically informed theory of self-regulation or intrinsic control may be able to ground our most ardently held ideas associated with freedom and preserve many of moral and social practices with minimal violence.

5. MORAL COGNITION

We care about freedom mainly because we care about moral responsibility. Constructing a moral theory that accords with our moral intuitions has been one of the central goals of philosophical thought. Given the reliance we place on intuition, understanding why and how we have the moral views that we do may provide us some meta-level moral insight. Until recently, the only way to study moral cognition was to probe it behaviorally: observe people's actions or note their answers to questions about situations requiring moral judgments. However, with the prevalence of neuroimaging and its application to increasingly abstract domains of cognition, a new way of probing moral cognition has emerged. We are beginning to get the first glimpses into the brain networks that subserve our moral reasoning, and these have proven very enlightening. Other publications have reviewed what has been learned about the neural basis of moral cognition (Greene, 2003; Moll, Zahn, de Oliveira-Souza, Krueger, and Grafman, 2005), so I do not attempt that here. I am concerned mainly with the ethical implications of what has been learned.

The relative roles of emotion and cognition in moral judgment have long been a question of interest. A number of neuroimaging studies have been undertaken that indicate that some of our moral judgments (those in response to what Greene calls "personal" moral dilemmas) naturally excite areas involved in emotion, thus conforming to a sentimentalist view of moral judgment (Greene, Nystrom, Engell, Darley, and Cohen, 2004; Greene, Sommerville, Nystrom, Darley, and Cohen, 2001; Moll et al., 2005). In other situations, our reasoning is more analytical or cognitive, employing regions typically associated with deliberation and rational thought (Greene et al., 2004). Greene has argued that the presence of both these modes of moral cognition may correspond to the long-standing debates in moral philosophy between deontologists and utilitarians (Greene, 2003). Casebeer, in contrast, argues that moral cognition is more Aristotelian than Kantian or Millian, and that virtue ethics is therefore superior to the other ethical theories (Casebeer, 2003). With Greene, I am suspicious that a descriptive fact about how we do reason can give us reason to think that is how we should reason. However, I also agree with him that the descriptive information that neuroscience yields can affect our moral views. As he aptly puts it, "I view science as offering a 'behind the scenes' look at human morality...the scientific investigation of human morality can help us to understand human moral nature, and in so doing change our opinion of it" (Greene, 2003, p. 847).

In addition, our ability to probe the brain's response to different moral scenarios and to see various patterns so reflected raises the question of what it is that the brain is responding to. Are we in contact with objective moral truths about the world? Or are we taking our relatively automatic and reliable responses to reflect truths that aren't there? Greene, for example, thinks that recognition of the way our brains were wired by evolutionary influences suggests that our intuitive position as moral realists is mistaken: "Understanding where our moral instincts come from and how they work can, I argue, leads us to doubt that our moral convictions stem from perceptions of moral truth rather than projections of moral attitudes" (2003, p. 850). Thus, although it has been argued that universalism in moral intuitions is evidence that there we are responding to deep or universal truths, brain science may help us see that universalism in moral judgments (which is questionable on the face of it) may not be due to perception of some objective moral truths, but rather may reflect our common neural structures and their functions. Whether this is indeed the case and how we should respond to it are questions for neuroethics.

Finally, the neurosciences (construed broadly), may give us insight into why we have the particular moral intuitions we do. Are there relevant neural and evolutionary facts to consider? How deeply involved is our emotional brain? If indeed our intuitions are largely driven by emotional reactions, we may question whether principlism, the dominant view in bioethics, is an accurate reflection of those intuitions. And if it isn't, should we reject the view or embrace it as a rich and superior normative framework, not subject to the vagaries of biology? The way we answer these latter questions may be influenced by neuroscience, but they are supremely philosophical, and they may have an effect on applied ethics across the board.

6. Summary

So what's "neu" in neuroethics? Despite the significant areas of overlap between questions raised by genetics and those raised by neuroscience, there are areas in which the ethical issues raised by the two diverge. Here I have focused on the ability of neuroscience to illuminate issues involving consciousness, the self, personhood, decision making and freedom of the will, and moral cognition. For the most part, I have only raised questions, but I have also tried to give a sense of how current and future research might inform and shape those questions. The rest is up to future neuroethicists to tackle.

In closing, I note that even were we ultimately to concede that the questions in neuroethics and genethics were not distinct, or that neuroethics merely appropriates problems already recognized by genethics or bioethics in general, it would be a fallacy to conclude that there is no need for neuroethics or that it needlessly complicates our professional ontology. Our response to various bioethical problems often depends not just on a general understanding of the philosophical question at issue but also on a detailed understanding of the biological organ or mechanism in question, the methods or techniques employed for generating the data, a sense of what data are in fact relevant, knowledge of how to properly interpret scientific results, and a sophisticated appreciation of treatments currently or conceivably available. To the extent that proper bioethical analysis depends on a deep understanding of the science as well as the philosophy, we need people with training in both neuroscience and philosophy to engage with neuroethical questions, just as we need people with training in genetics and philosophy to tackle the problems raised by genethics. Neuroethics meets a new and current need.

ACKNOWLEDGMENT

The author was supported in part by an APD fellowship from the Australian Research Council and the University of Sydney.

NOTE

1. I have claimed that there is overlap between genethics and neuroethics, and that neuroethics raises some questions that genethics does not. Genethics likewise has its own proprietary issues, among them questions raised by the potential of altering the genetic sequence of a germ line or of choosing to gestate or terminate the gestation of a zygote with a particular genetic makeup. These are changes that affect not only the person whose genome is manipulated but potentially future generations as well and, in unlikely scenarios, the entire human race. There are a host of ethical and policy issues stemming from this possibility. Because the knowledge neuroscience yields (with the exception of neuroscientific studies of the genetic basis of the nervous system) tends to be about physiology, anatomy, or neurochemistry of an organ composed of already differentiated cells, it does not raise this same constellation of worries about paternalism with respect to future generations. Thus, genethics and neuroethics treat of distinct, but largely overlapping, sets of questions.

REFERENCES

Ayer, A. J. (1954). *Philosophical Essays*. New York: St. Martin's Press.
Barr, C. S., Newman, T. K., Becker, M. L., Parker, C. C., Champoux, M., Lesch, K. P., et al. (2003). The utility of the non-human primate model for studying gene by environment interactions in behavioral research. *Genes, Brain and Behavior* 2: 336–340.
Burley, J., and Harris, J. (Eds.). (2002). *A Companion to Genethics*. Malden, Mass.: Blackwell.
Casebeer, W. D. (2003). Moral cognition and its neural constituents. *Nature Reviews Neuroscience* 4: 841–846.
Chalmers, D. J. (1996). *The Conscious Mind: In Search of a Fundamental Theory*. Oxford: Oxford University Press.
Crick, F. (1995). *The Astonishing Hypothesis: The Scientific Search for the Soul*. New York: Simon and Schuster.
Dehaene, S. (Ed.). (2001). *The Cognitive Neuroscience of Consciousness*. Cambridge, Mass.: MIT Press.

Dehaene, S., Changeaux, J.-P., Naccache, L., Sackur, J., and Sergent, C. (2006). Conscious, preconscious, and subliminal processing: A testable taxonomy. *Trends in Cognitive Sciences* 10: 204–211.

Dehaene, S., Naccache, L., Cohen, L., Le Bihan, D., Mangin, J.-F., Poline, J.-B., et al. (2001). Cerebral mechanisms of word masking and unconscious repetition priming. *Nature Neuroscience* 4: 752–758.

Dehaene, S., Naccache, L., Le Clec, H. G., Koechlin, E., Meuller, M., Dehaene-Lambertz, G., et al. (1998). Imaging unconscious semantic priming. *Nature* 395: 597–600.

Farah, M. J., and Haberlein, A. (2007). Personhood and neuroscience: Naturalizing or nihilating? *American Journal of Bioethics* 7(1): 37–48.

Greene, J. (2003). From neural "is" to moral "ought": What are the moral implications of neuroscientific moral psychology? *Nature Reviews Neuroscience* 4: 847–850.

Greene, J., and Cohen, J. D. (2004). For the law, neuroscience changes nothing and everything. *Philosophical Transactions of the Royal Society of London, B: Biological Sciences* 359: 1775–1785.

Greene, J. D., Nystrom, L. E., Engell, A. D., Darley, J. M., and Cohen, J. D. (2004). The neural bases of cognitive conflict and control in moral judgment. *Neuron* 44: 389–400.

Greene, J. D., Sommerville, R. B., Nystrom, L. E., Darley, J. M., and Cohen, J. D. (2001). An fMRI investigation of emotional engagement in moral judgment. *Science* 293: 2105–2108.

Illes, J., and Racine, E. (2005). Imaging or imagining? A neuroethics challenge informed by genetics. *American Journal of Bioethics* 5: 5–18.

Kim, J.-N., and Shadlen, M. N. (1999). Neural correlates of a decision in the dorsolateral prefrontal cortex of the macaque. *Nature Neuroscience* 2: 176–185.

Koch, C. (2004). *The Quest for Consciousness: A Neurobiological Approach*. Englewood, Colo.: Roberts.

Kotz, S. A., Cappa, S. F., von Cramon, D. Y., and Friederici, A. D. (2002). Modulation of the lexical-semantic network by auditory semantic priming: An event-related functional MRI study. *Neuroimage* 17: 1761–1772.

Leon, M. I., and Shadlen, M. N. (1999). Exploring the neurophysiology of decisions. *Neuron* 21: 669–672.

Locke, J. ([1694] 1975). *Essay Concerning Human Understanding*. P. Nidditch (Ed.). Oxford: Clarendon Press.

Mazurek, M. E., Roitman, J. D., Ditterich, J., and Shadlen, M. N. (2003). A role for neural integrators in perceptual decision making. *Cerebral Cortex* 13: 1257–1269.

Moll, J., de Oliveira-Souza, R., Eslinger, P. J., Bramati, I. E., Mourao-Miranda, J., Andreiuolo, P. A., et al. (2002). The neural correlates of moral sensitivity: A functional magnetic resonance imaging investigation of basic and moral emotions. *Journal of Neuroscience* 22: 2730–2736.

Moll, J., Zahn, R., de Oliveira-Souza, R., Krueger, F., and Grafman, J. (2005). The neural basis of human moral cognition. *Nature Reviews Neuroscience* 6: 799–809.

Naccache, L., and Dehaene, S. (2001). Unconscious semantic priming extends to novel unseen stimuli. *Cognition* 80: 223–237.

Owen, A. M., Coleman, M. R., Boly, M., Davis, M. H., Laureys, S., and Pickard, J. D. (2006). Detecting awareness in the vegetative state. *Science* 313: 1402.

Parfit, D. (1986). *Reasons and Persons*. Oxford: Oxford University Press.

Portas, C. M. (2000). Auditory processing across the sleep-wake cycle: Simultaneous EEG and fMRI monitoring in humans. *Neuron* 28: 991–999.

Rissman, J., Eliassen, J. C., and Blumstein, S. E. (2003). An event-related fMRI investigation of implicit semantic priming. *Journal of Cognitive Neuroscience* 15: 1160–1175.

Roskies, A. L. (2002). Neuroethics for the new millennium. *Neuron* 35: 21–23.

Roskies, A. L. (2006). Neuroscientific challenges to free will and responsibility. *Trends in Cognitive Sciences* 10: 419–423.

Roskies, A. L. (2007). The illusion of personhood. *American Journal of Bioethics* 7: 55–57.

Roskies, A. L., and Nichols, S. (2008). Bringing moral responsibility down to earth. *Journal of Philosophy* 105: 371–388.

Schiff, N. D., Rodriguez-Moreno, D., Kamal, A., Kim, K. H. S., Giacino, J. T., Plum, F., et al. (2005). fMRI reveals large-scale network activation in minimally conscious patients. *Neurology* 64: 514–523.

Smilansky, S. (2000). *Free Will and Illusion*. Oxford: Oxford University Press.

Steinberg, D. (2005). Consciousness is missing—and so is research. *EMBO Reports* 6: 1009–1011.

Stoljar, D. (2006). *Ignorance and Imagination: The Epistemic Origin of the Problem of Consciousness*. Oxford: Oxford University Press.

PART VI

NEUROPHILOSOPHY AND PSYCHIATRY

CHAPTER 19

CONFABULATIONS ABOUT PEOPLE AND THEIR LIMBS, PRESENT OR ABSENT

WILLIAM HIRSTEIN

1. A THEORY OF CONFABULATION

The word *confabulate* is descended from the ancient Latin term *confabulari*, which means to talk with. *Con* means with, and *fabulari* means to talk, but the noun *fabula* also means tale or fable, and it was perhaps this that German neurologists Bonhoeffer (1901), Pick (1905), and Wernicke (1906) had in mind when they began referring to false memory reports made by their amnesic patients as *konfabulationen*. Most of these patients suffered from a syndrome that later came to be known as Korsakoff's amnesia. When asked what he did yesterday, a typical Korsakoff's patient has no memory at all, but instead of admitting ignorance will confidently report events that either did not happen (or at least did not happen to him) or happened to him long ago. A man might claim that he was at work at his supermarket, finishing up the year-end inventory, for example, when he had been in bed at the hospital the entire time. Through the early part of the twentieth century, then, it was assumed that a confabulation was simply a false memory report—or more precisely, a false claim alleged to be a memory report—and the term was restricted to these uses. But there was something more contained in the initial concept of confabulation that enticed people to apply it to more than just memory reports. During the remainder of the twentieth century the use of *confabulation* was gradually expanded to cover claims made by other types of patients, including patients who deny that they are injured, paralyzed, or even blind. Split-brain patients who make false claims about why they did certain things were also said to confabulate, as well as patients with misidentification disorders, who make false claims about the identities of people. More recently, it has been found that children up to a certain age tend to confabulate when asked to recall events, and some writers have argued that even normal people will confabulate in certain contexts.

Because of the recent proliferation of confabulation syndromes, contemporary writers attempting to construct a definition of confabulation have despaired of the fact that some of these syndromes involve memory disorders (Korsakoff's, and aneurysm of the anterior communicating artery, a similar syndrome), whereas others involve problems of perception (denial of paralysis or blindness, split-brain syndrome, misidentification disorders) (e.g., Johnson, Hayes, D'Esposito, and Raye, 2000). Because both memory and perception are knowledge domains, however, perhaps the broader sense of confabulation applies to knowledge itself, or more specifically, to the making of knowledge claims. According to this approach, to confabulate is to unintentionally make an ill-grounded (and hence probably false) claim that one should know is ill-grounded (Hirstein, 2005).

Confabulations are the result of two different phases of error. The first occurs in one of the brain's epistemic systems, either mnemonic or perceptual. This produces an ill-grounded memory or perception. These malfunctioning perceptual or mnemonic processes tend to be located in the back half of the brain's cortex, in the temporal or parietal lobes. Second, even with plenty of time to examine the situation and with urging from doctors and relatives, the patient fails to realize that the response is flawed, due to a malfunction of higher level brain processes located toward the front of the brain, in the prefrontal lobes. Nonconfabulating brains sometimes create flawed responses, but we are able to correct them, using these different prefrontal processes. If I ask you whether you have ever seen the Eiffel Tower, for instance, your brain is happy to provide an image of the tower, even if you've never been near it. But you are able to reject this as a real memory. You catch the mistake at the second phase. Thus, the typical etiology of confabulation involves damage in the posterior of the brain to some perceptual or mnemonic process, causing the first error stage, coupled with damage to some prefrontal process, causing the second error stage. The two events of damage need not occur at the same time; there are numerous cases in the literature in which patients with an existing site of brain damage began confabulating after damage to a second site.

Capgras syndrome, one of the misidentification syndromes, and anosognosia, in which patients deny having a disability they obviously have, are the two oddest members of the family of confabulation syndromes and the most difficult to assimilate to what is known about the others. A comprehensive theory of confabulation that encompasses these syndromes as well as the other confabulation syndromes could shed a great deal of light on some extremely puzzling human responses to brain injury. Neurologist Todd Feinberg has recently proposed a theory designed to encompass both the misidentification syndromes and asomatognosia, and a related disorder, anosognosia (Feinberg, 2001), according to which they are disorders of the patient's sense of personal relatedness to other people and to his or her own body.

In the subsequent sections, this view is examined and extended in a way that clearly brings these two types of syndrome under the tent of the two-phase theory. Aside from showing that these two syndromes fit the suggested definition of *confabulation*, my point in this chapter is that we can understand why people have these strange beliefs if we understand the nature of the representation systems that, when damaged, produce them. Once we understand how these representation systems are structured and how they operate, we will find that this helps us understand the rest of the confabulation syndromes as well. There are also broader implications. The phenomena and hypotheses described here are quite relevant to certain philosophical questions, about how humans identify people and objects and about how our knowledge in general is structured and grounded. They indicate that our ways of representing people and objects are more complex than had been thought, but any modifications these complexities force in our philosophical theories can also bring great increases in their explanatory power. They can allow us to understand the claims of people suffering from delusions.

If we understand confabulation as an epistemic problem, the confabulation syndromes can be categorized as disorders of the brain's knowledge domains:

1. Knowledge of the body and its surroundings (denial of paralysis).
2. Knowledge of recent events involving oneself, that is, autobiographical memories (Korsakoff's syndrome; anterior communicating artery syndrome).
3. Knowledge of other people (the misidentification syndromes).
4. Knowledge of our minds (split-brain syndrome).
5. Knowledge derived from visual perception (Anton's syndrome).

Stated in term of individually testable criteria, the recommended definition of *confabulation* is: S confabulates (that p) if and only if (1) S claims that p; (2) S believes that p; (3) S's thought that p is ill-grounded; (4) S does not know that his or her thought is ill-grounded; (5) S should know that his or her thought is ill-grounded; (6) S is confident that p. The concept of *claiming* (rather than, for instance, *saying* or *asserting*) is broad enough to cover a wide variety of responses by subjects and patients, including nonverbal responses, such as drawing and pointing. The second criterion captures the sincerity of confabulators. If explicitly asked, "Do you believe that p?," they invariably answer "yes." The third criterion refers to the problem that caused the flawed response to be generated: Processes within the relevant knowledge domain were not acting optimally. Criterion number four refers to a cognitive failure at a second phase, the failure to check and reject the flawed response. The fifth criterion captures a normative element in our concept of confabulation: If the confabulator's brain were functioning properly, he or she would know that the claim is ill-grounded and not make it. The claims made are about things any normal person would easily get right. The sixth and last criterion refers to another important characteristic of confabulators observed in the clinic, the serene certainty they have in their claims, even in the face of obvious disbelief by their listeners. This epistemic approach eliminates a problem endemic to the falsity criterion in the original definition, according to which confabulations are false memory reports: A patient might answer correctly out of luck. The problem is not so much the falsity of the patients' claims but their ill-groundedness and consequent unreliability, at least in the affected domain. In short then, in this epistemic view, to confabulate is to confidently make an ill-grounded claim that one should (but does not) know is ill-grounded.

1.1. Capgras Syndrome

Neurological patients with Capgras syndrome claim that people close to them, typically spouses, parents, or children, have been replaced by similar-looking impostors. When asked how they can tell that the person is an impostor, Capgras patients often confabulate. One patient claimed that she could tell her husband had been replaced because the new person tied his shoelaces differently, whereas another patient said that the impostor of her son "had different-colored eyes, was not as big and brawny, and that her real son would not kiss her" (Frazer and Roberts, 1994, p. 557). The patient's attitude toward the alleged impostor can vary. The majority of Capgras patients are suspicious of the "impostor" at the very least. Many are paranoid about the impostor, and attribute intent to harm to him or her, but there are also cases where the patient's attitude is positive.

Capgras syndrome patients thus misidentify people, including themselves (as seen in photos, or even in a mirror). Capgras syndrome fits the pattern of damage seen in the memory syndromes: damage to some knowledge system, in this case a perceptual one, paired with frontal damage. Several writers have hypothesized that the first damaged process is one that normally produces an emotion at the sight of a familiar person. One candidate for the second damaged process is one that detects conflicts among mental states and alerts other parts of the brain that initiate a resolution of the conflict. Confabulators in the clinic do seem bad at detecting and resolving conflicts in their claims. They are not bothered when the doctor points out they are contradicting themselves in what they say.

1.2. Anosognosia and Asomatognosia

Anosognosia means lack of knowledge or unawareness, of illness. First described in detail by Babinski (1914), this unawareness can accompany certain types of paralysis caused by damage to the right inferior parietal cortex and seems to play a role in causing an intriguing response known as *denial* in some patients. When asked about their disabilities, they will calmly and firmly deny that they are paralyzed or weakened. The typical denial patient, interviewed as he rests in bed after a stroke that has paralyzed his left arm, will claim that both arms are fine. When asked to touch the doctor's nose with his left arm, the patient will move his torso slightly, then stop. When asked whether they touched the doctor's nose, some patients will say that they did, whereas others will admit that they didn't but confabulate a reason for it, such as that they are tired, don't feel like following commands right now, always had a weak left arm, and so on. Some of these patients further deny that their brain injury has hampered them in any way. These patients are said to suffer from *neglect*—they neglect their arms as well as the space on their left by never attending to that space or initiating actions with that arm.

Although there is evidence that some anosognosic patients have some types of somatosensation (see Davies, Davies, and Coltheart, 2005), typically important higher-level somatosensory areas are damaged. These posterior areas of damage, especially in the inferior parietal cortex, create the first malfunction needed for confabulation, but until very recently no clear pattern of frontal damage had emerged in the study of anosognosia. In 2005, however, Berti et al. showed that patients who denied paralysis differed from those with paralysis but no denial in that the denial patients had additional damage in the frontal portions of a large brain network involved in the planning of motor actions. These frontal areas are directly connected to the damaged inferior parietal areas. Apparently, the frontal areas are capable of monitoring intended actions generated by posterior areas in the same network. As Berti and colleagues say, "monitoring systems may be implemented within the same cortical network that is responsible for the primary function that has to be monitored" (2005, p. 488). Some patients with anosognosia also manifest an even more curious condition known as *asomatognosia*. They deny ownership of their own limbs, almost always the left arm or leg. The patient typically confabulates that the limb belongs to the doctor, or sometimes to a spouse or relative, or even that it was left behind by a previous patient. Patients tend not to bother to elaborate these claims into more coherent stories, about how exactly a limb came to be left in bed, for instance. They are more likely to simply lose interest in the conversation and stop talking.

2. PHILOSOPHY AND COGNITIVE NEUROPSYCHOLOGY

The subject matter of philosophy is the set of intractable questions that are important to us as human beings. They are intractable in the sense that we do not know even what *sort* of theory might allow us to answer them. They are often the only problems of their type (as far as we know), so that the possibility of applying some theory from some other problem domain seems remote. The goal of philosophers is to answer these questions or show that they are ill-formed or meaningless. Beyond that, there are historically no specific restrictions on the sort of evidence that may be used in attempts to answer these questions, and a glance back at the history of philosophy shows that a wide variety of data sources have been considered relevant to these problems. There is, however, a quite recent conception of philosophy according to which its goal is more specific, to answer these questions using only a priori techniques, such as conceptual and logical analysis. This definition explicitly rules out a posteriori, empirical, or scientific techniques. This conception is, one suspects, ultimately an artifact of the separation into academic disciplines that occurred in the early twentieth century. Philosophers, wrongly I think, believed that they needed to clearly distinguish their discipline from the sciences in the same way that the subject matters of most of the other academic disciplines can be exclusively delineated. At the same time, early analytic philosophy was showing how powerful sheerly logical techniques are, and how many interesting problems needed to be solved and seemingly could be solved within this realm.

There is a potentially serious problem, however, with believing that solving a problem using only a priori techniques does not involve observation of the physical world. This commits one to the claim that one's mind is not part of the physical world, that is, dualism, something most philosophers reject. If we go further back into the history of philosophy, we see that philosophers have always thought about and observed the world to pose and solve their problems—Aristotle, Descartes, Berkeley, and Kant are four prime examples. Conversely, scientists frequently encounter and must solve conceptual problems, for example, Einstein's work on the concept of simultaneity. Even if we could devise a workable version of the a priori/a posteriori distinction, knowledge about facts is so thoroughly and densely interconnected with "conceptual" knowledge that it would still be clear we really do very little purely a priori thinking.

Once we reject this stifling and insufficiently motivated conception of philosophy, it is clear that neuroscience at all its levels of inquiry can inform the philosophy of mind. The new science of neurocomputation, for instance, has forced several important questions about the nature of mental representations and mental operations, about whether folk psychology will be eliminated, and others (P.S. Churchland, 1986; Churchland and Sejnowski, 1992). The approach taken here involves connecting philosophy with a branch of neuroscience operating several levels up from neurocomputation: cognitive neuropsychology. Much of the data we examine is from an era before there was anything known as cognitive neuropsychology, when our phenomena of interest were the province of either psychology or neurology. Neurologists have always attempted to discern brain function by studying patients with brain lesions, and now cognitive neuroscience has provided a new level of theory of brain structure and function to aid in this process. These neurologists and cognitive neuropsychologists work at one of the highest levels of brain structure, employing these new theories in efforts to understand behaviors and symptoms. One indication of this is that most of the behaviors and symptoms of interest to them are described in everyday folk-psychological terms, "I can't see out of my left eye," "I can't move my right arm," or, "I can't recognize people." Approaching the brain from this level allows one the great luxury of continuing to use the folk idioms, concepts, and beliefs, something that has many benefits, including making the writer's task of explanation vastly simpler. It also makes hypotheses easier to state, test, and refute if need be.

Philosophy can play a valuable role here, by building thought bridges between what the cognitive neuropsychologists are finding and what philosophy has uncovered in its long investigation of the mental, both via introspection and the observation of behavior. The British empiricists, especially Locke (1690/1959) and Hume (1777/1975), constructed elaborate theories of the mental, employing folk concepts such as *idea, sensation, thought*, and *understanding*. Kant (1787/1929) added entirely new dimensions to this system, such as a catalog of the thought patterns we naturally meet the world with. After Kant, the strand was lost, and for a time philosophy went into a period of that baroque overcomplexity that it had entered before Descartes, as generations struggled to understand and then modify the work of Hegel. Momentum was also lost during the final parts of the nineteenth century due to a debate that now seems quaint and difficult to capture, in which a position called psychologism was supposed to have been refuted. Psychologism has several versions, but it is fundamentally the view that logic is reducible to psychology, as opposed to the idea that logic and psychology are two separate realms, in the same way that math and science are. Defenders of the latter view won the debate, and the view is still orthodoxy. But this view leaves us with a troubling metaphysical dichotomy between the logical and the empirical. This dichotomy also was partly responsible for splitting philosophy off from the sciences, because it is clear that logic and philosophy are closely connected.

Behaviorism, the view that mental states such as believing and desiring are reducible to patterns of behavior, and eliminativism, the view that "belief" and "desire" don't refer to anything real, have also threatened to break this historical link. Despite their externalist approaches, the fine-grained conceptual analyses of mental state terms by Ludwig Wittgenstein (1953) and Gilbert Ryle (1949) showed that our ordinary mental terms concealed great complexity and sensitivity. Philosophy's other post-Kantian strand, phenomenology, devoted itself to intricate descriptions of conscious states, using introspection (Husserl, 1913/1973; Merleau-Ponty, 1962). John Searle (1983) made the fateful step, however, of building a philosophical theory—the theory of intentional states—which regimented our ordinary concepts of the mental into a philosophical theory that described our mental states as biological processes and events.

The task of those pursuing this line of inquiry is to design a philosophical theory of the mind that has all the right sockets and connectors to plug into a science, specifically contemporary neuroscience. While Paul and Patricia Churchland have broken links to the philosophical tradition by renouncing folk psychology and producing a robust version of eliminativism, their other great contribution, opening lines of communication and inquiry between philosophy and neuroscience, moves this historical dialectic forward. What is so vital about the connection the Churchlands pioneered to neuroscience is that it offers the possibility of connecting philosophical thought not with current paradigms or models in the mental sciences, some of which we saw in the last century, including psychoanalysis, behaviorism, and artificial intelligence, but rather with the much more sober and certain discipline of neurobiology itself. Those paradigms were more like metaphors for the mind than real theories of it. Of course, future modifications even in basic levels of neuroscience will occur, but the bet is that *neuron* will be a far more enduring concept than, say, *superego*.

2.1. Identification

Currently, a lively debate exists in philosophy between several competing theories about the nature of our ability to identify and think about people and objects of interest (e.g., Evans, 1982; McDowell, 1996). Specific questions in this debate are: What criteria must someone meet before she can be truly said to have a concept of x? When has someone correctly reidentified x? How does the ability to reidentify relate to our linguistic ability to refer to the same object or person on multiple occasions? And so on. The use of misidentification patients to study how we represent and think about people has great potential to inform this debate. One important question here is about our mental representations of other people—our concepts of individuals. The common assumption in the philosophical literature is that recognition of people normally occurs via a sheerly visual route. Our perception of someone's face may be bolstered by our perception of the sound of his or her voice in a judgment of identity, of course, but the philosophical discussions of identification have focused on visual identification via external appearance. The behavior of both Capgras patients and the other misidentification patients suggests, however, that there is something more involved in identification of people than how a person appears externally or sounds. Our brains do not treat having a certain face as a sufficient condition for the identity of a person. None of the existing philosophical theories takes account of this however, so none of them has the resources to explain why Capgras patients do not acknowledge the identities of their loved ones. Similarly, seeing that an arm is attached to one's own shoulder is not by itself enough to convince us that the arm is ours, in certain situations. What the misidentification syndromes and anosognosia show is that the way we identify people and their limbs is roughly twice as complicated as we thought. Even if I am incorrect about this, if the philosophical question is "How do we identify people?" we need to know about what goes wrong in Capgras and the other misidentification syndromes, as well as those cases in which the identity of body parts is denied.

2.2. Knowledge

Another part of philosophy that could benefit from a look at the phenomena described here is epistemology. Confabulation itself is of interest philosophically because of what it indicates about the ways in which people construct knowledge (or fail to) and make claims based on that knowledge. Our knowledge of our bodies has traditionally been treated as a paradigm case of knowledge and sometimes as an example of something indubitable. When G. E. Moore (1939) was searching for a fact about the external world that we are entirely certain of, and that can be easily demonstrated by a speaker, he chose the existence of his own hands, saying, "Here is one hand, and here is another," while holding them up. Wittgenstein was troubled by Moore's attempt to respond to the philosophical skeptic about the external world merely by holding up his hands and insisting on knowledge about them, and his last work, the posthumously published *On Certainty* (1969) is devoted to ruminations about the meaning of Moore's act. One thing that bothered Wittgenstein was the question of what it would even mean to doubt that *this* is one's hand. "The propositions presenting what Moore '*knows*' are all of such a kind that it is difficult to imagine *why* anyone should believe the contrary" (1969, p. 93). How can there be any question of knowledge, when there is no question of doubt, wondered Wittgenstein. Perhaps a study of people who do believe the contrary, that *this* is not their hand, might help us understand our knowledge of these basic facts about ourselves and the world. Looking at this most fundamental type of knowledge can help us understand how our knowledge systems are structured and how reliable they actually are.

The asomatognosic does not experience doubt, he is quite certain that this thing he sees is not his arm. Wittgenstein was also concerned to make the point that knowledge is not established by our degree of certainty, for example, how certain Moore feels when he looks at his hand, or how difficult Moore finds it to doubt the presence of his hand. One can feel extremely certain yet still be wrong; one can be completely uncertain and be right. Even though this feeling of certainty directed at basic facts such as the existence of our arms does not guarantee knowledge, we need to understand it. One hypothesis available here is that our propositional knowledge, that is, semantic memory, is grounded on our nonpropositional knowledge, knowledge kept in analog rather than conceptual form. The brain represents the body using not (just) concepts but analog maps, somatotopic maps scattered throughout the dorsal portions of the cortex.

2.3. Rationality

All of the syndromes discussed here are caused by focal brain damage or lesions, although some can also be caused by pervasive brain damage—misidentification syndromes are relatively common among Alzheimer patients, for instance. The patient's behavior is also only disrupted in domain-specific ways. Even though the Capgras patient and the asomatognosic might seem irrational when they discuss their loved ones or their arms, they behave quite rationally in other domains. They are able to answer all sorts of questions involving general knowledge, geography, cities, famous people, animals, and so on. They have what are called content-specific delusions, as opposed to the large systems of delusions constructed by some schizophrenics, for instance. The focal nature of the lesions in these patients, and the specificity of the domains in which they are confabulatory, make them of great interest to researchers, because they offer the tantalizing possibility of learning about the functions of previously mysterious brain areas, their areas of damage.

The specificity of the patients' problem thus makes them good objects of study, but it creates another problem. To state, as many clinicians do, that these patients are otherwise rational is to beg the question against holistic theories of rationality, according to which isolated islands of irrationality are impossible. According to the holist, our beliefs are so thoroughly and densely interconnected that any irrational beliefs would immediately infect huge numbers of other beliefs with their irrationality, making the person more globally irrational. Quine (1953) spoke of a web of belief; one cannot pull on one part of a spider web without bringing the rest of the web along. Some of the beliefs in the web, those toward the center are more basic and foundational than the others. They are less likely to be changed by experience, but Quine insisted that experiences could still come along that would change even them. These holists agree, however, that changing the more basic beliefs should force great changes in the entire web. Yet somehow these patients accomplish this odd specificity, even though the beliefs in question are among the most basic a person can have: This is my arm, this person is my father. The patient is not concerned when he is confronted with patent contradictions between the delusional belief and other firmly held beliefs. The patients' abilities to think and reason run into a firmly held but irrational belief; curiously, the reasoning system meekly defers to the irrational belief. A study of all of these phenomena might reveal hidden features of human rationality and help us get a better grasp on this vital concept.

Whether or not philosophy should be delineated as a purely conceptual enterprise, the philosopher's training in dealing with concepts can be useful at the early stages of scientific theory formation to forestall certain errors, clarify concepts and distinctions, and, again in this particular case, bring a huge historical body of thought and research to bear on the new discoveries. In the same way the perceptual system gets its best grasp on reality by letting the incoming energy flow reverberate all the way up to the top levels of the perceptual system, all the way into the cognitive system, then back down, and back and forth until a stable and sensible percept can be developed, cognitive science needs to reverberate all the way from the neuroscientist's findings made with a microscope to the philosopher's findings made with logic and thought experiments.

3. Three Theories

In the cases of both Capgras syndrome and asomatognosia, something very close and very familiar, a loved one or a body part, is claimed to be unfamiliar. Just as some patients with asomatognosia will claim that the arm they see is someone else's arm, the Capgras patient will claim that people who should be very familiar to him have actually been replaced by someone else. French neurologist Jacques Vié (1930) was the first to explicitly mention this similarity. In this section, I examine three candidate explanations for the misidentification syndromes and asomatognosia.

3.1. The Emotional Theory

According to the emotional theory of Capgras syndrome, the patient fails to experience the normal emotional reaction to the sight of a familiar person, and this causes him or her to form the belief that the person is an impostor. This theory seems to originate with Capgras and Reboul-Lachaux's seminal article, in which they write that "the delusion of doubles is not...really a sensory delusion, but rather the conclusion of an emotional judgment" ([1923] 1994, p. 128). Many subsequent writers have argued that in Capgras syndrome there is a disconnection between the representation of a face and what Ellis and Young refer to as "the evocation of affective memories" (1990, p. 243) (see also Bauer, 1986; Hirstein and Ramachandran, 1997; Staton, Brumback, and Wilson, 1982). The patients recognize a face, but do not feel the expected emotions, and confabulate to explain this: "When patients find themselves in such a conflict (that is, receiving some information which indicates the face in front of them belongs to X, but not receiving confirmation of this), they may adopt some sort of rationalization strategy in which the individual before them is deemed to be an impostor, a dummy, a robot, or whatever extant technology may suggest" (Ellis and Young, 1990, p. 244).

The weak link in the emotional theory is the connection between the absence of an emotion and the creation of the impostor story. Why doesn't the patient merely say that people seem strange or unfamiliar? Stone and Young (1997, p. 344) add another ingredient, the patient's prior personality, suggesting that once the patient loses the normal affective reactions to faces, "because of a co-existing suspicious mood, or maybe a premorbid disposition, the person arrives at the idea that the source of these strange experiences must lie in a change in the external world, and the possibility of some kind of a trick, perhaps involving a substitution presents itself." But why would so many different patients with different personalities, and different premorbid dispositions arrive at the same highly unlikely story about the same trick? The emotional theory also seems not to be a good candidate for expansion into a more comprehensive theory that could also be applied to asomatognosia. When applied to asomatognosia, the emotional theory would generate the claim that we normally experience an emotional reaction at the sight of our arms and then confabulate that the arm is not our own to explain the absence of this emotion, and this seems extravagant.

3.2. The Personal Relatedness Theory

The patient who says, "That's not my father," and the one who says, "That's not my arm," have the same basic problem, according to Feinberg and colleagues (Feinberg and Roane, 1997). "Asomatognosia can be understood as a Capgras syndrome for the arm in which the personal relationship with the body part is lost" (Feinberg, DeLuca, Giacino, Roane, and Solms, 2005, p. 103). The Capgras patient has lost his sense of personal relatedness to his father, whereas the asomatognosic has lost his sense of personal relatedness to his arm. Feinberg then sets up a fascinating comparison between Capgras and asomatognosia on one hand, and another mis-identification syndrome, Fregoli syndrome: Both Capgras patients and asomato-gnosic patients claim that something or someone personally related to them is unfamiliar and distant. In contrast, the patient with Fregoli syndrome sees unfa-miliar people as familiar, or more broadly, falsely sees people as being personally related to him. These patients will claim that certain people they know are capable of manifesting different physical appearances, so the patients might complain that a certain person is following them or spying on them while taking on the outward appearance of different people. Feinberg argues that this distinction, between see-ing something as personally related and seeing something as distant and foreign, is of use in forming a taxonomy of the misidentification disorders. As he puts it, "the essential dichotomization of these various disorders is on the basis of an altera-tion in personal relatedness or significance" (Feinberg and Roane, 1997, p. 80). Syn-dromes such as Capgras and asomatognosia, which involve a decreased sense of relatedness in the patient, "should be thought of as a disavowal, estrangement, or alienation from persons, objects, or experiences." Syndromes such as Fregoli are on the "the opposite side of the spectrum" and "are manifestations of an over-related-ness with persons, objects, or experiences" (ibid.).

Not all patients can be described as claiming either under- or overrelatedness to people and things, Feinberg and colleagues acknowledge. Some of them do both at the same time, with the same person. "Many of the important misidentifications seen in neurological patients actually represent a *co-occurrence* of both Capgras and Fregoli types of misidentifications" (Feinberg and Roane, 1997, p. 80). Many con-fabulations by asomatognosics do not involve the patient claiming that the arm or person is completely unrelated to him. One patient of Feinberg's said that her hands were not hers but her husband's, saying that "He left them…just like he left his clothes" (2006, p. 74). Because of this third, mixed type, Feinberg and colleagues phrase their hypothesis in its final form as follows: Syndromes such as Capgras, Fregoli, and asomatognosia "represent either an increase, a decrease, or simultane-ous increase and decrease in the patient's personal relatedness to objects, persons, places, or events in the patient's environment" (ibid.).

3.3. A Representational Theory

Personal relatedness is an extremely broad concept, perhaps too broad to be of explanatory value in this context. A very high percentage of the representations in our brains are of things personally related to us, for obvious reasons. The entirety of episodic-autobiographical memory, for instance, contains representations of events personally related to us. There are many different ways we represent things, prop-erties, and facts that are important to us. In addition to episodic memory, we use somatotopic maps to represent several different properties of our bodies, and our semantic memories contain a self-concept that knits together all sorts of biographi-cal information about us and is immediately connected to our concepts of peo-ple and things of significance to us. A second criticism of the personal relatedness theory arises from the presence of "mixed" patients, who show both an increase and a decrease in their senses of personal relatedness for an object or person, because this indicates that the patients do not line up neatly on a single personal relatedness continuum.

The following hypothesis offers a more specific explanation of Capgras syndrome, Fregoli syndrome, asomatognosia, and other disorders of person and limb recognition that fits the basic two-phase approach that has been taken with the other confabulation syndromes. It provides an alternative account for why these syndromes exhibit the interesting variations in personal relatedness that Feinberg and colleagues observed. Our brains represent people both allocentrically and egocentrically. Allocentric representations of people are viewpoint-independent representations of their external bodily features. Our representations of peoples' faces are a paradigmatic example of allocentric representations. One sign that they are viewpoint-independent is that we can recognize people from many different angles. Egocentric representations encode the positions of things and spaces relative to a central "ego." Our representations of the spaces we inhabit are usually egocentric; they represent the distances of objects from us, the trajectories of objects with regard to our location, the possible effects on us of nearby objects, and so on. Egocentric representations contain an intrinsic point of view, whereas allocentric representations are viewpoint-independent. When I represent you from my perspective, I represent you allocentrically. When I represent you from your perspective, I typically represent you egocentrically. Egocentric representations give the ego a privileged place in the representational system, whereas a person's allocentric system can represent him as one person among many. Among the faces we are able to visually recognize is our own, usually seen in a mirror, but the same allocentric visual recognition processes are used whether we are looking at ourselves or at our friends.

One type of egocentric representation of an agent is a (spatial) analog representation from the unique point of view of that agent, from inside that agent's head, of processes and events within that agent's body, including that person's thoughts. We represent people egocentrically by simulating their current experiences from their points of view. The brain achieves this with an egocentric representation system that functions to represent a mind situated in a body, which is in turn situated in an environment, according to the representational theory. The egocentric system is responsible for part of our normal sense that we are embodied minds, moving about an environment. This system does not always represent us, however. It has two modes of functioning that I will call self-mode and other-mode. In self-mode, this system represents my mind, situated in my body, situated in my environment. When this system functions in other-mode, it represents other people as minds situated in bodies situated in environments. In either mode, the system is egocentric; different individuals can occupy the ego position in the system. In self-mode, I am the ego at the center of this system, in other-mode the egocentric system represents or simulates the egocentric system of a person of interest. Interestingly, the entire egocentric system functions as a representation in other-mode, but only the body and space portions of the egocentric system function as representations in self-mode, because the mental part of the egocentric system literally is part of our minds, rather than being a representation of them.

The allocentric system represents people from the outside, including detailed facial representations as well as representations of entire bodies or characteristic modes of dress. The skin seems to mark the boundary of what the allocentric system represents, and the mental component of the egocentric system represents events occurring inside the skin, as experienced from the point of view of that body's owner. Egocentric representations involve somatosensory representations, but also involve our awareness of our conscious perceptions, thoughts, and emotions. Allocentric representations are primarily visual but also involve auditory representations, as well as representations generated by other sense modalities. The egocentric system may well have other modes, including what we might call an alternative self-mode, which we use to imagine ourselves in the future or in other possible scenarios.

One possible area of weakness in the representational view is its extravagance. It posits an entire type of representation, these egocentric representations of others, in addition to the known allocentric representations. But we should not be surprised that a species whose success is so tied to its social nature has representation systems this elaborate for perceiving and understanding others. Social factors have been more important to individual humans' survival and flourishing than the mere pragmatics of obtaining food and shelter for some time now. The average contemporary person supports him- or herself not by knowledge of how to grow food and weave clothes, but by knowledge of other people, and how and when to interact with them.

4. Representations of Minds

We perceive personality by representing moods, emotions, and character. We read several different features of minds using several different brain processes, one of which, I suggest, is the egocentric mind-reading system described here. The problem of the misidentification patients on this hypothesis is due to a failure of their brains to activate the correct egocentric representation of the person they are seeing. Once we get to know a person well, we develop an individualized egocentric representation of his or her mind. I suggest that we also possess generic egocentric representations that can be applied to people we do not yet know well. These generic representations show themselves in our psychologies as character stereotypes. We observe a person for a few moments, then conclude, "Ah, he's one of *those* kinds of people," calling the appropriate generic egocentric representation into play in our attempt to understand him.

We employ or own egocentric representation system in other-mode, or as a simulation, to understand the actions of other people. This is a variety of simulation theory (Goldman, 2006) in which an egocentric representation system is employed as an analog model of that same system in another person. One piece of data that is at least consistent with the claim that malfunction exists in a system that is involved in representing both ourselves and others is the regular occurrence of self-misidentifications along with misidentifications of others. The misidentification syndromes can be understood as caused by damage to the mind-representing part of this large egocentric representation system. Analogously, asomatognosia can be understood as due to damage in the body-representing part of the egocentric representation system. According to this hypothesis both Capgras and Fregoli syndromes are mind-reading disorders, due to failures of one of our mind-reading systems (Hirstein, 2005), a set of brain processes we use to understand and predict the behavior of others. Capgras syndrome occurs when egocentric representations of a particular person are damaged or inaccessible and are replaced by other, incorrect egocentric representations.

The representational theory of misidentification takes what the patients say seriously, unlike the other approaches, which dismiss it as a convenient creation. There is nothing specific about an absence of emotional arousal, for instance, that would lead someone to posit an impostor. But the experience of an unfamiliar mind situated within a familiar body, with a familiar face, is exactly what would lead to assertions about impostors. According to Feinberg's theory, the Capgras patient experiences a lack of personal relatedness, and this causes him to claim that the person he sees is an impostor. But the patient does not merely see someone familiar as unfamiliar, he perceives that person as having a *different identity* from the person he knows. The patient does not merely treat the impostors as less related than before but as no longer having the same mind, the same motives, moods, and emotions (e.g., paranoid Capgras patients attribute evil intentions to the impostors). According to the representational theory, the Capgras patient perceives his father as having a foreign mind, and this makes him claim that he is an impostor.

To claim that someone is not in fact your father but some stranger pretending to be your father is to make a claim about the identity of that person and also to disavow the personal relatedness of that person. Logically, the identity of someone is independent of that person's degree of personal relatedness to us, but in practicality, when the identity of loved ones is at stake, alterations in perceived identity will also involve alterations in perceived personal relatedness. Conversely, alterations in the patient's sense of personal relatedness need not also involve alternations in perceived identity. One might experience a loss in the sense of personal relatedness to a person, yet not doubt the identity of that person, even if that person is one's father, so that the person might say, "Dad seems like a stranger to me," but be speaking metaphorically, not literally, as the Capgras patient does. If I perceive my wife as having an alien mind, that alters my sense of her personal relatedness to me, but if she seems strange to me, this need not alter my perception of her identity. Thus an alteration in one's sense of personal relatedness alone is not sufficient to produce a misidentification disorder.

I suspect that the personal relatedness factor one sees in the misidentification syndromes is due to the way the egocentric system is not merely egocentric and typically used to represent ourselves but also used to represent people, objects, and events of personal significance. Rather than explaining the patient's beliefs by way of a malfunction in her person-representation systems, Feinberg attributes them partly to emotional/motivational factors. The tendency of patients to cling strongly to the delusional belief, according to Feinberg, "suggests that there is an impediment or resistance to the truth" (Feinberg et al., 2005, p. 115). Feinberg posits various motivational factors as a way to this tenacity, but another explanation for the patients' insistence on their beliefs is that they experience a pronounced perception of an unfamiliar person. This perception is coming from a normally trustworthy source, and the patients lack the ability to critically assess its groundedness.

According to the representational theory, these syndromes are not disorders of personal relatedness, but rather disorders caused by damage to an egocentric representation system. We normally use this system to represent ourselves and our surroundings, but it can also be used as a simulation (in what I am calling other-mode) to understand others. There is truly an ego at the center of this system, in the sense of ego that means mind. We use this system to construct full-blown representations of the minds of people close to us. To produce an accurate simulation of another person, we need an extensive and detailed representation. We need to build a complete scale model of an airplane to test it in a wind tunnel, for example, because of the holistic way changes in one property of the airplane affect others. If we change the airflow over one part of the plane, we have then changed the airflow over the parts of plane behind this part. Similarly, we need a full model of a minded, embodied person in an environment to perform effective simulations of people in alternative situations.

The way we know what to expect from a person is to create a simulation of him or her. But how do we represent the personalities of the people we know? As we watch the angry person, livid that his car won't start, we don't just understand his angry actions, the slamming of doors and hoods. We understand how the anger was generated. We know how our own anger generates angry actions because we experience this causation directly. We can also understand why someone does not act. When we understand someone's pain, we understand how the pain restricts her actions and depresses her moods. Representations of personalities also include representations of that person's characteristic emotions and moods. Some types of simulations of minds can be thought of as functions from perceptions to actions. Two different people will respond differently to the same perceptions. One person may do what another merely considers then inhibits, because of differences in the way that prefrontal processes filter contemplated actions. There are also cases in which a perception causes a certain emotion, which in turn causes an action. To represent these personalities, these functions, we would also need to simulate these emotions. Knowing someone means knowing what makes her happy and what makes her angry, as well as how she behaves when she's angry or happy. We are not normally aware of our mind representations as representations because we simply see ourselves as perceiving people with emotions and personalities and characters.

We do not realize that we are not actually seeing their emotions, intentions, or motives, we are reproducing them within ourselves.

5. Executive Processes

According to the two-phase theory of confabulation I am working within here, once a person or limb is misidentified (phase one), the brains of the patients fail to employ executive processes to correct the error (phase two). What exactly are executive processes, though? Cognition requires both representations and processes for manipulating those representations—these latter are executive processes. Executive processes perform many different operations on representations. One clear illustration of executive processes at work managing representations occurs when we recall some past event from our lives. Your memory itself is just a huge collection of representations; executive processes must control the search and reconstruction processes that take place when we remember. Executive processes control mental activity by allowing us to shift our focus from perception to memory or back or rearrange items held in working memory (e.g., in the digit span task, where a sequence of numbers is read out loud to the subject, who must then report the sequence in reverse order) (Shimamura, 2002).

Marcia Johnson's theory of memory confabulations is that they are caused by a deficit in a general executive function she calls "reality monitoring"—the ability to distinguish real from imagined events (Johnson, 1991). Real memories, according to Johnson, can often be distinguished from mere imaginings by the amount of perceptual detail they contain, as well as by the presence of supporting memories, including information about where and when the remembered event occurred—known as source memory. Normal people are able to differentiate real from spurious information at high success rates by employing executive processes. This seems to be a learned or at least a developed ability. Small children often have trouble drawing the line between the real and the merely imagined until their frontal lobes develop. When the relevant executive processes are damaged, mere imaginings can be mistaken for actual visual experiences. In the early days of psychosurgery, Whitty and Lewin (1957) described a condition they called "vivid daydreaming," that appeared in 8 of 10 patients who had undergone an anterior cingulectomy (removal of a portion of cortex in the medial prefrontal lobes) in an attempt to control severe obsessive compulsive disorder. The patients would claim odd things happened to them in the hospital—a man said his wife had stopped by for tea, and a woman claimed she saw the nurses putting pins in her food—and then admit that they could not tell whether they had imagined them or whether the events had really happened.

A great deal of what we normally call thinking, deciding, planning, and remembering is accomplished primarily by the brain's executive processes. One introspectively accessible measure of the amount of executive activity is our sense of mental effort. Increased mental effort correlates with increased usage of oxygen by executive areas, which is detectable by brain imaging. In such studies, tasks are devised that require the intervention of executive functions, then brain activity is monitored as the subject attempts the task. Most executive processes reside in the prefrontal lobes, including the dorsolateral frontal lobes on the side of the brain, the ventrolateral frontal lobes below them, and the orbitofrontal lobes located on the brain's undersurface just above the eye sockets (Moscovitch and Winocur, 2002). One area that is frequently active during effortful processing is the aforementioned anterior cingulate. The anterior cingulate is thought to play a role in resolving conflicts between routine actions that are not relevant to the present task and novel actions that are relevant. It also activates strongly when the subject detects an error in his or her response (Carter, Botvinick, and Cohen, 1999). Imaging studies show that the prefrontal executive processes become less active during routine actions, while we are dreaming, and during certain meditative states.

Another source of information about executive processes is the study of neurological patients who have lost one or more executive functions due to brain damage. A favorite test of planning ability is the Tower of Hanoi puzzle, in which several stacked disks of gradually larger sizes must be transferred from one peg to another, obeying the rule that a larger disk may never be put on a smaller one. Patients with damage to the dorsolateral prefrontal cortex are at a loss in this task. Some of these patients will also perseverate, causing them to fail another standard test, the Wisconsin Card Sorting Test. Here the subject must sort cards, each of which contains one or more colored shapes. First the subject is instructed to sort the cards by the shape of their figures. Then the rule is changed, and the subject is told to sort the cards by the color of their figures. The patients will not be able to change, even though many of them remark that they know they are sorting incorrectly. They have lost the ability to disengage ongoing behavior, another executive process.

According to several theorists, the prefrontal cortex does not contain our conscious mental representations. They reside in posterior cortical regions, in the temporal and parietal lobes. The prefrontal lobes contain the processes that monitor and manipulate these representations. Thus the function of the prefrontal cortex (PFC) and its executive processes is "modulatory rather than transmissive. That is, the pathway from input to output does not 'run through' the PFC. Instead, the PFC guides activity flow along task-relevant pathways in more posterior and/or subcortical circuits" (Miller and Cohen, 2001, p. 184). More specifically, the dorsolateral prefrontal cortex is responsible for "the monitoring of multiple events within working memory, regardless of the nature of the stimulus...rather than the maintenance of the stimuli *per se*," which occurs in posterior temporal and parietal areas (Petrides, Alivisatos, and Frey, 2002, p. 5649).

It is important to note that the executive processes can participate in the act of recognition itself, and they normally have the power to overrule initial perceptual identifications. We all experience strange perceptions at times, but we are able to correct them using executive processes. I believe I see my friend during a trip to Nepal, but then I realize how improbable that is—this friend never travels, has no interest in Nepal, and so on—so I do not allow myself to recognize that person as my friend. As Rapcsak, Polster, Comer, and Rubens note, "the frontal lobes are also likely to be responsible for detecting and resolving potential ambiguities arising in connection with the operations of perceptual recognition systems" (1994, p. 577). When a person encounters an object, x, what he or she identifies as x is a product of three dissociable factors: the state of the allocentric representation system, the state of the egocentric representation system, and the state of the person's executive processes. When we first become aware of a person's presence, two different streams of processing commence their work. Failure of either the allocentric stream or the egocentric stream, coupled with the relevant executive failure, should produce a confabulation if the patient is asked the right question, which in the case of Capgras syndrome is simply a question about the identities of the people standing at his or her bedside. The decision must be made at the executive level as to whether the presence in consciousness of a given representation truly means that the represented object is there. For example, the existence of phantom limbs involves (I will argue shortly) an active egocentric representation of the missing limb, but at the executive level that activity is not taken as a veridical representation (mainly because the allocentric system strongly confirms the absence of the limb). Conversely, severing of the nerve to an arm can produce the impression that the arm is not there, due to the removal of somatosensation, which is part of the egocentric system. But executive processes are able to let the continued correctness of the external, allocentric representations of the arm overrule this impression: The arm is still there, merely numb. The executive systems apparently have the ability to let either the allocentric system or the egocentric system win out over the other, in the event of discord between their representations of the object confronting one.

6. Anomalies of Person Recognition

Neurological patients with prosopagnosia can no longer visually recognize the people they know, but they continue to attribute the same personalities and other mental traits to them once they recognize them via some other means, such as by their voices. Sometimes a prosopagnosic may succeed in a certain type of effortful visual recognition by depending on specific clues, such as a person's distinctive nose or ears, or even the type of glasses or necktie someone typically wears, as opposed to normal face perception, which is done holistically rather than in such piecemeal fashion and much more quickly. The prosopagnosic cannot easily recognize friends and family by their external appearances, their faces are not familiar. But once the patient hears his mother speak, he recognizes her, and will treat her as his mother. For the prosopagnosic, the familiar face is not present, but the person is.

For the Capgras patient, the familiar face is present, but the person is not. The Capgras patient's relevant executive processes are malfunctioning, and this prevents him from realizing how implausible the impostor claim is and rejecting it. The typical prosopagnosic does not have executive damage, but according to the theory described here, a prosopagnosic with executive damage should confabulate when asked to identify people. The two patients of Rapcsak et al. (1994) seem to fit this profile. They were both unable to recognize familiar faces, and when asked to identify faces in photographs, they employed the style typically seen in prosopagnosics of attempting to identify faces by focusing on features. The use of this strategy, together with executive failure, caused the patients to confabulate that unfamiliar people were familiar, because the unfamiliar person shared some facial feature with the familiar person. One of the patients pointed to a fellow patient on the ward, for example, and exclaimed, "There's my father! I'd recognize that hooked nose anywhere!" (Rapcsak et al., 1994, p. 569). Both patients had suffered massive right hemisphere strokes that produced fronto-temporal-parietal areas of damage that perhaps were extensive enough to produce both the required damage to the face perception system as well as to a related prefrontal executive area. The authors support the idea of frontal executive damage by noting that "the dysfunction of the decision making process in our patients was evidenced by the fact that they rarely if ever attempted to verify the correctness of their initial impressions regarding a person's identity. Instead, they seemed to accept the output generated by the impaired face recognition system unconditionally" (Rapcsak et al., 1994, p. 576). We might call this syndrome *dysexecutive prosopagnosia*. It causes misidentifications based on superficial similarities of facial features that patients lack the executive processes to correct.

The patient with Cotard syndrome says that he and/or others are dead, hollow, or empty beings. These patients perceive bodies and faces well enough but see no persons at home in them, rather like a dense neurological version of the psychiatric notion of depersonalization. Cotard himself reported that his patient said she had "no brain, nerves, chest, or entrails, and was just skin and bone" (Berrios and Luque, 1995, p. 185). One Cotard patient described "feeling nothing inside" (Wright, Young, and Hellawell, 1993); another patient "felt that her brain was dead" (Young, Leafhead, and Szulecka, 1994). In 1788, Charles Bonnet described a patient who, after what appears to have been a stroke, "demanded that the women should dress her in a shroud and place her in a coffin since she was in fact already dead" (Förstl and Beats, 1992). According to the representational theory, Cotard syndrome is caused by destruction of the mind-representing part of the egocentric representation system. Patients with Cotard and Capgras syndromes recognize familiar people externally but attribute either no mind at all to them, and hence speak of them as "dead" or "robots" (Cotard), or they perceive them to have strange, unknown minds, and hence speak of them as "impostors" (Capgras).

The Fregoli syndrome patient sees a certain significant person as somehow inhabiting several different bodies. According to the representational theory, what happens in Fregoli syndrome is that the patient's egocentric representation of a familiar person is paired with allocentric representations of unfamiliar faces and bodies. This produces in the patient the impression of a single person disguising him- or herself as a succession of strangers. Intermetamorphosis is an especially odd misidentification syndrome in which the patient perceives someone as changing from one identity to another, including changes in that person's face. People sometimes appear to metamorphose into other people right before their eyes. Courbon and Tusques's (1932) original patient was a woman who said that her husband's face could change to look exactly like that of a neighbor and that many other people took on the appearance of her son. Intermetamorphosis apparently involves activation of both the allocentric and egocentric components of incorrect person representations. These disorders are summarized in table 19.1.

6.1. Mild Variants of the Clinical Syndromes

All of the misidentification disorders involve compromised executive processes, but what happens when only the first phase malfunctions and the person's executive processes are intact? We should expect this to produce mild anomalies of person recognition that all of us might experience during our lifetimes (summarized in table 19.2). The mild variant of Capgras in the person with intact executive processing might be a feeling that one does not know a person one thought one knew, that the person's psychology might be quite different from what one had thought. The mild variant of Cotard syndrome might be depersonalization, where the person sees others as empty but does not confabulate about them being dead. Stories of zombies in folklore and cinema indicate an experience on the part of the viewer that might be categorized as another mild variant of Cotard syndrome: One experiences an animate but mentally empty person. Similarly, some theorists have argued that at least some autistic people see others as objects, without an inner mental life. The mild variant of Fregoli syndrome would be a feeling that a certain person bears a strong psychological similarity to another person one knows well, a condition we might call inner resemblance, to contrast it with a common experience we can call outer resemblance, in which one judges a person to outwardly resemble someone familiar. The mild variant of the state of intermetamorphosis in which someone appears to have both the outer and inner identity of another would be a case in which someone resembles a familiar person both outwardly and mentally (called strong resemblance in table 19.2).

7. Anomalies of Limb Recognition

Feinberg and colleagues tested 12 patients with right hemisphere stroke damage for asomatognosia (Feinberg, Haber, and Leeds, 1990). Their test consisted simply of holding up the patient's left hand and asking, "What is this?" Within the asomatognosia group, the most common misidentification was calling the limb "your [the doctor's] hand" or "your arm." Several of these patients also referred to the limb as

Table 19.1. Severe disorders of person recognition

Condition	Object	Allocentric System	Egocentric System	Executive Processes	Person's Report
Correct recognition	x	x	x	yes	That is x.
Failure to recognize	x	none/x'	none	yes	I don't recognize that.
Capgras syndrome	x	x	y'/none	no	x is an impostor.*
Cotard syndrome	x	x	none	no	x is dead/empty.*
Intermetamorphosis	x	y	y	no	x changed into y.*
Fregoli syndrome	y	none/y'	x	no	x is disguising himself as y.*
Prosopagnosia	x	none	x	yes	x looks unfamiliar.
Dys. prosopagnosia	y	none	x	no	y is my father.*

*Indicates confabulation.
' Indicates a newly-created representation.

"the doctor's" hand. One patient referred to the limb as "a breast" and a "deodorant." One patient called it "my mother-in-law's" hand (Feinberg et al., 1990, p. 1391).

Asomatognosics may claim that the arm "belongs to a fellow patient previously transported by ambulance, or that it had been forgotten in bed by a previous patient" (Bisiach and Geminiani, 1991). One of Feinberg's other patients called his left arm "a useless piece of machinery" (Feinberg, 2001). As the tone of these responses implies, patients may display dislike or even hatred of the paralyzed limb, a condition known as misoplegia. Another patient called his arm a piece of "dead wood" (Weinstein, 1991); yet another called his "a piece of dead meat" (Critchley, 1974). "Actually, the theme of the arm as being 'dead' in some sense, literally or figuratively, is common in asomatognosic patients" according to Feinberg (2006, p. 4). Some patients claim that their flesh is rotting away (Fine, 2006, p. 52). The arm involved is almost always the left arm, and asomatognosia also occurs at a high frequency among patients whose right hemisphere is temporarily anesthetized. Meador, Loring, Feinberg, Lee, and Nichols (2000) found that 88 percent of 62 epileptic patients (without any specific right hemisphere damage) whose right hemispheres were temporarily deactivated by an amobarbital injection could not recognize their own left hands.

If Capgras syndrome is the opposite of Fregoli syndrome, then what is the opposite of asomatognosia? The vast majority of people who undergo amputation of a limb have a clear sensation that the limb is still there—a phantom limb. So vivid is this impression that many patients, on regaining consciousness after the operation, do not realize that the limb is gone until they lift the covers and see.

Their experience of the limb seems to be the same as before. They experience it as being in a certain position, as being hot or cold, as being in pain, as being paralyzed, and sometimes even as moving in response to their intentions, for instance as reaching out to shake hands with someone (Ramachandran and Hirstein, 1998). Conversely, one account of the problem in anosognosic patients is that they have lost the capacity to represent the arm as something with which they can accomplish tasks. We accomplish tasks with tools, but we move them from the outside, whereas we move our arms and legs from the inside. Our limbs respond not to our actions, as tools do, but to our wills. In the asomatognosic patient the amputation, performed by nature itself, is a sort of inner amputation. For humans, the arms are the primary executors of the will. In them, a portion of the will's domain has been cut off. The asomatognosic's arm is there, but it seems to him that it is not; the phantom limb patient's arm is not there, but it seems to him that it is. The arms of phantom limb patients feel the same from the inside, as it were, but obviously do not look the same on the outside. Asomatognosia is just the opposite: The patient's limb looks the same externally but lacks certain internal sensations.

There is a great difference in conviction, of course. The asomatognosic is certain that the arm is not his arm, whereas the phantom limb patient is able to overrule the vivid impression and acknowledges that his limb is gone. If the two-part theory of confabulation is correct, however, the difference between the two is that the asomatognosic has damaged frontal processes—processes that could prevent his odd belief from establishing itself—and this explains the difference in conviction. But what would a phantom limb patient *with* compromised executive processes say about his limb? There is an analogy here with dysexecutive prosopagnosia in the realm of limbs. Amputee patients with phantom limbs have not normally also sustained brain damage, but if a person lost a limb *and* damaged the relevant frontal processes, would he actually deny that his limb was gone? The Capgras patient D.S. described in Hirstein and Ramachandran (1997) was just such a person. D.S.'s right arm needed to be amputated, just below the elbow, and at several points after his car accident that resulted in both the amputation and brain damage, he denied that his arm was gone.

The analogy—prosopagnosia is to Capgras what phantom limb is to asomatognosia—is not perfect. There is a significant difference between the sort of representation failure that occurs with phantom limbs and the failure in prosopagnosia. In the prosopagnosic, (allocentric) face representations are damaged or inaccessible, whereas in the phantom limb patients, (allocentric) representations of the missing limb are presumably intact but not satisfied. Perhaps then, an even closer analog of phantom limb applied to the person is a case in which the interior, the mind, of a person is somehow there without a body. Claims about ghosts, imaginary friends, and some conceptions of gods and spirits may be cases of this.

7.1. Mild Variants of the Clinical Syndromes

What a person considers to be herself depends on how she represents herself. Apparently some of the brain's body-representing areas employ the following rule:

Something is a part of you if and only if it moves in response to your will and you feel what happens to it. When the asomatognosic patient's arm is numb and does not respond to his will, he concludes that it is not his arm. Another rule devised by Dennett (1991) to capture these phenomena is, "I am what I control and care for." The patient can no longer control the limb and cares nothing for it. Botvinick and Cohen (1998) discovered a fascinating way to trick the brain's somatosensory processes into representing something alien as part of oneself, called the rubber hand illusion. The subject is seated with his right hand on a table, but hidden from his view by an occluder. In full view, however, is a realistic-looking rubber hand. The experimenter is seated across the table from the subject, and touches the subject's real hand (out of the subject's view) and the rubber hand (in view of the subject) in the same way at the same time. This causes the subject to feel exactly what he sees happening to the rubber hand. The synchrony of touching very quickly produces a powerful illusion in the subject that the rubber hand is his hand. One piece of evidence for this is the presence of a strong emotional response (as measured by increases in skin conductance) when the rubber hand is pricked with a pin or a finger is bent way back (Armel and Ramachandran, 2003). We might modify Dennett's maxim as follows: I am what I control and feel (because I automatically care for the things I feel).

Conversely, if I cannot control something and feel nothing that happens to it, those posterior brain processes seem to conclude that it is not part of me. If the representational account proposed here is correct, asomatognosia is due to two factors: destruction of an egocentric representation of the limb involved together with damage to executive processes capable of correcting the impression that the limb is not their own. Patients who suffer only the first type of damage while possessing intact executive processes might experience the strong impression that the affected limb is not their own but be able to correct it. Writer Oliver Sacks suffered a bad fall while hiking in the mountains of Norway, breaking his leg at the femur. The break almost severed a nerve in his leg, causing a complete loss of somatosensation together with paralysis of the leg for several weeks. He describes his impressions as he sat in bed looking down at his leg in its cast.

> It was utterly strange, not-mine, unfamiliar. I gazed upon it with absolute non-recognition. I have had—we all have had—sudden odd moments of non-recognition, jamais vu; they are uncanny while they last, but they pass very soon, and we are back in the known and familiar world. But this did not pass—it grew deeper and deeper—and stronger, and stronger.
> The more I gazed at that cylinder of chalk, the more alien and incomprehensible it seemed to me. I could no longer feel it as "mine," as part of me. It seemed to bear no relation whatever to me. It was absolutely not-me—and yet, impossibly, it was attached to me—and even more impossibly, "continuous" with me. (Sacks, 1984, p. 72)

This may be the sort of experience that could lead a person without intact executive functioning to simply accept it on face value: This thing is not my leg. Sacks concludes by emphasizing the role of somatosensation in producing the sense that the leg is ours. "One may be said to 'own' or 'possess' one's body—at least its limbs and moveable parts—by virtue of a constant flow of incoming information, arising ceaselessly, throughout life, from the muscles, joints and tendons. One has oneself, one *is* oneself, because the body knows itself, confirms itself, at all times, by this sixth sense" (1984, p. 71). Alternatively, the phantom limb patient with intact executive processes still has these egocentric processes operating. This allows her to maintain a rational attitude toward her predicament and, more practically, the intactness of the egocentric representation system is an important factor in the success of prosthetic devices. The patient comes to accept the device as part of her because the egocentric representation of her former arm successfully inhabits it.

8. CLASSIFYING DISORDERS OF LIMB AND PERSON RECOGNITION

On the conception defended here, our analog representations of persons are compounds of egocentric representations and allocentric representations. If we take a given person, x, in the patient's circle of friends, relatives, and acquaintances, complete recognition of that person occurs when both the allocentric and the egocentric parts of the subject's representation of x are intact, active, and functioning properly (which includes being properly connected to each other), and the patient's executive processes are functioning correctly. The disorders and anomalies of person and limb recognition we have discussed are summarized in tables 19.1–19.3. The status of the allocentric, egocentric, and executive systems are indicated for each condition. At the top, x is correctly recognized by the patient when the patient's existing allocentric and egocentric representations of x are activated by the perception of x.

What the person ultimately reports, the rightmost columns of these tables, is a product of the allocentric and egocentric representation systems together with any executive activity. Notice that where there are no executive processes (because there is already an anomaly present), what the person says is a confabulation, marked by an asterisk (∗). The entries in this column describe the basic form a person's claims might take when asked about a person or arm. In the case of the confabulations, these basic forms are more like confabulation templates than actual confabulations, which tend to be more detailed and interesting. The tables also encode two types of representational mismatches. What we might call semantic mismatches occur when either an allocentric or an egocentric representation fails to match its real-world object. Two examples of this are Fregoli syndrome (table 19.1) and the rubber hand illusion (table 19.3). The egocentric representation of x is activated in the presence of another person, y, in Fregoli syndrome, and the egocentric representation of my hand, s, is activated by the sight of the rubber hand, r, being touched. All of the

Table 19.2. Anomalies of person recognition

Condition	Object	Allocentric System	Egocentric System	Executive Processes	Person's Report
Correct recognition	x	x	x	yes	That is x.
Failure to recognize	x	none/x'	none	yes	I don't recognize that.
Depersonalization	x	x	none	yes	x seems empty.
"Seeing" zombies	x	x	none	yes	x is a mindless body.
Autism	x	x	none	?	x seems like an object.
Inner resemblance	x	x	y	yes	x thinks like y.
Outer resemblance	x	y	x	yes	x looks like y.
Strong resemblance	x	y	y	yes	x looks and thinks like y.
"Seeing" ghosts	none	none/x	x	yes	It feels like x is still here.

abnormal conditions above contain either a semantic mismatch or a missing object (the "none" entries, we might call these semantic failures). Some of the conditions also contain what we might call a cognitive mismatch, cases in which the allocentric and egocentric representations are mismatched to each other. Fregoli's syndrome also contains one of these. For instance, a stranger's face (allocentric) is mismatched to my brother's mind (egocentric).

Table 19.3 affirms the analogy between asomatognosia and Capgras syndrome for oneself by giving the two a similar profile; they both involve an intact allocentric system and a damaged egocentric system. The analogy can be developed further if we take the patient's emotional response to the person or limb into account (table 19.4). In the second line of the table, the negative reactions toward previously loved and familiar people correspond to the asomatognosic's misoplegia for her newly unfamiliar and unloved arm. In the third line, the Capgras patient who has no suspicion or other ill feelings toward the impostor is analogous to the asomatognosic patient who is completely neutral about her arm while firmly insisting it is not hers. The patients who call their disowned arms by pet names (e.g., "Little Suzie," "a pet rock," or "a clumsy cat"; Paulig, 2000) fall into this category. In the bottom line, the patient with Cotard syndrome for himself is analogous to the asomatognosic who claims that his arm is "a useless piece of machinery," "dead wood," or "dead meat." The analogy continues: The same question arises in the study of both Capgras and asomatognosia about whether the egocentric representation system is not functioning, or functioning with the wrong representation. My claim that in Capgras the egocentric system is functioning but with the wrong representation (possibly a generic one), if true, would work to clearly differentiate Capgras from Cotard

Table 19.3. Disorders and anomalies of limb recognition

Condition	Object	Allocentric System	Egocentric System	Executive Processes	Person's Report
Correct recognition	s	s	s	yes	That is my arm.
Failure to recognize	s	none/s'	none	yes	I don't recognize that.
Asomatognosia	s	s	r'/none	no	That is not my arm.*
Denervation	s	s	none	yes	It feels like s is not my arm.
Rubber hand illus.	r	r	s	yes	It feels like r is my arm.
Phantom limb	none	none	s	yes	It feels like s is still there.
Dys. phantom limb	none	none	s	no	My arm is still there.*

*Indicates confabulation.
¹ Indicates a newly created representation.

syndrome; the egocentric system of the Cotard patient is not functioning at all. One might use the same principle to distinguish between the asomatognosic who says his arm is his brother's (incorrect egocentric representation) and the asomatognosic who says that his arm is dead (no egocentric representation). The reason for the analogies between person and arm representation in this account is that we use the same egocentric system to represent both people and limbs, including ourselves and our limbs.

One might augment table 19.1 to include a treatment of places, where one sees the same sort of misidentifications, places that are present are represented as absent (this is not my house), and places that are absent are represented as present (this is my office [said of the hospital room]). The egocentric representation system, as a whole, represents a mind in a body in a place, so it is natural that there would be patients who show different combinations of delusions about minds and bodies, bodies and places, and so on. The patient of Paulig (2000) had anosognosia for hemiplegia and also misidentified her daughter. The patient of Staton et al. (1982) claimed that people, buildings, and even his cat had been replaced by impostors. The Cotard patient of Young, Robertson, Hellawell, de Pauw, and Pentland (1992) believed that he was dead and also had trouble recognizing buildings and other places. The patient of Frazer and Roberts (1994) claimed that both her husband and her house were duplicates. Neglect itself ranges from neglect of the body (personal neglect), to neglect of nearby objects (peripersonal neglect) (Halligan and Marshall, 1991), to neglect of distant objects (extrapersonal neglect) (Cowey, Small, and Ellis, 1994).

Table 19.4. Analogies between variants of Capgras/Cotard syndromes and asomatognosia

People	Limbs	Confabulations
Capgras for self	asomatognosia	That is not me/mine.
Capgras with suspicion	misoplegia	That person/limb is bad.
Capgras without suspicion	asomatognosia	That limb is not mine.
Cotard for self	"dead" arm	I am (my limb is) dead.

9. EPISODIC MEMORIES OF OTHERS

A person's episodic memories are memories of that person from her point of view. The representations that are stored in episodic memory are egocentric in the sense that they represent events as we experienced them, hence they are also called autobiographical memories. Autobiographical episodic memories combine several different subrepresentations, including representations of our bodies moving through different spaces and environments and representations of the people and objects with which we have had significant interactions. We carefully represent each aspect of a particularly significant interaction, exactly what was said, and in which tone of voice. In addition to representations of emotions, episodic memories may also contain representations of other conscious states, such as our thoughts, motives, and intentions at the time of the event. The typical autobiographical memory representation is of a person with a conscious mind, moving through space, interacting with people and objects.

The episodic memory system is also able to aggregate its information into our existing concepts of important people and things. Once this information enters the system of concepts, it becomes part of the semantic memory system and is then accessible to the process of thinking itself. Thus, the episodic memory system can feed the semantic memory system. For instance, if I travel to Paris, the episodic memories I amass as I see important sites in the city also add information to my semantic representation of Paris, the Eiffel Tower, the Arc de Triomphe, and so on. All of this information tends to be either conceptual or allocentric in form, but I suggest that the egocentric realm has its own ability to aggregate its representations into a full-blown simulation of persons' minds. As I accumulate information about someone over the course of many interactions with her, I also accumulate information about her thoughts, moods, and emotions, using the egocentric representations system in other-mode. We might call such memories "biographical memories." These accumulations of simulated mental states constitute representations of the minds of the significant people in our lives. If this is right, our representation of a significant person would contain an allocentric component with representations of how he looks and sounds, and an egocentric representation of his mind, body, and environments from his viewpoint. Our awareness of the minds of others when the egocentric system is operating in other-mode is nonexplicit and faint in our minds. Perhaps this is a reason that distinguishing whether an emotion or a simulation of a mind is missing (as may happen in Capgras syndrome) is difficult for the patients. Perhaps another reason why the activity level of the egocentric system needs to be low when it is operating in other-mode is because full-blown conscious representation leads to actual external actions, not merely to represented actions, in much the same way the dreaming mind malfunctions during REM sleep disorder, when dreamed perceptions cause real actions. Simulations cannot fully employ this representation system without danger of causing real actions with potentially disastrous consequences.

The experimental and clinical data show that this biographical memory system may have a special fragility in the way it sorts incoming memories according to persons' identities. The system needs to be able to create new concepts when new people are encountered and properly segregate this concept from its concepts of other people. For instance, if I start a new job and spend several hours with a new co-worker, my brain will begin creating a representation of this person. But when this person leaves and another new co-worker enters, my brain needs to close the first file it opened and start another one. There needs to be a firm partition between these two representations, so that I do not confuse the identities of my co-workers. In many of the syndromes we have examined, this partitioning system seems to be overfunctioning. As we tested one Capgras patient's ability to discern gaze direction by showing him 30 photos of a model looking either directly at the camera or various degrees off center, an interesting thing happened. After the 11th slide, he claimed that the identity of the model had changed and the photos were actually of a different but similar looking woman (Hirstein and Ramachandran, 1997). A partition had been made in his memory, as if a file had been closed and a new one opened. It is also frequently reported in the literature that Capgras patients create several doubles for a person. In their original article, Capgras and Reboul-Lachaux say that "more often than not it is one and the same person who changes successively into the first double, the second, the third, etc., at intervals of a few hours, a few days, or a few weeks" ([1923] 1994, p. 127). This partitioning phenomenon can produce the appearance of two people, two arms, or two places where there is only one by drawing an arbitrary boundary in the brain's system of filing memories. In doing so, it appears to the patient to confirm his impressions that the person, arm, or place is not his own.

The memory system of the misidentification patient can also lose large portions of information accumulated about a person or thing, which the patient perceives as a strange, sudden aging of the thing represented. One Capgras patient expressed amazement that his leather boots were well worn because he remembered them as looking new (Staton et al., 1982), as if the memories of those boots over a certain time span had been lost. The original intermetamorphosis patient of Courbon and Tusques complained that "They have changed my hens, they've put two old ones in the place of two young ones" (1932, p. 139). Another patient said that that "old man" could not be his father. It seems too strong to claim that this filing problem is the cause of the misidentifications, as for example, Staton et al. (1982) do. If it were just a memory problem, the patients would say, "Dad, what happened to you? You've *really* aged!" But the patient does not say this. He says, "You are not my father, you are someone else." There may be a connection between the filing problem and the problem of identity. Based on what has been reviewed here, one would expect both these segregation phenomena and the loss of time interval phenomena to be caused by malfunctions in the egocentric system.

We possess representations of specific individual minds, if the ideas here are right, but there is also evidence that we possess generic mind representations that we use to understand strangers. We create generic representations of other significant things. All of my episodic memories of visits to grocery stores, for instance, organize themselves into generic memories of certain grocery store types, which I access when I decide where to go to purchase certain foods or where to look for what I want once I'm in a grocery store. If the Capgras patient has lost his representation of his father's individual mind but uses a generic representation when he now looks at him, this is precisely what would produce the impression of an impostor—his father's body and face, alloyed with the mind of some other person. One Capgras patient we saw believed his father was an impostor, and referred to him as "that nice Jewish gentleman." He also tended to categorize other people by religion (Hirstein and Ramachandran, 1997). Perhaps this patient's generic egocentric representations were organized according to religions. Some people also associate personality types with certain races, a raw but regrettable fact that is perhaps more revealing of the mechanics of racism than talk about external differences. On this hypothesis, then, when both individual and generic egocentric representations are unusable, Cotard syndrome results. The patient can only represent people externally, using the allocentric system, and this causes him to see them as empty and without minds. This can also explain why some patients, such as that of Wright et al. (1993) alternate between Cotard and Capgras syndromes: The patient's egocentric representations of individuals are inaccessible, whereas his generic egocentric representations are intermittently on- and off-line, perhaps due to irregular blood flow or to remapping of the damaged neural networks. When they are online, the patient has Capgras syndrome. When they are off-line, he has Cotard syndrome.

10. Neuroscientific Findings

Theories of the crucial neural locus for asomatognosia have focused on the inferior parietal lobes, particularly on the right side. The inferior parietal lobes are constituted by two gyri, the supramarginal gyrus (Brodmann area 40) and the angular gyrus (Brodmann area 39) (see figure 19.1). Nielsen (1938) was the first

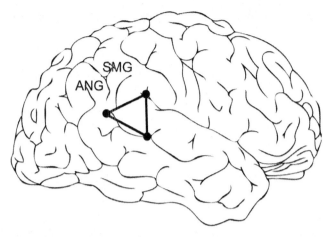

Figure 19.1. Cortical areas of interest. Triangle encloses the temporo-parietal junction. ANG: angular gyrus; SMG: supramarginal gyrus. Diagram after Mort et al. (2003); Saxe demarcates the TPJ as slightly anterior to this location (e.g., Saxe, 2005, p. 176).

argue that the crucial site of damage leading to asomatognosia is the right supramarginal gyrus or its connections to subcortical areas. The study mentioned earlier by Feinberg et al. (1990) involving 12 asomatognosic patients also supported this localization.

In 2003, Rizzolatti and Mattelli argued that the traditional division of visual streams leaving the occipital lobe into a ventral and a dorsal one (Ungerleider and Mishkin, 1982) is inadequate and that the dorsal stream of visual processing should be divided into two separate streams, which they call the dorsodorsal stream and the ventrodorsal stream. The dorsodorsal stream has all of the characteristics traditionally attributed to the dorsal stream: It involves the superior parietal lobe and functions to provide information required to execute actions involving, for example, reaching for nearby objects. The idea of a ventrodorsal stream is a new concept, however, and the stream has been found to have some interesting characteristics. Area PF in the Rhesus monkey, which corresponds to the supramarginal gyrus in humans, is the primary recipient of visual input for this stream. The inferior parietal lobe receives input from the superior temporal polysensory area, an area that merges input from several different sense modalities (Desimone and Gross, 1979). Area PF is now known to contain mirror neurons, neurons that respond when the subject executes a particular, say, arm action, or when the subject sees another person execute that same action (Rizzolatti and Craighero, 2004). In my earlier terminology, PF is able to operate in both self-mode and other-mode. Ramachandran and Rogers-Ramachandran (1996) found that patients with anosognosia who falsely claimed they had moved their hands in response to a request also (falsely) claimed that *other* patients they observed had moved their arms in response to the same request. The simplest explanation of this is that the same damaged system is responsible for both the confabulations about whether the patients moved and the confabulations about whether the people they were observing moved.

The crucial posterior damage site for misidentification syndromes (in addition to frontal damage causing executive failures) may be a cortical area just inferior to the supramarginal gyrus, the temporoparietal junction (TPJ). Two Cotard patients studied by Young and his colleagues (Young et al., 1992; Young et al., 1994) had temporoparietal contusions along with bilateral frontal damage. The Capgras patient of Staton et al. (1982) showed "moderate atrophy...at the temporo-parietal junction." Similarly, a Capgras patient seen by Johnson and Raye (1998) had a right temporoparietal hematoma. A Fregoli patient described by Feinberg, Eaton, Roane, and Giacino (1999) also had damage at the TPJ. The TPJ has been found to be active during several "theory of mind" tasks, in which subjects need to understand the actions and motives of others. Saxe has recently undertaken a series of fMRI studies designed to clarify the role played by the right TPJ in understanding the minds of others. In a typical task, the brain of a subject is scanned as she observes people performing certain actions or displaying certain emotions. Saxe describes the TPJ as an "area for representing mental states" (2006, p. 235) that responds selectively to "the attribution of mental states" (Saxe and Wexler, 2005) and plays a role in developing an "integrated impression" of people. This may be the sort of area that when damaged affects our representations of the minds of other people, producing (along with executive failure) the misidentification disorders. I have also postulated that these separate events of representing peoples' minds are accumulated in episodic memory—biographical memories. There is evidence of a TPJ link to the autobiographical memory system (Maguire, 2001), and Fink et al. (1996) found TPJ activity during a task in which subjects recalled emotional autobiographical events from their pasts.

Damage to this complex of areas should produce problems in the patient's egocentric representation of himself as well as in his egocentric representations of others. Adolphs, Damasio, Tranel, and Damasio (1996) found activity in the right parietal cortex during a task in which subjects attributed mental states to other people. This caused them to suggest in a subsequent work that

> in addition to retrieval of visual and somatic records, the difficulty of the particular task we used may make it necessary for subjects to construct a somatosensory representation by internal *simulation*. Such an internally constructed somatic activity pattern—which could be either covert or overt—would simulate components of the emotional state depicted by the target face. In essence, the brain would reconstruct a state akin to that of the person shown in the stimulus. (Adolphs, Tranel, and Damasio, 2001, p. 101)

Representations of emotional states would be part of the egocentric representation system; they are a way of representing the mind of the person of interest.

One phenomenon that is capable of yielding more clues about how to unite our understandings of asomatognosia and the misidentification syndromes such as Capgras and Cotard is called "mirror agnosia." Ramachandran and colleagues discovered that certain anosognosic patients have lost their ability to interpret mirror images. Their test is simple: A mirror is held in front of the patient so that he can see himself from the torso up. As he watches, an assistant holds a pen just above the patient's left shoulder, so that the pen is visible to him only in the mirror. The patient is then told to grab the pen with his right hand. Amazingly, some patients will repeatedly bump their hands into the mirror, or try to reach behind it rather than simply reaching back toward their left to grasp the pen (Ramachandran, Altschuler, and Hillyer, 1997).

Some Capgras patients experience the impostor delusion when they look at themselves in a mirror. The patient of Silva, Leong, Wine, and Saab "developed the delusion that his facial reflection in mirrors and other glass surfaces was no longer his own face but the work of an autonomous evil being. The image of his face was identical to his own face except that the image appeared to be very sinister and aggressive" (1992, pp. 574–575). Breen, Caine, Coltheart, Hendy, and Roberts (2000) describe a patient with "marked right hemisphere dysfunction" who came to believe that his mirror image was actually another person. He did not believe that the person in the mirror wanted to hurt him, though, and his egocentric representation of the man seemed to be generic. When asked what the man in the mirror thought, the patient answered that he hadn't been able to get him to talk. The patient was not shocked by these events and impassively noted that the man shaved when he shaved and dressed as he dressed. When Breen and colleagues tested the patient for mirror agnosia, he repeatedly bumped his hand against the mirror. Breen, Caine, and Coltheart (2004) also report a second patient who misidentified himself in mirrors and had temporoparietal damage.

Understanding how to interpret mirrors requires knowledge of how to move from the default origin of the egocentric representation system, our own minds, out into the world, reflected at the appropriate angle off the mirror. We also need to shift the origin of the egocentric representation system when we observe other people, from our own minds to that of the person of interest. Damage to the egocentric representation system compromises both of these abilities. Saxe notes that "the TPJ region is also selectively recruited for determining how the spatial relations between two objects would appear from a character's point of view versus the subject's own position" (2006, p. 236). Blanke and colleagues have found that one can produce a vivid out-of-body experience involving what they refer to as an "abnormal egocentric visuospatial perspective" (Blanke et al., 2005) by electrically stimulating the TPJ (Blanke and Arzy, 2005), something that again is consistent with its use to represent not only our own location in space but also locations we are not currently in. This suggests that Blanke is able to produce out-of-body experiences by stimulating the right TPJ not because we evolved a brain area that lets us have such experiences but because Blanke and colleagues are stimulating an area that is capable of representing nonactual egocentric situations, primarily so that it can function in other-mode to simulate other people. In another experiment, Arzy and colleagues stimulated the left TPJ and found that it produced in their subjects "the strange sensation that somebody is nearby" who imitated the subject's own body position and posture (Arzy, Seeck, Ortigue, Spinelli, and Blanke, 2006, p. 287).

Perhaps the stimulation produced an odd mix of the TPJ's other-representing functions (the sense that someone is nearby) but with the body-representing areas continuing to represent the subject's own body positions while also representing those as body positions of another person, producing the sense of doing something in unison with another.

The areas in and around the TPJ participate in several diverse and fascinating mental functions, and just as in the case of the prefrontal lobes, we are still in the process of developing conceptual schemes that adequately classify and describe both the functions and the systems responsible for them. Aichhorn, Perner, Kronbichler, Staffen, and Ladurner (2006) recommend that the TPJ be divided into two areas, arguing that its dorsal portion is "responsible for representing perspective differences and making behavioral predictions," whereas its ventral region—along with the medial prefrontal cortex—is responsible for "predicting behavioral consequences" of another person's mental states. The brain's right hemisphere appears to contain areas, such as the inferior parietal cortex and the TPJ just below it, that serve the dual function of representing ourselves on certain occasions and other people on other occasions. I suggest that areas such as the supramarginal gyrus and the TPJ, working in concert with interconnected areas in the temporal and prefrontal lobes, are responsible for the sense of oneself as an embodied being with a mind situated in an environment. Out-of-body experiences, for instance, contain representations of what one's phenomenology, one's mental life, would be like, as well the changes in one's body and its environment. We represent our minds as directing intentional activity into this spatial milieu via the body. Alternatively, when we understand the intentional actions of others, this area serves as an egocentric representation of them.

We represent animate limbs with additional types of representations that we do not employ when we look at dead limbs. We normally represent our limbs as the business end of our bodies, the executors of our wills in the world. We also represent the arms of others as executors of actions. Sometimes when we know that arms will be acting toward us, we focus our attention on them, as do boxers, for instance (the attention, not the eyes, which are typically directed at the opponent's head). But even in these cases, we do not represent the arms as the real initiators of the actions. We are also tracking the mental states of the owner of those arms, and we represent the actions of the arms as caused by his mental states.

11. CONCLUSION

The account here, if correct, brings the misidentification syndromes and asomatognosia into line with the rest of the confabulation syndromes by showing how they also fall under the two-factor theory. Confabulation is caused by two events: (1) damage to some perceptual or mnemonic process in the posterior of the brain, typically the cortex; and (2) damage to some prefrontal process that monitors and can manipulate and/or correct the output of that perceptual or mnemonic process. In the case of neglect and asomatognosia, the posterior lesion tends to occur in the inferior parietal lobe, often in the supramarginal gyrus. The lesion that produces misidentifications seems to be just below that one, in the TPJ. Damage to these egocentric representation systems alters, sometimes quite subtly, the way a person perceives herself and her body, as well as other people and their bodies. But instead of saying that her limb doesn't feel the same, or that something is different about her father, the patient with damage to these structures, as well as to their allied prefrontal structures, will claim that the limb is not her limb, and the man at her bedside is not her father. When the patient's executive processes are intact, however, she can overrule mere appearances: Even though it feels as if my arm is still there, it isn't (phantom limb); even though that person seems like a stranger, he isn't (prosopagnosia).

Their ability to detect and reject or repair ill-grounded representations positions the executive systems as a second line of defense against candidate beliefs that are false because of malfunctions in the posterior representation systems. But they are apparently the second and final line of defense, so that when they fail, irrationality and its errors can manifest. The ability to be rational depends fundamentally on the ability to correctly identify people and objects on multiple occasions. A person contradicts herself when she claims that the same thing both has and lacks the same property at the same time. Contradiction is the arch-enemy of rationality, but contradiction only exists when the *same* thing is referred to or thought of in both instances. How much of the (local) irrationality of the patients is traceable to their identification problems? In a normal person, acceptance of these mistaken identifications will quickly run into large numbers of contradictory beliefs, strongly alerting the person that some serious rethinking is in order. Clinical confabulation patients of all sorts are simply not alarmed by contradictions, however, and are not led by them into the rethinking process.

If the approach described here is correct, we build large, detailed representations of the minds of those close to us. These representations are exquisitely sensitive to changes in the beliefs or personalities of the people they are directed at. We create these representations so automatically, and they operate so subtly, that when they are damaged we have trouble understanding what has happened. The damage leads in some minds to the creation of confabulations about who these people are. If this approach is right, these syndromes, as well as asomatognosia and other allied syndromes, can be understood as responses to damage of certain types to a representational system with a certain structure. The personal element in the misidentification syndromes observed by Feinberg and colleagues is a byproduct of the operation of the egocentric representation system. This system either represents me or things and people of interest to me. The change in personal relatedness does not offer a very specific explanation of the contents of the confabulations, however. It is not just that the person seems to the Capgras patient not to be personally related to him (or that the sight of the person fails to produce an emotional response, as in the emotional theory). The representational theory described herein provides an account that explains what the patients explicitly say. Having egocentric representations of people and things of interest might seem counterproductive, if it is true that damage to such a system can produce such debilitating consequences as Capgras and asomatognosia, but this disadvantage is vastly outweighed by the increase in predictive power the ability to apply an egocentric representation system to others allows.

One of my goals here has been to present the empirical phenomena in such a way that makes their relevance to philosophical questions obvious. There are some concrete hypotheses suggested by what we have reviewed here that are of relevance to philosophy. First, identification of people and body parts involves egocentric and allocentric representations together with executive processes. If this is correct, it needs to be taken into account in the philosophical discussions of how humans identify objects and people. Second, contrary to what Wittgenstein (see Rhees, 2003) and others have indicated, if the evidence given here is correct, there can be local irrationality, cases in which people are only irrational in certain topic domains. Third, our explicit, conceptual knowledge of our bodies in an important way rests on this set of allocentric and egocentric analog representations. For instance, when the asomatognosic claims that arm is not his, he is using concepts such as *arm* and *mine*, but his error occurred at the lower, analog level, not at this conceptual level, which merely faithfully carries through the error. If this is right, it seems vital to the discussion in epistemology of Moore's claim to know that his hand exists, because it indicates that knowledge expressed in concepts ("Here is my hand") rests on knowledge embodied in analog form. More broadly, these phenomena would be strongly relevant to many discussions in epistemology concerning foundationalism. Finally, the phenomena reviewed here do support Wittgenstein's separation of knowledge from feelings of certainty. The patients are quite certain of their (false) identity claims, because they no longer have the executive processes to produce and sustain doubt.

Although the person with a phantom limb has lost something of great value, the limb itself, she retains something of even greater value, the egocentric representation of the limb. This representation easily and naturally comes to inhabit the prosthetic arm as the patient recovers. The prosopagnosic has lost his ability to identify people by their faces, but he has not lost the people themselves. He retains his representations of their minds, and these minds can reinhabit the visually unfamiliar people around him. The patients suffering from Capgras and Cotard syndromes have in a very real sense lost their loved ones, because they have lost their grasps of their mental lives, their minds. The patients are surrounded instead by empty people, or strangers, some of whom mimic or menace them from behind mirrors. The patient with asomatognosia has an alien, unwanted appendage, someone else's arm, or a dead or empty arm, dangling from her own shoulder. The approach taken here explains these strange symptoms not as the result of deep and mysterious psychiatric conflicts as had been thought, but rather of the way our representational systems are organized, and the way they respond to damage.

ACKNOWLEDGMENTS

Thanks to Xavier Arko, Todd Feinberg, Thomas O'Donnell, V. S. Ramachandran, Katie Reinecke, and Katrina Sifferd for helpful feedback and other contributions.

REFERENCES

Adolphs, R., Damasio, H., Tranel, D., and Damasio, A. R. (1996). Cortical systems for the recognition of emotion in facial expression. *Journal of Neuroscience* 16: 7678–7687.

Adolphs, R., Tranel, D., and Damasio, A. R. (2001). Neural systems subserving emotion: Lesion studies of the amygdala, somatosensory cortices, and ventromedial prefrontal cortices. In G. Gainotti (Ed.), *Handbook of Neurophysiology*. New York: Elsevier.

Aichhorn, M., Perner, J., Kronbichler, M., Staffen, W., and Ladurner, G. (2006). Do visual perspective tasks need theory of mind? *Neuroimage* 30: 1059–1068.

Armel, K. C., and Ramachandran, V. S. (2003). Projecting sensations to external objects: Evidence from skin conductance response. *Proceedings of the Royal Society of London, Series B* 270: 1499–1506.

Arzy, S., Seeck, M., Ortigue, S., Spinelli, L., and Blanke, O. (2006) Induction of an illusory shadow person. *Nature* 443: 287.

Babinski, J. (1914). Contribution a l'etude des troubles mentaux dans l'hemiplegie organique cerebrale (anosognosie). *Revue Neurologique* (Paris) 27: 845–848.

Bauer, R. M. (1986). The cognitive psychophysiology of prosopagnosia. In H. D. Ellis, M. A. Jeeves, F. Newcombe, and A. Young (Eds.), *Aspects of Face Processing*. Dordrecht: Nijhoff.

Berrios, G. E., and Luque, R. (1995) Cotard's syndrome: Analysis of 100 cases. *Acta Psychiatrica Scandia* 91: 185–188.

Berti, A., Bottini, G., Gandola, M., Pia, L., Smania, N., Stracciari, A., et al. (2005). Shared cortical anatomy for motor awareness and motor control. *Science* 309: 488–491.

Bisiach, E., and Geminiani, G. (1991). Anosognosia related to hemiplegia and hemianopia. In G. P. Prigatano and D. L. Schacter (Eds.), *Awareness of Deficit after Brain Injury: Clinical and Theoretical Issues*. Oxford: Oxford University Press.

Blanke, O., and Arzy, S. (2005). The out-of-body experience: Disturbed self-processing at the temporo-parietal junction. *Neuroscientist* 11: 16–24.

Blanke, O., Mohr, C., Michel, C. M., Pascual-Leone, A., Brugger, P., Seeck, M., et al. (2005). Linking out-of-body experience and self processing to mental own-body imagery at the temporoparietal junction. *Journal of Neuroscience* 25: 550–557.

Bonhoeffer, K. (1901). *Die Akuten Geisteskrankehiten der Gewohnheitstrinke*. Jena: Gustav Fischer.

Botvinick, M., and Cohen, J. (1998). Rubber hands "feel" touch that eyes see. *Nature* 391: 756.

Breen, N., Caine, D., and Coltheart, M. (2004). Mirrored-self misidentification: Two cases of focal onset dementia. *Neurocase* 7: 239–254.

Breen, N., Caine, D., Coltheart, M., Hendy, J., and Roberts, C. (2000). Towards an understanding of delusions of misidentification: Four case studies. In M. Coltheart and M. Davies (Eds.), *Pathologies of Belief*. Oxford: Blackwell.

Capgras, J., and Reboul-Lachaux, J. (1923). L'illusion des "sosies" dans un délire systématisé chronique. *Bulletin de la Société Clinique de Médecine Mentale* 11: 6–16. Reprinted in Ellis, H. D., Whitley, J., and Luauté, J. P. (Eds.). (1994). Delusional misidentifications: The three original papers on the Capgras, Fregoli and intermetamorphosis delusions. *History of Psychiatry* 5: 117–146.

Carter, C. S., Botvinick, M. M., and Cohen, J. D. (1999). The contribution of the anterior cingulate cortex to executive processes in cognition. *Reviews in the Neurosciences* 10: 49–57.

Churchland, P. S. (1986). *Neurophilosophy: Toward a Unified Science of the Mind/Brain.* Cambridge, Mass.: MIT Press.

Churchland, P. S., and Sejnowski, T. (1992). *The Computational Brain.* Cambridge, Mass.: MIT Press.

Courbon, P., and Tusques, J. (1932). L'illusion d'intermetamorphose et de charme. *Annals of Medical Psychology* 90: 401–406.

Cowey, A., Small, M., and Ellis, S. (1994). Left visuo-spatial neglect can be worse in far than near space. *Neuropsychologia* 32: 1059–1066.

Critchley, M. (1974). Misoplegia or hatred of hemiplegia. *Mt. Sinai Journal of Medicine* 41: 82–87.

Davies, M., Davies, A., and Coltheart, M. (2005). Anosognosia and the two-factor theory of delusions. *Mind and Language* 20: 209–236.

Dennett, D. (1991). *Consciousness Explained.* Boston: Little, Brown.

Desimone, R., and Gross, C. G. (1979). Visual areas in the temporal cortex of the Macaque monkey. *Brain Research* 178: 363–380.

Ellis, H. D., and Young, A. W. (1990). Accounting for delusional misidentifications. *British Journal of Psychiatry* 157: 239–248.

Evans, G. (1982). *The Varieties of Reference.* Oxford: Oxford University Press.

Feinberg, T. E. (2001). *Altered Egos: How the Brain Creates the Self.* Oxford: Oxford University Press.

Feinberg, T. E. (2006). Our brains, our selves. *Daedalus* 135(4): 72–80.

Feinberg, T. E., DeLuca, J., Giacino, J. T., Roane, D. M., and Solms, M. (2005). Right hemisphere pathology and the self: Delusional misidentification and reduplication. In T. E. Feinberg and J. P. Keenan (Eds.), *The Lost Self: Pathologies of Brain and Identity.* Oxford: Oxford University Press.

Feinberg, T. E., Eaton, L. A., Roane, D. M., and Giacino, J. T. (1999). Multiple Fregoli delusions after brain injury. *Cortex* 35: 373–387.

Feinberg, T. E., Haber, L. D., and Leeds, N. E. (1990). Verbal asomatognosia. *Neurology* 40: 1391–1394.

Feinberg, T. E., and Roane, D. M. (1997). Anosognosia, completion and confabulation: The neutral-personal dichotomy. *Neurocase* 3: 73–85.

Fine, C. (2006). *A Mind of Its Own: How Your Brain Distorts and Deceives.* New York: Norton.

Fink, G. R., Markowitsch, H. J., Reinkemeier, M., Bruckbauer, T., Kessler, J., and Heiss, W. D. (1996). Cerebral representation of one's own past: Neural networks involved in autobiographical memory. *Journal of Neuroscience* 16: 4275–4282.

Förstl, H., and Beats, B. (1992). Charles Bonnet's description of Cotard's delusion and reduplicative paramnesia in an elderly patient (1788). *British Journal of Psychiatry* 160: 416–418.

Frazer, S. J., and Roberts, J. M. (1994). Three cases of Capgras' syndrome. *British Journal of Psychiatry* 164: 557–559.

Goldman, A. (2006). *Simulating Minds: The Philosophy, Psychology, and Neuroscience of Mindreading*. Oxford: Oxford University Press.

Halligan, P. W., and Marshall, J. C. (1991). Left neglect for near but not far space in man. *Nature* 350: 498–500.

Hirstein, W. (2005). *Brain Fiction: Self-Deception and the Riddle of Confabulation*. Cambridge, Mass.: MIT Press.

Hirstein, W., and Ramachandran, V. S. (1997). Capgras syndrome: A novel probe for understanding the neural representation of the identity and familiarity of persons. *Proceedings of the Royal Society of London, Series B* 264: 437–444.

Hume, D. (1777/1975). *Enquiries Concerning Human Understanding*. Oxford: Clarendon Press.

Husserl, E. (1913/1973). *Logical Investigations*. London: Routledge.

Johnson, M. K. (1991). Reality monitoring: Evidence from confabulation in organic brain disease patients. In G. P. Prigatano and D. L. Schacter (Eds.), *Awareness of Deficit after Brain Injury: Clinical and Theoretical Issues*. Oxford: Oxford University Press.

Johnson, M. K., Hayes, S. M., D'Esposito, M. D., and Raye, C. L. (2000). Confabulation. In J. Grafman and F. Boller (Eds.), *Handbook of Neuropsychology*. New York: Elsevier.

Johnson, M. K., and Raye, C. L. (1998). False memories and confabulation. *Trends in Cognitive Sciences* 2: 137–145.

Kant, I. (1787/1929). *Critique of Pure Reason*. New York: Macmillan.

Locke, J. (1690/1959). *An Essay Concerning Human Understanding*. New York: Dover.

Maguire, E. A. (2001). Neuroimaging studies of autobiographical memory. In A. Baddeley, J. Aggleton, and M. A. Conway (Eds.), *Episodic Memory: New Directions in Research* Oxford: Oxford University Press.

McDowell, J. (1996). *Mind and World*. Cambridge, Mass.: Harvard University Press.

Meador, K. J., Loring, D. W., Feinberg, T. E., Lee, G. P., and Nichols, M. E. (2000). Anosognosia and asomatognosia during intracarotid amobarbital inactivation. *Neurology* 55: 816–820.

Merleau-Ponty, M. (1962). *Phenomenology of Perception*. London: Routledge.

Miller, E. K., and Cohen, J. D. (2001). An integrative theory of prefrontal cortex function. *Annual Reviews of Neuroscience* 24: 167–202.

Moore, G. E. (1939). Proof of an external world. *Proceedings of the British Academy* 25: 273–300.

Mort, D. J., Malhotra, P., Mannan, S. K., Rorden, C., Pambakian, A., Kennard, C. et al. (2003). The anatomy of visual neglect. *Brain* 126: 1986–1997.

Moscovitch, M., and Winocur, G. (2002). The frontal cortex and working with memory. In D. T. Stuss and R. T. Knight (Eds.), *Principles of Frontal Lobe Functions*. Oxford: Oxford University Press.

Nielsen, J. M. (1938). Gerstmann syndrome; finger agnosia, agraphia, confusion of right and left, acalculia; comparison of this syndrome with disturbances of body scheme resulting from lesions of right side of brain. *Archives of Neurological Psychiatry* 39: 536–560.

Paulig, M. (2000). Somatoparaphrenia: A positive variant of anosognosia for hemiplegia. *Nervenarzt* 71: 123–129.

Petrides, M., Alivisatos, B., and Frey, S. (2002). Differential activation of the human orbital, midventrolateral, and mid-dorsolateral prefrontal cortex during the processing of visual stimuli. *Proceedings of the National Academy of Sciences USA* 99: 5649–5654.

Pick, A. (1905). Zür Psychologie der Confabulation. *Neurologische Centralblatt* 24: 509–516.

Quine, W. (1953). *From a Logical Point of View*, 2nd ed. Cambridge, Mass.: Harvard University Press.

Ramachandran, V. S., Altschuler, E. L., and Hillyer, S. (1997). Mirror agnosia. *Proceedings of the Royal Society of London, Series B* 264: 645–647.

Ramachandran, V. S., and Hirstein, W. (1998). The perception of phantom limbs: The D. O. Hebb lecture. *Brain* 121: 1603–1630.

Ramachandran, V. S., and Rogers-Ramachandran, D. (1996). Denial of disabilities in anosognosia. *Nature* 382: 501.

Rapcsak, S. E., Polster, M. R., Comer, J. F., and Rubens, A. B. (1994). False recognition and misidentification of faces following right hemisphere damage. *Cortex* 30: 565–583.

Rhees, R. (2003). *Wittgenstein's On Certainty: There—Like Our Life*. Oxford: Blackwell.

Rizzolatti, G., and Craighero, L. (2004). The mirror neuron system. *Annual Reviews of Neuroscience* 27: 169–192.

Rizzolatti, G., and Mattelli, M. (2003). Two different streams form the dorsal visual system: Anatomy and function. *Experimental Brain Research* 153: 146–157.

Ryle, G. (1949). *The Concept of Mind*. New York: Barnes and Noble.

Sacks, O. (1984). *A Leg to Stand On*. New York: Summit Books.

Saxe, R. (2005). Against simulation: The argument from error. *Trends in Cognitive Sciences* 9: 174–179.

Saxe, R. (2006). Uniquely human social cognition. *Current Opinion in Neurobiology* 16: 235–239.

Saxe, R., and Wexler, A. (2005). Making sense of another mind: The role of the right temporo-parietal junction. *Neuropsychologia* 43: 1391–1399.

Searle, J. R. (1983). *Intentionality: An Essay in the Philosophy of Mind*. Cambridge: Cambridge University Press.

Shimamura, A. P. (2002). Memory retrieval and executive control processes. In D. T. Stuss and R. T. Knight (Eds.), *Principles of Frontal Lobe Functions*. Oxford: Oxford University Press.

Silva, J. A., Leong, G. B., Wine, D. B., and Saab, S. (1992). Evolving misidentification syndrome and facial recognition deficits. *Canadian Journal of Psychiatry* 37: 239–241.

Staton R. D., Brumback R. A., and Wilson, H. (1982). Reduplicative paramnesia: A disconnection syndrome of memory. *Cortex* 18: 23–36.

Stone, T., and Young, A. W. (1997). Delusions and brain injury: The philosophy and psychology of belief. *Mind and Language* 12: 327–364.

Ungerleider, L. G., and Mishkin, M. (1982). Two visual streams. In D. J. Ingle, M. A. Goodale, and R. J. W. Mansfield (Eds.), *Analysis of Visual Behavior*. Cambridge, Mass.: MIT Press.

Vié, J. (1930). Un trouble de l'identification des personnes: L'illusion des sosies. *Annals of Medical Psychology* 88: 214–237.

Weinstein, E. A. (1991). Anosognosia and denial of illness. In G. P. Prigatano and D. L. Schacter (Eds.), *Awareness of Deficit after Brain Injury: Clinical and Theoretical Issues*. Oxford: Oxford University Press.

Wernicke, K. (1906). *Grundriss der Psychiatrie*, 2nd ed. Leipzig: Thieme.

Whitty, C. W., and Lewin, W. (1957). Vivid day-dreaming: An unusual form of confusion following anterior cingulectomy in man. *Brain* 80: 72–76.

Wittgenstein, L. (1953). *Philosophical Investigations*. New York: Macmillan.

Wittgenstein, L. (1969). *On Certainty*. New York: Harper and Row.

Wright, S., Young, A. W., and Hellawell, D. J. (1993). Sequential Cotard and Capgras delusions. *British Journal of Clinical Psychology* 32: 345–349.

Young, A. W., Leafhead, K. M., and Szulecka, T. K. (1994). Capgras and Cotard delusions. *Psychopathology* 27: 226–231.

Young, A. W., Robertson, L. H., Hellawell, D. J., de Pauw, K. W., and Pentland, B. (1992). Cotard delusion after brain injury. *Psychological Medicine* 22: 799–804.

CHAPTER 20

DELUSIONAL EXPERIENCE

JENNIFER MUNDALE
AND SHAUN GALLAGHER

ONE of the central debates concerning delusion has to do with the role played by faulty hypothesis formation and other cognitive errors. Top-down models assign causal power to such errors in generating delusions, whereas bottom-up models regard these same cognitive errors as at least secondary to (and in some cases derivative from) the delusional experience. We support a bottom-up model of delusion, one that holds that delusional experiences are immediate and noninferential. With respect to the noninferential character of delusion, our approach is similar to that espoused by Gold and Hohwy (2000) in which delusions are referred to as "disorders of experience." At the same time, however, we also acknowledge the explanatory appeal of top-down models of delusion, in which delusions are thought to derive from predictable, cognitive errors. Rather than accept that delusions are the result of higher-order cognitive mistakes, however, we argue that the kinds of errors to which such top-down models typically appeal may themselves be understood, in certain crucial respects, in a bottom-up way or as part of the immediate experience of the delusional subject. This view is supported by Kapur's (2003) work in which schizophrenic delusion is understood in terms of aberrant salience, which in turn is explained at the neurological level as a disorder of the dopaminergic system. Thus, our model of delusion provides an integrated approach in which aberrations at the neurological level are directly related to a "disorder of experience," at the phenomenological level, without recourse to mistaken inferences at the cognitive level. Though we acknowledge that delusions are, of course, associated with higher order cognitive effects, we argue that these are not the proper locus for the explanation of the delusional experience itself.

To further contrast bottom-up versus top-down views of delusion, a typical example of the top-down approach is the two-factor or two-stage model of delusion. In a two-stage model, delusions are seen as an erroneous, cognitive attempt to explain an anomalous experience. The first stage consists of the anomalous experience, such as a hallucination, and the second stage consists of the cognitive or reasoning error that, in attempting to explain the anomalous experience, generates the delusion.

Ramachandran's (1998) explanation of Capgras's delusion illustrates this top-down, two-stage approach. In his account, the first stage is the anomalous perceptual experience of seeing one's parents or other loved ones without simultaneously experiencing an emotional response to them. This sets the stage for the second factor, which is the attempt to rationalize this experience by regarding the loved one as an impostor. The second factor generates the delusional component, and it is either immune or very resistant to revision.

Not all two-stage models consist purely of neurological and cognitive deficits. McKay, Langdon, and Coltheart (in press) have recently argued for including motivational factors in the two-stage model, either as stage 1 or stage 2 factors, noting that "desires are powerful doxastic forces." Though we disagree with certain features of the two-stage model, we support the view that desires, appetites, wishes, and other motivational factors have something important to contribute to our understanding of delusion, perhaps especially in understanding the theme and maintenance of a delusion.

Alternatively, the key feature of bottom-up theories, sometimes referred to as empiricist theories, is the denial of the claim that delusions are cognitively derived, second-order processes. Gold and Hohwy (2000) have recently offered an especially innovative example of a bottom-up model, one that provides a useful starting point for the discussion of our own account. One of the central features of Gold and Hohwy's model has to do with what they call "experiential irrationality," something they regard as "a new department of rationality." In their view, this new category of rationality is needed because neither the standard categories of content rationality nor procedural rationality adequately capture the irrational nature of schizophrenic delusion. As they explain:

> We claim...that the source of thought insertion and related delusions is the experience itself of the schizophrenic subject, and, in particular, its alien quality. The elaboration of the delusion in hypotheses and ancillary beliefs should be understood to be derivative from, or secondary to, this experience. Thus the violation of egocentricity does not merely produce strange experiences that form the basis of delusional beliefs as the result of pathological processes of thought or reasoning. Rather, it is *the experience of non-egocentric thought as alien* that is the delusion itself. The alien quality of the delusional experience is part of its content, and it is the content of experience that is the locus of the delusion and thus of the irrationality. At least some delusions, therefore, are best explained as *disorders of experience* rather than disorders of belief, desire, or reasoning. (Gold and Hohwy, 2000, p. 160)

"Experiential irrationality" itself is an intriguing concept, as it suggests the non-derivative immediacy of at least some forms of delusion, an approach we find not only empirically convincing but intuitively appealing as well. As Gold and Hohwy further note, the subject is not led *into* a deluded hypothesis, his experience is itself delusional. Subjects experience certain thoughts as *intrinsically* alien. In contrast with top-down models, they insist that "A hallucination is an unusual form of experience, but no subsequent judgment is required on the part of the subject for the experience to become delusional" (2000, p. 162).[1] This insistence on the first-order immediacy of the delusion is one of the key features of the bottom-up model we advocate and to which we now turn.

On this bottom-up model, we can distinguish between (1) first-order experience, that is, the phenomenological level of immediate, prereflective, lived-through experience of the world; and (2) higher order cognition, a reflective experience that supports the ability to make attributive judgments about one's own first-order experience. Both first-order experience and second-order cognition depend on a third level of the cognitive system, (3) the nonconscious, subpersonal processes that are best described as neuronal or brain processes. As Gallagher has previously argued (2000a, 2004, 2007), schizophrenic delusions, such as thought insertion, alien control, and other misattributions of agency, are experienced by the subject at the first-order phenomenological level. They are immediate, noninferential, and nonintrospective. This is especially clear starting with prodromal symptoms, that is, early symptoms that precede the characteristic manifestations of the fully developed illness. Though the higher order, cognitive report of the delusional experience may be confused, it is *not* necessarily mistaken; the subject is merely recounting what he or she is experiencing at the phenomenological level.

Furthermore, the problems that manifest themselves at the level of first-order experience are not explained by misguided beliefs, dysfunctional introspective processes, or pathological self-referential narratives, as top-down models would suggest (e.g., Graham and Stephens, 1994; Hoffman, 1986), rather, they are the result of dysfunctions at the neuronal level. For example, in schizophrenia, neurological problems may cause the tacit sensory-motor processes that are normally implicit in first-order phenomenal experience to become abnormally explicit (Sass, 1998, 2000; Sass and Parnas, 2003). Accordingly, what is normally the tacit integration of cognitive, emotional, and motivational factors is disrupted at the level of first-order experience; the implicit unity of the self breaks down, and one begins to feel alienated from one's thoughts and actions.

On this kind of account, for example, problems with self-agency that manifest themselves in the first-order phenomenology of thought insertion and delusions of control are generated on a neurological level. Farrer and Frith (2002; Farrer et al., 2003), for example, have shown contrasting activation in the right inferior parietal cortex for perception of action caused by others, and in the anterior insula bilaterally when action is experienced as caused by oneself. The role of the anterior insula in providing a sense of self-agency involves the integration of three kinds of signals generated in self-movement: somatosensory signals (sensory feedback from bodily movement, e.g., proprioception), visual and auditory signals, and corollary discharge associated with motor commands that control movement. They suggest that a "close correspondence between all these signals helps to give us a sense of agency" (Farrer and Frith, 2002, 602). That is, a disruption in one or more of these signals, a disruption in their integration, or some other kind of malfunction in the anterior insula or the right inferior parietal cortex may generate a loss of the sense of self-agency or a sense of alien control at the level of first-order experience. Indeed, in schizophrenic patients, the feeling of alien control (delusions of control) during a movement task has been associated with an increased activity in the right inferior parietal lobe (Spence et al., 1997). There may be a more general or basic disruption of neuronal processes that affect not just the sense of agency for motor action but also disrupt the sense of agency for cognitive processes, resulting in symptoms of thought insertion. The sense of agency for thought may depend on the anticipatory aspect of working memory (Gallagher, 2000b, 2004), something that may also malfunction in schizophrenic subjects with delusions of control (see Daprati et al., 1997; Franck et al., 2001; Singh et al., 1992; Vogeley, Kurthen, Falkai, and Maier, 1999).

The delusional experiences (of control and thought insertion) may then motivate second-order introspective processes, which may be playing a defensive role in an attempt to explain or justify the alien experience. In this way, higher order processes are reiterating and perhaps enhancing problems first manifested at the experiential level. Thus, a key point of contrast between bottom-up and top-down models concerns the location of causal power. According to the top-down approach, the misattribution of agency to someone or something else is caused by a cognitive error, which becomes the explanans rather than the explanandum (Gallagher, 2007). According to the bottom-up approach, the primary cause of delusional experience is to be found in the brain pathology; at best, whatever higher order cognition does is secondary to the alien experience.

Although we deny that the delusional experience is primarily the product of faulty reasoning at the cognitive level, we also acknowledge the heuristic appeal of various mental errors commonly associated with delusion. Unlike top-down models, however, we do not locate the primary influence of these errors at the cognitive level (as far as the delusional experience is concerned). Thus, one can retain the explanatory value of certain kinds of mental errors within a bottom-up model of explanation. More specifically, we claim that there are very basic kinds of mental errors that, though often *referred* to as cognitive errors, are so deeply entrenched in us and so automatic that they are an integral part of our *immediate, phenomenological experience*. Well-known examples of such errors may include salience effects, attribution errors, primacy and recency effects, contrast effects, and various other biases and distortions. Salience effects pertain to causal attribution: observers consistently attribute greater causal influence to those objects (and persons) in their immediate environment that are most salient, not necessarily the most causally influential (Taylor and Fisk, 1975). Attribution errors come in many forms, but the most common—the so-called "fundamental error of attribution"—consists of overattributing the cause of others' behavior to internal, dispositional factors, such as character, abilities, and motivations, and underattributing their behavior to external, situational factors (Ross, 1977). More is said below about salience, attribution, and the relation between them. Such biases are commonly regarded as having a top-down influence and to be operative primarily at the cognitive level. Although no one is denying that these *can* have higher order, cognitive influences, biases such as these also exert a bottom-up or background influence on first-order experience. In other words, their influence can be precognitive and noninferential. If this is so, then it would allow for some of the appeal of the cognitive approaches to delusion, while preserving the position, which we think is fundamentally correct—that the delusional experience is immediate and not derived from faulty inference.

Salience effects and their role in misattribution, for example, are prime examples of the sort of effect that, in the case of schizophrenic delusion, exerts important precognitive, or background effects. The association between schizophrenic symptoms and dopaminergic dysfunction has been studied and generally accepted for decades, though there is still considerable controversy over the exact role played by dopaminergic excess. Drawing from the contributions of such researchers as Bindra, Toates, Panksepp, DiChiara, and others, Kapur (2003) expands on the so-called motivational salience hypothesis, that is, the view that dopamine mediates the qualitative (attractive or aversive) "valence" that attaches to an external stimulus. Overall, Kapur seeks to explain schizophrenic delusion as a state of abnormal salience. He arrives at this conclusion by combining a modified version of the motivational salience hypothesis with the dopamine hypothesis, that is, the hypothesis that schizophrenia is associated with the faulty dopamine regulation.

For Kapur, the motivational salience hypothesis helps explain the heightened significance that schizophrenics may attach to ordinary objects, sensations, events, or ideas. He speculates that prior to a psychotic episode, patients experience an abnormal dopamine release, which in turn leads to an experience of the exaggerated and contextually unmotivated importance of ordinary stimuli. In the psychotic state, Kapur insists, it is not just that dopamine mediates salience but that the rush of dopamine "becomes a creator of saliences, albeit aberrant ones" (2003, p. 15). As he points out, this fits well with first-person reports of the psychotic experience. Patients report such things as having a new awareness of their surroundings, a heightened sense of consciousness, unusually sharp sensory abilities, newfound clarity of thought, and so on. This exaggerated sense of significance is the catalyst for the delusion. Motivational salience may also help explain the problem of specificity (Gallagher, 2004), that is, the fact that in the case of thought insertion, specific kinds of thought contents (but not all kinds) appear to be inserted. In terms of content, these experiences are very specific and are often associated with specific others. In effect, schizophrenics may experience a certain semantic or content consistency amid the agentive inconsistency of their inserted thoughts. It is difficult to explain the problem of specificity in purely subpersonal terms (e.g., Frith's [1992] suggestion about the dysfunction of a subpersonal comparator). Salience effects at the first-order level of experience, however, may contribute to an explanation.

Somewhat surprisingly, at this point, Kapur largely invokes a two-stage, top-down process for completing the full-blown generation of the delusion, claiming that "once symptoms are manifest, delusions are essentially disorders of inferential logic" and that delusions are "a 'top-down' cognitive explanation that the individual imposes on these experiences of aberrant salience in an effort to make sense of them" (2003, p. 15). It is not clear, however, where Kapur divides the cognitive from the precognitive influences on the delusion, in that he accounts for the variable form of expression of the delusion partly in cultural terms. For example, he notes that a patient in one context may impute evil intentions to a local shaman, whereas in another, more modern context, the patient may implicate the local police (2003, p. 15). We don't dispute the cultural variability that one sees in the expression of delusions, or the cognitive contributions that may later reverberate through the patient's altered epistemological framework, coloring each psychotic episode. Rather, we argue that these cognitive factors are not, in the first instance, responsible for the delusional experience itself.

To recap Kapur's contribution, however, and to return to our main focus, he argues that (1) schizophrenics suffer from aberrant dopamine regulation, (2) dopamine mediates salience, and therefore, (3) schizophrenics suffer from aberrant salience effects. Additionally, Kapur notes that psychotic schizophrenics suffer from "alterations in attributional styles," among other biases and distortions, which is not surprising if salience mediates attribution. Next, we examine this link between causal attribution and salience, adding another link between lower order, neurological phenomena and first-order, phenomenological experience.

Several authors have touched on the relation between salience and attribution. Heider (1958) is often credited as the earliest, but the work of Taylor and Fisk (1975, 1978) is widely cited as the most central and detailed work in substantiating the relation between salience and attribution. In one well-known experiment, Taylor and Fisk (1975) set up a two-man conversation, watched by six silent observers arrayed in different positions around the two men. The two men in the center (call them A and B) sat facing each other as they conversed, and the observers were arranged around them as follows: two observers sat to the north of the conversation, behind A, with a direct view of B's face (and no view of A's face); two observers sat to the south of the conversation, behind B with a direct view of A's face (and no view of B's face); one observer sat to the east of the conversation, with an equal view of both A and B; and one sat to the west of the conversation, also with an equal view of both A and B. Thus, during the conversation, two people observed only A's face, two observed only B's face, and two had equal views of both men's faces. Though the six observers were naive participants, the two conversationalists were trained to engage in a standard, scripted conversation that lasted approximately 5 minutes. During this conversation, A and B made roughly equal contributions, exchanging "the same amount of information of approximately equivalent social desirability" (Taylor and Fisk, 1975, p. 441). After the conversation, the observers were asked to rank A and B according to the role each had taken in setting the tone of the conversation, influencing the course and content of the conversation, and causing the other man to behave as he did. As Taylor and Fisk predicted, perceptions of causal agency varied according to the position of the observers. Those who could see the face of A judged him to have exerted more causal influence than B; those who could see the face of B judged him to have more causal influence than A; those with an equal view of both judged that each had displayed roughly equal causal influence over the conversation. Salience, in this case, was a matter of which man's face each observer could see; other things being equal, an actor whose face we can see is more salient to us than an actor whose face we can't see. That which is more salient, in turn, is judged to have greater causal effect. As Taylor and Fisk conclude,

> Perceptually salient information is subsequently overrepresented when one imputes social or causal meaning to one's perceptual experience. Thus a perceiver, even a highly sophisticated adult perceiver, is to some extent bound by the literal nature of the sensory experience he seeks to transcend when he is interpreting the environment of which he is a part. (1975, p. 445)

Coupling this with Kapur's work, if psychosis is a state of aberrant salience, and salience governs causal attributions, it is not surprising that psychotics should exhibit certain kinds of attribution errors. Furthermore, this matter of being "bound" by our sensory experience, in this context, may help explain the stubborn, nearly inescapable nature of errors of attribution, as well the precognitive level at which their influence operates.

In an appropriately titled paper, "Swimming Upstream against the Fundamental Attribution Error," Pietromonaco and Nisbett (1982) show how attribution errors are resistant to change, even for normals (nonpsychotics), even under circumstances in which subjects are aware of the pitfalls of misattribution. In an experiment that has since become a classic, Pietromonaco and Nisbett employed another famous experiment, the Darley and Batson (1973) study concerning the helping behavior of seminary students. In this 1973 study, seminary students were asked to give a short talk on the parable of the Good Samaritan. While on their way to their talk, they were lead by an experimental assistant down an alley where they encountered a shabbily dressed man, slumped over and groaning in distress (actually, an actor planted by the experimenters). Darley and Batson then observed whether the seminary students would stop to help. They found that the extent to which the students helped was related to how hurried they were to get to their talk. If the experimental assistant rushed them along, telling them they were running late and so better hurry, they were less likely to help or even acknowledge the man in the alley. But if they weren't rushed along, and told they had a few minutes to spare, they were more inclined to assist the man. The fact that the students were giving a talk on the parable of the Good Samaritan seemed to have no effect on their behavior. The lesson of this study, for the purposes of the later Pietromonaco and Nisbett experiment, was that helping behavior was related to the external situation of hurriedness, rather than on the internal or dispositional factor of religiosity.

Pietromonaco and Nisbett used this earlier study in the following way: They presented about half of their subjects with a summary of it, but withheld it from the other half. They then presented all subjects with a scenario similar to the one described in the Darley and Batson study, and asked them to predict the helping behavior of the seminary students. Not surprisingly, the group that had not read about the Darley and Batson study relied on religiosity, a dispositional factor, in predicting helping behavior, thus repeating the fundamental error of attribution. What was surprising, however, was that the students who had read the Darley and Batson study—those who were already aware of the tendency toward misattribution—did the same thing! In fact, they were not significantly less inclined to repeat the error than the naive group. These and similar experiments support our view that attribution errors can and do exert a precognitive, noninferential influence on our experience.

Through following out the neurological and phenomenological underpinnings of misattribution, we hope to have given a plausible, bottom-up account of the genesis of schizophrenic delusions, particularly those involving misattributions of agency. In our account, there is no need to appeal to any cognitive-level mistakes in reasoning to explain how delusions arise. Though we do grant that many cognitive-level effects are commonly observed in schizophrenic psychosis, we deny that they should be regarded as the causal catalyst for the delusion.

NOTE

1. In later work, Hohwy (2004) appears to favor a combination of bottom-up and top-down models and thinks neither is adequate alone. But he does not appear to revoke his claim about the nonderivative nature of (at least some) forms of schizophrenic delusion.

REFERENCES

Darley, J. M., and Batson, C. D. (1973). From Jerusalem to Jericho: A study of situational and dispositional variables in helping behavior. *Journal of Personality and Social Psychology* 27: 100–108.

Daprati, E., Franck N., Georgieff, N., Proust J., Pacherie E., Dalery J., et al. (1997). Looking for the agent: An investigation into consciousness of action and self-consciousness in schizophrenic patients. *Cognition* 65: 71–86.

Farrer, C., Franck, N., Georgieff, N., Frith, C. D., Decety, J., and Jeannerod, M. (2003). Modulating the experience of agency: A positron emission tomography study. *Neuroimage* 18: 324–333.

Farrer, C., and Frith, C. D. (2001). Experiencing oneself vs. another person as being the cause of an action: The neural correlates of the experience of agency. *Neuroimage* 15: 596–603.

Franck, N., Farrer, C., Georgieff, N., Marie-Cardine, M., Daléry, J., d'Amato, T., et al. (2001). Defective recognition of one's own actions in patients with schizophrenia. *American Journal of Psychiatry* 158: 454–59.

Frith, C. (1992). *The Cognitive Neuropsychology of Schizophrenia*. Hillsdale, N.J.: Erlbaum.

Gallagher, S. (2000a). Philosophical conceptions of the self: Implications for cognitive science. *Trends in Cognitive Sciences* 4: 14–21.

Gallagher, S. (2000b). Self-reference and schizophrenia: A cognitive model of immunity to error through misidentification. In D. Zahavi (Ed.), *Exploring the Self: Philosophical and Psychopathological Perspectives on Self-Experience*. Amsterdam: John Benjamins, 203–239.

Gallagher, S. (2004). Neurocognitive models of schizophrenia: A neurophenomenological critique. *Psychopathology* 37: 8–19.

Gallagher, S. (2007). Sense of agency and higher-order cognition: Levels of explanation for schizophrenia. *Cognitive Semiotics* 0: 32–48.

Gold, I., and Hohwy, J. (2000). Rationality and schizophrenic delusion. In M. Coltheart and M. Davies (Eds.), *Pathologies of Belief*. Oxford: Blackwell, 145–165.

Graham, G., and Stephens, G. L. (1994). Mind and mine. In G. Graham and G. L. Stephens (Eds.), *Philosophical Psychopathology*. Cambridge, Mass.: MIT Press, 91–109.

Heider, F. (1958). *The Psychology of Interpersonal Relations*. New York: Wiley.

Hoffman, R. (1986). Verbal hallucinations and language production processes in schizophrenia. *Behavioral and Brain Sciences* 9: 503–517.

Hohwy, J. (2004). Top-down and bottom-up in delusion formation. *Philosophy, Psychiatry and Psychology* 11: 65–70.

Kapur, S. (2003). Psychosis as a state of aberrant salience: A framework linking biology, phenomenology, and pharmacology in schizophrenia. *American Journal of Psychiatry* 160: 13–23.

McKay, R., Langdon, R., and Coltheart, M. (in press). Models of misbelief: Integrating motivational and deficit theories of delusions. *Consciousness and Cognition*.

Pietromonaco, P. R., and Nisbett, R. E. (1982). Swimming upstream against the fundamental attribution error: Subjects' weak generalizations from the Darley and Batson study. *Social Behavior and Personality* 10: 1–4.

Ramachandran, V. S. (1998). Consciousness and body image: Lessons from phantom limbs, Capgras syndrome and pain asymbolia. *Philosophical Transactions of the Royal Society B: Biological Sciences* 353: 1851–1859.

Ross, L. (1977). The intuitive psychologist and his shortcomings: Distortions in the attribution process. In L. Berkowitz (Ed.), *Advances in Experimental Social Psychology*, vol. 10. New York: Academic Press, 174–177.

Sass, L. (1998). Schizophrenia, self-consciousness and the modern mind. *Journal of Consciousness Studies* 5: 543–65.

Sass, L. (2000). Schizophrenia, self-experience, and the so-called negative symptoms. In D. Zahavi (Ed.), *Exploring the Self*. Amsterdam: John Benjamins, 149–182.

Sass, L., and Parnas, J. (2003). Schizophrenia, consciousness, and the self. *Schizophrenia Bulletin* 29, 427–444.

Singh, J. R., Knight, T., Rosenlicht, N., Kotun, J. M., Beckley, D. J., and Woods, D. L. (1992). Abnormal premovement brain potentials in schizophrenia. *Schizophrenia Research* 8: 31–41.

Spence, S. A., Brooks, D. J., Hirsch, S. R. Liddle, P. F. Meehan, J., and Grasby P. M. (1997). A PET study of voluntary movement in schizophrenic patients experiencing passivity phenomena (delusions of alien control). *Brain* 120: 1997–2011.

Taylor, S. E., and Fiske, S. T. (1975). Point of view and perceptions of causality. *Journal of Personality and Social Psychology* 32: 439–445.

Taylor, S. E., and Fiske, S. T. (1978). Salience, attention, and attribution: Top of the head phenomena. *Advances in Experimental Social Psychology* 11: 249–288.

Vogeley, K., Kurthen, M., Falkai, P., and Maier, W. (1999). The human self construct and prefrontal cortex in schizophrenia. *Association for the Scientific Study of Consciousness: Electronic Seminar*. Available at: www.phil.vt.edu/assc/esem.html.

CHAPTER 21

THE CASE FOR ANIMAL EMOTIONS: MODELING NEUROPSYCHIATRIC DISORDERS

KENNETH SUFKA, MORGAN WELDON, AND COLIN ALLEN

1. INTEREST IN ANIMAL EMOTIONS

There is considerable interest from a diversity of fields in questions surrounding animal emotions. One such question is whether some nonhuman animals experience emotions similar in kind to those of humans. If the answer is affirmative, it seems likely that some nonhuman animals are capable of experiencing suffering that is similar to what humans experience when subjected to noxious (i.e., tissue-damaging) stimuli or nonnoxious stressful conditions. Indeed, nonhuman animals are widely used in neuroscientific research, some of which involve studies of nociception. Though all animals display escape and avoidance behaviors in response to noxious stimuli, any evidence that justifies the additional claim that some nonhuman animals may also experience suffering as part of their pain response raises a number of moral concerns (Allen, 2004; Clark, 1977; Degrazia, 1996; Robinson, 1997; Shriver, 2006).

The widespread international concern for animal welfare is evidenced by the enactment of laws and the establishment of governing institutions. These include the Canadian Animal Welfare Law, the European Union Panel on Animal Health and Welfare, the Indian Prevention of Cruelty to Animals Acts and Animal Welfare Board, the Australian Prevention of Cruelty to Animals Act and Bureau of Animal Welfare, and the U.S. Animal Welfare Act and Office of Laboratory Animal Welfare, among others. These animal welfare regulations indicate that a public intuition exists that some nonhuman animals possess internal subjective experiences that are similar to our own. Although such a claim has potential moral implications for animal welfare, discussion of these implications is beyond the scope of this chapter. Rather, we seek to evaluate some of the evidence that underlies the claim that nonhuman animals indeed suffer. We describe some potential confounds affecting the kinds of evidence usually cited, and we end by describing evidence from animal models of neuropsychiatric disorders that may circumvent some of these problems.

2. Evidence of Animal Emotions from Human Pain and Suffering

2.1. What Is Pain?

The International Association for the Study of Pain (IASP) defines pain as "an unpleasant sensory and emotional experience associated with actual or potential tissue damage, or described in terms of such damage" (IASP Task Force on Taxonomy, 1994). This definition references both the sensory and affective dimensions of pain (Melzack, 1973). The sensory dimension of pain provides quantitative nociceptive information, such as its location, intensity, modality, and duration. For example, if one spills very hot coffee on one's right hand, the sensory dimension of the pain provides the knowledge that the right hand (location) has been exposed to a noxious (intensity) thermal (modality) stimulation for a short period of time (duration). The affective dimension provides qualitative information about a pain's valence, or the subjective feeling that painful stimulation is incredibly unpleasant. On spilling hot coffee on one's hand, the affective pain dimension is the emotional distress experienced afterward.

In sum, the phenomenology of pain includes both sensory and affective components. The former constitutes information about a pain's location, intensity, modality, and duration, and the latter refers to the emotional valence of the experience. Evidence outlined in the next section suggests these phenomenological distinctions in humans are subserved by distinct neural systems.

2.2. Cortical Substrates of Pain Phenomenology

Numerous studies demonstrate that noxious stimulation activates several distinct regions of the cortex, including primary somatosensory (S1), secondary somatosensory (S2), anterior cingulate (ACC), insula, and medial prefrontal cortical areas. Several studies by Catherine Bushnell and colleagues have seemingly dissociated the sensory and affective dimensions of pain perception, localizing these dissociable processes to activity in distinct brain areas. In one positron emission tomography (PET) study, regional cerebral blood flow (rCBF) levels were obtained during a thermal grill illusion task. This is an illusion in which contact with spatially alternating warm and cool thermal stimuli leads to reports of pain and unpleasantness, despite neither stimulus producing pain or unpleasantness when presented alone (Craig, Reiman, Evans, and Bushnell, 1996). Using a subtraction technique to compare the two conditions (pain versus no pain perception), only increased activity in the ACC seemed to account for participants' reported pain experience.

In another study, these researchers used hypnotic suggestion to manipulate participants' pain affect, holding pain intensity perception constant while their hands were submerged in hot water. Verbal reports confirmed that hypnotic suggestion was successful in dissociating pain unpleasantness and intensity. Participants' verbal ratings of pain unpleasantness increased and decreased with the appropriate hypnotic suggestion, while their pain intensity ratings did not. Again, rCBF results show a significant increase in ACC activity that parallels participants' level of pain unpleasantness ratings (Rainville, Duncan, Price, Carrier, and Bushnell, 1997). A similar study that attempted to hold participants' perception of pain unpleasantness constant while manipulating perception of pain intensity produced strikingly different results. Here, the strongest change in pain-intensity–evoked activity was localized to S1 (Rainville, Carrier, Hofbauer, Bushnell, and Duncan, 1999). However, there were also findings in this experiment that may weaken the "dissociation argument," and these are discussed later in the chapter.

One interesting case report is that of a 57-year-old male who suffered a stroke affecting the hand region of his right S1 and S2 cortex (Ploner, Freund, and Schnitzler, 1999). Noxious cutaneous laser stimulation presented to his left foot produced a well-localized pain sensation; however, the same stimulus presented to his left hand at three times the intensity failed to evoke a pain sensation. Interestingly, the patient "spontaneously described a 'clearly unpleasant' intensity dependent feeling emerging from an ill-localized and extended area 'somewhere between the fingertips and shoulder' that he wanted to avoid" (Ploner et al., 1999, p. 213). Furthermore, this patient was "completely unable to describe quality, localization and intensity of the perceived stimulus." Case studies like this, as well as the PET studies described earlier, provide compelling evidence for the differential involvement of cortical structures in our sensory and affective dimensions of pain experiences.

2.3. Do Animals Suffer When in Pain?

The question of whether some nonhuman animals experience some emotions similar to those of humans, such as suffering associated with pain, has been approached using a comparative biology argument (Clark, 1977; Degrazia, 1996; Robinson, 1997; Shriver, 2006). The notion behind this approach is that if sufficient similarity exists between the anatomical and physiological pain mechanisms of a human and an animal, then it is likely that their affective experiences in response to noxious stimuli are similar (Allen, 2004; Clark, 1977; Degrazia, 1996; Robinson, 1997; Shriver, 2006). As a side note, some philosophers and scientists go further to claim that not only do some animals experience the negatively valenced state of pain affect, they also experience an emotional awareness (Bekoff, 2006) that a particular stimulus is causing their negative internal state. Shriver (2006) goes even further in using this comparative biological approach to make the claim that animals suffer. He notes that humans and rats both possess an ACC, and he highlights recent empirical data (LaGraize, Labuda, Rutledge, Jackson, and Fuchs, 2004) that selective modulation of a rat's ACC seems to alter the animal's pain behavior in ways suggestive of an alteration in the animal's affective processing of noxious stimuli. Before discussing these data, it is important to consider the methodology underlying such approaches to studying pain in animals.

The study of the neural substrates of pain in animals requires some combination of neurophysiological and nonverbal behavioral methods. Typical neurophysiological manipulations include promoting or interfering with normal neural communication through electrolytic or chemical lesions, electrical stimulation, and/or drug agonist or antagonist administration (Carlson, 2007). Other neurophysiological approaches include recording neural activity through a number of methods ranging from single cell recording (Carlson, 2007) to optical imaging (Gibson, Hebden, and Arridge, 2005). Behavioral approaches to the study of pain in animals typically rely on an animal's reflex response to noxious stimulation (Sufka, 1996; see also chapter 5 in this volume). Among these reflex responses are the hotplate and tail-flick tests with thermal stimuli, the toe pinch and paw pressure tests with mechanical stimuli, and the formalin, capsaicin, and acetic acid tests with chemical stimuli. Several animal models of chronic pain conditions have also been developed. Two of the most commonly used chronic pain models are the rat peripheral neuropathy model, involving damage to the sciatic nerve, and the rat arthritic model, involving administration of complete Freund's adjuvant, carrageenan, or urate crystals, to a paw, joint, or base of the tail to produce chronic inflammation.

One novel approach to the study of pain behavior is the conditioned place preference (CPP) paradigm (Sufka, 1994). This procedure is commonly used to evaluate the affective/motivational properties of drugs (Carr, Fibiger, and Phillips, 1989; van der Kooy, 1987) and is based on traditional learning principles whereby animals approach or avoid environments previously paired with reinforcing or aversive stimuli, respectively. In a series of experiments (Sufka, 1994; Sufka and Roach, 1996), arthritic rats given different classes of analgesic drugs in one environment spent more time in that environment compared to a second environment paired with saline during a subsequent preference choice test. The authors argued that such a paradigm is capable of quantifying an animal's affective/motivational response to pain-relieving drugs that avoids the potential confounds of alterations in simple pain reflex behaviors that may or may not be indicative of pain relief. Whether the behavior of these rats reflected a change in their affective response to pain is unknown, because each of the drugs tested has also been shown in other studies to reduce pain sensation, as indicated by alterations in the animal's reflex responses to noxious stimuli.

In a somewhat different kind of paradigm, Perry Fuchs's lab (LaGraize et al., 2004) used a modified open field apparatus in an attempt to dissociate pain affect from pain sensation. In their place escape/avoidance paradigm, rats are tested in a small enclosure situated on a wire mesh floor in which half the chamber is painted black and the other half white. Rats normally prefer the dark half of the compartment and tend to spend about 70 percent of their time on that side of the apparatus. Surgical ligation of the left L5 nerve was performed to induce a neuropathic chronic pain state. This procedure produces a hyperalgesic response (i.e., heightened sensitivity to noxious stimuli) in the affected hind limb and paw. Testing in the place escape/avoidance paradigm involved delivery of suprathreshold mechanical stimulation to the hyperalgesic hindpaw via von Frey monofilament (a kind of flexible pin that allows the experimenter to precisely control the force of a pin prick) when rats crossed into the black side of the chamber, and delivery of the same noxious stimulus to the unaffected (right) hindpaw when they entered the white side. Because the black side of the apparatus was now associated with painful stimulation to their hyperalgesic hindpaw, rats spent more time on the white side. A separate group of rats received electrolytic lesions to the ACC prior to the same place escape/avoidance paradigm test trial. Relative to the sham lesion control group, these animals spent more time in the black side despite mechanical stimulation to their hyperalgesic hindpaw. Interestingly, while these ACC-lesioned animals now tolerated noxious stimulation to their hyperalgesic hindpaw by showing the black side preference, they continued to show the same paw withdrawal reflex response to the probe as sham-lesioned animals. From these data, one can infer that ACC lesions selectively alter the negative affective response to painful stimulation without removing the sensory response. These findings lend support to the notion that, like humans, the ACC selectively processes the aversive qualities of painful conditions.

In a follow-up dissociation study (LaGraize, Borzan, Peng, and Fuchs, 2006), Fuchs's group used the same model of neuropathic pain and the place escape/avoidance paradigm, but instead of altering ACC functioning via electrolytic lesion they administered morphine directly (i.e., intracranially via cannula) to the ACC. Morphine, an opioid agonist, is the gold standard analgesic whose pain-relieving effects are thought to involve, in part, modulation of ACC activity through mu-opioid receptor binding. The results of these experiments parallel their earlier findings in that morphine-treated neuropathic rats spent more time in the black side despite mechanical stimulation to their hyperalgesic hindpaw than saline-treated neuropathic rats. Once again, both groups of rats continued to show the same paw withdrawal reflex response to the von Frey mechanical probe. Dissociation studies like these lend support to the notion that some nonhuman animals are capable of experiencing emotions similar to those of humans, such as suffering.

2.4. Potential Confounds of Pain Studies

The argument that some nonhuman animals experience some emotions similar to those of humans is based on the notion that if there are homologies in neural structures across species and similar physiological responses in these structures, then emotional homology is likely to exist across species. In the case of pain and suffering in humans, there exist distinct pathways and cortical regions for process- ing the sensory (i.e., S1) and affective (i.e., ACC) components of pain. Similar path- ways and structures exist in rodents that seem to share functional homologies to humans in response to painful conditions. However, data show that the ACC and S1 cortical regions may not be entirely dissociable, and worse, the ACC may possess other functions that confound the notion of its role in pain affect. This last point is important because changes in behavior that are correlated to alterations ACC func- tion may represent a confound between affective processing and other functions of the ACC.

One hint that the sensory and affective dimensions of pain processing are not completely dissociable in neural structures comes from one of the hypnotic induc- tion studies described earlier (Rainville et al., 1999). In this experiment, readers will recall that hypnotic induction altered participants' affective experience (and altered ACC activity) to a noxious stimulus of fixed intensity but did not change their ver- bal rating of the intensity of that noxious stimulus. However, this dissociation did not occur when experimenters attempted to alter through hypnotic induction their participants' sensory (i.e., intensity) dimension of pain processing. That is, hyp- notic induction that altered participants' pain intensity ratings also resulted in cor- responding changes in their pain unpleasantness ratings. This experiment indicates that these pathways cannot be fully dissociated because changes in sensory pain perception produce corresponding changes in the affective dimension of pain pro- cessing. This absence of a double dissociation between pain affect and pain sensa- tion may confound the overall argument about animal emotion and suffering, as we explain shortly.

There are compelling data to suggest that a subset of ACC neurons code for noxious stimulus type, which is clearly a sensory component of pain sensation. A study by Hutchinson and colleagues (Hutchison, Davis, Lozano, Tasker, and Dostrovksy, 1999) recorded individual neurons from approximately 400 recording sites in and around the ACC in awake patients undergoing cingulotomies. Just over 100 of these sites were monitored for changes in activity while the patients were sub- jected to noxious (heat, pinprick, or cold) and nonnoxious mechanical and thermal stimuli. None of the ACC neurons responded to nonnoxious stimuli. Most cells did respond to the presentation of noxious stimuli, thus confirming a role for the ACC in pain processing. However, responses in these neurons carried modality informa- tion. Some responded to only one type of noxious stimuli, others to two, and still others to three. These are the kinds of response patterns seen in neurons in S1 and suggest that at least part of the ACC may code for pain sensory information rather than pain affect.

That the ACC may not selectively code for pain affect comes, surprisingly, from a third study by Fuchs (LaBuda and Fuchs, 2005). Using the same neuropathic model of chronic pain and place escape/avoidance paradigm outlined earlier, these researchers attempted to stimulate ACC neurons rather than lesion them in an attempt to selectively modulate pain affect in their paradigm. Given that their earlier studies showed attenuation of negative pain affect by both ACC lesions (LaGraize et al., 2004) and ACC morphine administration (LaGraize et al., 2006), which facilitates local inhibitory circuits, one might predict that stimulation of this area would increase negative pain affect in rats and lead to an enhanced avoidance of the dark side of the chamber. In fact, ACC stimulation produced a decreased avoidance of the dark side of the chamber in a manner similar to ACC lesions and ACC morphine administration.

LaBuda and Fuchs note that the mechanisms by which ACC stimulation leads to outcomes similar to their ACC lesion study in the place and escape/avoidance paradigm are unknown. Although there is evidence that ACC circuitry is involved in associative learning and memory tasks (Koyama, Kato, and Mikami, 2000; Takenouchi et al., 1999), the authors explain that impairments in these general learning and memory processes were unlikely as animals continued to show some discriminative functions. They speculate about the existence of a "behavioral suppression system" operating in the ACC circuitry. Such a system would be responsible for environmental threat evaluation and would coordinate appropriate behavioral responses in the organism. If true, this leaves open the possibility that in animals ACC circuitry may play a role other than pain affect. Without the functional homology, it weakens the comparative biological argument that some nonhuman animals experience emotions similar in kind to humans.

3. Animal Modeling of Neuropsychiatric Disorders

3.1. An Alternative Strategy

In this section, we suggest an alternative strategy for making the claim that some nonhuman animals experience emotions similar to those of humans. We believe this strategy avoids the confounds outlined earlier. The approach is drawn from the fields of neuroscience and psychopharmacology whereby animal researchers use animals to develop and validate animal models of human neuropsychiatric disorders. Their purpose for doing so varies depending on the specific research questions posed. These may include attempts to provide a better understanding of the pathogenesis of the syndrome or its response to a novel pharmacotherapy, among others. Whatever the research question, the implicit assumption is that the animal model itself displays important features that are valid representations of a given clinical syndrome. Therefore, if one identifies a specific clinical syndrome that involves pronounced changes in a person's emotional state and that syndrome can be effectively simulated in an animal model, then it is very likely that the animal experiences an emotional state similar to that of the human.

For an animal model to be considered a valid simulation of a neuropsychiatric disorder, it must meet a number of specified criteria that are, not surprisingly, the same as those outlined for describing and validating human clinical syndromes offered by Emil Kraepelin over 100 years ago. Kraepelin, who is considered the founding father of modern psychiatry, believed that syndromes should cluster along the lines of their signs and symptoms. More important, he argued that any given syndrome should be validated by consideration of etiological origins, pathophysiological course, and progression and response to various treatments. Although animal researchers often discuss the validity of their models in terms of face, construct, and predictive validity (terms to be explained), the actual indexes used to establish each of these come from the criteria originally outlined by Kraepelin, as we explain next.

3.2. Validity Criteria for Animal Models

McKinney and Bunney (1969) provided the first and most influential parameters for establishing animal model validity. They called for a neo-Kraepelinian approach in which the validity of an animal model was considered on the basis of how well it represented the syndrome's (1) etiology, (2) symptomatology, (3) physiological basis, and (4) treatment of a human psychopathological condition. This approach fared well in the literature as many subsequent critiques have used some variation of these evaluation criteria (e.g., Abramson and Seligman, 1977; Bond, 1984; Kalueff, Wheaton, and Murphy, 2007; Murphy, 1976).

Building on this early work, Willner (1986) argued that McKinney and Bunney's evaluation criteria only assessed a paradigm's face validity, which refers to the surface-level similarities between the animal model and the human psychopathology. Willner contended that models of neuropsychiatric disorders should be evaluated on two additional dimensions: predictive validity and construct validity. Predictive validity assesses the performance of a model, which is typically accomplished by demonstrating a similarity in treatment efficacy between an animal model and the human clinical condition (e.g., examining them for drug false positives and false negatives and for similarity in pharmacological treatment potencies). Construct validity assesses the theoretical rationale of the animal model. Willner argued that for an animal model to have a construct validity, it must be evaluated on two criteria. "Firstly it must be established that homologous constructs are being studied in animals and people.... Secondly, it must be shown that a change at the level of the construct being modeled is in fact central to the disorder" (1986, p. 684). Thus, construct validity is established by the demonstration of similar theoretical underpinnings between the paradigm and the clinical condition. An excellent example of a clinical syndrome's theoretical foundation being used to establish a paradigm's construct validity is the learned helplessness theory of depression (Vollmayr and Henn, 2001).

Following Willner's contribution, theorists began to argue about the importance of each type of validity for simulations of neuropsychiatric disorders (Kalueff and Tuohimaa, 2004; van der Staay, 2006). Most authors agree that each validity type is not of equal value. For example, face validity is often characterized as being too superficial and limited due to species-specific behavioral repertoires. Some authors have proposed hierarchies that list the three validity types in order of increasing importance; typically in the order of face, predictive, and construct validity with the last being considered of primary importance (Kalueff and Tuohimaa, 2004; van der Staay, 2006).

Van der Staay (2006) agrees that construct validity is the primary criterion by which an animal model should be judged. However, instead of advocating Willner's concept of construct validity, van der Staay argues that both face and predictive validity can play an important role in establishing a model's construct validity. He says that construct validity is established by the network of associations of the neuropathological signs and behavioral symptoms, etiologies, and drug effects between the human clinical syndrome and the animal model. Thus, construct validity is established by assessing the degree of linkage in similarity between the animal model and clinical disorder in terms of their etiologies, biochemical signs, behavioral symptoms, and drug treatment effect profiles.

3.3. Anxiety–Depression Continuum as a Clinical Syndrome

The next step in the project of validating animal models of suffering is to select and describe the details of a clinical condition that entails some change in a person's emotional state and involves subjective feelings of distress, despair, and suffering. The hope is to link this syndrome to a valid animal simulation. Two clinical syndromes that come to mind are anxiety disorder and the mood disorder of major depression. The current *Diagnostic and Statistical Manual of Mental Disorders* (DSM-IV), which uses symptom expression alone as its taxonomic principle, categorizes anxiety and depression as separate Axis I clinical syndromes (American Psychiatric Association, 1994). Such a taxonomy, as originally outlined by Kraepelin's criteria, implies that these syndromes have distinct etiological origins, symptom expression, pathophysiological substrates, and treatment response outcomes.

Evidence is mounting, however, to suggest that anxiety and depressive disorders have more in common than previously thought. For example, anxiety and depressive disorders share many signs and symptoms (Watson, 2005) and present comorbidity rates ranging from 50 percent to 90 percent (Kessler et al., 1994; Kessler et al., 2005). Structural equation modeling suggests a direct correlation between anxiety disorders and depression with the factors of high negative affect and low positive affect being significant contributors to both syndromes (Brown, Chorpita, and Barlow, 1998). From an etiological perspective, three interacting vulnerabilities have been identified as important contributors to the expression of negative affect in anxiety and depressive disorders: (1) general biological vulnerabilities, such as genetic contributions; (2) general psychological vulnerabilities, such as early life experiences of unpredictability and uncontrollability; and (3) specific psychological vulnerabilities, such as faulty associative learning experiences (Barlow, 2000). Although the underlying pathophysiological processes of anxiety and depression are diverse and complex, common biological markers exist and include dysregulation of glucocorticoids (Arborelius, Owens, Plotsky, and Nemeroff, 1999), monoamines (Ressler and Nemeroff, 2000), and neurotrophic factors (Jiang et al., 2005). Furthermore, anxiety and depression share similar response rates to various classes of pharmacological agents, notably antidepressants (Feighner, 1999). Collectively, these findings argue that genuine boundaries may not actually exist between these clinical disorders and are better served by a single overarching construct (Watson, 2005). One model suggests that anxiety and depression may represent different temporal facets of a single syndrome, the anxiety–depression continuum, where the expression of the depressive state follows the anxiety state to an unresolved stressor (Kasper, 2001).

3.4. The Chick Anxiety–Depression Continuum Model

The next question to address is whether an anxiety–depression continuum can be modeled in an animal simulation. Although numerous animal paradigms exist that model anxiety-like syndromes (see Green and Hodges, 1991, for review) and depression-like syndromes (see Willner, 1991, for review), no rodent models have been integrated in such a way as to model an anxiety–depression continuum. However, anxiety-like states have been modeled in domestic fowl chicks in response to very brief social separation (for review, see Panksepp, 2003). Furthermore, depression-like states have been modeled in chicks in response to longer periods of isolation stress (Lehr, 1989). Two recent studies incorporate features of the aforementioned assays in an attempt to model an anxiety–depression continuum in chicks (Sufka et al., 2006; Warnick, Huang, Acevedo, and Sufka, in press) and these findings are summarized next.

In the chick anxiety–depression model, socially raised 4–6-day-old chicks are placed into isolation chambers for a 2-hour test session in which distress vocalizations are recorded in 5-minute blocks. Social separation initially elicits high distress vocalization rates that decline over the course of the 2-hour isolation test period. During the first 5-minute block, vocalization rates are at their highest. This appetitively motivated behavioral response aimed at reestablishing social contact is, much like a panic response, elicited by the sudden onset of the social-separation stressor. Evidence that this initial phase models an anxiety-like state is provided by the observation that a broad class of pharmacological compounds effective in treating human anxiety (Baldessarini, 2001) decreases distress vocalizations during this time block. Among these include meprobamate, pentobarbital, chlordiazepoxide, alprazolam, lorazepam, phenelzine, imipramine, maprotiline, and clonidine (for review, see Feltenstein and Sufka, 2008). What is particularly interesting about this phase of the model is its sensitivity to compounds that are used clinically in the treatment of panic disorder (e.g., phenelzine, imipramine, alprazolam, and clonidine) but not generalized anxiety disorder (e.g., buspirone and trazodone). This pharmacological pattern of effects, along with the symptom onset being rapid, intense, and brief with clear etiological origins, suggest that the anxiety portion of the simulation most closely resembles situationally bound panic disorder (Warnick, Wicks, and Sufka, 2006).

During the course of the next 15–20 minutes, rates of distress vocalizations show a steady decline to about 40–50 percent of the initial rate. After this transitional phase, chicks enter the depression phase of the model. This depressive-like state is characterized by a reduced and stable pattern of distress vocalization throughout the remainder of the 2-hour test session. The behavioral response in chicks (drop in vocalization rates) to a prolonged stressor resembles behavioral despair that is commonly associated with depressive states and well linked to learned helplessness theories of depression (Katz, 1981; Seligman, Maier, and Geer, 1968). Evidence that this phase models a depression-like state is provided by the observation that a broad class of pharmacological compounds effective in treating human depression (Baldessarini, 2001) attenuates this behavioral despair response, including the antidepressants imipramine, maprotiline, and fluoxetine (Sufka et al., 2006; Warnick et al., in press).

To further establish this chick procedure as a valid simulation of an anxiety–depression continuum, levels of corticosterone and the cytokine interleukin-6 (IL-6) were assayed at varying time points across the separation-stress period. Corticosterone, a neuroendocrine marker of many stress responses, increased over the first 15 minutes of isolation and declined thereafter (Sufka et al., 2006). This pattern is typical of stress-provoking stimuli and reflects a negative feedback process of the glucocorticoid system (Keller-Wood and Dallman, 1984). Cytokines are proteins involved in a wide range of immunological, neurophysiological, and neuroendocrine functions and are a major contributing pathological feature underlying the anxiety–depression continuum hypothesis (Kim et al., 2007). In the chick model, plasma IL-6 concentration was elevated after 120 minutes of social-separation stress (Warnick et al., in press). Interestingly, increased production of cytokines has been linked to changes in glucocorticoid levels that accompany anxiety states (O'Brien, Scott, and Dinan, 2004). This fits well with the observation that corticosterone levels are elevated early in the test session (Sufka et al., 2006) followed by increased IL-6 production at the end of the test session, and it appears to mirror the pathophysiological response of an anxiety–depression continuum.

As a simulation of a neuropsychiatric disorder, the chick anxiety–depression continuum model appears to possess face, construct, and predictive validity in that (1) the procedure involves a potent identifiable stressor, (2) the pattern of distress vocalizations sequentially models a anxiety-like state resembling panic followed by a depressive-like state resembling learned helplessness, (3) the dependent measure of distress vocalizations shows appropriate sensitivity to anxiolytic and antidepressant probes, and (4) the biomarkers of stress and depression (i.e., corticosterone and IL-6) show patterns of release that parallels that produced by emotional stressors in human. Taken together, these data go far in establishing the validity of the chick anxiety–depression continuum as a simulation of a neuropsychiatric disorder.

4. Conclusion

The purpose of this chapter was (1) to examine critically the evidence that philosophers have used to justify the claim that some nonhuman animals experience emotions similar to those of humans, such as pain and suffering; and (2) to provide an alternative strategy to making similar claims but to do so in a manner that avoids the possible confounds present in the existing pain literature. Although neuroscientific findings show that nonhuman animals share structural homologies with humans in neural systems responsible for pain processing, evidence that the ACC in animals solely processes pain affect is questionable. The alternative approach we propose draws from animal modeling research in which animals are used to simulate a neuropsychiatric disorder. The premise is that if the animal simulation is valid—that is, it compares well with its corresponding human neuropsychiatric disorder in terms of etiology, symptomatology, pathophysiology, and response to treatments—one is entitled to argue that the animal shares an emotion similar in kind to the human counterpart. In this approach we selected the anxiety–depression continuum, whose core symptoms involve changes in emotional processing in response to stress, and we presented data bearing on the chick anxiety–depression continuum model to demonstrate that the model possesses face, construct, and predictive validity. With these homologies present, the case for emotional homology between the animal model and clinical syndrome is strengthened.

One might argue that the great phylogenetic distance between humans and *Aves* makes it unlikely that emotional states such as anxiety and depression can be properly modeled in chicks. However, the strength of our argument is not in the specific example but in the approach or methodology. Furthermore, animal models exist outside human psychiatric disorders and cover a wide variety of human cognition, behavior, and emotions. So if the avian model of anxiety and depression is unattractive for running the argument, then perhaps a nonhuman primate model of drug addiction and its withdrawal syndrome will suffice. Indeed, the method we advocate should provide a supportive framework for philosophers and scientists to discuss not only the existence but also the extent of animal emotional experiences. Doing so will have both practical and theoretical implications for scientists and philosophers, starting with the context of advancing biomedical research in the most humane and ethical manner.

REFERENCES

Abramson, L. Y., and Seligman, M. E. P. (1977). Modeling psychopathology in the laboratory: History and rationale. In J. D. Maser and M. E. P. Seligman (Eds.), *Psychopathology: Experimental Models*. San Francisco: Freeman, 1–26.

Allen, C. (2004). Animal pain. *Noûs* 38: 617–643.

American Psychiatric Association. (1994). *Diagnostic and Statistical Manual of Mental Disorders*, 4th ed. Washington, D.C.: American Psychiatric Press.

Arborelius, L., Owens, M. J., Plotsky, P. M., and Nemeroff, C. B. (1999). The role of corticotropin-releasing factor in depression and anxiety disorders. *Journal of Endocrinology* 160: 1–12.

Barlow, D. H. (2000). Unraveling the mysteries of anxiety and its disorders from the perspective of emotion theory. *American Psychologist* 55: 1247–1263.

Bekoff, M. (2006). Animal emotions and animal sentience and why they matter: Blending "science sense" with common sense, compassion and heart. In J. Turner and J. D'Silva (Eds.), *Animals, Ethics and Trade*. London: Earthscan, 28.

Bond, N. W. (1984). Animal models in psychopathology: An introduction. In N. W. Bond (Ed.), *Animal Models in Psychopathology*. Sydney: Academic Press, 1–21.

Brown, T. A., Chorpita, B. F., and Barlow, D. H. (1998). Structural relationships among dimensions of the DSM-IV anxiety and mood disorders and dimensions of negative affect, positive affect, and autonomic arousal. *Journal of Abnormal Psychology* 107: 179–192.

Carlson, N. R. (2007). Methods and strategies of research. *Physiology of Behavior*, 9th ed. Boston: Pearson Education, 135–160.

Carr, G. D., Fibiger, H. C., and Phillips, A. G. (1989). Conditioned place preference as a measure of drug reward. In J. M. Liebman and S. J. Cooper (Eds.), *The Neuropharmacological Basis of Reward*. Oxford: Clarendon Press.

Clark, S. R. L. (1977). *The Moral Status of Animals*. Oxford: Oxford University Press.

Craig, A. D., Reiman, E. M., Evans, A. C., and Bushnell, M. C. (1996). Functional imaging of an illusion of pain. *Nature* 384: 258–260.

Baldessarini, R. J. (2001). Drugs and the treatment of psychiatric disorders. In J. G. Hardman and L. E. Limbird (Eds.), *Goodman & Gilman's: The Pharmacological Basis of Therapeutics*, 10th ed. New York: McGraw-Hill.

Degrazia, D. (1996). *Taking Animals Seriously*. New York: Cambridge University Press.

Feighner, J. P. (1999). Overview of antidepressants currently used to treat anxiety disorders. *Journal of Clinical Psychiatry* 60: 18–22.

Feltenstein, M. W., and Sufka, K. J. (2008). Development and validation of alternative models of anxiety and depression using domestic fowl. In A. V. Kalueff and J. L. LaPorte (Eds.), *Behavioral Models in Stress Research*. Hauppage, N.Y.: Nova Science, 35–65.

Gibson, A. P., Hebden, J. C., and Arridge, S. R. (2005). Recent advances in diffuse optical imaging. *Physics in Medicine and Biology* 50: R1–R43.

Green, S., and Hodges, H. (1991). Animal models of anxiety. In P. Willner (Ed.), *Behavioral Models in Psychopharmacology: Theoretical, Industrial and Clinical Perspectives*. Cambridge: Cambridge University Press.

Hutchison, W. D., Davis, K. D., Lozano, A. M., Tasker, R. R., and Dostrovksy, J. O. (1999). Pain-related neurons in the human cingulate cortex. *Nature Neuroscience* 2: 403–405.

IASP Task Force on Taxonomy. (1994). Part III: Pain terms, a current list with definitions and notes on usage. In H. Merskey and N. Bogduk (Eds.), *Classification of Chronic Pain*, 2nd ed. Seattle: IASP Press, 209–215.

Jiang, X., Xu, K., Hoberman, J., Tian, F., Marko, A. J., Waheed, J. F., et al. (2005). BDNF variation and mood disorders: A novel functional promoter polymorphism and Val66Met are associated with anxiety but have opposing effects. *Neuropsychopharmacology* 30: 1353–1361.

Kalueff, A. V., and Tuohimaa, P. (2004). Experimental modeling of anxiety and depression. *Acta Neurobiologiae Experimentalis* 64: 439–448.

Kalueff, A. V., Wheaton, M., and Murphy, D. L. (2007). What's wrong with my mouse model? Advances and strategies in animal modeling of anxiety and depression. *Behavioral Brain Research* 179: 1–18.

Kasper, S. (2001). Depression and anxiety—separate or continuum? *World Journal of Biological Psychiatry* 2: 162–163.

Katz, R. (1981). Animal models and human depressive disorders. *Neuroscience and Biobehavioral Reviews* 20: 231–246.

Keller-Wood, M. E., and Dallman, M. F. (1984). Corticosteroid inhibition of ACTH secretion. *Endocrine Reviews* 5: 1–24.

Kessler, R. C., Berglund, P., Demleer, O., Jin, R., Merikangas, K. R., and Walters, E. E. (2005). Lifetime prevalence and age-of-onset distributions of DSM-IV disorders in the national comorbidity survey replication. *Archives of General Psychiatry* 62: 593–602.

Kessler, R. C., McGonagle, K. A., Zhao, S., Nelson, C. B., Hughes, M., Eshleman, S., et al. (1994). Lifetime and 12-month prevalence of DSM-III-R psychiatric disorders in the United States. Results from the national comorbidity survey. *Archives of General Psychiatry* 51: 8–19.

Kim, Y., Na, K., Shin, K., Jung, H., Choi, S., and Kim, J. (2007). Cytokine imbalance in the pathophysiology of major depressive disorder. *Progress in Neuropsychopharmacology and Biological Psychiatry* 31: 975–1152.

Koyama, T., Kato, K., and Mikami, A. (2000). During pain-avoidance neurons activated in the macaque anterior cingulate and caudate. *Neuroscience Letters* 283: 17–20.

LaBuda, C. J., and Fuchs, P. N. (2005). Attenuation of negative pain affect produced by unilateral spinal nerve injury in the rat following anterior cingulate cortex activation. *Neuroscience* 136: 311–322.

LaGraize, S. C., Borzan, J., Peng, Y. B., and Fuchs, P. N. (2006). Selective regulation of pain affect following activation of the opioid anterior cingulate cortex system. *Experimental Neurology* 197: 22–30.

LaGraize, S. C., Labuda, C. J., Rutledge, M. A., Jackson, R. L., and Fuchs, P. N. (2004). Differential effect of anterior cingulate cortex lesion on mechanical hypersensitivity and escape/avoidance behavior in an animal model of neuropathic pain. *Experimental Neurology* 188: 139–148.

Lehr, E. (1989). Distress call reactivation in isolated chicks: A behavioral indicator with high selectivity for antidepressants. *Psychopharmacology (Berlin)* 97: 145–146.

Melzack, R. (1973). The physiology of pain. In *The Puzzle of Pain*. New York: Basic Books, 95–96.

McKinney, W. T., and Bunney, W. E. (1969). Animal model of depression. I. Review of evidence: Implications for research. *Archives of General Psychiatry* 21: 240–248.

Murphy, D. L. (1976). Animal models for human psychopathology: Observations from the vantage point of clinical psychopharmacology. In G. Serban and A. Kling (Eds.), *Animal Models in Human Psychobiology*. New York: Plenum Press, 265–271.

O'Brien, S. M., Scott, L. V., and Dinan, T. G. (2004). Cytokines: Abnormalities in major depression and implications for pharmacological treatment. *Human Psychopharmacology* 19: 397–403.

Panksepp, J. (2003). Can anthropomorphic analyses of "separation cries" in other animals inform us about the emotional nature of social loss in humans? *Psychological Reviews* 110: 376–388.

Ploner, M., Freund, H. J., and Schnitzler, A. (1999). Pain affect without pain sensation in a patient with a postcentral lesion. *Pain* 81: 211–214.

Rainville, P., Carrier, B., Hofbauer, R., Bushnell, M. C., and Duncan, G. H. (1999). Dissociation of sensory and affective dimensions of pain using hypnotic modulation. *Pain* 82: 159–171.

Rainville, P., Duncan, G. H., Price, D. D., Carrier, B., and Bushnell, M. C. (1997). Pain affect encoded in human anterior cingulate but not somatosensory cortex. *Science* 277: 968–971.

Ressler, K. J., and Nemeroff, C. B. (2000). Role of serotonergic and noradrenergic systems in the pathophysiology of depression and anxiety disorders. *Depression and Anxiety* 12: 2–19.

Robinson, W. S. (1997). Some nonhuman animals can have pains in a morally relevant sense. *Biology and Philosophy* 12: 51–71.

Shriver, A. (2006). Minding mammals. *Philosophical Psychology* 19: 433–442.

Seligman, M. E., Maier, S. F., and Geer, J. H. (1968). Alleviation of learned helplessness in the dog. *Journal of Abnormal Psychology* 73: 256–262.

Sufka, K. J. (1994) Conditioned place preference paradigm: A novel approach for analgesic drug assessment against chronic pain. *Pain* 58: 355–366.

Sufka, K. J. (1996). Novel approaches for analgesic drug assessment: New animal paradigms. *Expert Opinion on Investigational Drugs* 5: 421–428.

Sufka, K. J., Feltenstein, M. W., Warnick, J. E., Acevedo, E. O., Webb, H. E., and Cartwright, C. C. (2006). Modeling the anxiety-depression continuum hypothesis in domestic fowl chicks. *Behavioral Pharmacology* 17: 681–689.

Sufka, K. J., and Roach, J. T. (1996). Stimulus properties and antinociceptive effects of bradykinin B_1 and B_2 receptor antagonists in rats. *Pain* 66: 99–103.

Takenouchi, K., Nishijo, H., Uwano, T., Tamura, R., Takigawa, M., and Ono, T. (1999). Emotional and behavioral correlates of the anterior cingulate cortex during associative learning in rats. *Neuroscience* 93: 1271–1287.

van der Kooy, D. (1987). Place conditioning: A simple and effective method for assessing the motivational properties of drugs. In M. A. Bozarth (Ed.), *Methods for Assessing the Reinforcing Properties of Abused Drugs*. New York: Springer.

van der Staay, F. J. (2006). Animal models of behavioral dysfunctions: Basic concepts and classifications, and an evaluation strategy. *Brain Research Reviews* 52: 131–159.

Vollmayr, B., and Henn, F. A. (2001). Learned helplessness in the rat: Improvements in validity and reliability. *Brain Research Protocols* 8: 1–7.

Warnick, J. E., Huang, C.-J., Acevedo, E. O., and Sufka, K. J. (in press). Modeling the anxiety-depression continuum in chicks. *Journal of Psychopharmacology*.

Warnick, J. E., Wicks, R. T., and Sufka K. J. (2006). Modeling anxiety-like states: Pharmacological characterization of the chick separation stress paradigm. *Behavioural Pharmacology* 17: 581–587.

Watson, D. (2005). Rethinking the mood and anxiety disorders: A quantitative hierarchical model for DSM-V. *Journal of Abnormal Psychology* 114: 522–536.

Willner, P. (1986) Validation criteria for animal models of human mental disorders: Learned helplessness as a paradigm case. *Progress in Neuropsychopharmacology and Biological Psychiatry* 10: 677–690.

Willner, P. (1991). Animal models of depression. In P. Willner (Ed.), *Behavioral Models in Psychopharmacology: Theoretical, Industrial and Clinical Perspectives*. Cambridge: Cambridge University Press.

PART VII

NEUROPHILOSOPHY

CHAPTER 22

LEVELS, INDIVIDUAL VARIATION, AND MASSIVE MULTIPLE REALIZATION IN NEUROBIOLOGY

KENNETH AIZAWA AND CARL GILLETT

> No one supposes that all the individuals of the same species are cast in the very same mould. These individual differences are highly important for us, as they afford materials for natural selection to accumulate.... These individual differences generally affect what naturalists consider unimportant parts; but I could show by a long catalogue of facts, that parts which must be called important, whether viewed under a physiological or classificatory point of view, sometimes vary in the individuals of the same species.
>
> Charles Darwin, *On the Origin of Species*

Neuroscientists, like all biologists, hold two fundamental beliefs about nervous systems. First, they believe that nervous systems can be studied at any number of distinct but interdependent levels of organization in which entities at one level are explained by the qualitatively different entities at one or more lower levels that are taken to compose them. Neuroscientists study structures as large as communities of interacting organisms and as small as individual proteins. There are thus a number of neurobiological levels.

The second fundamental belief is that nervous systems display individual variation. Subsequent research has shown that Darwin (1964) surely understated the case, especially with the subject matter of the neurosciences, when he observed that not all individuals of a species are cast from the same mold. Organisms obviously vary in their genetic makeup, but given distinct histories of interaction with their environments even genetically identical individuals will diverge in their phenotypic details. In truth, no two organisms are exactly alike, molecule for molecule, cell for cell, or organ for organ—especially when the molecules, cells, and organs in question are those studied by the neurosciences.

Combining these two fundamental beliefs, we may say that as far as can currently be determined, individual variation appears at every level of neurobiological organization. As a result, because component entities such as realizer properties vary at particular levels, we contend that we have overwhelming scientific evidence for what we call the massive multiple realization (MMR) hypothesis about psychological properties:

> (MMR) Many human psychological properties are multiply realized at many
> neurobiological levels.

Putting the thesis in other words, MMR is the claim that for many human psychological properties, the instances of these properties are realized by different lower level properties at many of the levels studied in neuroscience.[1]

As our opening points suggest, and as the evidence we highlight supports, the MMR hypothesis is uncontentious for many working neuroscientists (although they obviously do not refer to the relevant phenomena in the terms used in the thesis). In contrast, the existence of *any* multiple realization of psychological properties by neuroscientific properties, let alone *pervasive* or *massive* multiple realization, has been bitterly fought over by philosophers. To understand these differing reactions of neuroscientists and philosophers, it is important to briefly lay out the recent background to debates in general philosophy of science, the philosophy of psychology, and the philosophy of neuroscience. Setting the scene in this manner allows us to better situate our work in the chapter and the overall position we ultimately defend in relation to recent philosophical battles.

All areas have narratives (stories, if you prefer) about the present issues and competing positions. Though obviously a caricature, the following is hopefully a useful sketch of one common narrative current in much philosophy of neuroscience about the recent dialectical state-of-play and philosophical battle lines. (We should note that researchers in philosophy of psychology obviously have different stories to tell, but one of these narratives does reflect this understanding of the debate.[2])

On one side, so the story goes, we find proponents of cognitive science (the name of Jerry Fodor is often dropped at this point) who are taken to endorse the existence of multiple realization. These defenders of cognitive science are also taken to use multiple realization to establish the autonomy of cognitive science from neuroscience, where the latter is read as the claim that neuroscience and cognitive science do not intertheoretically constrain each other. On the other side, the story continues, we find those who emphasize the importance of neuroscience and defend the existence of intertheoretic constraints between cognitive sciences and neuroscience, and who consequently use such intertheoretic constraint to attack the existence of multiple realization. (Writers offering such arguments include Bechtel and Mundale, 1999, Shapiro, 2004, and others.) Along with these opposing commitments, our two camps are also read as having conflicting views about the possibility of Nagelian reduction (Nagel, 1961), and the existence of univocal realizations and/ or species-specific identities between neuroscientific and psychological properties. The defenders of cognitive science are taken to reject such claims, and those sympathetic to neuroscience are interpreted as defending them.

This narrative obviously posits a range of ongoing disputes that have implications far beyond the philosophy of psychology and the philosophy of neuroscience, because the questions putatively at issue concern the status and importance of various scientific disciplines. It is thus only a small step from these scholarly discussions about the nature and appropriate relations of neuroscience and psychology, and their respective entities, to more pragmatic debates over the appropriate funding levels for these scientific areas and particular approaches within them. Unsurprisingly, as is often the case when funding discussions become public, the resulting debates in philosophy have been heated and hard-fought. Our goal in this chapter is to engage these philosophical disputes over multiple realization from some fresh directions and attempt to reconnect the concerns of philosophers with the frameworks that working neuroscientists take to be mundane.

First, though passion has not been lacking in recent discussions in philosophy, what has been missing is any precise philosophical framework for a key element of these debates in the compositional relations between the levels of entities in neuroscience, including realization relations between properties. Our initial attempt to freshen the recent debates focuses on addressing this deficit. We begin by using a concrete, well-understood case from neurobiology, in section 1, to highlight variation and levels in neurobiology and also to sketch the general nature of the concepts of composition routinely posited in explanations in the sciences. Using these more general observations as a platform, we then provide precise theory schemata for both the realization relations between properties and multiple realization itself.[3]

Our framework for realization and multiple realization provides new theoretical resources, and we also seek to freshen the debate in a second way by using our framework to examine a selection of empirical evidence to highlight the nature of a number of neurobiological levels. We therefore give a brief sampling of scientific findings in section 2, illuminating the variety of such levels, and show that there is plausibly important individual variation at every physiologically significant level of organization in the nervous system—from proteins to whole brains. Applying this theoretical work on realization and multiple realization, we consequently show that such evidence about individual variation provides a prima facie plausible case for MMR. Our more detailed theoretical frameworks for scientific composition thus illuminate why working scientists apparently find multiple realization, though described in different terms, to be so mundane.

Since so many philosophers have thought that multiple realization is far from trivial, perhaps even being scientifically damaging, we finish, in section 3, by exploring philosophical concerns about the MMR hypothesis. We show that our more precise theoretical framework for realization, in combination with neurobiological evidence, establishes that a range of common objections to the existence of multiple realization are mistaken. For example, we show that multiple realization simply does not establish the methodological autonomy of cognitive science and other branches of psychology, but actually supports the utility of a coevolutionary research strategy based around methodological interactions between the psychological and neurobiological sciences.

One of our goals in the chapter is therefore to show that the lack of a theoretical framework for scientific composition has been highly damaging, because we demonstrate that with a precise account of realization relations in the sciences one can establish the error of *both* of the sides commonly taken to be battling in recent philosophical debates. With better accounts of scientific composition, realization, and multiple realization in hand, we show that the empirical evidence underpinning the standard neuroscientific belief that nervous systems have individual variation at many levels of organization supports *both* MMR *and* intertheoretic constraint between cognitive science and neuroscience. As we suggested, such a combination of multiple realization and methodological interaction between neuroscience and psychology has been anathema to many philosophers, though it appears mundane to working scientists in both disciplines. Our hope is that getting clearer about scientific composition generally, and realization and multiple realization in particular, restores a balance between the outlooks of philosophers and neuroscientists, not least by challenging a number of mistaken and damaging positions that have recently taken root in the philosophies of neuroscience and psychology.

1. Composition in the Sciences: Understanding Realization and Multiple Realization

In this section we seek to give a clearer picture of the compositional concepts posited in mechanistic explanations in the sciences, some of which are summarized in table 22.1.[4]

We should remark that terms like *realization, constitution,* and *implementation* have been used in all manner of ways by theoreticians, whether metaphysicians, logicians, or philosophers of science. For example, the word *realization* has been used by philosophers and scientists to refer to a number of very different concepts

Table 22.1. Compositional Relations in the Sciences

Type of Entity as Relata	Compositional Relation
Processes	Lower level processes *implement* a higher level process
Individuals	Lower level individuals *constitute* a higher level individual
Properties	Lower level properties *realize* a higher level property
Powers	Lower level powers *comprise* a higher level power

in a range of distinct projects. However, given the focus here, we exclusively use these terms to refer to the relevant compositional relations posited in the sciences and thus offer a view of realization that seeks to capture the compositional relations between properties posited in mechanistic explanations.[5]

Although we are concerned with scientific compositional relations in general, we focus most of our attention on individuals and properties and their compositional relations in constitution and realization. In treating properties, we assume a weak version of the "causal theory of properties." This is a variant of Shoemaker's (1980) account under which a property is individuated by the causal powers it *potentially* contributes to the individuals in which it is instantiated. On this view, two properties are different when they contribute different powers under the same conditions.

To concretely anchor our work and aid the explication of our accounts of realization and multiple realization, we focus on a familiar case from neurobiology, where our explanations are well confirmed, in recent mechanistic explanations of color processing in the human retina at a number of neurobiological levels. The sciences provide mechanistic explanations of the retina that take it to be constituted by individuals at cellular, biochemical, and atomic levels and take the chromatic processing properties of the human retina to be correspondingly realized by properties and relations at the cellular, biochemical, and atomic levels, among others.

Focusing on individuals (as shown in figure 22.1), the sciences now take the retina to be constituted by, among other things, rods and cones; take rods and cones to be constituted by, among other things, complex light-sensitive protein molecules; and take such molecules of photopigment to be constituted by various atoms. Turning to properties and relations, as we relate in more detail as we progress through this section, the sciences also provide mechanistic explanations of the properties of the individuals at higher levels in terms of the properties of individuals at lower levels. For instance, the sciences take the retina's property of processing color to be realized by, among other properties/relations, the light absorbing and signaling properties of retinal cells and their pattern of synaptic connections; take the phototransducing property of cones (the property of releasing neurotransmitters in response to light) to be realized by, among other properties/relations, the light absorbing property of photopigment molecules; and take the property of absorbing light of a certain spectrum, of individual photopigment molecules, to be realized by,

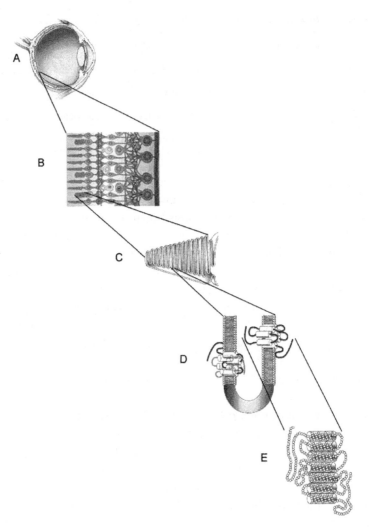

Figure 22.1. (A) The eye. (B) A Cross-section of the retina showing the principal cell types (including the rods and cones). (C) The outer segment of a cone. (D) Photopigments embedded in the membrane of the cone outer segment. (E) The amino acid chain of a cone photopigment.

among other properties/relations, the valence properties of the constituent atoms and their bonds.

Our approach is to work our way up through the mechanistic explanations offered at successively higher levels, starting with how atoms and their properties/relations constitute and realize photopigments and their properties—thus working from the bottom of figure 22.1 upward through the associated layers of explanations. By working through these various levels, we develop our various points in stages. First, we illustrate some general features of scientific composition, and then we articulate precise schemata for the realization and multiple realization of properties. In addition, our work also highlights the type of evidence that grounds the twin beliefs of neuroscientists that there are many neurobiological levels and individual variation at each of them. Last, and perhaps most important, we use our scientific examples to illuminate the reasons we contend that the evidence supporting these neuroscientific beliefs also underpins pervasive or "massive" multiple realization in neurobiology.

To start, let us consider an atomic-to-molecular case, where the lower level individuals are atoms of hydrogen, carbon, oxygen, nitrogen, and so on, and the higher level individual is a molecule of normal human green photopigment.[6] The relevant lower level properties and relations of the atoms include charge and bonding relations; the relevant higher level property of the photopigment is the property of being maximally sensitive to light of about 530 nm, with a bell-shaped distribution of sensitivity around that peak (see figure 22.2).[7] The sciences provide a clear mechanistic explanation of why a normal human green photopigment has the latter property under the normal physiological background conditions in a cone.

The sciences distinguish two portions of the cone photopigments: an 11-*cis*-retinal element and an opsin protein. The individual atoms in the retinal element have properties such as size and valence, which give them the powers to form certain types of bonds in response to various situations. For instance, the bonded and spatially aligned carbon, hydrogen, and oxygen atoms in a molecule of 11-*cis*-retinal form a long chain of alternating single and double carbon bonds (see figure 22.3). In this chain, the bond between the 11th and 12th carbon atoms of the 11-*cis*-retinal contributes the power of capturing a photon of light of a certain kind to these atoms. As a result, the powers contributed by the atoms' properties and relations noncausally result in the green photopigment having the property of absorbing a particular spectrum of light with a maximum sensitivity at 530 nm. The properties and relations of the individual atoms thus together realize the photopigment's property.

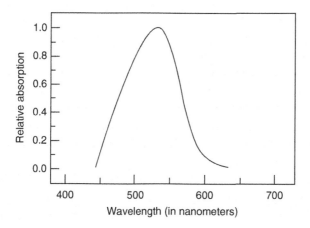

Figure 22.2. M-cone photopigment sensitivity curve. Modified from Sekular and Blake (2002, figure 2.23, p. 74).

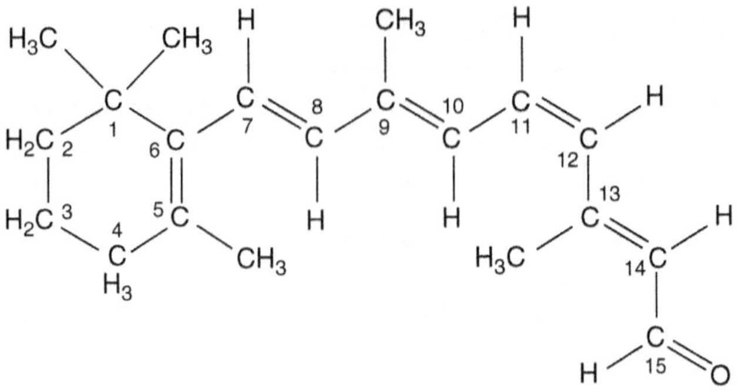

Figure 22.3. 11-cis-retinal. Modified from Casiday and Frey (1998).

In this and other mechanistic explanations, we have compositional relations posited between powers, properties, individuals, and processes. Individual atoms of carbon, nitrogen, hydrogen, and so forth constitute the photopigment molecule. The powers of the atoms to capture certain photons comprise the power of a photopigment molecule. The properties and relations of these individual atoms together realize the light sensitivity of the photopigment molecule and the processes of assimilating photons into a particular electronic configuration implement the process of absorbing light of a certain spectrum. Though such complexity is daunting, we can begin to understand such compositional notions if we use our example to draw out what appear to be some of their general features.

First, we note that the various compositional relations in our example are a species of determination relation, but one that is rather different from causal determination—such "horizontal" causal determination is temporally extended, relates wholly distinct entities, and often involves the transfer of energy or the mediation of force. In contrast, the vertical determination involved with compositional relations is synchronous. For example, it takes no time for the atoms to constitute the photopigment molecule or for the properties and relations of the constituent atoms to realize the property of absorbing light of 530 nm. Compositional relations also do not relate wholly distinct entities, because it is the individual atoms that constitute the photopigment molecule and the properties of the atoms (such as their size, charge, polarity, bonding relations, etc.) that realize the higher level property (such as a green photopigment molecule's light sensitivity). Finally, compositional relations do not involve the transfer of energy and/or the mediation of force between composing and composed entities. Compositional relations in the sciences are thus very different from causal relations and are a variety of what we call noncausal determination.

Second, compositional relations in the sciences usually relate qualitatively different kinds of entity. For example, the green photopigment has the property of being maximally sensitive to light of 530 nm, but no atom in the photopigment has such a property. We thus have individuals that constitute other individuals with which they need share no properties. Similar points hold for the relevant powers, properties, and mechanisms. A quick examination of cases of compositional relations posited in the special sciences shows that this feature is pervasive—entities usually compose entities of *qualitatively different* kinds.

Initially, it might seem surprising that entities of one kind could compose and explain entities of completely different kinds. Third, and perhaps most important for our purposes, we should mark that compositional relations are usually "many-one" in the sense that *many* component entities compose some higher level entity. Thus a number of atoms constitute the molecule of photopigment, and a number of properties and relations of the atoms realize the property of absorbing light of 530 nm. This feature is important because it dispels any mystery about how relations of composition in the sciences can relate qualitatively different entities. Even though the composing entities are individually different from the composed entity, nonetheless the composing entities *together* noncausally result in the composed entity. This distinctive feature of such composition relations consequently allows one to mechanistically explain powers, properties, individuals, and processes of one kind using, *together*, powers, properties, individuals, and processes of very different kinds.

As we will see shortly, the latter mundane feature also underlies the phenomenon of multiple realization, but before we turn to multiple realization, let us now more carefully articulate the nature of scientific realization. In our case, the photopigment's property of being maximally sensitive to light of 530 nm is individuated by the power of absorbing light in the neighborhood of 530 nm. As we outlined, the mechanistic explanation of why the photopigment has this property is that its constituent atoms have properties, such as valence and charge, which contribute the powers of capturing photons and changing their electronic configurations to form new sets of bonds. As a result, the sciences tell us that the photopigment molecule has a specific property of absorbing light of 530 nm, G, because its constituent atoms have properties and relations, $F_1–F_n$, that can change their energy levels in a very particular way on absorption of certain photons. The powers contributed by and individuative of the properties and relations of the constituent atoms in this manner noncausally result in the powers contributed by and individuative of the property of the photopigment.

Using these observations as a guide, we offer this thumbnail account of realization in the sciences (elsewhere dubbed the Dimensioned view):[8]

> (Realization) Property/relation instance(s) $F_1–F_n$ realize an instance of a property G, in an individual s under conditions \$, *if and only if*, under \$, $F_1–F_n$ together contribute powers, to s or s's part(s)/constituent(s), in virtue of which s has powers that are individuative of an instance of G, but not vice versa.

A number of features of the Dimensioned view, mirroring the common characteristics of scientific composition noted earlier in our example, are worth emphasis. First, the Dimensioned view accommodates realization as a species of noncausal determination. Second, it permits realizer and realized properties to be qualitatively distinct, allowing that these properties may contribute no common powers and be instantiated in different individuals. Perhaps most important, the Dimensioned account implicitly acknowledges that realization is usually a many-one relation, for it allows that many realizer properties may contribute powers that *together* determine that the relevant individual has the qualitatively different powers individuative of the qualitatively different realized property.

Our work understanding the common features of composition in the sciences obviously underpins this view of realization and it again offers help if we turn to the phenomenon of multiple realization. Recall the second and third of the general features of scientific composition, which are shared by realization relations. Given the characteristic that scientific realization often relates qualitatively different kinds of property, and the feature that many properties together realize other properties, then a variety of realizer properties that are qualitatively distinct from other realizers and the realized property can each *together* realize instances of the same special science property. The result is *multiple* realization—instances of the same higher level property realized by distinct lower level properties and relations that together noncausally result in the powers of the same special science property, despite being different from each other and the realized property in the powers they individually contribute.

We can give substance to these abstract points if we again return to the concrete example of the green photopigment and its property of maximally absorbing light of 530 nm. For the sciences have now identified two chemically distinct molecules, constituted by two distinct combinations of atoms, that current evidence indicates have the same peak sensitivity as the normal human green photopigment (see, for example, Merbs and Nathans, 1993). In addition to the normal amino acid sequence of the green opsin, there is another sequence produced by a homologous recombination of the first two exons of the gene for the normal human red photopigment with the last four exons of the gene for the normal green photopigment. As a result, given the differing properties and relations of the atoms in these two molecules, there are two known combinations of atomic properties and relations that noncausally give rise to the same property of maximally absorbing light of 530 nm.[9] We thus have different realizations of the standard green peak light sensitivity. This should be unsurprising, for we have seen that because realizers usually compose a qualitatively different realized property, this opens the space for *distinct* combinations of realizers to noncausally result in instances of the *same* higher level property. In just this fashion, we have multiple realizations at the atomic level of the property of maximally absorbing light of 530 nm.

(As an aside, because this type of point will be important later, notice that the multiple realization of the property of being maximally sensitive to light of 530 nm is not simply a function of our attending to a property using a relatively coarse "grain" of description at the higher level, such as being light sensitive, rather than a relatively fine "grain" of description, such as being maximally sensitive to light of 530 nm. Even the relatively fine grain of description of the higher level property allows for its multiple realization. Anyone familiar with the recent literature will recognize that we are reacting to concerns raised by Bechtel and Mundale, 1999. In section 3, we return to Bechtel and Mundale's point about grains of description and directly address objections that may be based on their concerns.)

We can use these points to frame a precise, abstract account of multiple realization in the sciences as follows:

> (Multiple Realization) A property G is multiply realized *if and only if* (i) under condition \$, an individual s has an instance of property G in virtue of the powers contributed by instances of properties/relations F_1–F_n to s, or s's constituents, but not vice versa; (ii) under condition \$* (which may or may not be identical to \$), an individual $s*$ (which may or may not be identical to s) has an instance of a property G in virtue of the powers contributed by instances of properties/relations F^*_1–F^*_m of $s*$ or $s*$'s constituents, but not vice versa; (iii) F_1–$F_n \neq F^*_1$–F^*_m; and (iv), under conditions \$ and \$*, F_1–F_n and F^*_1–F^*_m are at the same scientific level of properties.[10]

Overall, the theory schema is fairly obvious. Conditions (i)–(iii) simply frame the demand for distinct sets of realizer properties for instances of the same realized property. However, the final condition deserves more comment.

Implicitly, philosophers have always had something like condition (iv) in mind when discussing multiple realization in the sciences. To see why one needs (iv), either implicitly or explicitly, consider the following common situation. Properties and relations of certain atoms realize the property of maximally absorbing a certain frequency of light; but obviously properties and relations of certain fundamental microphysical properties realize the properties and relations of these atoms and hence *also* realize this instance of the property of the photopigment of maximally absorbing that frequency of light. But since the properties and relations of the atoms $\neq$ properties and relations of fundamental microphysical individuals, it appears that in such cases if we only use conditions (i)–(iii), then this entails we have a case of multiple realization. But we obviously do not want to treat the difference between realizers at the physical and chemical levels as sufficient for multiple realization. What has gone awry is that the two sets of properties are not at the same level and are implicitly excluded as candidates to ground a case of multiple realization. Addition of condition (iv) explicitly resolves this problem, though we suggest the condition is usually implicitly accepted as a shared background condition in earlier discussions of multiple realization in the sciences.[11]

An advantage of using (iv) is that it also combats a common philosophical practice that can cause problems. The practice in question is that of talking simply about the multiple realization of some property, whether psychological, biological, or whatever, and saying nothing further. Often, given the context, this may be a harmless way of talking, but we should note how it may be damaging. Given the nature of the realization relation, claims about realization and hence multiple realization are always relative to *particular* properties and levels—as both of our schemata now make explicit. Thus, property instance G is not simply realized; rather, it is realized by instances of certain lower level properties F_1–F_n. And instances of property G are multiply realized by instances of properties F_1–F_n and instances of properties F^*_1–F^*_m, when F_1–F_n and F^*_1–F^*_m are at the same level, as condition (iv) now makes clear. Thus, claims of realization and multiple realization are always indexed to particular levels and specific properties at these levels. We can quickly see the importance of this point.

Suppose that some higher level property G is multiply realized by microphysical properties of fundamental particles and hence multiply realized at the microphysical level. This does not, of course, mean that G is multiply realized in, say, distinct physiological properties. After all, it is logically possible to have G be univocally realized in the same physiological properties of two organisms and also have these properties in turn be univocally realized in the same biochemical properties of these organisms, but then have these biochemical properties be multiply realized by the microphysical properties of the fundamental particles that constitute these two organisms. So our two instances of G might be univocally realized at level X (the physiological level) and level X − 1 (the biochemical level), and still be multiply realized at level X − 3 (the microphysical level). We can thus see that a property is not simply *either* univocally realized *or* multiply realized. This is a false dichotomy, for such ascriptions are indexed to levels, and a property may be univocally realized at one level and multiply realized at another. To avoid confusion in talking about multiple realization, one therefore needs to be careful to make claims about realization, and hence multiple realization, indexed to particular realizers and levels.

If we return to our general accounts of realization and multiple realization, we can further illustrate their character if we consider another layer of mechanistic explanation we find for color processing in the retina. We have already noted how properties and relations of atoms can realize and multiply realize a molecular property. So let us move to a molecular-to-cellular case in our molecular explanations of the properties of a human cone at the cellular level, where we again consider how molecular properties and relations realize and multiply realize a cellular property.

In this case, at the lower level the relevant individuals are water molecules, ions (such as Ka^+, Na^+, and Ca^{++}), phospholipids, proteins, and so on, and at the higher level the individual under consideration is obviously a human cone (see figures 22.4 and 22.5). The higher level property of the cone that is mechanistically explained in this case is its property of releasing a neurotransmitter, in this case glutamate, in response to the absorption of light. The lower level properties and relations used to explain this property include having a charge, light sensitivity, polarity, and spatial arrangement.

In this case, our mechanistic explanations are more complex, but consider some of the highlights of these accounts of how the lower level entities compose (and hence explain) the higher level entities in question. Phospholipid molecules have both a hydrophilic and a hydrophobic region. Given this configuration, they

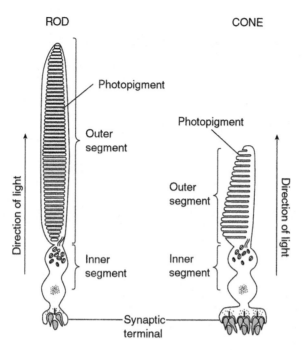

Figure 22.4. Structure of human rods and cones. From Sekular and Blake (2002), figure 2.29, p. 69.

spontaneously form a bilayer structure in which the hydrophilic regions face outward to an external aqueous environment in either the extracellular space or the cytoplasm, while the hydrophobic tails of the molecules cluster together inside the bilayer. This phospholipid bilayer constitutes the cell membrane, illustrated in the right half of figure 22.5. Proteins, for their part, also have hydrophobic and hydrophilic portions that help embed them in the cell membrane (see again the right half of figure 22.5). Human cone opsins, for example, have an evolutionarily well-conserved set of seven transmembrance amino acid sequences (see figure 22.6). Ion channels have amino acid sequences that enable them to span the cell membrane and provide bindings sites on one or another side to regulate the flow of ions through the channel. Cytoskeletal proteins, also partially embedded in the cell membrane, shape a cell into exotic configurations, such as those of the rods or cones.

Photopigment molecules are embedded in the cell membrane in the outer segment of the cone (recall figure 22.5). On absorption of a photon, a single photopigment molecule will change conformation and release into the cytoplasm a molecule of all-*trans*-retinal leaving an activated opsin molecule in the membrane. One activated opsin molecule binds to a single G protein molecule located on the inner surface of the cell membrane. This G protein molecule, in turn, activates a molecule of an enzyme, cGMP phosphodiesterase, which breaks down cGMP. When

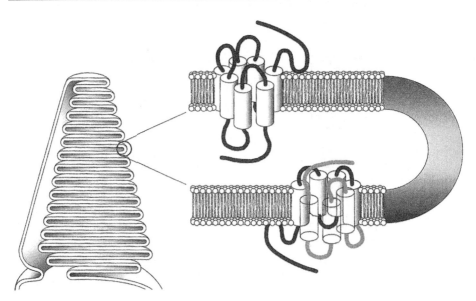

Figure 22.5. Photopigment molecule embedded in the cell membrane and phospholipid molecules of the membrane constituting a cone. Modified from Sharpe, Stockman, Jägle, and Nathans (1999), figure 1.2, p. 6.

intracellular cGMP concentrations subsequently decrease, cGMP is removed from a cGMP-gated Na^+ channel, leading to the closure of the channel. Closing the channel blocks the influx of Na^+ into the cell. In concert, vast numbers of photopigment molecules, G protein molecules, ion channels, and Na^+ ions go through this process, leading to the hyperpolarization of the cell. This hyperpolarization propagates from the outer segment to the synaptic contact of the cone, where it reduces the rate

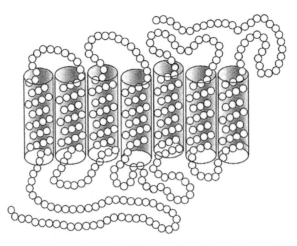

Figure 22.6. Schematic of an opsin embedded in the cell membrane. The seven cylinders represent portions of the opsin spanning the cell membrane. Based on Sharpe et al. (1999), figure 1.17A, p. 43.

of release of the neurotransmitter glutamate. This reduction in neurotransmitter release is the cone's signal that the cell has been illuminated. The foregoing lower level processes may be summarized schematically as follows.

Photon capture → all-*trans*-retinal release → G protein activation →
cGMP phosphodiesterase activation → cGMP decrease →
cGMP released from ion channels → ion channel closure →
cone hyperpolarization → decreased glutamate release.

Obviously a large number of these molecular processes occur together, and these lower level processes implement the cellular process of signaling the presence of light by release of glutamate. Consequently, we can thus also see that the cone's property of releasing a neurotransmitter in the presence of light is evidently realized by the properties and relations of the molecular individuals within the cell.

Our molecular-cellular example illustrates exactly the same features of the realization relation we described in the atomic-to-molecular example. First, the lower level properties and relations of the molecules stand in a synchronous, noncausal determination relation to the higher level property of releasing a neurotransmitter in the presence of light. There is no transmission of energy or mediation of force between the lower level properties and relations and the higher level property, where these properties are also not wholly distinct. Second, the relata in this realization relation are once more qualitatively distinct. The relevant determining properties and relations of the molecules are their charges, polarity, and light-absorbing capacity, where the determined property of the cell is its releasing glutamate in response to the presence of light. (With regard to individuals, the particular molecules in a cone do not release glutamate in response to light, whereas the cone does have this property. Similar points hold for the relevant higher and lower level powers and processes.) Third, the property of releasing a neurotransmitter in response to light is realized by *many* molecular properties and relations. It is the properties and relations of the individual molecules that *together* result in the cell's property of releasing glutamate in response to illumination.

The foregoing explains how a cone's property of signaling is realized by the lower level properties of ions, phospholipids, proteins, and so on. Now, however, we can see how distinct sets of molecular-level properties can provide for multiple realizations of a cone's property of transducing light into glutamate release. To do this, we might focus on any of the differing relevant properties of any of the different protein molecules in the biochemical cascade already described. We might focus on the different molecules of cGMP phosphodiesterase. Still, the clearest case of multiple realization emerges from the research on the most studied components in the cascade, namely, the photopigments. These photopigments differ in one of their molecular level properties, namely, their absorption spectra.[12] We can thus see in this case that there are distinct molecular-level properties, that is, distinct absorption spectra, that give rise to the same cellular property of transducing light into a neurochemical currency of glutamate release. Once again, we have a case of multiple realization, in this example of a cellular property by molecular properties.

At this point, it is worth stepping back from our examination of concepts of scientific composition to note some related methodological practices. Working scientists move freely between appealing to entities at different levels, for instance, switching from focusing on atomic-level properties, in the differences in amino acid sequences, to appealing to molecular-level properties, in the differences in absorption spectra. In fact, working scientists often freely move up or down through a number of levels of compositionally related entities to get explanatory help. What underpins this amazingly fruitful methodological maneuver? Briefly put, researchers pursue this methodological strategy because they recognize that when entities bear compositional relations, the nature of component entities at one level has ramifications for the entities at some other level that they compose. For example, working scientists clearly appreciate the potential ramifications of differences in atomic-level properties for the molecular-level properties they are taken to realize.

It is worth marking that our schemata for realization and multiple realization provide a ready explanation for this common feature of actual science. Although we have not explicitly noted this feature so far, we should mark that our schemata take realization to be a *transitive* relation—a feature that it shares with other scientific composition relations. Thus if property instances F_1–F_m realize G_1–G_n, in certain individuals and under specific conditions, and G_1–G_n realize property instance H, then F_1–F_m realize H. Consequently, under our schema for scientific realization, it makes as much sense to say that an instance of the property of releasing a neurotransmitter in response to illumination (by light in the neighborhood of 530 nm) is realized by molecular-level properties as it does to say that this instance of the property of releasing glutamate in response to illumination (by light in the neighborhood of 530 nm) is realized by certain atomic level properties.[13] Given the transitivity of compositional relations like realization, we can thus see how working scientists can successfully move up or down through levels of compositionally related entities to provide explanatory gain in their work at some other level of entities. In section 3, we explore this important point further, but at the risk of belaboring the case of color processing in the retina, we wish to advance to yet one more layer of mechanistic explanation and another level of entities.

The last case we consider is a cell-to-tissue case that concerns how a certain property of the retina, basically the property of signaling a pattern of color in the visual field, is realized and multiply realized by cellular level properties. In this example, the lower level individuals are the particular photoreceptor cells, the amacrine cells, bipolar cells, horizontal cells, and retinal ganglion cells (see figure 22.7). The higher level individual is a retina. The lower level properties and relations of the cells include releasing glutamate in the presence of light within a given band of frequencies, releasing certain neurotransmitters, binding certain neurotransmitters, having certain electrochemical synapses, and certain patterns of connectivity. The higher level property of the retina that is mechanistically explained is the retina's property of signaling a pattern of color in the visual field.

Once again, we have mechanistic explanations of the relevant properties that are highly detailed and rather complex in nature, so we only briefly review some of the

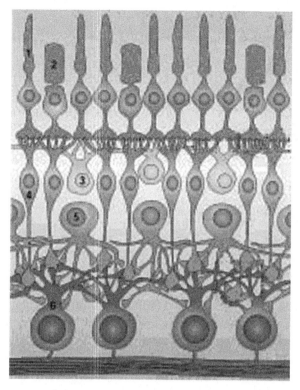

Figure 22.7. Cells constituting the human retina. (1) Rods, (2) cones, (3) horizontal cells, (4) bipolar cells, (5) amacrine cells, and (6) retinal ganglion cells. Modified from Wässle (2004), figure 1, p. 2.

highlights of our explanations of the retina's property in terms of the properties and relations of the cells that are taken to compose it. When introducing our molecular-cellular-level example, we already briefly described the nature of the biochemical cascade involved in translating photon capture into changes in glutamate release. Given only a single photopigment, a single cone can release glutamate in response to a relatively narrow band of light frequencies, but it is unable to signal the specific frequency of the incoming light. A given decrease in glutamate release may equally result from either a high-intensity light at a frequency to which the photopigment is relatively insensitive, or a low-intensity light at a frequency to which the photopigment is relatively sensitive. If processes of glutamate release from cones are going to implement a retina's process of signaling distinct patterns of color in the visual field, there is an obvious problem. However, this difficulty is resolved by the ratio of glutamate release in cells containing photopigments of different sensitivities. The three types of cones in the normal human eye, S-, M-, and L-cones, process short-, medium-, and long-wavelength frequencies of light. That is, each changes its glutamate release in response to a different band of frequencies of incident light (see figure 22.8). Each type of cone releases glutamate as it does in virtue of containing a chemically distinct photopigment. That is, each photopigment consists of a protein component, an opsin,

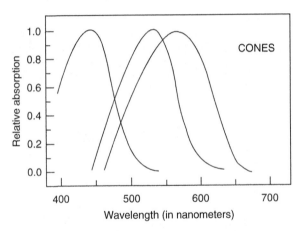

Figure 22.8. Absorption spectra of the S-, M-, and L-cones. From Sekular and Blake (2002), figure 2.23, p. 74.

covalently bonded to an 11-*cis*-retinal component, and the opsin components vary from cone to cone. The amacrine, bipolar, horizontal, and ganglion cells, of course, contribute to the retina as well, but for simplicity we set their role to one side.

This cell-to-tissue example again supports the existence of the features of the realization relation we described in our previous cases. First, the lower level properties and relations of the cells stand in a synchronous, noncausal determination relation to the higher level property of signaling patterns of color in the visual field. There is no transmission of energy or mediation of force between the lower level properties and relations of the cells to the higher level property of the retina, where the relevant properties, and the individuals that have them, are not wholly distinct. Second, the relata in this case of realization are again qualitatively distinct. The relevant determining properties and relations of the cells include their capacity to release glutamate in response to illumination, releasing certain neurotransmitters, binding certain neurotransmitters, having certain electrochemical synapses, having certain patterns of connectivity, and so on; in contrast, the determined property of the retina is its signaling patterns of color in the visual field. Third, in the case of the retina, once again *many* properties and relations of individual cells *together* noncausally result in the retina's property of signaling a pattern of color in the visual field.

There are many ways the property of signaling a pattern of color in the visual field is multiply realized by properties at the cellular level. The simplest examples stem from some of the principal forms of color blindness in which one type of cone is missing. The retinas of so-called dichromats are not completely insensitive to color; it is not as though they can make no color discriminations. Instead, they are able to make fewer color discriminations than can the retinas of normal humans. So these retinas are still color processors. There are, however, three ways of being a dichromatic retina, each corresponding to the loss of a distinct photopigment. The retina of a protanope lacks red cones, the retina of a deuteranope lacks green cones, and the retina of a tritanope lacks blue cones. Each form of dichromacy corresponds to a distinct realization of an instance of the property of signaling patterns of color in the visual field.

Less dramatic, and perhaps somewhat less familiar, are the cases of what are called anomalous trichromats. These individuals possess three distinct types of cones, but their sensitivities are not those of normal cones. For example, in one of the most common forms of red-green colorblindness, the red cones and the green cones release glutamate in response to relatively similar bands of electromagnetic radiation, hence there is not enough difference in the properties of the red and green cones to implement a higher level process that can signal differences between certain patterns of color. This gives rise to color-sensitivity "blind spots." Anomalous trichromacy is, of course, a kind of color processing, and its subjects do realize instances of the property of signaling patterns of color in the visual field, but in addition it grades off into normal color vision. There is no sharp dividing line between normal trichromacy and anomalous trichromacy. To take just one well-known example in the biochemistry of vision literature, the human red cone appears to be polymorphic. That is, it comes in two forms. One form of the red cone has the photopigment with an amino acid sequence with a serine amino acid at position 180, and the other photopigment has alanine at that position. Both forms are quite common in the human population. One has the multiple realization of normal human color vision by having some individuals with cones containing one red photopigment and other individuals with cones containing the other.[14]

Recent work on the biochemistry of opsins has suggested an even more radical form of multiple realization of the property of signaling patterns of color. In a classic paper, Nathans, Thomas, and Hogness (1986) identified the gene sequences, hence the amino acid sequences, of the three opsin components of the photopigments. In addition, they found that normal humans vary in the number of genes coding for the green pigment. In other words, there are multiple loci each coding for a green photopigment. Subsequent research has also found that normal humans vary in the number of genes coding for the red pigment (Neitz and Neitz, 1995). This suggests the possibility that a given individual can possess distinct versions of the gene for the green and red photopigments at the different loci, and hence can possess distinct green and red photopigments and distinct green and red cones. Furthermore, it is hypothesized that part of the reason for individual variation in color sensitivity within humans is due to differences in the number of different kinds of cones. Some individuals might have, say, only one type of green cone and one type of red cone, and other individuals might have, say, two different green cones and seven different types of red cone.[15]

To summarize, by examining a number of connected examples of mechanistic explanations from a familiar and well-confirmed area of research in neurobiology, we have supported a number of claims. First, we have shown that the compositional relations posited in such explanations have some important common features in being transitive, noncausal determination relations that are usually many-one and relate qualitatively different entities at distinct levels. Second, building on these observations about the common features of scientific composition generally, we have provided precise accounts of both scientific realization and multiple realization. As we have seen, once one gets a better grip on scientific composition, the character of multiple realization becomes more understandable. For we have seen that a number of component entities usually together compose some qualitatively different entity. As a result, diverse kinds of component entities can together, usually on separate occasions, compose instances of the same composed entity. The result, in the case of properties, is multiple realization of instances of the same higher level property by different lower level realizers.

In addition to articulating a theoretical framework for realization and multiple realization, our work surveying these concrete scientific examples also supported our specific claims about neurobiology. In the case of color processing in the human retina, we have shown that there are a number of neurobiological levels relevant to our mechanistic explanations. This supports the first belief we have attributed to working neurobiologists. Furthermore, at the atomic-to-molecular, the molecular-to-cellular, and cell-to-tissue cases, we have also shown that we find individual variation among the relevant entities at the lower level, thus supporting the second belief of neurobiologists that we find individual variation at all levels. Finally, applying the theoretical framework to the empirical evidence that underlies scientists' commitments to multiple levels and individual variation in each of them, we have also shown how a strong case can be made for multiple realization of molecular properties by properties at the atomic level, cellular properties by properties at the molecular level, and tissue properties by properties at the cellular level. Given the transitivity of scientific relations of realization, in our concrete scientific case we have thus found plausible evidence for the multiple realization at many neurobiological levels of the relevant human psychological properties in this example, such as the property of signaling patterns of color in the visual field.

2. Levels, Individual Variation, and Multiple Realization in Nervous Systems

With our theoretical framework in place, we now wish to widen our focus and examine evidence about a still wider range of entities in various neurobiological levels. Obviously we cannot attempt anything like a comprehensive survey of the relevant empirical findings; in fact, we can only highlight a fraction of these results. However, our initial goals will be to note the apparently wide body of evidence supporting the twin claims of working neuroscientists: that there are a number of neuroscientific levels and that individuals at each of these levels vary in their properties. Our work in the previous section highlights why such findings plausibly underpin multiple realization, so our approach is to survey the evidence for individual variation at each level and then conclude the section by returning to the issue of why such evidence provides support for multiple realization. Given the recent and rapidly growing resistance of so many philosophers to the existence of multiple realization in psychology and neuro-science, we hope that our work, however rough and incomplete, provides a clear and bold statement of the type of evidence that such critics need to address.

We begin, for obvious reasons, with lower neuroscientific levels, where our accounts are more mature and work through progressively higher levels, where our understanding becomes steadily less developed. As the reader will clearly see, a pattern of individual variation is obvious across these levels. Given our focus on multiple realization and the relative stages of development of various areas of research, our focus in each case is on showing that at the level in question there is variation across individuals where, very roughly, we have the following situations. Either (i) the properties of one level are known to be realizers of properties at the next higher neuroscientific level; (ii) our present accounts suggest that the properties of one level are likely to be realizers of properties at the next higher neuroscientific level; or (iii) our accounts of the properties of one level do not yet enable us deter-mine which specific properties at the lower level are likely to be realizers of proper-ties at the next higher neuroscientific level. Our focus on (i), (ii), or (iii) obviously results from the very different stages of development of both our accounts of the entities within different levels of neuroscientific organization and/or our intralevel mechanistic explanations of entities at differing levels using compositional rela-tions between these entities. In concluding the section, we argue that the pattern of pervasive individual variation, in situations (i), (ii), or (iii), nonetheless grounds a plausible case that the relevant neuroscientific properties are multiply realized.

In section 1, we reviewed the scientific case for the view that there is multiple realization by properties at the atomic level of a molecule of photopigment's prop-erty of having a particular light sensitivity. Now we wish to draw attention to the fact that the properties of human cone photopigments are unlikely to be unique in this regard and that many molecular properties are likely to be similarly multiply realized at the atomic level. Consider a hemoglobin molecule's property of bind-ing oxygen with such and such an affinity, or a protein kinase A (PKA) molecule's property of phosphorylating cAMP response element binding protein (CREB) with such and such a rate constant, or an alcohol dehydrogenase molecule's property of oxidizing ethanol to acetaldehyde at such and such a rate. Each of the forego-ing molecular properties is likely to be realized by distinct combinations of atomic level properties. Thus, one instance of the property G of binding oxygen with such and such an affinity will be realized by one set of atoms bearing properties/relation F_1–F_n (such as valence and bonding), where another instance of G will be realized by another set of atoms bearing properties/relations F^*_1–F^*_m, where F_1–F_n and F^*_1–F^*_m are at the same level, and F_1–$F_n \neq F^*_1$–F^*_m. Similar points hold mutatis mutandis for other properties such as G_1 of phosphorylating CREB.[16]

We can quickly identify some of the reasons for such widespread multiple realization at the atomic level. Any given type of protein varies in its amino acid sequence across different individual organisms, so that any given type of protein varies in the numbers and arrangements of atoms of carbon, hydrogen, nitrogen, oxygen, and so on. Along with this variation in individuals comes variation in their properties. Atoms of carbon, hydrogen, nitrogen, oxygen, and so forth differ in (most notably) their valence, which confers on them different powers to bind to other atoms. The properties/relations of the atoms give proteins such properties as their size, shape, and charge distributions. Properties like size, shape, and charge distribution confer on proteins their powers to bind substrates and catalyze biochemical reactions. Finally, along with this variation in properties/relations comes variation in powers. The different binding powers of a protein's atoms comprise the different powers for such things as binding substrates and catalyzing biochemical reactions.[17] The foregoing is a more general outline of the underlying factors we found for the cone photopigments examined in section 2, and we have now seen that such factors appear to apply quite generally for properties of complex proteins at the biochemical level. We have thus found strong evidence for both individual variation at the biochemical level and multiple realization of the properties at this level by atomic properties, thus indicating this is an example of type (i).

Move, now, to a slightly higher level of neurobiological organization, where we find dendritic spines. Dendritic spines are individual finger-like to mushroom-like extensions on the dendrites of neurons to which synapses connect (see figure 22.9). Individual dendritic spines are constituted by various types of individuals, including phospholipid molecules, water molecules, various individual ions, various cytoskeletal protein molecules that support the spine's shape and function, and various proteins embedded in or attached to the membrane surface. Properties such as a given size and shape of an individual dendritic spine are realized by various properties of the spine's constituents. The individual constituents of a dendritic spine bear such properties as having a hydrophobic segment (the phospholipids),

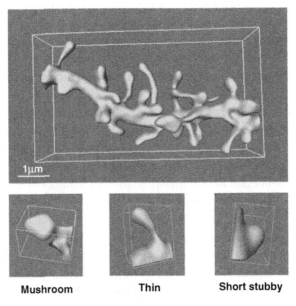

Mushroom   **Thin**   **Short stubby**

Figure 22.9. Dendritic spines and some of their common shapes. No synapses from other neurons are shown. McKinney (2005), figure 1, p. 1300. Reproduced with permission.

having a hydrophilic segment (the phospholipids), being polar (water), bearing a positive charge (K^+, Na^+, Ca^{++} ions), gating ions (K^+ and Na^+ channels), and so on. Most relevant for determining, say, the shape of the spine might be certain cytoskeletal proteins. These cytoskeletal proteins multiply realize the shape of a dendritic spine insofar as different protein molecules contribute different properties that noncausally determine the shape of the spine. Applying our schemata for realization and multiple realization, we would say that in some cases it is the instances of properties/relations F_1–F_n of the individual proteins of a dendritic spine that together realize some of the instances of the properties G of having a mushroom shape, where in other cases it is the instances of properties/relations F^*_1–F^*_m of the individual protein molecules of the spine that realize other instances of G.[18]

We have now seen that the properties of a dendritic spine might be multiply realized by lower level properties and that we presently have a case of type (ii) with such properties. But at the still higher level neuronal level of properties, dendritic spines are still more interesting for their apparent role in multiply realizing properties of neurons. An individual neuron is, of course, constituted by numerous subcellular components, such as dendritic spines, dendrites, axons, Golgi apparati, endoplasmic reticuli, and so forth. These individuals bear all manner of properties, such as size and shape, and we might, in principle, look to the properties of any of these constituents for sources of multiple realization of a neuronal property G, such as a V1 neuron's property of responding maximally to a line of a particular orientation. To illustrate our points, however, we focus on the properties of individual dendritic spines to illuminate sources of multiple realization at the neuronal or cellular level.

Dendritic spines differ in size and shape as measured in terms of such things as the size of the neck, their length, total volume, and head volume (see table 22.2 for data on hippocampal dendritic spines). Differences in these properties confer different electrical powers on these spines. For example, a spine's property of having a long neck and large head confers on it the power to limit the effects of the neurotransmitter released onto that spine to that spine. Furthermore, a spine's property of having a long neck and large head confers on it the power to limit any firing-dependent chemical changes in the synapse to that spine. If we consider the properties of all the dendritic spines on a given neuron, one can expect them to be such that there is one set F_1–F_n that will in part

Table 22.2. Variation in Functionally Significant Properties of Dendritic Spines: Ranges in Dimensions of Hippocampal Dendritic Spines and Their Synapses

	Dentate Gyrus	Area CA3	Area CA1
Neck diameter (μm)	0.09–0.54	0.20–1.00	0.038–0.46
Spine length (μm)	0.20–1.78	0.60–6.50	0.160–2.13
Spine volume (μm^3)	0.003–0.23	0.13–1.83	0.004–0.56
Head volume (μm^3)			0.003–0.55

Source: Sorra and Harris, 2000.

realize, say, a V1 neuron's property G of responding maximally to a line of a particular orientation, where another set of properties F^*_1–F^*_m of all the dendritic spines on another neuron will also realize that neuron's instance of property G.[19] Recent work on dendritic spines supports this view. Many of the basic features of dendritic spine morphology have been revealed by electron microscopic investigations of serial sections of fixed tissues, but more recent work has made it possible to make in vivo observations of changes in spine morphology over periods of days and weeks.

Scientists can insert genes that code for fluorescent proteins into mice. These genes produce fluorescent proteins in neurons that can be reliably reidentified day after day through fluorescence microscopy. With this technique, a large majority of dendritic spines have been found to be stable over the course of days and weeks, but nevertheless there remain, even in adult mice, changes in the number, size, and shape of dendritic spines.[20] In other words, this technique has revealed that even in adults there remains some degree of plasticity in spine morphology. Insofar as spine morphology varies in a single individual over time, it is highly likely that there will be variation in spine morphologies in different individuals of a given species at a given time.

Here we maintain that we have an example of type (ii), wherein the properties of one level are likely to be realizers of properties at the next higher neuroscientific level. What remains open for future investigation is the extent to which distinct properties/relations of distinct numbers and configurations of dendritic spines can be said to realize, at least in part, different properties of neurons.

Next consider a series of larger neural structures, where we think we can be less confident about which lower level properties realize which higher level properties. Thus we do not provide the level of detail given in earlier examples in this section where we plausibly had cases of types (i) or (ii). For example, consider cortical columns. Each individual column consists of a set of neurons that are relatively densely connected among themselves, but relatively less densely connected to neurons outside the column.[21] Many of the properties of individual columns, thus, appear to be realized at least in part by the properties/relations of individual neurons. Consider the finding by Kaschube, Wolf, Geisel, and Löwel (2002), using radiographic imaging techniques, that there is a high degree of individual variation in the size and shape of orientation columns in a population of 31 animals, some of which came from the same litter. Here we have a case of type (iii), but nonetheless we have strong evidence for individual variation at the level and the likelihood that the properties that are realizers will also be varied, hence making multiple realization likely.

Continue to another higher level of organization. In area V1, cortical columns are organized into still larger structures, ocular dominance columns. Ocular dominance columns are regions of layer IVc of area V1 that respond preferentially to inputs from one or another eye. Cytochrome oxidase staining enables the columns associated with one eye to be stained and the columns associated with the other remained unstained. In a study of six macaques, Horton and Hocking (1996) found numerous dimensions of variability in the ocular dominance columns. They found that the number, or periodicity, of ocular dominance columns in V1, varies by something on the order of 50 percent, and this variation is independent of the surface area of V1. Increased periodicity is, however, correlated with the complexity of the columnar mosaic. That is, monkeys with relatively few columns have longer and smoother columns, where monkeys with relatively more columns also had shorter columns with more frequent bifurcations and islands (see figure 22.10). Using radiographic techniques, Kaschube et al. (2003) quantified the interindividual variability in the spacing of ocular dominance columns of cat primary visual cortex in 39 animals from three colonies. Once again, we have powerful evidence for individual variation in the properties at the relevant levels despite this being a case of type (iii) where we do not know which specific properties at this level are likely to be the realizers of particular higher level properties.

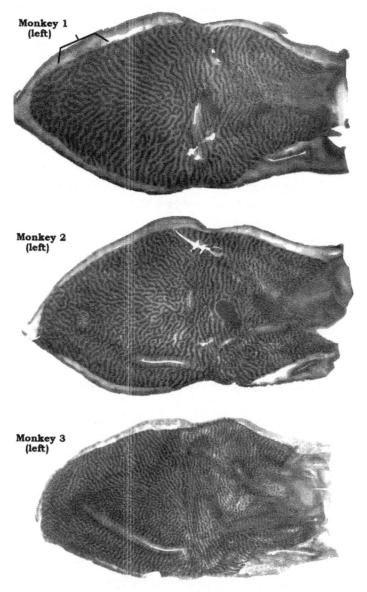

Figure 22.10. Intraspecific variance in ocular dominance columns of macaques. From Horton and Hocking (1996), figure 2, p. 7232.

Next consider some of the larger brain regions and collections of brain regions so convincingly described by Korbinian Brodmann (1909). Over the past century, a variety of methods have revealed individual variations in these structures made up of cortical columns. Stensaas, Eddington, and Dobelle (1974) found the human area V1 to vary in surface area by a factor of up to three.[22] Furthermore, some of these variations are highly correlated. Using structural and functional MRI, Dougherty et al. (2003) found that when V1, V2, and V3 are functionally delimited, the central 12° of the visual fields of V1 and V2 vary in surface area by a factor of about 2.5, where the central 12° of the visual field of V3 displays somewhat more limited variability. In addition, they found correlations in the variation of the surface area of V1 and V2 but weaker correlations between V1/V2 and V3. In primary auditory cortex, Rademacher et al. (2001) found that like V1, regions Te1 and Heschel's gyrus could vary by a factor of up to three across individuals. Penfield and Boldrey (1937) and Woolsey, Erickson, and Gilson (1979) used evoked potentials and electrical stimulation of the brain to find that human somatosensory and motor cortices vary by up to 100 percent.

Combinations of Brodmann's brain regions also show individual variation. Using morphometric and cytoarchitectonic techniques, Andrews, Halpern, and Purves (1997) found that the volume of the lateral geniculate nucleus, the cross-sectional area of the optic tract, and the surface area and volume of V1 all varied by about a factor of 2.5 across individuals.[23] The optic nerve, the optic tract, and areas V1, V2, and V3 reveal cortical magnification. That is, this portion of the visual system devotes disproportionately more cortex to the foveal regions of the retina than to the parafoveal regions. For areas V1, V2, and V3, as the distance from the fovea (eccentricity) increases, the surface area of the cortex dedicated to one degree of visual arc decreases. Dougherty et al. (2003) used fMRI data to document individual variation in the degree of cortical magnification. This suggests, as did the previous case, that properties of functionally significant combinations of brain regions, such as the "early visual system," might be multiply realized by properties/relations of different combinations of cells or perhaps by properties/relations of distinct combinations of cortical columns. Once again, though we have a case of type (iii), we nonetheless have strong evidence for individual variation at the level and the likelihood that the properties that are realizers will also be varied, hence making multiple realization likely.

Finally, there are apparent variations in whole brains. Individual variations in the weights, areas, and volumes of large brain structures have long been documented using postmortem analyses. More recently, however, MRI techniques have enabled investigators to measure individual variation in areas and volumes of brain regions in vivo, thereby avoiding confounding factors, such as variations due to differences in postmortem preservation techniques. Allen, Damasio, and Grabowski (2002) reported the results of MRI of brain volumes in normal subjects. All subjects, 23 male and 23 female, were right-handed with no left-handedness in first-degree relatives. There were healthy, with no history of neurological or psychiatric illness. They were primarily of European descent recruited primarily from the Iowa City community. The principal results regarding individual variation are shown in the table 22.3.

Table 22.3. Variations in Brain Dimensions in Humans

Region	Side	Male Mean cc (range)	s.d.	Female Mean cc. (range)	s.d.
Hemisphere (including cerebellum)					
	Left	618.9 (512.2-722.9)	54.7	547.0 (472.6-674.3)	47.8
	Right	621.7 (513.5-733.9)	58.3	552.7 (475.8-688.3)	49.5
Frontal					
	Left	205.2 (163.4-286.9)	25.8	182.8 (157.0-228.0)	17.0
	Right	208.3 (170.0-263.8)	24.0	186.2 (162.4-228.5)	17.2

The last four cases, at the very highest levels of organization, were of type (iii), where we lack detailed accounts of the specific lower level properties that realize properties at the particular higher level in question. However, as we have briefly noted in our discussion, it should now be clear that such examples still support the likelihood of multiple realization. However, to further illustrate how such examples support multiple realization, let us consider in more detail how the case at hand provides such evidence. Our examples of cortical columns, ocular dominance columns, Brodmann's brain regions and combinations of them, entire lobes, and entire brains have a common feature. The structures vary in size. This suggests that these structures differ in the number of neurons they contain.[24] Bare differences in numbers of cells might give rise to different combinations of properties/relations that realize properties at the level of cortical columns, ocular dominance columns, and so forth, and hence might well suffice for multiple realization. In addition, differences in the number of cells in a given region are also likely to induce or be correlated with new properties/relations among the cells. Differences in the numbers of cells will not necessarily be "just more of the same, only bigger." The latter point is rather speculative neuroscience which is why we have chosen to put the case into category (iii), wherein the properties of one level do not yet enable us to determine which properties are likely to be realizers of properties at the next higher neuroscientific level. However, once again, we have strong evidence for individual variation at this level and the levels below it, and thus the likelihood that the properties that are realizers will also be varied, hence making multiple realization likely.

Our brief sampling of empirical findings makes it plausible that there is a wide base of evidence supporting working neuroscientists in their twin commitments that there are a variety of neurobiological levels and that we find individual variation at many of these levels. Let us now briefly explain why these two commitments provide evidence for multiple realization, drawing together our foregoing points about the particular examples of types (i)–(iii).

As we have seen, depending on whether the examples are instances of cases (i), (ii), or (iii), the strength of evidence for multiple realization varies. Some psychological properties, such as being a deuteranope, are instances of situation (i) and sometimes (ii), and in these cases we have clear and compelling evidence for multiple realization. For other properties, we have found that our understanding is still in situations (ii) or (iii), and we are much less sure what the realization bases of these properties might be. Nonetheless, we have seen that even in cases of type (ii) and (iii) we still have evidence, albeit weaker in nature, for individual variation in the properties that are candidates for being realizers at the neurobiological levels below the relevant realized properties. Because the lower neurobiological levels displaying such individual variation supply the realizers for the psychological properties in question, and because we have found with our type (i) examples that in neurobiology individual variation favors multiple over univocal realization, such examples provide indirect support for the multiple realization of the relevant psychological properties. We can see that cases of type (i) strongly support the existence of multiple realization and that situations of type (ii), depending on their maturity, strongly or more weakly support multiple realization. Furthermore, we have now also seen that examples of type (iii) provide weaker support for multiple realization, within the context of our wider evidence that all higher level scientific properties are realized and our findings in cases of type (i) from neurobiology that individual variation at a level grounds multiple realization at that level.

Despite the differences in the strength of evidence the kinds of case supply, we have thus found that cases of types (i), (ii), and (iii) in neurobiology all provide support for the multiple realization of psychological properties at the relevant level. How one uses this evidence is a delicate issue. It should be obvious that potentially we have the grounds for a very blunt enumerative induction to the conclusion that *all* human psychological properties are multiple realized at *all* neurobiological levels. However, we should also be clear that such a blunt enumerative induction to such a strong conclusion is questionable, especially given the rough-and-ready nature of our sampling of empirical evidence and because as different areas become more mature we may well discover that *some* human psychological properties are univocally realized by the properties at *some* neurobiological levels. We therefore put this stronger conclusion to one side. A weaker conclusion, we contend, can be safely supported by such an induction and challenges the recent philosophical skepticism that there is *any* multiple realization in neurobiology. For given the evidence we have seen that cases of types (i)–(iii) provide for multiple realization we suggest an enumerative induction, or other argument, can be safely constructed to ground a very plausible case for MMR—that is, the claim that *many* human psychological properties are multiple realized at *many* neurobiological levels.

To summarize, we applied our more precise theoretical framework for scientific realization and multiple realization to a brief sampling of some of the evidence about individual variation in humans at the various levels of neuroscientific organization, from the biochemical to the entirety of the brain. We argued that our framework shows that the nature of our empirical evidence provides prima facie plausible reasons to believe that many human psychological properties are multiply realized at many neuroscientific levels. One might not think that such a conclusion is particular noteworthy or surprising given the nature of the empirical evidence so commonly found in neurobiology at all levels. But given the increasingly widespread contention of philosophers that there is *no* multiple realization in neurobiology, we hope our admittedly rough-and-ready defense of MMR is dialectically useful.

To put the point in Darwin's favored terminology: One can show, by a long catalog of facts, that parts whose properties must be called important for the realization of a psychological property often vary in the individuals of the same species. Consequently, we have evidence for multiple realization of many psychological properties, at many neurobiological levels, in different organisms of a single species. There presently look to be few levels of neuroscientific organization that are simple or uniform enough to provide for a univocal realization of many psychological properties. We thus have prima facie plausible empirical reasons to accept the truth of MMR.

3. MMR: Philosophical Objections and Wider Implications

As suggested in our introduction, the conclusions of the last section are not news to working scientists. For reasons that should now be clear, we contend that many neuroscientists find pervasive multiple realization to be a common and uncontentious feature of their subject matter (though obviously they do not use the phrase "multiple realization" to describe this phenomenon). However, because many philosophers deny the existence of multiple realization in neuroscience and argue that it is has radical or dangerous implications for scientific methodology, we want to conclude this chapter by considering some important philosophical objections to multiple realization. We hope to both further illuminate the nature and implications of MMR and also assess the substance of such concerns. We begin by considering older objections to multiple realization and work our way through more recent critiques.

3.1. Objection 1: The Evidence Used to Establish Multiple Realization Does Not Preclude Univocal Realization or Species-Specific Narrow Identities

This type of objection comes in two related flavors, based on a defense of either a species-specific univocal realization base for psychological properties or a so-called species-specific narrow identity between neural and psychological properties. Given the focus of the discussion on multiple realization, we structure our discussion around the former version of such an objection, though we finish by showing how our response also applies to the narrow identity version.

Crucially, such older objections were mounted in response to defenses of multiple realization, primarily some arguments of Hilary Putnam (1967), based around so-called philosophical thought experiments, such as imagining a silicon-based life form or robots, designed to show the possibility of multiple realization bases for psychological properties. However, in response, critics responded that they could just as easily imagine that psychological properties were uniquely realized by *some* lower level properties in a certain species.

This is apparently one of the points Jaegwon Kim is concerned to highlight when he observed that the existence of some diversity in lower level properties does not automatically preclude a univocal realization of higher level properties at some level:

> The fact that two brains are physico-chemically different does not entail that the two brains cannot be in the "same physico-chemical state."... To argue that the human brain and the canine brain cannot be in the same brain state because of their different physico-chemical structure is like arguing that there can be no microphysical state underlying temperature because all kinds of objects with extremely diverse microphysical compositions can have the same temperature; or that water-solubility cannot have a microstructural "correlate" because both salt and sugar which differ a great deal from each other in atomic composition are soluble in water. If the human brain and the reptilian brain can be in the same "temperature state," why can they not be in the same "brain state," where this state is characterized in physico-chemical terms? (Kim, 1972, pp. 189–190)

Here we take two points to be at work. First, Kim presses the general point that if imagined possibilities guide us in such cases, the critics of multiple realization can also avail themselves of the possibilities we can conceive. Building on this general point, second, Kim presses that although we can imagine multiple realization, we can also further imagine that among this multiplicity at some neuroscientific level there is a *shared* neuroscientific base across these differences that allows for a univocal realization (and/or the base for a so-called narrow, species-specific identity) at this neurobiological level.

We agree with this much of Kim's view. Our earlier work highlighting the fact that all claims of multiple realization are indexed to particular realizer properties and levels supports Kim's conclusion. In earlier debates, defenders of multiple realization wished to use this phenomenon to undermine type-type identities between neural and psychological properties. However, to establish that there are no such identities, one needs to show that psychological properties are multiply realized by the properties *at all neuroscientific levels* and not just some. As Kim presses, although psychological properties might be multiply realized at neuroscientific level N the multiplicity of neuroscientific levels of organization still allows that at neuroscientific level (N − 1) there is a univocal realization for the diverse neuroscientific entities at level N and hence, by the transitivity of realization, for the relevant psychological properties. Exploiting this conclusion, Kim presses his first point about the methodology of imagined cases to suggest that because we can imagine such a situation, arguments from imagined cases of multiple realization actually fail to support the existence of the kind of multiple realization that would preclude any neural-psychological identities.

Looking more widely, as an overall strategy one can see the appeal of defending narrower claims about univocal realization or identities (see, e.g., Churchland, 1986, pp. 356–357). If we move from species-generic psychological properties to species-specific psychological properties, we are more likely, in a purely logical sense, to find univocal realizations. However, this logical point notwithstanding, we have now shown that our *empirical* evidence about individual variation within the human population plausibly undermines this route to univocal realization. Individual variations are variations among individuals of the same species, variations that are likely to be found even within much more narrowly circumscribed subpopulations of any species. The evidence for individual variations in neurophysiological and biochemical properties that we have used to support the MMR of psychological properties thus consequently provides prima facie plausible reasons to reject univocal realizations or species-specific narrow identities, even within organisms of a species.

The points that Kim makes about what we may or may not be able to imagine apparently does little to undermine the kind of argument from empirical evidence we have presented here. We happily admit that it is an open epistemic possibility that the MMR hypothesis may be undermined by future scientific discoveries, for like all claims supported on scientific grounds, we take this hypothesis to be empirically defeasible. In fairness, we should also emphasize that Kim's objection was originally directed against the very different, conceivability style defense of multiple realization presented by Putnam and not the type of argument we have built around actual empirical evidence. However, other defenses of univocal realization, both within organisms of certain species and across different species, have been defended by a variety of writers over the years (see, e.g., Bechtel and Mundale, 1999; Bickle, 2003; Braddon-Mitchell and Jackson, 1996; Churchland, 1986). At least some of these writers make claims about the actual world, and we suggest that our present evidence undermines their claims for species-specific (let alone transspecies) univocal realizations or narrow identities between human psychological and neural properties.[25]

3.2. Objection 2: The Dimensioned Accounts of Realization and Multiple Realization Trivialize the Issues

A rather different kind of objection comes from recent philosophical debates over the proper understanding of realization, and hence multiple realization, in the sciences. This objection claims that because the Dimensioned view of realization leads us to recognize the empirical support for MMR and hence endorse this thesis, this trivializes the whole question of multiple realization and undermines the Dimensioned view of realization itself. For these accounts obviously lead to accepting that there is far more multiple realization in the world than many philosophers of mind intuitively expected, and, the objection concludes, given these counterintuitive results we should therefore should abandon the Dimensioned view of realization and a key part of our argument for MMR.[26]

In response, it is worth marking that we have offered our accounts of scientific composition generally, and realization relations in particular, as parts of a wider understanding of the compositional concepts used in the sciences, in particular as views of the concepts deployed in mechanistic explanations in the special sciences. We suggest that the success of such accounts should consequently be judged by how well they do in capturing the features of the concepts actually used in such scientific explanations, and we have defended our theoretical framework with this point clearly in mind. What if the resulting account does not accord with some philosopher's intuitions or prior expectations about the nature or implications of compositional concepts? As in so many other cases where the sciences have surprised philosophers, we do not see why such a conflict would pose a problem for the success of our theoretical framework—for our work would simply highlight how our pretheoretic intuitions clash once again with the findings of the sciences and should be revised accordingly.

Furthermore, we should also emphasize that we take it to be a thoroughly empirical matter both whether we find multiple realization in some area of the sciences, and, if there is any, how much multiple realization there is. There may well be areas of the sciences where the properties of this area, Y_1-Y_n, are rarely if ever multiply realized by the properties, X_1-X_n, of the relevant lower level science. In such cases, the evidence, largely in the shape of the nature of the well-confirmed mechanistic explanations offered in these areas, will determine what one is justified in saying about these issues. What if such an examination of the relevant mechanistic explanations justified us in thinking that Y_1-Y_n are multiply realized, or even *pervasively* or *massively* multiply realized, by the properties X_1-X_n of the lower level science, and this was in conflict with some philosopher's prior expectations about the extent of multiple realization in this area of the sciences? Once again, we simply do not see why this would pose a problem, for it seems to be one more example in which the sciences have corrected a mistaken belief about the structure of the natural world.

Given these points, and our foregoing accounts of scientific realization, as well as our survey of the empirical evidence for individual variation at all neuroscientific levels, we suggest that the trivialization worry fails to pose a substantive difficulty for our argument for MMR.

3.3. Objection 3: The Present Immaturity of the Psychological Sciences Means That We Are Unable to Usefully Assess Whether Multiple Realization Exists

This objection begins from the present immaturity of many areas of the psychological sciences where it is still a legitimate question which kind of psychological entity figures in successful explanations. What higher level psychological properties are supposed to be the same in the face of all the lower level biological, chemical, and physical diversity? Are the properties supposed to include both cognitive and qualitative properties? Are they supposed to be those borrowed from folk psychology or those legitimated by scientific psychology? Are the psychological properties that form the basis of such a scientific psychology likely to be local, embedded properties or so-called extended properties? And so on. Given all these open questions, proceeds the objection, we cannot be sure whether psychological properties are indeed multiply realized, because we lack a well-confirmed account of the nature of such properties to begin with.

Our simplest response here is that almost however one answers these questions about the relevant psychological properties, one still arrives at the multiple realization of the posited psychological properties. If individual variation is a pervasive feature of nervous systems at virtually all levels, then many legitimate kinds of psychological property will turn out to be multiply realized at many neuroscientific levels. If, say, a putative property of suffering a particular kind of pain is realized in certain kinds of neuronal activities, and those neurons or their activities display individual variation in the ways in which they still each give rise to one and the same kind of pain, then that pain will be multiply realized. Similarly, mutatis mutandis for a putative property of believing that 2 + 2 = 4. The qualification "almost" is meant to mark that our claim is obviously empirically defeasible once more, thus there could be developments in the psychological sciences or neurosciences that would establish univocal realizations. However, our point is that given our present evidence such eventualities appear unlikely.[27]

3.4. Objection 4: The Worry about "Grains"—Arguments from Multiple Realization Only Succeed by Typing Neural and Psychological Entities Using Different Grains of Description

Bill Bechtel and Jennifer Mundale provide arguments against the existence of multiple realization, the most important of which we examine shortly. Having argued that psychological properties are not multiply realized, Bechtel and Mundale then take on the further burden of explaining why so many writers have mistakenly thought they were. They tell us:

> one diagnosis of what has made the multiple realizability claim as plausible
> as it has been is that researchers have employed different grains of analysis in
> identifying psychological states and brain states, using a coarse grain to identify
> psychological states and a fine grain to differentiate brain states. Having invoked
> different grains, it is relatively easy to make a case for multiple realization. But if
> the grain size is kept constant, then the claim that psychological states are in fact
> multiply realized looks far less plausible. One can adopt either a coarse or a fine
> grain, but as long as one uses a comparable grain on both the brain and mind
> side, the mapping between them will be correspondingly systematic. (1999, p. 202)

The diagnosis Bechtel and Mundale offer is that recent defenders of multiple realization have been careless with their use of descriptions of the relevant cases from the neurosciences and hence been led astray.

We can begin to appreciate the basis of their diagnosis by noting that for any state of affairs there are obviously a range of descriptions that all truly hold of it. For example, we always have descriptions truly applying more general predicates as well as other descriptions truly applying more specific predicates. Determinable and determinate predicates present one obvious case among many others: As we saw in section 1, it is true, for instance, that both "the cone has the property of releasing a neurotransmitter in response to light" and also that "the cone has the property of

releasing a neurotransmitter in response to light in the neighborhood of 530 nm."
Because it will be important shortly, we also note that there is a very strong prima
facie case, primarily based on considerations of ontological parsimony, that rather
than these true sentences each picking out distinct properties, that is, the property
of releasing a neurotransmitter in response to light *and* the property of releasing
a neurotransmitter in response to light in the neighborhood of 530 nm, we should
take both of these descriptions to be about the same property, in the property of
releasing a neurotransmitter in response to light in the neighborhood of 530 nm.
Some care needs to be used in discerning which of the true descriptions associated
with our successful scientific explanations provide the most veracious guide to the
relevant entities.

Bechtel and Mundale suggest that proponents of multiple realization may have
been less than careful in addressing these kinds of issues in the scientific cases they
use to support their claims. Defenders of multiple realization, these authors propose, may have gotten confused by using more specific descriptions with the lower
level properties that are realizers but more general descriptions when describing
the psychological properties they realize. The resulting diagnosis is thus that the
appearance of homogeneity at the psychological level, in combination with heterogeneity at the level of the realizers, is merely an artifact of choosing different grains
of description to apply to the properties at these levels, rather than an actual feature
of the properties illuminated by our scientific explanations.

Against the background of Bechtel and Mundale's arguments against multiple
realization, the grains diagnosis obviously has an important dialectical role. However, we must be careful to note that Bechtel and Mundale do not themselves use the
grains point itself to argue against multiple realization, though such an argument is
increasingly offered in conversation. The reader will already have appreciated that
our response to the last criticism, underpinned by our earlier work, provides the
basis of a blunt reaction to use of the grains point as an independent objection to
multiple realization. Current neuroscience strongly suggests that at almost every
level of organization the nervous systems of individuals in any significantly large
population will display individual variation and hence we will have heterogeneity
among the component entities that compose the same higher level entities. To see
how the evidence we have laid out grounds such a response in detail, let us consider one body of findings outlined earlier, in the recent evidence about changes in
dendritic spine structure within the same individual over time—though we should
emphasize that similar problems arise with a wide range of different findings as we
already illustrated in section 1 for the cone's properties.

In such cases, it is plausible that the relevant lower level realizer properties do
indeed change, because these changes are tracked in the innovative experimental
methodology. The proponent of such a grains critique might nonetheless respond
that the relevant realizers across time are always instances of some common, general property, for example, the property of being a property of a dendritic spine.
However, as the point about ontological parsimony makes plausible, this suggestion should be rejected on general grounds. For it would lead us to posit *two* sets of

properties, the specific properties of dendritic spines outlined and also some further general property, such as the property of being a property of a dendritic spine or the like. There are obvious reasons from ontological parsimony to deny that there are such general properties, for instead we may simply assume there are two sets of specific and general predicates we may use to refer to the property referred to by the specific predicate.

Though we appear to have good reason to posit heterogeneity among the realizers, perhaps the proponent of such a grains critique may have better luck denying the needed homogeneity with the higher level property instances. Once again, however, our empirical evidence poses a problem for any such claim, because the cases at hand occur within the same individual who often appears to persist in having an instance of some specific psychological property. Thus unlike cases involving organisms of different species or victims of trauma, where one may raise real concerns about sameness of psychological property, there is far less scope for arguing that the psychological property must change as its realizers change. Absent some background theoretical reason for the assumption that realized property instances with differing realizers must be themselves instances of distinct properties, it thus appears that the nature of our empirical evidence in this kind of example supports the same psychological property being realized in the individual by different realizers over time.

Our brief examination of one body of empirical evidence highlights how the nature of such findings often frustrates the easy use of concerns about grains of descriptions as an independent argument against the existence of multiple realization. However, as we emphasized, Bechtel and Mundale only use the grains point *after* presenting their arguments against multiple realization, so let us finally turn to the most important of these criticisms.

3.5. Objection 5: The Existence of Multiple Realization Would Entail the Methodological Isolation of Psychology

This final objection has recently become quite influential (see Bechtel and Mundale, 1999, and Shapiro, 2004, among others). Such objections start by assuming that multiple realization entails that there is no intertheoretic constraint between the sciences studying realizer and realized properties. But it is then plausibly shown, using real examples, that neuroscience and psychology do intertheoretically constrain each other. Thus it is concluded that multiple realization does not exist for neural and psychological properties.

Elsewhere we dub this the methodological argument against multiple realization and critically examine it at length (Aizawa and Gillett, "Multiple realization and methodology in neuroscience and psychology," unpublished working paper). Of all the recent objections to multiple realization, we suspect this has been the most persuasive, not least because it links so seamlessly with the heated philosophical discussions of methodology and funding priorities for neuroscience and psychology. However, we believe that our earlier work quickly shows that the key premise of such objections is mistaken—it is simply false that multiple realization entails that there is no intertheoretic constraint between the sciences studying realizer and realized properties. In fact, the reverse is true, as our earlier remarks about the methodological implications of the transitivity of scientific realization suggested.

As we have seen from our examination of concrete scientific cases, certain properties are realizers of other properties *only if* the powers of these properties together noncausally determine the powers of the realized property instance. There are other important features of realization relations, but given only the latter aspect, we can see that there are very clear and tight constraints on which types of property are such that their instances can realize some other instance together. As a result of this ontological point, there are strong reasons to expect that under certain circumstances (such as having sufficiently well-confirmed theories), the nature of realization relations will ground intertheoretic constraints between the disciplines studying realizer and realized properties.

For example, if one has a very well-confirmed theory of the nature of some realized property, that is, an account of its individuating powers, then this theory can be used top-down to guide and even constrain research about the realizers of this property given other information about them. These realizers must result in the known powers of the realized property, so one can exclude certain hypotheses about the realizers or prioritize others, depending on whether these hypotheses make claims about the realizers' powers that together allow them to noncausally result in the powers of the realized property. In the reverse direction, working bottom-up, if one has a well-confirmed account of the nature of the realizer properties of some realized property, this constrains theories of the realized property in various ways. For instance, precise knowledge of the realizers' powers can exclude or prioritize certain hypotheses about the individuating powers of the realized property. Theories of the realized property's nature are in part plausible to the degree to which we can see that the powers the hypothesis accords to the realized property are such that they can noncausally result from the powers attributed to the realizers by our well-confirmed account of the latter.

Such conclusions are startling to many philosophers. Nonetheless, these abstract points ground a persuasive case that under certain conditions, because the properties involved in realization relations ontologically determine each other there will consequently be a range of obvious intertheoretic constraints between the disciplines studying realizer and realized properties. Because cases of multiple realization all involve realization relations, the obvious conclusion is that multiple realization, under the appropriate conditions (such as having suitably confirmed theories, etc.), actually results in the disciplines studying realizer and realized properties intertheoretically constraining each other. Given this point, rather than undermining the existence of multiple realization, all the evidence for intertheoretic constraint between neuroscience and psychology looks very different—such evidence is compatible with or even further supports the existence of multiple realization!

We can thus see that the methodological argument against multiple realization is ultimately unsound. Perhaps more important, we can take the sting out of recent concerns about the implications of multiple realization. For multiple realization, as a species of realization, simply does not entail, if it exists, that psychology will be methodologically isolated. In fact, the reverse is true. The existence of multiple realization increases the likelihood that one of the most fruitful approaches to research is a coevolutionary research strategy, where neurobiology and psychology each constrain each other in a mutually beneficial dance of fit and adjustment. We can therefore see that mistaken assumptions about the methodological implications of multiple realization have led to ungrounded fears about the impact of multiple realization and have apparently blinded many philosophers to what we have suggested is the wealth of evidence for MMR.

4. CONCLUSION

To finish, consider this passage, in which William Wimsatt bemoans the approach that has recently characterized specific areas of philosophy of science and wonders whether we can do better as philosophers. He states:

> We show our own disciplinary biases and force them on others: the various "philosophies of X" often seem to be more about arguments internal to philosophy than "of" anything....
>
> *Can we still be recognizably philosophical while letting the subjects of "philosophies of" shine through much more clearly and inspire new philosophies, rather than merely exporting the same old "philosophical" disputes to these new territories?* (Wimsatt, 2007, p.7; emphasis in original)

Though the focus of Wimsatt's remarks is slightly different than our own, we hope our work not only illuminates some of Wimsatt's concerns but also provides one positive answer to his important question.

We began the chapter by noting that researchers in the philosophy of psychology, and those in the philosophy of neuroscience, each have very different views about the existence of multiple realization and its methodological implications, as well as endorsing differing positions about connected issues such as the possibility of reduction. However, just as Wimsatt suggests, we have found that in this case the clashing positions in these two "philosophies of" appear to be philosophical artifacts, rather than being underpinned by the relevant areas of science. We have shown that neither the position in philosophy of neuroscience that there is no multiple realization nor the view in philosophy of psychology that multiple realization grounds the strong methodological autonomy of psychology is correct.

As we have seen, driven by the empirical findings they routinely confront, working neuroscientists endorse the existence of a range of neurobiological levels and the variation of individuals at all of these levels. By finally applying a more precise framework for realization and multiple realization to the empirical evidence that underpins the latter commitments of scientists, we have shown that many psychological properties of humans are plausibly multiply realized by properties at many neuro-biological levels. In addition, however, we have also noted that such multiple realization produces intertheoretic constraint, rather than methodological autonomy, between the sciences that study realizer and realized properties—including psychology and the swath of disciplines that study neurobiological levels. Our work thus illuminates one important example where Wimsatt is correct in chiding researchers in "philosophies of," for we have shown that philosophers of neuroscience and philosophers of psychology have defended positions that fail to reflect either the nature of the disciplines they study or the commitments of the workers in these areas.

In addition, we hope that our substantive work here has been recognizably *philosophical* and provides one answer to Wimsatt's important question about how we may still pursue philosophy while being guided by scientific findings and commitments. Providing an abstract framework for scientific composition, as well as schemata for realization and multiple realization in the sciences, is a recognizably philosophical project—though clearly informed and guided by the sciences themselves—and one we have seen can produce substantive philosophical conclusions. We suggest that philosophers of science generally can profit by pursuing similar projects in what has come to be called the metaphysics of science: the careful, abstract investigation of ontological issues as they arise *within* the sciences and their findings, models, explanations, and so on. Our conclusion is therefore that even philosophers of science engaged in "philosophies of" this or that science may benefit by adding the tools of the metaphysics of science to their methodological armory.

Acknowledgments

Thanks to Marica Bernstein for comments on an earlier draft of this chapter.

NOTES

1. There are, of course, a number of stronger but related versions of this hypothesis. For example, one can change the two "many" quantifiers to "most" or "all" and not limit the hypothesis merely to human psychological processes. For the space of the present discussion, however, we defend only this weaker hypothesis. Furthermore, as we see later, properties usually come along in packages with distinctive powers, individuals, and processes. Consequently, as well as the multiple realization of properties, we also endorse the multiple constitution and multiple implementation of psychological individuals and processes in humans. Once again, however, we leave that claim to one side here. Finally, we also note that we defend multiple realization, constitution, and implementation for the psychological properties, individuals, and processes found in most terrestrial species, but again we limit our focus to humans here.

2. Exactly which researchers hold which views, and hence narratives, is a very contentious issue in this area, for reasons that will become apparent. However, though we accept that some philosophers of psychology have defended strong methodological autonomy for psychology, and hence endorse this narrative, we argue in Aizawa and Gillett ("Multiple realization and methodology in neuroscience and psychology," unpublished working paper) that this was plausibly not the position of Fodor (1968), or other writers defending the received view of special sciences such as William Wimsatt or Philip Kitcher.

3. Historically speaking, philosophers of mind have more often discussed multiple realizability, rather than multiple realization. Here we limit our attention to multiple realization, because it allows us to sidestep issues about the proper modality, it simplifies and abbreviates further discussion, and once multiple realization is established, the multiple realizability follows rather easily.

4. For a more extensive exposition of the nature of these compositional concepts, see Gillett ("Making sense of levels in the sciences: Composing powers, properties, parts, and processes," unpublished working paper).

5. It is worthwhile marking some of the distinct notions of realization current in recent philosophical discussions and that the parties to the present debate only defend variants of one of these concepts. (See Endicott, 2005, for a survey of some of main varieties of the concept of realization.) Some writers fail to appreciate the variety of concepts of realization, and hence confuse them, so it is worth distinguishing three kinds of notion of realization.

First, there is a group of semantic notions that we term *Linguistic*, or L-realization and that hold between entities in the world and some set of sentences. Famously, for example, the work of David Lewis on topic-neutral Ramseyfication and theoretical terms uses a notion of L-realization. Basically, on Lewis's view of realization it holds between entities in the world and the set of Ramseyfied sentences putatively defining some theoretical term F—crudely put, an entity X L-realizes F when the entity X satisfies the relevant Ramsey sentences for F.

Second, there is a kind of computational or mathematical relation commonly referred to as realization and used in both the sciences and philosophy, which we call *Abstract* or A-realization. Very crudely, X is taken to A-realize Y if the elements of X map onto or are isomorphic with the elements of Y. This notion of realization is commonly utilized with formal models and hence with work using such models, for example in computational accounts of cognitive processes. Note that here the relata of such realization relations are largely unconstrained because A-realization simply holds in virtue of a mathematical mapping, or isomorphism, which can obviously hold between all manner of entities.

Finally, the third kind of notion of realization is what we may call *Causal-Mechanist* or M-realization. The latter contrasts with L- and A-realization by having as relata causally individuated entities in the world, often (though not exclusively) property instances. M-realization has been the focus of many writers, and in particular philosophers of science have been especially interested in such relations, which they take to be posited in so-called mechanistic explanations in a range of the special sciences. In our discussion, for obvious reasons, we focus exclusively on a notion of M-realization when we discuss realization.

6. There are three types of cone photopigments. Sometimes they are classified as blue, green, and red and sometimes they are classified as short wavelength, middle wavelength, or long wavelength (S, M, and L), respectively.

7. In actual neuroscience, it is common to decompose a cone photopigment molecule into a protein component and a nonprotein chromophore. The protein component might then be decomposed into distinct amino acids. We skip these intermediate levels between

the entire cone photopigment molecule and the individual atoms primarily because of the greater familiarity of atomic-molecular relations and to simplify the exposition.

8. This thumbnail account is defended in Gillett (2002, 2003). A full account of the Dimensioned view of realization, as a part of integrated view of the compositional relations posited in the sciences between packages of powers, properties, individuals and mechanisms, is offered in Gillett ("Making sense of levels in the sciences," unpublished working paper).

9. Scientific purists will no doubt observe the simplification we have been working with in referring to the property of being maximally sensitive light of 530 nm. Distinct experimental methods yield slightly different values for maximal sensitivity. Moreover, these methods include one or another measure of error. What remains through this simplification is that current science takes the maximum absorption spectra of distinct amino acid sequences to be the same up to experimental error.

10. To avoid confusion, we reiterate what might seem obvious: Our theory schema is intended to follow the usual convention and illustrate how properties are multiply realized—for if two instances of the same property are differently realized at the same level, then the property is *multiply* realized. However, as we see in examples to follow, an instance of a higher level property may itself also be multiply realized over time by distinct lower level realizers. In such cases we thus have both a higher level property and also a single instance of this property that are multiply realized. However, for simplicity, we focus primarily on properties as the entities that are multiply realized.

11. Some readers may be concerned that adding (iv) leaves us with a dangerously imprecise notion in that of a level of entities. However, as William Wimsatt and others have argued (Wimsatt, 1976, 1994), there is a reasonably clear scientific notion of a level of entities, under some condition, as entities that do or can participate in the same causal mechanisms under those conditions (or which participate in processes that together implement other processes). This scientific concept of a level can underwrite (iv), and elsewhere one of us has also outlined a precise definition of this notion of a level (Gillett, "Making sense of levels in the sciences," unpublished working paper).

12. As we mentioned, distinct sets of atoms with distinct properties can give rise to distinct molecules with instances of the same property of absorbing a certain spectrum.

13. The methodological implications of realization, and other compositional relations in the sciences, are also explored in more detail in Aizawa and Gillett ("Multiple realization and methodology in neuroscience and psychology," unpublished working paper).

14. See Sharpe et al. (1990).

15. The astute reader will no doubt again anticipate the concerns that arise about these examples with regard to which grains of description, specific or general, one should take to pick out the actual properties. We happily agree that these are substantive issues, and interesting cases can be presented for a number of interpretations. However, given the range of lower level individual variation, in the same manner that we highlighted in the molecular-to-cellular example, we suggest that it is highly plausible that in the final analysis at least *some* of these findings will again ultimately support multiple realization in the cell-to-tissue example.

16. This is one of the central contentions of Aizawa (2007).

17. As suggested previously in note 7, in actual practice it is common enough for neuroscientists to relate amino acid sequences and their properties/relations and powers, on the one hand, to proteins and their properties/relations and powers, on the other, rather than relating atoms, atomic-level properties/relations, and atomic-level powers to proteins, protein-level properties/relations, and protein-level powers. However, this practice changes nothing philosophically relevant to our concerns.

18. For simplicity, we set aside properties that other components of a dendritic spine contribute to the shape of the spine.

19. Of course, we are setting aside mention of the contributions of other properties of the subcellular components of the neuron. This is merely for expository simplicity.

20. See, for example, Zuo, Lin, Chang, and Gan (2005) and Majewska, Newton, and Sur (2006).

21. Perhaps glial cells should be included as part of the realizer of a cortical column, but merely for the sake of simplicity of exposition we set the consideration aside. Nothing of philosophical import appears to turn on it.

22. Van Essen, Newsome, and Maunsell (1984) found almost as much variation in the surface area of V1 in the macaque. These variations appear to be independent of body weight. In a study with only six macaques, Horton and Hocking (1996) found much less variability.

23. Of course, the optic tract and lateral geniculate nucleus are not cortical structures.

24. Here we again set aside complications regarding the possible role of glial cells.

25. Aizawa (2007) further defends the claim that essentially all psychological properties are multiply realized in virtue of the variations in amino acid sequences that are components of all nerve cells, and indeed all major tissues of the body. That paper presupposes something like the Dimensioned view of realization and theory of multiple realization advanced here.

26. A number of philosophers have pressed concerns of this kind in conversation and talks.

27. As a side note, it is worth examining a related worry analytic philosophers often raise: Why doesn't the logical possibility of individuating psychological properties just as finely as their putative realizers immediately falsify our claim? Once again, we note that we take successful scientific explanations to be our guide to the entities that exist, whether powers, properties, individuals, or processes, and whether such entities should be taken to be psychological. Thus, although individuating psychological properties so finely might be thought to be possible, this would still be a long way from showing properties individuated in such a manner underlie successful scientific explanations. Thus, by itself, the possibility does not pose a problem for our claim.

REFERENCES

Aizawa, K. (2007). The biochemistry of memory consolidation: A model system for the philosophy of mind. *Synthese* 155: 65–98.

Aizawa, K., and Gillett, C. (unpublished working paper). Multiple realization and methodology in neuroscience and psychology.

Allen, J. S., Damasio, H., and Grabowski, T. J. (2002). Normal neuroanatomical variation in the human brain: An MRI-volumetric study. *American Journal of Physical Anthropology* 118: 341–358.

Andrews, T., Halpern, S., and Purves, D. (1997). Correlated size variations in human visual cortex, lateral geniculate nucleus, and optic tract. *Journal of Neuroscience* 17: 2859–2868.

Bechtel, W., and Mundale, J. (1999). Revisiting multiple realization. *Philosophy of Science* 66: 175–205.

Bickle, J. (2003). *Philosophy and Neuroscience: A Ruthlessly Reductive Account*. Boston: Kluwer.

Blake, R., and Sekuler, R. (2002). *Perception*, 4th ed. Boston: McGraw-Hill.[a]

Braddon-Mitchell, D., and Jackson, F. (1996). *Philosophy of Mind and Cognition: An Introduction*. Oxford: Blackwell.

Brodmann, K. (1909). *Vergleichende Lokalisationslehre der Grosshirnrinde in ihren Principien, dargestellt auf grund des Zellenbaues*. Leipzig: Johann Ambrosius Barth Verlag. 2nd ed., 1925. English translation by Laurence J. Garey, *Brodmann's 'Localisation in the Cerebral Cortex'* (Smith-Gordon, 1994); new impression, Imperial College Press, 1999.

Churchland, P. S. (1986) *Neurophilosophy: Towards a Unified Science of the Mind/Brain*. Cambridge, Mass.: MIT Press.

Darwin, C. (1964). *On the Origin of Species. A Facsimile of the first edition*. Cambridge, Mass.: Harvard University Press.

Dougherty, R., Koch, V., Brewer, A., Fischer, B., Modersitzki, J., and Wandell, B. (2003). Visual field representations and locations of visual areas V1/2/3 in human visual cortex. *Journal of Vision* 3: 586–598.

Endicott, R. (2005). Multiple realizability. In *The Encyclopedia of Philosophy*, 2nd ed. New York: Macmillan.

Fodor, J. (1968). *Psychological Explanation*. New York: Random House.

Gillett, C. (2002). The dimensions of realization: A critique of the standard view. *Analysis* 62: 316–323.

Gillett, C. (2003). The metaphysics of realization, multiple realizability and the special sciences. *Journal of Philosophy* 100: 591–603.

Horton, J., and Hocking, D. (1996). Intrinsic variability of ocular dominance column periodicity in normal macaque monkeys. *Journal of Neuroscience* 15: 7228–7339.

Kaschube, M., Wolf, F., Geisel, T., and Löwel, S. (2002). Genetic influence on quantitative features of neocortical architecture. *Journal of Neuroscience* 22: 7206–7217.

Kaschube, M., Wolf, F., Puhlman, M., Rathjen, S., Schmidt, K., Geisel, T., et al. (2003). The pattern of ocular dominance columns in cat primary visual cortex: Intra- and interindividual variability of column spacing and its dependence on genetic background. *European Journal of Neuroscience* 18: 3251–3266.

Kim, J. (1972). Phenomenal properties, psychological laws, and identity theory. *Monist* 56: 177–192.

Majewska, A. K., Newton, J. R., and Sur, M. (2006). Remodeling of synaptic structure in sensory cortical areas in vivo. *Journal of Neuroscience* 26: 3021–3029.

McKinney, R. A. (2005). Physiological roles of spine motility: Development, plasticity, and disorders. *Biochemical Society Transactions* 33: 1299–1302.

Merbs, S., and Nathans, J. (1993). Absorption spectra of the hybrid pigments responsible for anomalous color vision. *Science* 258: 464–466.[b]

Nagel, E. (1961). *The Structure of Science*. New York: Harcourt, Brace, and World.

Nathans, J., Thomas, D., and Hogness, D. S. (1986). Molecular genetics of human color vision: The genes encoding blue, green, and red pigments. *Science* 232: 193–202.

Neitz, M., and Neitz, J. (1995). Numbers and ratios of visual pigment genes for normal red-green color vision. *Science* 267: 1013–1016.

Penfield, W., and Boldrey, E. (1937). Somatic, motor and sensory representation in the cerebral cortex of man as studied by electrical stimulation. *Brain* 60: 389–443.

Peters, M., Jänke, L., Staiger, J. F., Schlaug, G., Huang, Y., and Steinmetz, H. (1998). Unsolved problems in comparing brain sizes in *Homo sapiens*. *Brain and Cognition* 37: 254–285.

Putnam, H. (1967). Psychological predicates. In W. H. Capitan and D. D. Merrill (Eds.), *Art, Mind, and Religion*. Pittsburgh: University of Pittsburgh Press, 37–48.

Rademacher, J., Morosan, P., Schormann, T., Schleicher, A., Werner, C., Freund, H.-J., et al. (2001). Probabilistic mapping and volume measurement of human primary auditory cortex. *NeuroImage* 13: 669–683.

Shapiro, L. (2004). *The Mind Incarnate*. Cambridge, Mass.: MIT Press.

Sharpe, L. T., Stockman, A., Jägle, H., and Nathans, J. (1999). Opsin genes, cone photopigments, color vision, and color blindness. In K. R. Gegenfurtner and L. T. Sharpe (Eds.), *Color Vision: From Genes to Perception*. Cambridge: Cambridge University Press.

Shoemaker, S. (1980). Causality and properties. In P. van Inwagen (Ed.), *Time and Cause*. Dordrecht: Reidel.

Sorra, K., and Harris, K. (2000). Overview on the structure, composition, function, development, and plasticity of hippocampal dendritic spines. *Hippocampus* 10: 501–511.[c]

Stensaas, S. S., Eddington, D. K., and Dobelle, W. H. (1974). The topography and variability of the primary visual cortex in man. *Journal of Neurosurgery* 40: 747–755.

Van Essen, D., Newsome, W., and Maunsell, J. (1984). The visual field representation in striate cortex of the macaque monkey: Asymmetries, anisotropies and individual variability. *Vision Research* 24: 429–448.

Wässle, H. (2004). Parallel processing in the mammalian retina. *Nature Reviews Neuroscience* 5: 1–11.[d]

Wimsatt, W. (1976). Reductionism, levels of organization and the mind-body problem. In G. Globus, I. Savodnik, and G. Maxwell (Eds.), *Consciousness and the Brain*. New York: Plenum, 199–267.

Wimsatt, W. (1994). The ontology of complex systems: Levels of organization, perspectives and causal thickets. *Canadian Journal of Philosophy*, supplement 20: 207–274.

Wimsatt, W. (2007). *Re-Engineering Philosophy for Limited Beings*. Cambridge, Mass.: Harvard University Press.

Woolsey, C., Erickson, T., and Gilson, W. (1979). Localization in somatic sensory and motor areas of human cerebral cortex as determined by direct recording of evoked potentials and electrical stimulation. *Journal of Neurosurgery* 51: 476–506.

Zuo, Y., Lin, A., Chang, P., and Gan, W. (2005). Development of long-term dendritic spine stability in diverse regions of cerebral cortex. *Neuron* 46: 181–189.

CHAPTER 23

NEURO-EUDAIMONICS OR BUDDHISTS LEAD NEUROSCIENTISTS TO THE SEAT OF HAPPINESS

OWEN FLANAGAN

Neuro-Eudaimonics

Eudaimonics is naturalistic inquiry into the constituents and causes of happiness, which Aristotle wisely said is what everybody wants more than anything else (Flanagan, 2007). Most people think Aristotle was right that the one (perhaps only) universal truth about *Homo sapiens* is that at every time and in every place people wish to be happy, to flourish, to achieve eudaimonia. So it would be good to know what it is, where it is kept, and how to get some of it. Neuro-eudaimonics, if there is or can be such a thing, claims that neuroscience can advance our understanding of the constituents and causes of happiness. Here I examine what some early forays into neuro-eudaimonics have actually delivered and discuss the promise and prospects of this research program. Eudaimonics is promising, but the neuroscientific contribution to the study of the nature, causes, and constituents is easily overrated (Flanagan, 2007).

"The Colour of Happiness" was the title of an article I wrote for *New Scientist* in May 2003 that reported on two preliminary studies of "positive affect" in (as revealed in the brain of) exactly one meditating monk (Flanagan, 2003b). To my chagrin, news agencies such as Reuters, the BBC, and Canadian and Australian Public Radio were quick to sum up the message of my essay with hyperbole of this sort: "Buddhists Lead Scientists to 'Seat of Happiness'" (a Japanese website put it this way which I found especially compelling:

性格・幸福感・感情：昔の記事 書庫館（進化研究と社会>

I did (too) many media interviews in a futile attempt to quell or at least rein in the ridiculous enthusiasm for the idea that the brains of Buddhists were extremely frisky in the happiness department, and thus the owners of these brains were unusually happy people, perhaps the happiest of all, and that, in addition, meditation (whatever that is) was responsible for the very happy brains inside the very happy people. I was asked when I had discovered that Buddhists were the happiest people who ever lived and where exactly in the brain the happiness spot was. *Dharma Life* magazine, in an amusing headline of its own, called the scientists, Richie Davidson and Paul Ekman, who performed the early studies on the meditating monk, "Joy Detectives."

I had joked for years about the way, for example, the *New York Times* Tuesday Science Section reported neuroscientific discoveries. Like most of my neurophilosopher friends, I thought most of the hyperbolic hoopla foolish but harmless. But this Buddhism stuff was not funny. First, it was happening to me. Second, the situation felt Orwellian and thus vaguely dangerous. Most Buddhists I know are sweet and dear, but I sensed that many of the Buddhists I knew and respected were all too ready to buy into the hyperbole and sell their own Buddhist brand of snake oil claiming for it certification by neuroscience as *the* way to happiness and goodness. Being allergic to magic univocal spiritual solutions, I had to play skeptic.[1] Even if neuroscientists are generally responsible in reporting results (although it is worth noting that neuroimaging especially allows reports on very small *n*'s), the neuro-journalists are not. So a certain neuro-skepticism is warranted (see Harrington, 2008, for a compelling, suitably skeptical, history of mind–body medicine).[2]

What is the evidence for the claim that there is a connection between Buddhism and happiness? The claim that there is some such connection is very much (still) out there. The first point or observation is that there are several different claims that, to my eye, are being conflated:

1. There is a connection between being a Buddhist (what counts as being-a-Buddhist? what are the membership properties?) and being happy (which kind? how defined?).
2. There is a connection between meditating (which way, among the 84,000 types?) in a Buddhist way and feeling good (feeling good = being happy?).

3. There is a connection between being-in-Buddhist-frame-of-mind and being good (what is the connection between happiness and goodness?).
4. There is a connection between being a Buddhist and physical heath and well-being (what is the connection between health and happiness?).
5. There is a connection between being a Buddhist and possessing certain kinds of unusual autonomic nervous system control, such as being able to control the startle reflex (what is the connection between happiness and this sort of autonomic control?).
6. Experienced Buddhist practitioners are very good face readers (what is the connection between face reading and happiness?).
7. Experienced Buddhist meditators have lots of synchronized global brain activity (so did Timothy Leary and other acid trippers).

There are more, but 1–7 provide a sense of the distinct hypotheses being bandied about and conflated as if they express some well-founded scientific consensus that Buddhists are unusually happy.

Happiness and the Brain

At the time I wrote "The Colour of Happiness" article, the only completed brain study I discussed actually on the connection between Buddhism and happiness had an $n = 1$, that is, exactly one experimental subject had his brain scanned by an fMRI. This is not ordinarily considered a good sample size. However, this first exemplary individual, Matthieu Ricard, was an experienced Buddhist monk (born and bred in France) and his left prefrontal cortex (the area just behind the forehead), an area well established to be reliably correlated with positive emotion, lit up brightly (thus the editor's choice of "colour" in the title).[3] Indeed, the left side lit up brightly and more leftward than any individual tested in previous studies (approximately 175 subjects). However, none of these prior studies involved people meditating while the scanning was under way (in the monk's case, most meditation was on compassion and loving kindness). But as I have said, these scientific problems did not prevent various media sources from announcing that scientists had established that Buddhist meditation produces (a high degree of) happiness. I do not know whether the "joy detectives," who, unlike me, were actually doing the preliminary studies, cautioned the neuro-journalists or not. I guess not, because they are enthusiasts for the hypothesis that was receiving media confirmation, if not its empirical equivalent.

Fortunately (for science), prior to the study of the meditating monk, there had been a number of excellent studies on positive affect and the brain (Davidson, 2000; Davidson and Hugdahl, 2002; Davidson and Irwin, 1999; Davidson, Scherer, and Goldsmith, 2002), which the 14th Dalai Lama (using his given name, Tenzin Gyatso), alluded to in an op-ed piece for the *New York Times* (Gyatso, 2003a), I reported on in *New Scientist,* and Dan Goleman (2003b) wrote about in the *New York Times.* Davidson and colleagues' experiments revealed that when subjects are shown pleasant pictures (say, sunsets), scans (PET or fMRI) or skull measurements of activity (EEG) reveal increased left side activity in the prefrontal cortex. When subjects see unpleasant pictures (say, a human cadaver), activity moves rightward. Furthermore, people who report themselves generally to be happy, upbeat, and the like, show more stable left side activity than those who report feeling sad or depressed, in whom the right side of prefrontal cortex is more active.

Positive mood, we can say, has two faces. This makes a neurophenomenological approach possible. Subjectively, phenomenologically, or first-personally positive mood reveals itself in a way that an individual feels and about which he or she typically can report on (although subjects commonly report difficulty describing exactly what the positive state is like). Objectively, the subjective feeling state is reliably correlated with a high degree of leftward prefrontal activity (the neuro-part). Thus we can say that *if* a subject is experiencing happiness or, what is possibly different, is in a good mood, then left prefrontal cortex is or gets frisky, or bright, or even colorful depending on whether you use EEG, fMRI, or PET.

It is important to emphasize that the prefrontal cortices are involved in more than emotion, affect, and mood. The prefrontal lobes are relatively recently evolved structures (in ancestors of *Homo sapiens*) and have long been known to play a major role in foresight, planning, and self-control. The confirmation of the fact that prefrontal cortices are also crucially implicated in emotion, mood, and temperament is exciting because it lends some insight into where—one place where—a well-functioning mind coordinates cognition, mood, and emotion. How exactly the coordination is accomplished is something about which little is known at this time.[4]

Davidson found that in a normal population (of undergraduates) prefrontal lobe activity is distributed in a bell-shaped curve fashion. If the curve were entirely normal and assuming that the undergraduate population is representative, we would expect 67 percent of the population to show mixed left and right activity with roughly 16 percent showing predominantly left side activity and 16 percent showing predominantly right side activity. If the curve were normal, we might use alleged neurophenomenological background knowledge and say one-sixth of ordinary Americans are "very happy," two-thirds feel mixed or average ("okay," as we say), and one-sixth feel "on the low side." However, Davidson's bell curve was not quite normal. It bulged some toward the happy side. This is consistent with data that claim that 30 percent of Americans are very happy (= say so), 60 percent are okay, and 10 percent are "not too happy" (Flanagan, 2007, pp. 150–159).

Given these data, I take it that any finding to the effect that Buddhist practitioners are happier than most would be a statistical finding that significantly more than 30 percent would be in the first group. A representative sample of Buddhist practitioners with 40 percent in the first group would be statistically astounding. A somewhat lower percentage would still be impressive. No such data exist—not even data showing that Buddhists hit the average (American) population score of 30 percent.

Putting this important point about the hoopla given the evidence aside, we still might wish to ask this about the one meditating monk studied: Was the meditating monk who was "off the charts" the happiest subject ever tested? Saying "yes" is tempting, and many of my interviewers assumed that this was part of the message, as if being "leftmost" is like being the tallest. But this is crazy. At best, being leftward is correlated with being happy or with, what is different, good mood. There is no evidence that (x) $(y)(L)(H)$ if $Lx > Ly$ then $Hx > Hy$. Nothing that is known about brains and the ways subjective states are realized or subserved neurally would make the hypothesis that the meditating monk is the happiest person ever tested worth taking seriously.

Consider this sort of familiar example: Suppose two people think [that patch is red] in response to the exact same red patch stimulus. Assume that both are having the exact same thought, although it must be said even this assumption is controversial. We might after all experience red a bit differently, perception of red things might cause different associations, and so on. Bracket these worries. Assume that whatever else goes on when each of these two individuals think [that is a red patch], both think that much and each thinks the thought in the same way as far as that red patch goes. If so, there will be brain activation in each individual that is that thought or is the neural correlate of that thought. But no one expects two different brains to have exactly the same thought in a way that is subserved by perfectly identical neural activation. The consensus is that the exact same thought can be realized (indeed is likely to be realized) in different brains in somewhat different ways. We expect the same for phenomenologically identical or very similar emotional states. There is always a level of grain at which (or so most think) some nontrivially different set of neural conditions will, or at least can, realize or subserve mental states that are functionally or phenomenologically indistinguishable.

One upshot is this: For all we currently know, the subject who tests 25th or 35th from the leftmost point so far plotted might be, according to all the evidence taken together—phenomenological, behavioral, hormonal, neurochemical—the happiest person ever tested. Left side prefrontal activity may be a reliable measure of positive affect, but no respectable scientist has asserted, let alone confirmed, that among "lefties," the further left you are, the happier you are.

There are some other problems. First, the concepts of "positive mood" and "positive affect" and "happiness" are not the same concepts. Running them together is not permitted. Furthermore, none of these concepts are fine-grained enough, or sufficiently well operationalized by the scientists who use them, that we know what specific kind of positive mood or emotional state is (allegedly) attached to a lit-up area. (Seligman, 2002, is exceptional among mind scientists in trying to sort out the constituents and components of our ordinary conception of happiness.) A second problem is that there is little effort being expended to distinguish among the neural realizer(s) of happiness, and its *content* and *causes*. For all anyone knows at this point, a happy life (assuming we have a genuine case) whose causal source is family might light up the brain in the same way as a happy life whose source is virtue or even money. For all anyone knows, a state of happiness whose contentful character is a meditation on nothingness may light up the same way as the state of happiness whose contentful character involves solving quantum physical equations. On the other side, one might wonder why we should seriously expect phenomenological states as different as hedonistic happiness and Buddhist happiness to be realized the same way in the brain. Consider that many contemplatives, for example, Christian Trappist, Cistercian, and Carthusian contemplatives believe in and meditate on a personal deity. Personal faith and a relationship with God are almost certainly thought to be constitutive of the kind of happiness they seek. This difference in the content of their mental states—from Buddhists, for example—is one that ought to (it better) reveal itself when and if brain scans reach a point that they can deliver fine-grained understanding of different kinds of mental states, including happiness. Scientists can look for mental states that take a deity as their foci (mental content) without believing that there really are deities. But if thinking starts to go in this credible direction, then the fact that the happy hedonist and the happy Buddhist brains light up the same way might make us think that the lit-up stuff isn't really illuminating what we want to see more clearly.

Buddhist Happiness

These difficulties about the concepts being used and about content and causes suggest that anyone who aims to study the relations among a life form such as Buddhism and happiness ought to look carefully at the concept of happiness that the tradition claims to offer. Buddhism doesn't say much about happiness. It says a lot about suffering and its causes. But not suffering is not the same as being happy. You have a headache. You are suffering. I give you aspirin. Are you happy?[5]

Buddhism claims, first and foremost, to offer a solution, so far as one is possible, to what it claims is the main existential problem faced by all humans: how to minimize suffering. Happiness, not being possible, is not much, or at least not the main thing, on offer in classical Buddhism (at least not until one has lived uncountable lives at which point if happiness is conceived as reaching nirvana, one becomes happy by becoming nothing, nothing-at-all). However this situation has changed recently. The 14th Dalai Lama says repeatedly in recent writings that happiness is the sole universal aim of humans. He and several Western collaborators have been charting out approaches, which might help us overcome suffering—this is the aspirin part (Flanagan, 2000; Goleman, 2003a)—and then to help us find the way to "true happiness," as conceived in a Buddhist way, what I call happiness[buddha] (Dalai Lama, 1999; Dalai Lama and Cutler, 1998; Flanagan, 2006, 2007).

So we might wonder, given the hoopla over happy Buddhists, (1) what kind of happiness does Buddhism offer (happiness[buddha] I claim, but what is that?); and (2) is there any reason to think that Buddhists are happy in the same first-personal (phenomenological) way and neural way that Trappist monks or hedonists or University of Wisconsin undergraduates are happy? Or is it that many more Buddhists are happy in this presumably neurally shared way? But then again, given that Buddhists seek the kind of happiness Buddhism promises and not the kind that Trappist monks, hedonists, or Wisconsin undergraduates seek, it seems very odd to think that happiness across these traditions or life forms would show up "the same way" in brains.

Like every other moral tradition, Buddhism distinguishes between worthy pleasures and base ones, between things we ordinarily think bring happiness and things that really do bring happiness. Money doesn't bring happiness, at least not true happiness (although it might help some), but wisdom *and* virtue do. Buddhism is, at a most fundamental level, a practical philosophy that claims that wisdom and virtue are their own reward. Wisdom and virtue constitute liberation. By achieving wisdom and virtue, we overcome suffering and unsatisfactoriness and gain (maybe) happiness[buddha]. What is happiness[buddha]?

Here's a credible answer. A person who is happy[buddha] is conventionally moral, so he or she doesn't lie, steal, cheat, gossip, or work for nonpacifistic organizations (the noble eightfold path). In addition, he or she works to develop four virtues, compassion (wishing to alleviate suffering), loving kindness (wishing to bring happiness in its stead), sympathetic joy (joy about the successes of others), and equanimity. These four virtues are necessary for happiness[buddha], but they are not sufficient. Happiness[buddha] also requires wisdom where the wisdom consists of knowing such truths as that everything is impermanent and that I, being one of the things in the everything, am impermanent, too. This is wisdom. Taken together the four great virtues and a wise assessment of the nature of reality and oneself will bring happiness[buddha]. Will these virtues and this wisdom bring the same sort of happiness the hedonist seeks, or the same sort of happiness a Jewish mystic seeks or a liberal twenty-first-century American seeks? It would be odd to think that the answer is yes because each of these conceptions of happiness claims for itself very different causes and contents. It is logically possible that everyone in fact seeks the same kind of happiness, but it doesn't seem likely. If this is right, then there is a major but unnoticed conceptual problem facing the happiness researchers who seem to assume that what are multifarious conceptions of happiness with distinctive causes and constituents can be measured against each other by looking at or for a single type of brain activity.

What Does Happiness Have to Do with It?

Even if this problem of looking for a univocal marker for what could seem to be unitary (it's happiness we are talking about) phenomena but isn't can be solved, there are other matters about the interpretation of the research. Specifically, there is research that is interpreted by the "Buddenthusiasta" (some neuro-journalists but also some of the researchers) as reinforcing the happiness hypothesis but that doesn't.

Consider Paul Ekman's work. Before the meditating monk's brain was scanned in Davidson's lab in Wisconsin, he spent several days with Ekman in San Francisco. Ekman is the world's leading authority on the basic emotions (fear, anger, sadness, surprise, disgust, contempt, and happiness) and on the universal facial expressions that accompany them (Ekman, 2003; Ekman, Campos, Davidson, and De Waal, 2003; Flanagan, 2003a). With his longtime colleague and collaborator, Robert Levenson, who works across San Francisco Bay at the University of California, Berkeley, the two set to work at studying the effects of long-term Buddhist practice on evolutionarily basic emotional responses and on individual differences in ability to read emotions from faces. Thus, one study focused on the startle response, which is thought to be essentially a mental reflex (i.e., virtually automatic). The other looked at face reading.

When I tell people about this research, there is often a presumption that Buddhist practice is known to result in unusual abilities, such as the ability to control anger or read faces more sensitively than normal people. But this is not known. It is what Buddhism advertises about itself. It hasn't been tested systematically to this day, because Ekman and Levenson's experiments were only pilot studies and thus it could be (still might be) mere Buddhshit. I mention this because I myself was initially too naive in interpreting the results I revisit here, being caught up until recently (2007) in the hype (for a form of life I very much admire) and not always being careful enough to mark the paucity of evidence for the happiness hypothesis (Flanagan, 2000, 2002, 2003b, 2006). As I report on the Ekman and Levenson pilot studies, ask yourself this question: What does this research have to do with testing the connection between Buddhism and happiness? The right answer is that although the pilot studies were done on a small number ($n = 4$, as I recall) of Buddhist practitioners, what they test has *nothing* obvious to do with the happiness hypothesis.

First the startle results. The amgydala, twin almond-shaped organs, as well as adjacent structures in the forebrain beneath the cerebral cortex, are part of quick-triggering machinery for fear, anxiety, and surprise. I see a fierce, snarling wolf and—without any forethought—head for the hills in fear. Lightning strikes in my vicinity—I am scared and anxious and seek lower ground. The amygdala and associated structures are key components of this affective response system. It is likely (but not yet confirmed) that areas in these very old brain structures (fish have amygdala-like structures) are involved in other evolutionarily basic emotions such as anger and, more controversially, in certain pleasant feelings associated with good meals or good sex. Although the amygdalae lie beneath the cerebral cortex, they require cortical processing for activation. I need to see the bear (visual cortex) or hear the thunder (auditory cortex) before I feel frightened.

Much of what we know about the amygdala is due to path-breaking work by Joseph LeDoux (1996) at New York University, who instigated work throughout the world on these structures. We know, among other things, that a person, via the amygdala and thalamus, can be classically conditioned so that things that really aren't worth being scared of or anxious about can become fear- or anxiety-inducing. We also know that although the prefrontal cortices and amygdala interact, what the amygdala "thinks" and "feels" is extraordinarily hard to override simply by conscious rational thought.

Ekman found some confirmation in the pilot study for the hypothesis that experienced meditators don't get nearly as flustered, shocked, or surprised as ordinary folk by unpredictable sounds, such as loud gunshots. Indeed, there is some reason to believe that one subject, our friend the meditating monk, in addition to not showing signs of being flummoxed, did not even move the five facial muscles that always move (at least a little) when the startling sound occurred. According to the standard protocol in such experiments, he was told that a loud noise would occur when the count backward from 10 reached 1. He chose "one-pointed concentration" in one test and "open state" meditation in another. The monk reported the biggest experienced effect in the open state where he "moved" the expected loud noise far away so when it came, it seemed a faint noise.

Interestingly, during one-pointed concentration mediation the most interesting physiological surprise occurred. The monk's heart rate and blood pressure, contrary to all expectations and unbeknownst to him, actually decreased. Of course, these results need to be replicated with larger populations, but again the preliminary findings are really interesting because gaining control over autonomic processes is thought by some to be nearly impossible (without extensive cognitive-behavioral therapy).

Next consider the face-reading results. The face-reading system is very complicated, brain-wise. It involves the amygdala, visual cortex, frontal cortex, and more and is not reflexive in the way the startle response operates. We may well be innately biased to accurately read basic emotions off faces. But proficiency at doing so takes time and experience. Children of severely depressed and/or alcoholic parents confuse angry and sad faces. However, because the facial muscles move in essentially the same ways across all cultures (modulated by local display rules), most of us (if we are paying attention) become pretty good at detecting the emotions expressed facially for the emotions actually being experienced. This is especially so when we are presented with photos in which various emotions are displayed or in simple one-on-one conversational settings.

At first it looked to Ekman's team as if no one ever studied ($n > 5,000$) was any good at the following: show a fleeting image of a person displaying a basic emotion for long enough that it is detected and processed in the brain (between one-fifth and one-third of a second), but not long enough so that the person looking at it can report what he or she saw. Then ask the subject to pick out (i.e., "guess") which face from an array of pictures matches what was just flashed. The normal score is at random, that is, one in six correct answers/guesses. This is somewhat surprising because the literature on what is called implicit memory or subliminal perception often shows that people respond above chance with similarly short, below-threshold stimuli in other domains, but not with faces. However, to everyone's great surprise, the meditating monk and two other experienced meditators scored at 2 standard deviations above the norm, getting three or four out of six right! Ekman hypothesizes that some combination of meditative work on empathy and concentration explains these unusual results. If so, we have no clue as to how meditation causes such remarkable powers. Before we try to answer how the remarkable power is caused, we need to replicate the very small sample evidence that such powers reliably exist among experienced meditators. That has not been done.

There is reason to worry about the hypothesis. The word was that no one had ever done as well as the adepts. This turns out to be false. There were a few others in the big database Ekman had who achieved similar scores. There is no way to know whether these individuals were skillful face readers or just lucky. That aside, Ekman has developed techniques that can train anyone to be as good as the four adepts at reading micro-expressions. (You can purchase it at www.paulekman.com/training_cds.php if you have the proper certification and $175.)

What remains very interesting is why, if it is so easy to learn this skill, everyone hasn't done so—after all, there is an arm's race to detect liars and cheaters. Ekman (personal communication) has no answer yet. The fact remains that the adepts naturally developed the skill, but not as far as we know by trying to do so for faces. My best guess is that what is called insight (*vipassana*) meditation where concentration and skills of analytic attention are honed (often primarily on one's own sensations, mental states, etc.) result in good analytic skills in interpersonal situations. Ekman's first surmise was that it might have to do with skills that come from *metta* (loving kindness) meditation, where empathy and compassion are honed. We may both be right. But as of now, we just don't know why or how these adepts developed the skill.

It is worth emphasizing—returning to the question "what does this have to do with happiness?"—that Ekman's own work on Buddhist practitioners, aside from his collaboration with Davidson on the left prefrontal cortex study, has nothing directly to do with measuring happiness—happiness either as understood in ordinary language or as defined by Buddhism or some other ethical or spiritual tradition. Perhaps being unusually calm when a loud noise occurs relates to feelings of well-being. For now, all we can say is that certain kinds of meditation can be used to screen the effects of normally unpleasant stimuli. Regarding face reading, no evidence exists relating the ability to read below conscious-threshold facial stimuli and good feelings, happiness, let alone happiness[buddha]. If the results are replicated, the enhanced empathy hypothesis (probably combined with the enhanced attentiveness hypothesis) is a contender, but again empathy can, in certain individuals, be a source of some distress. In fact, Buddhist practitioners have long recognized this problem, so that there are techniques to ward off being afflicted by negative emotions that are not one's own. At this point, there are no data on the effectiveness of such techniques.

BUDDHISM AND INFLUENZA

There are several other studies that examine potential links between Buddhism and things other than happiness. A group at Emory University, led by Guiseppe Pagnoni, is comparing Zen meditators with at least 3 years' experience against controls with no such experience to measure attention, concentration, and problem-solving ability. If Zen meditators are better than the controls at these tasks, then perhaps Zen meditation techniques can be used on persons with attentional disorders (ADHD, e.g.) and possibly even for those in the early stages of Alzheimer disease.

Meanwhile, a collaboration between Richie Davidson and Jon Kabat-Zinn (Davidson et al., 2003; Rosenkrantz et al., 2003), with an $n = 25$, found that as little as 8 weeks of 1 hour daily meditation and 3 hours of weekly training produced positive effects on mood (as measured by leftward movement in prefrontal cortical activity) in the meditators (all of whom worked in stressful high-tech jobs), as well as increased immune function as measured by the number of influenza antibodies in meditators versus the nonmeditating controls, where both groups had taken the flu vaccine.

The important point for now is that the Davidson and Kabat-Zinn study examined the link between Buddhism and both positive affect and positive immune system effects. Measuring changes in the immune system and changes in cognitive performance among those who practice one-pointed meditation and those who do not are completely tractable using existing psychophysical tools. However, studies allegedly establishing links between meditation and positive affect have yet to become sophisticated enough to tell us much about the kind of positive affect experienced, and whether and how positive affect connects with the kind of happiness that is alleged to come from wisdom and virtue. Our ways of measuring brain function in a fine-grained manner that correlates activity with specific and various types of mental states are in their infancy. Note, for example, the debate over whether (and if so how and where) the amygdala processes positive basic emotions (left or right, anterior or posterior). In 1999, Davidson and Irwin pointed out that resolving this question requires more powerful fMRI magnets than existed at the time. Now a few sufficiently powerful magnets exist and are coming on line, but they are being used on scientific issues other than whether Buddhist brains are particularly frisky in the happiness department.

Even now with magnets powerful enough to plot activity in the prefrontal cortex, we understand almost nothing about how to distinguish among the myriad specific states that fall under the very general categories of positive affect or good mood. That said, the meditating monk did show different kinds of neural activity when he was engaged in different kinds of meditation. It is far too early to know, however, whether the brain processes involved, say, in his meditation for compassion, correspond to the brain processes of other meditators engaged in compassion meditation and whether (and if so, how) these are the same or different from the neural activity of nonmeditators who experience or embody compassion.

In any case, it is completely unclear at this time whether and in what ways better immune function and better capacities to pay attention link up with happiness. They obviously link up to better health (a lower chance of catching the flu) and possibly with better school and job performance. It is easy to see how these might lead to a better life than the alternative. What link if any these things have to happiness in the relevant sense(s) remains obscure.

I don't mean to be understood as saying that the scientific work just described is not interesting. My point so far is to emphasize that the extant research on Buddhism and happiness is heterogeneous in terms of what states of body or mind it targets. The work just discussed connects Buddhism to effects on the immune system or on attention; concentration, and cognition; or on suppression of the startle response; or on face reading. This work is not about the effects of Buddhism on happiness. Even the work that claims to be on happiness is not, in every case, at least obviously, about happiness. This is because positive mood or positive affect does not obviously equal happiness, even in the colloquial sense(s). The tools that we currently use are simply not powerful enough to yield fine-grained descriptions of the mental states of subjects that would enable us, for example, to say, "Look, there is the compassion. Notice how it looks different from loving kindness." Combining various existing technologies, including doing assays of neurochemicals, might enable us to make such assertions after studying large populations of subjects. But that is a long way off (meanwhile, see Ospina et al., 2007, for reasons to worry that what the Buddenthusiasta believe to be the case will be confirmed to be the case).

WHAT DOES METAPHYSICS HAVE TO DO WITH IT?

Now that we have examined an array of research that claims to measure a variety of states produced by Buddhist practice, I can express more clearly the problem that concerns me about brain studies of happiness. To make the concern as clear as possible, it is necessary to say something about the metaphysical background assumptions that guide this work.

Almost all neuroscientific work proceeds on either of two assumptions. The first view, *identity theory*, assumes that all mental states *are* in fact brain states. We access the surface structure of our minds first-personally, in a phenomenological manner, in terms of how a particular state seems or feels to us. But first-person access fails to get at the neural deep structure of our mental states. Only impersonal, or third person, techniques can do this. Suppose I see a red patch. According to identity theory, my brain will reveal activity in visual cortex in areas that specifically compute "redness" and "patchiness." There will also be some computation somewhere that marks, or is, the "I see." Then there will be some activity that is or represents where the components are bound (in psychology this is known as "the binding problem") or come together to produce my unified perception. The complete neuroscientific picture of my perception of the red patch will reveal everything that is true of my subjective perception, including causal and constitutive features of the perception that I am clueless about first-personally.

The second view, the *neural correlate view* (NCV) can be understood as quietistic or agnostic as far as commitment to metaphysical physicalism goes (the view that "what there is and all there is, is physical," i.e., matter and energy transfers). Although NCV claims that each and every mental state has certain distinctive neural correlates, it need neither endorse nor condemn the view that the subjective properties of every experience are reducible to or exhausted by the neural underpinnings of that experience. Perhaps subjectively experienced mental states have sui generis properties that are nonphysical.

In addition, although proponents of the NCV usually assume, as do proponents of identity theory, that there will be neural property correlates for all the features of mental states as detected first-personally, the view doesn't actually entail this. Because identity is not claimed, mental states might possibly be caused by or correlated with brain states, but the neural correlates do not contain specific matches (correlates) for each and every property revealed at the mental level.

In a piece, "On the Luminosity of Being," (Gyatso, 2003b), that appeared alongside my "Colour of Happiness," the Dalai Lama expresses doubt that at least in the case of states of "luminous consciousness," *any* neural correlates will be found for this extra-special conscious mental states. Luminous consciousness is an especially pure state of mind that involves getting in touch with one's purest essence, one's Buddha nature, whatever that is. His argument rests first on the rarity of this state; second, on the fact that luminous consciousness *seems* so very nonphysical; and third, on the fact that Buddhist philosophy claims that destructive mental states, afflictions, and poisons, such as delusion, avarice, and hatred—the three poisons—do not penetrate luminous consciousness. Or better, these three poisons penetrate all material nature (and thus the brain). But we can overcome the poisons, so we must have a part of mind that has no commerce, not even correlative commerce, with the material world. This is luminous consciousness. The argument is obviously unpersuasive (see Flanagan, 2007, chapter 3, for a discussion of Dalai Lama's views on testability and the nature of consciousness).

Mental Detection: Content and Causes

Whether one is an identity theorist or holds the weaker neural correlate view, NCV, one will need to do what Varela (1999) calls *neurophenomenology*. In the simplest terms, neurophenomenology is the strategy of trying to explain the activity of the mind–brain by carefully gathering sensitive first-person phenomenological reports from subjects, and then using whatever knowledge and tools we currently possess in cognitive psychology and neuroscience to locate how the brain is doing what the subjects report experiencing.

Neurophenomenology is the only game in town because when we explore the conscious mental, we must always use two kinds of probes. First, there is the subjective or phenomenological method of gathering first-person information about what an experience seems or feels like. First-personally, we only know and can report what content our state has—"I am happy because [my son graduated from college today]." Sometimes we make surmises about the causes of the states with particular contents. In the example, the cause might be identical to the content: "I'm so happy because my son graduated today." But often content and cause come apart. Suppose taking an antidepressant causes a person's mood to improve to the point that she finally appreciates good weather once again. She says, "What a beautiful sunny day." That [it is a beautiful sunny day] is the content of her mental state. But the cause of her positive mental state is due in some measure to the medication.

Do current techniques and technologies for studying the brain reveal any fine-grained details that correspond to what I call the content and the cause(s) of mental states as revealed first-personally? The answer is no. Even if we grant that current techniques can detect positive affect, there is no technique that can distinguish contents of "propositional attitude" states—states like I believe that [p], I expect that [q], I am happy that [r], where p, q, and r are the propositional contents of the states.

My brain may light up "happily," but no brain technology can reveal at present or in the foreseeable future that the content is that [my son is about to graduate] as opposed to that [it is a cool and sunny day]. First-person phenomenological reports or behavioral observation can lead us to distinguish between two individuals, one who is happy that [she is working for Doctors without Borders] and the other who is happy that [he just made a million dollars on insider trading]. Suppose, as is possible, that their happy centers light up in the same way and to the same degree, neuroscience will reveal no such content difference. So content is a big problem—terra incognita for contemporary brain science.

Similar problems arise regarding the causes of contentful mental states. When the cause of a mental state lies in the past, say, in one's upbringing or in many years of practicing meditation, brain scans can't reveal the actual distal cause(s) because these lie outside the brain and in the past. Even supposing, as is plausible, that distal external causes leave neural traces, these are probably global and no one has a clue as to how to study or detect them.

CONCLUSION: HOW MUCH NEW LIGHT IS BEING SHED?

One lesson about neurophenomenology and the study of happiness is that happiness[buddha] is characterized as having a certain cause and a certain content (with constituent structure, for example, the four required virtues of compassion, loving kindness, sympathetic joy, and equanimity). If there is such a thing as happiness[buddha], it is produced by distinctively Buddhist wisdom and virtues. And first-person detection (very humble detection) that one is enlightened and virtuous is at least part of the content of the happiness.

Assume that we gather a group of Buddhists of the same age, with the same amount of training, committed to the same kind of Buddhism, and so on. Can brain scans detect the "belief" states that constitute their enlightenment/wisdom? No. The problem could be due to current technologies or current psycho-neural theories of how, what, and where belief states are, or (most likely) both. In any case, we cannot presently see or measure or distinguish among such states. Can we distinguish among the virtues in the brain? No. Can we detect virtue, in general, in human brains? No. At present we are utterly clueless and without resources to do any such fine-grained analyses of the neural underpinnings of states of character. Here is the good news—if there is any prospect for doing so, it will come from using the method of neurophenomenology while we develop more sensitive methods, technologies, and theories for studying the brain.

It amuses me to think of Siddhartha Gautama looking down from nirvana, heaven, the true pure land, or wherever, and observing all the activity attempting to study, confirm, or disconfirm the relation between Buddhist practices and various goods. I think he would be pleased both that Buddhism has so many advocates and that the hope it brings to alleviate suffering and achieve true happiness is being taken very seriously. I picture him a bit befuddled by all the new gadgets being used to measure all sorts of mental and bodily states as well as by a Zeitgeist that so relishes empirical confirmation. But that aside, I like to think of Buddha as approving of what we are trying (still) to learn: how to end suffering, achieve enlightenment and goodness, and to find true happiness.

Now is a propitious time to proceed with scientific studies on the connections between Buddhist practices and the various positive mental and physical states these practices are hypothesized to engender. The good news is that for immune response, sensitivity of the virtually automatic amygdala-based emotional system, facial expression detection, and cognitive task performance guided by one-pointed meditation, there are reliable fine-grained physiological, behavioral, and, in some cases, neurological measures than can be used, even if these have not yet been used on sufficiently large populations to have really confirmed any of the hypotheses in the air.

As far as measuring and locating the neural correlates for the different types of happiness, we have a long and difficult row to hoe. We need to combine very sensitive phenomenological reports about the feeling and contours that comprise the heterogeneous kinds of happiness that ordinary speech picks out. Seligman's (2002) research on "authentic happiness"' holds promise for distinguishing among the multifarious kinds of happiness (as understood colloquially) by using questionnaires that try to get clear and nuanced reports from subjects on their mental states (see also Easterlin, 2003, 2004; Frank, 2004). I like to think that my own work introducing the research program of eudaimonics (Flanagan, 2007) advances the inquiry and shows that the study of happiness will get nowhere unless scholars who understand the history and philosophical texture of the multifarious wisdom traditions are involved. Indeed, without deep philosophical understanding of what various traditions promise in terms of virtue, wisdom, and happiness, including how these are alleged to interpenetrate, the neuroscientists don't know what they are looking for. This is, by and large, the case as I write.

It follows that for the promising program of eudaimonics to proceed, we will require thick descriptions of the multiplicity of theory and tradition specific conceptions that offer true happiness. We know that Aristotle, Epicurus, Buddha, Confucius, Mencius, Jesus, and Mohammed each put forward somewhat different philosophical conceptions of an excellent human life with somewhat different conceptions of what constitutes true happiness. With these different conceptions well articulated, we can look at brain activity within and across advocates of different traditions to see what similarities and differences our mappings reveal. The same strategy should work for negative emotions and destructive mental states. Get well-honed first-person reports from subjects on the negative states they experience, and then look for brain correlates. With such data in hand, we can test Buddhist techniques, say, meditation on compassion, which are thought to provide antidotes for anger, hatred, and avarice. Along with first-person reports on any experienced change in mood or emotion, we can look and see what, if anything, reconfigures itself brain-wise. We can do the same for practices from other traditions. Eventually, we will want to coordinate such studies with the ever-deeper knowledge of the connections among virtue, mental health, well-being, and human flourishing, allowing science and philosophy to speak together about what practices seem best suited to make for truly rich and meaningful lives. At this distant point, with an array of conceptions of excellent human lives before us, as well as deep knowledge of how the brains of devotees of these different traditions look and work, we should be able to speak much more clearly about the nature of happiness and flourishing.

I have offered several reasons for a somewhat cautious, even indirect approach to the study of happiness at the present time. For scientists, when studying a form of life or a practice that has its home in a form of life, specify very precisely what goods the life form or practice claims to offer and then explain in similarly precise detail what mental or bodily effects you claim to discover among practitioners. In concert with experts on the form of life, proceed to more completely articulate what exactly it is that is being seen or revealed.

For the time being, we might follow Seligman's attitude toward the scientific status of the terms *happiness* and *well-being*: "The word *happiness* is the overarching term that describes the whole panoply of goals of Positive Psychology. The word itself is not a term in the theory.... Happiness, as a term, is like *cognition* in the field of cognitive psychology or *learning* within learning theory. These terms just name a field, but they play no role in the theories within the field" (2002, p. 304).

The unease I have expressed about the theoretical usefulness (or lack thereof) of the colloquial concept of happiness ought to be shared by Buddhist practitioners and Buddhist studies experts. Unless the concept of happiness is being put forward in a theory-specific way, such as Buddhism and Aristotelianism both do (and as could be done for Trappist monks and the local hedonist club), then we might for now be best advised to stop talking about it, or at least to stop using the everyday term *happiness* in philosophical or scientific contexts. Scientists like Seligman are, of course, also entitled (indeed encouraged, if it is possible) to try to draw out and specify the ordinary understanding of the constituents of positive states of mind such as happiness. They will then have regimented, in a precise way or ways, the meanings of happiness according to folk psychology.

The more theory-specific conceptions of virtue, well-being, and flourishing that we have, so much the better will be our understanding of the constituents of happiness. Overlapping consensus on the components of these things will, hopefully, reveal itself. Importantly, differences in conceptions of virtue, well-being, and flourishing will also reveal themselves. The overlaps and the differences can be discussed and debated at the philosophical level from a normative ethical perspective, and the scientists can chime in, wearing philosophical hats if they wish but, equally important, telling us how the brains of practitioners from different traditions light up, which neurochemicals rise and fall, and so on.

Intertheoretical conversation such as I am envisioning will put us in the exciting position of being able (a) to have a better idea of the fine-grained states we are looking for, and (b) to compare different theories in terms of the goods they claim to produce and hopefully do in fact produce.

For those of us who are convinced that Buddhism is a noble path to wisdom, virtue, and happiness[buddha], and especially at this time when some scientists claim to be reaching pay dirt in the empirical exploration and confirmation of what many Buddhist practitioners already claim to know, it is necessary to speak with maximal precision about what practices, Buddhist and others, are thought to produce what sorts of specific positive states of mind and body. Overall, this sort of inquiry provides a truly exciting, unique, and heretofore unimagined opportunity for mind-scientists, practitioners, and philosophers from different traditions to join together in a conversation that combines time-tested noble ideals with new-fangled gadgetry to understand ourselves more deeply and live well, better than we do now. On the other hand, we need to beware of overrating brain imagery and what it shows. Some days when I think about brain imaging I am reminded of the following joke. "In the beginning there was nothing and then God said 'Let there be Light.' There was still nothing, but you could see it much better."

NOTES

1. My friend Rob Hogendoorn and I have coined the word *Buddshit*, which is simply self-serving, specifically Buddhist bullshit. Bullshit is universal. Buddhists are just lucky to have their own name for their kind of bullshit.

2. No investigation is required to find many examples of the hype that concerns me here. This week (March 2008) as I was completing this chapter, an article appeared in the *Shambala Sun*, a popular Buddshit magazine, called "Mindfulness of Mind," by Michael Stroud, which advertises itself as a report on "the growing evidence of meditation's helpfulness" on health. But it does no such thing. Instead, we get a report on what some people at good universities are studying about possible effects of meditation. There is reason for concern because a comprehensive meta-analysis for the U.S. Department of Health and Human Services (Ospina et al., 2007) of all the literature up to 2002 claims no significant results overall.

3. William James made the study of exemplary individuals, some of them genuine odd-ducks, respectable in his masterpiece *Varieties of Religious Experience: A Study in Human Nature* (1898/1982). *Varieties* is based on the Gifford Lectures, in Edinburgh, Scotland, delivered by James in 1898. But there is an important difference between this work on spirituality and the work I am discussing in eudaimonics. James's masterpiece emphasized the variety, the heterogeneity of states that all might be called "spiritual." The work on Buddhists and their brains seeks or is reported by the neuro-journalists as seeking general, univocal, shared features of happy people with happy brains.

4. Deficit studies are terrific ways to figure out how a complex system works, so looking at areas affected by stroke, tumors, and so on, has been very helpful in distinguishing among areas differentially involved in particular types of processing. Damasio's work (especially 1994) has gotten lots of attention. Phineas Gage is widely taken as an example of someone with a moral deficit, a "moral knockout," due to a brain deficit in medial frontal cortex. And he is. But the evidence from Phineas and contemporary patients involves gross anatomical problems. You knock out a big area, and you normally get big problems. But the Phineas cases as well as the more recent ones provide little information about the normal subtle communication between different brain areas involved in sociomoral cognition.

5. Actually, classical Theravadan Buddhism devotes considerable attention to the topic of happiness and its causes, although these mundane forms of happiness are always less good than nirvanic release. Theravadan Buddhism also involves fewer lives before nirvanic release than later Mayahana Buddhism, sometimes as few as seven. I thank Donald Lopez for asking me to be clear on this matter even though I am not concerned about delicate matters of Buddhology.

REFERENCES

Dalai Lama. (1999). *Ethics for the New Millennium*. New York: Riverhead Books.
Dalai Lama and Cutler, H. C. (1998). *The Art of Happiness: A Handbook for Living.* New York: Riverhead Books.
Damasio, A. (1994). *Descartes Error: Emotion, Reason, and the Human Brain*. New York: Avon.
Davidson, R. J. (2000). Affective style, psychopathology and resilience: Brain mechanisms and plasticity. *American Psychologist* 55: 1196–1214.
Davidson, R. J., and Hugdahl, K. (Eds.). (2002). *The Asymmetrical Brain*. Cambridge, Mass.: MIT Press.
Davidson, R. J., and Irwin, W. (1999). The functional neuroanatomy of emotion and affective style. *Trends in Cognitive Sciences* 3: 11–21.

Davidson, R. J., Kabat-Zinn, J., Schumacher, J., Rosenkrantz, M., Muller, D., and Santorelli, S. F., et al. (2003). Alterations in brain and immune function produced by mindfulness meditation. *Psychosomatic Medicine* 65: 564–570.

Davidson, R. J., Scherer, K. R., and Goldsmith, H. H. (Eds.). (2002). *Handbook of Affective Sciences*. New York: Oxford University Press.

Easterlin, R. A. (2003). Explaining happiness. *Proceedings of the National Academy of Sciences: Inaugural Articles by Members of the National Academy Elected on April 30, 2002.*

Easterlin, R. A. (2004). Money, Sex, and Happiness: An Empirical Study. National Bureau of Economic Research. Working Paper 10499. Available online: www.nber.org/papers/w10499.

Ekman, P. (2003). *Emotions Revealed*. New York: Times Books.

Ekman, P., Campos, J., Davidson R. J., and De Waal, F. (Eds.). (2003). *Emotions Inside Out*, vol. 1000. New York: Annals of the New York Academy of Sciences.

Flanagan, O. (2000). Destructive emotions. *Consciousness and Emotions* 1: 259–281.

Flanagan, O. (2002). *The Problem of the Soul: Two Visions of Mind and How to Reconcile Them*. New York: Basic Books.

Flanagan, O. (2003a). Emotional expressions. In *Cambridge Companion to Darwin*. Cambridge: Cambridge University Press.

Flanagan, O. (2003b). The colour of happiness. *New Scientist*, May 24.

Flanagan, O. (2006). The bodhisattva's brain. In D. K. Nauriyal, M. Drummond, and Y. B. Lal (Eds.), *Buddhist Thought and Applied Psychological Research*. London: Routledge, 149–174.

Flanagan, O. (2007). *The Really Hard Problem: Meaning in a Material World*. Cambridge, Mass.: MIT Press.

Frank, R. H. (2004). How not to buy happiness. *Daedelus* 133: 69–79.

Gyatso, T. (2003a). The monk in the lab. *New York Times*, April 26.

Gyatso, T. (2003b). On the luminosity of being. *New Scientist*, May 24.

Goleman, D. (2003a). *Destructive Emotions: How Can We Overcome Them?* New York: Bantam Books.

Goleman, D. (2003b). Finding happiness: Cajole your brain to lean left. *New York Times*, February 4.

Harrington, A. (2008). *The Cure Within: A History of Mind-Body Medicine*. New York: Norton.

James, W. (1898/1982). *The Varieties of Religious Experience*. New York: Penguin Books.

LeDoux, J. (1996). *The Emotional Brain*. New York: Simon and Schuster.

Ospina, M. B., Bond, K., Karkhaneh, M., Tjosvold, L., Vandermeer, B., Liang, Y., et al. (2007). Meditation practices for health: State of the research. Agency for Healthcare Research and Quality, U.S. Department of Health and Human Services, contract 290-0200023.

Rosenkrantz, M. A., Jackson, D. C., Dalton, K. M., Dolski, I., Ryff, C. D., Singer, B. H., et al. (2003). Affective style and in vivo immune response: Neurobehavioral mechanisms. *Proceedings of the National Academy of Sciences USA* 100: 11148–11152.

Seligman, M. E. P. (2002). *Authentic Happiness: Using the New Positive Psychology to Realize Your Potential for Lasting Fulfillment*. New York: Free Press.

Stroud, M. (2008). Mindfulness of mind. *Shambala Sun*, March.

Varela, F. J. (1999). The specious present: A neurophenomenology of time consciousness. In J. Petitot, F. J. Varela, B. Pachoud, and J.-M. Roy (Eds.), *Naturalizing Phenomenology: Issues in Contemporary Phenomenology and Cognitive Science*. Stanford, Calif.: Stanford University Press.

CHAPTER 24

THE NEUROPHILOSOPHY OF SUBJECTIVITY

PETE MANDIK

1. INTRODUCTION

Conscious experience, according to many philosophers, is subjective. Claims about the so-called subjectivity of consciousness are offered as apparently obvious facts about consciousness. Furthermore, in much philosophical literature, these supposedly obvious claims are exploited as the bases for some not-at-all-obvious conclusions, like, for instance, the conclusion that no neuroscientific theory could possibly explain consciousness. If such claims are correct, then the neurophilosophy of consciousness is somewhere between impossible and ridiculous.

In this chapter, I present a case that claims of the subjectivity of consciousness are far from obvious or innocent and are instead very strong empirical claims about the structure, acquisition, and content of concepts. As such, it is entirely appropriate to bring empirical considerations to bear on the question of whether experience is essentially subjective. I describe various neurophilosophical accounts of the relevant notions (concepts, consciousness, sensation, introspection, etc.) and build a case against the subjectivity of consciousness. Along the way I discuss the prospects of neurophilosophical accounts of subjectivity and argue for the superiority of subjectivity eliminativism over subjectivity reductionism.

My plan is as follows. First, I conduct a quick review of the notion of subjectivity as it figures in some classic discussions in the philosophy of mind, especially those surrounding the work of Nagel and Jackson. I develop the idea that in these contexts, subjectivity is one-way knowability. Next, I turn to discuss neurophilosophical perspectives on the topics of consciousness, phenomenal character, concepts, and "knowing what it is like." Then I examine the proposal that, due to the structure of the relevant concepts, one can only have the concept of what it is like to have certain experiences if one has had those experiences. Finally, I bring the insights developed in the previous sections to bear on the twin questions of whether (1) in perception we perceive properties that may be known in no other way and (2) in introspection we introspect properties that may be known in no other way. My conclusions are that both questions merit negative answers.

2. Subjectivity and the Philosophy of Mind

What, in the context of the philosophy of mind, is subjectivity? Subjectivity has something to do with consciousness, but it is not consciousness itself. Subjectivity has something to do with the so-called phenomenal character of conscious states, but it is not identical to phenomenal character. Subjectivity is an alleged property of phenomenal character, namely, the property of being one-way knowable. More specifically, the claim that phenomenal character is subjective is the claim that the only way to know some phenomenal character is by *having* a conscious experience that has that character. (This is a first pass and will be refined further later.) Whatever the relevant sense of "know" is here, it is the sense relevant to "knowing what it is like" to have some conscious experience.

Before we further refine these characterizations, some brief historical remarks are in order. Much contemporary discussion of the related notions of subjectivity and "what it is like" stem from the work of Thomas Nagel (1974). Nagel got philosophers worried about the question "what is it like to be a bat?" and urged that because bat experience must be so very different from our own, we could never know. He further suggested that no amount of knowledge about bat behavior or bat physiology could bridge the gap.

Though Nagel did not draw dualistic conclusions from these considerations, other philosophers did. In particular, Jackson (1982) and subsequent commentators developed an argument against physicalism based on the special ways in which what it is like to have conscious states with certain phenomenal characters must be known. The most famous version of Jackson's ensuing "knowledge argument" centered on a thought experiment about a woman, Mary, who somehow knows all of the physical facts, especially those about the neural basis of human color vision, without ever herself having seen red. On seeing red, Mary allegedly must necessarily be surprised and thus learns only then what it is like to see red. Because she knew all of the physical facts before coming to know what it is like to see red, knowing what it is like must be knowing something nonphysical.

At this point, we can attempt some further refinement of the subjectivity claim. At a first pass, we might try to characterize the key idea behind Nagel's and Jackson's arguments as

> K: For all types of phenomenal character, to know what it is like to have a conscious experience with a phenomenal character of a type, one must have, at that or some prior time, a conscious experience with a phenomenal character of the same type.

One appealing feature of K is that it would justify the claims that humans cannot know what it is like to have bat experiences, and people who have only seen black and white cannot know what it is like to see red.

However, even fans of Nagel and Jackson are likely to reject K on the grounds that there are many types of phenomenal characters for which K is highly implausible. Suppose that there was some shade of gray or some polygon that Mary had never seen before. Few philosophers are likely to suppose that Mary would be surprised on seeing a 65.5 percent gray or a 17-sided polygon for the first time. Similarly, such philosophers would think that one can extrapolate from relevantly similar experiences to knowledge of what it would be like to see Hume's missing shade of blue (*A Treatise of Human Nature*, Bk. I, Pt. I, Sec. I; Hume [1739] 1978).

Perhaps, then, the idea behind subjectivity considerations is better put by modifying K by replacing "the same" with "a relevantly similar" and replacing "all" with "at least one," resulting in the following.

> K+: For at least one type of phenomenal character, to know what it is like to have a conscious experience with a phenomenal character of that type, one must have, at that or some prior time, a conscious experience with a phenomenal character of a relevantly similar type.

Thus, we have, in K+, an explication of what it means to equate the subjectivity of phenomenal character with the one-way knowability of phenomenal character.

More remains to be said on what the sense of knowledge is that is most relevant here. Proponents of the knowledge argument against physicalism have interpreted knowing what it is like as a kind of propositional knowledge. Some physicalists have granted this assumption and others have questioned it, offering that a different kind of knowledge, such as know-how, constitutes knowing what it is like (Lewis, 1983, 1990; Nemirow, 1980, 1990).

In this chapter I simply grant, without further discussion, the propositional assumption, but for a longer discussion of this point see Mandik (2001). It is thus assumed that knowing what it is like to have a conscious experience with some phenomenal character C is the same as knowing some proposition P. It is further assumed that P is the proposition that having a conscious experience with some phenomenal character C is like such and such.

There are at least two general possible reasons that C would be one-way knowable, one having to do with belief and the other having to do with warrant. The belief reason says that one cannot know P without having C (I intend "having C" as shorthand for "having a conscious experience with phenomenal character C") because one is incapable of believing P without having C. The warrant reason grants that one can believe P without having C but claims that one's belief that P cannot have sufficient warrant to count as knowing P unless one has had C. Neurophilosophical work pertinent to subjectivity has mostly concerned the belief claim, and in this chapter my attention is similarly restricted.

We must turn now to ask why it would be the case that believing P requires having C. A natural kind of answer to such a question is one that appeals to concepts. What one can or cannot believe depends on what concepts one does or does not have. If one has no concept of, say, dark matter, then one cannot have beliefs about dark matter.

Several authors have proposed that we have special concepts—so-called phenomenal concepts—by which we think of the phenomenal characters of our conscious states. Part of what is supposed to be special about phenomenal concepts is that one can acquire a phenomenal concept of C only by having conscious experiences with phenomenal character C. Although there are various ways of construing phenomenal concepts, I focus here only on those construals whereby the assertion of the existence of phenomenal concepts is inconsistent with the falsity of K+ (for examples of such construals, see Papineau, 1999; Tye, 2000). If there are such things as phenomenal concepts, then they can explain the one-way knowability of C that is constitutive of the subjectivity of C: C's being subjective is due to C's being one-way conceptualizable. The phenomenal concept of C is the unique concept that picks out C as such.

I argue that when viewed from a neurophilosophical point of view, the phenomenal concepts proposal looks very strange indeed. For a brief sketch of how one might attempt to ground phenomenal concepts in neuroscience, we can turn to a recent proposal by Beaton:

> We would be wrong to think that, when Mary is released, just gaining the correctly configured sensory apparatus is sufficient for her to know what it is like to see red. Just picking out red—in V4 say—without any connection to the brain regions responsible for additional, more conceptual abilities, would be the equivalent of blindsight. In order for Mary to come to consciously see red, she has to be able to *report* that she is seeing red now, to be able to choose to remember and imagine it at will, and to act on her imagination as appropriate, after having seen it. It seems highly likely that these more complex, conceptual abilities are functions of the associative and frontal regions of the human brain...regions which are functionally distinct from lower level sensory cortex in the important sense that sensory cortex can continue to effectively carry out the vast majority of its tasks without the presence of higher brain regions, whilst the converse is not true....
>
> On the present view then, on exposure to colour, Mary gains a new configuration in her sensory cortex (specifically in the region dedicated to the processing of colour), but she additionally gains a new neural configuration in her associative and/or frontal cortical regions. This additional configuration corresponds to Mary's having gained a new concept, a concept which I will gloss as "*red_as_experienced.*"...She now possesses a new concept, of red as

experienced, grounded in the very sensory apparatus which enables her to detect and respond to red stimuli. (2005, pp. 13–14)

A neurophilosophical proposal such as Beaton's constitutes an attempt to provide a reduction of subjectivity to aspects of neurophysiology insofar as it seeks to identify properties such as one-way knowability with certain aspects of the functioning of the nervous system. A different neurophilosophical approach, the one advocated in this chapter, attempts to eliminate subjectivity by arguing that (1) there are no aspects of neural function with which so-called one-way knowability can plausibly be identified, and (2) there is no reason for maintaining a belief in the irreducible existence of subjectivity.

Before further developing neurophilosophical considerations appropriate for evaluating the phenomenal concepts proposal and its role in the debate between subjectivity reductionism and subjectivity eliminativism, it will be useful to sketch some neurophilosophical accounts of consciousness, character, concepts, and knowing what it is like.

3. Consciousness and Concepts

There is no shortage of philosophical theories of consciousness these days and several merit the label "neurophilosophical." Neurophilosophy is often distinguished from philosophy of neuroscience in that the former involves the application of neuroscientific concepts to philosophical problems and the latter is the philosophical examination of neuroscience (Bickle, Mandik, and Landreth, 2006). Neurophilosophical theories of consciousness bring neuroscientific concepts to bear on philosophical problems concerning consciousness. In Mandik (2006b) I review neurophilosophical accounts of consciousness due to Churchland, Prinz, and Tye, and in Mandik (2005, 2008) I present one of my own. Here I attempt a sketch of the main outlines of the latter theory, though the differences among these theories are negligible with respect to the issues of significance in the current chapter.

There are three main questions that philosophical theories of consciousness are concerned to answer. The first concerns the question of what the difference between conscious states and unconscious states amounts to. States of the retina carry information about the distribution of visible light arrayed in front of the organism, but retinal states are alone insufficient for consciousness. Higher level states, such as one's abstract knowledge that dogs are mammals, are likewise insufficient for consciousness—you have known for some time that dogs are mammals but were unlikely to be consciously thinking that dogs were mammals a few moments ago. The second question concerns what one is conscious of when one has conscious states. I have just now become conscious of the noise that my air conditioner makes, although I am quite sure it has been making that noise before I became conscious of it. In what does this aspect of consciousness consist? Finally, the third question of consciousness is the one that most preoccupies philosophers working on consciousness: the question of what phenomenal character consists in.

To convey the outlines of the neuroscience relevant to consciousness it will be useful to focus on just one kind of consciousness, namely, visual consciousness and the basic relevant neuroscience concerning vision. Visual information is processed through various levels in a visual processing hierarchy. The lowest levels are at the sites of transduction in the retina. Progressively higher levels of processing are located in (in order) the subcortical structures of the lateral geniculate nucleus (LGN), primary visual area (V1), various cortical areas in the temporal and parietal lobes, and, at the highest levels, areas in the frontal cortex and hippocampus.

Two main features of the hierarchy are especially worth noting. The first is that distinctive kinds of perceptual information are represented at distinct levels. The second is that information flows not only from lower to higher levels but also back down from higher to lower. This first point, concerning distinctive kinds of information, is especially useful for identifying which states of neural activation are most relevant to various conscious states. So, for example, one element of conscious visual perception involves subjective contour illusions such as Kanizsa triangles; however, neural activity in V1 does not reflect the presence of subjective contours, and activity in V2 does (von der Heydt, Peterhans, and Baumgartner, 1984).

One general remark that can be made about the difference in the information represented at the different levels is that at the lowest levels the information is very specific and is increasingly abstract at higher levels. For example, color constancy is registered at levels higher than V1 (Zeki, 1983). Very low levels are sensitive to the specific colors, viewer-relative locations, and orientations of specific stimuli. At higher levels, neural activity indicates less of a preference for such specificities.

These various facts about the representational contents of conscious experiences and the kinds of information present at the various levels of the hierarchy help locate conscious states at relatively intermediate levels of the hierarchy. However, simply being an intermediate-level state of neural activation does not suffice for being a conscious state, and this is where the second crucial fact about the processing hierarchy comes into play.

Conscious perceptual states are those involved in neural activations that involve the bottom-up activation of intermediate levels that are also undergoing modulation by various top-down influences. According to the neurophilosophical theory of consciousness spelled out in Mandik (2005, 2008), a conscious state is a hybrid composed of a pair of reciprocally interacting states, one of which is higher in the hierarchy than the other.

Evidence for the need for such reciprocal interaction includes results of transcranial magnetic stimulation experiments by Pascual-Leone and Walsh (2001) whereby V5 activity sufficed for conscious motion perception only if information was allowed to feed back down from V5 to V1. Another line of evidence for the reciprocity hypothesis comes from Lamme et al. (1998), wherein anesthetized animals show brain activity in response to stimuli, but only of a feedforward type that involved no feedback from higher to lower levels.

Regarding the three questions of consciousness, the question of what makes states conscious has already been addressed: States are conscious when they are intermediate-level hybrids, parts of which are reciprocally interacting representations. Moving on to the question of what we are conscious of when we have conscious states, the natural suggestion is that we are conscious of the representational contents of the reciprocally interacting states. The answer to this question is closely related to the question of phenomenal character: What constitutes what it's like to be in a conscious state is what the conscious state represents, that is, the character of a conscious state is one and the same as the way the state represents things to be. (This is not necessarily to adopt a first-order representationalist position such as Dretske, 1995, or Tye, 1995, 2000, for it is open that some of the things that are represented are other mental states and thus sometimes, though not always, the conscious states will involve higher order representations.)

Visual consciousness comes in two modes that are relevant to the present discussion: perception and introspection. The following account is adapted from Mandik (2006a, in press), which builds on Churchland (1979). First, we can characterize perception in a way that is neutral with respect to whether the perception in question is conscious perception. Thus, the account of perception is that it is the automatic conceptual exploitation of the information sensations carry about events in the external world (in exteroception) and in the body (in interoception). Thus, when one sees a coffee mug, one has a sensation that carries information about the mug, and this sensation in turn elicits the automatic (noninferential) application of certain concepts, such as the concept of a mug. Introspection is the automatic (noninferential) conceptual exploitation of the information that mental states carry about themselves.

In terms of the visual processing hierarchy, we can identify the concepts in question with representational states that are relatively high in the hierarchy and the sensations with states relatively low in the hierarchy. Unconscious perception takes place when a sensation elicits the application of a concept without feedback from the conceptual level back down to the sensational level. A conscious perception occurs when the feedback occurs in addition to the processes that alone would suffice for unconscious perception.

The account of introspection is modeled on the account of perception. Where perception of external events is the automatic conceptual exploitation of information that sensations carry about those events, the introspection of sensation is the automatic conceptual exploitation of information that sensations carry about themselves. When the sensations are in appropriately reciprocal interactions with the elicited concepts, the introspection involved is the kind relevant to discussions of knowing what it is like.

Perception and introspection are ways of getting knowledge. But the open question is whether the knowledge thereby gotten can only be gotten in those ways. To address the question, it will be helpful to give a characterization of what the knowledge consists in that is relatively neutral on the question at hand. Leaving aside knowledge of what it is like for a moment, let us consider some general remarks about knowledge and some prototypical instances of knowledge.

Consider, for example, your knowledge of how tall you are. There was a time at which you acquired that knowledge, and it was likely when you were undergoing a conscious occurrent mental state, the content of which is that your height is such and such. This information was stored to be available for later retrieval. You may very well be retrieving it right now and thus undergoing another conscious occurrent mental state—this time, the conscious thought that your height is such and such. However, in the expanse of time between acquisition and retrieval, you did know what your height was even though you were not undergoing an occurrent conscious mental state with that content. Your stored knowledge over the intervening period may or may not count as an occurrent mental state, but clearly it does not count as a conscious mental state. As such, you can have that knowledge even at times that you are subject to no conscious states at all (as in, perhaps, when you are in a deep sleep).

Putting this in terms of concepts, one can have a concept at a time (in at least some cases) in which one is not at the same time making use of that concept in an occurrent conscious mental state. Another point this example allows us to highlight is that even though the knowledge of your height was acquired by having a conscious experience, no particular kind of conscious experience was required to learn that your height was such and such. You could have equally well learned that fact even if you were color blind or totally blind. Putting this in terms of concepts, the concepts involved in knowing that your height is such and such can be acquired regardless of which particular type of conscious experience concerned your height being such and such.

Let us return now to the question of knowing what it is like. The intuition, K+, lying behind the subjectivity claim entails that there is at least one kind of knowledge that can be had only if one has had or is having an experience of a certain type. The phenomenal concepts strategy under discussion is making a claim about the relevant concepts in question, namely, that the concepts constitutive of knowing what it is like cannot be acquired without undergoing, now or previously, an experience with the phenomenal character in question. This is a claim made by physicalists as well as antiphysicalists, so it is fair to ask whether a neurophilosophical defense of the claim can be given.

There are two general strategies one might pursue in defending the claim about concepts. The first defends it in terms of the structure of the concepts themselves. The second defends it in terms of the semantic facts about the representational contents of the concepts. I address these strategies in sections 4 and 5, respectively.

4. The Structure of Concepts Defense of Subjectivity

There are various things that the postulation of concepts is supposed to explain, but for current purposes we can focus on just two: categorization and inference. When I categorize diverse visual stimuli, say, those involved in seeing a China pug and those involved in seeing a Doberman, as both indicating examples of dogs, it is my concept of dogs that allows me to do this. When I draw an inference, for example, that this China pug is a mammal, on the basis of my prior belief that all dogs are mammals, the inference is enabled by me possessing, among other things, a concept of mammals. Often, inferences are spread out over time, involving chains of thought with distinct mental events constituting the contemplation of various premises and the reaching of a conclusion. A neurophilosophical account of concepts must, at a minimum, provide for an account of what concepts are such that they can play these roles in categorization and inference.

For a relatively simple neural model of how concepts figure in categorization, we can look to Churchland's (1989) account of concepts in terms of feedforward neural networks. In the neural models in question, the networks consist in a set of input neurons, a set of output neurons, and a set of "hidden" neurons intervening between the inputs and outputs. Neurons are connected by various connections that can be "weighted," meaning that the connections may be assigned values that determine how much influence the activation of one neuron can have on the activation of another. Information flows through the network along the connections.

A network is a strictly feedforward network if information flows only from input neurons to hidden neurons and from hidden neurons to output neurons. In a massively connected feedforward network, each input neuron is connected to every hidden neuron, and each hidden neuron is connected to every output neuron.

Learning takes place by making adjustments to the connection weights. To consider an example of the learning of a categorization task, consider a network trained to visually discriminate cats from dogs. The inputs are an array of retinal cells on which black and white bitmapped photographs of dogs and cats may be projected. The output units are two units, labeled "dog" and "cat," respectively. Initially, the connection weights are set to random values, and the network is expected to be at chance for correctly identifying a given photograph as being of a dog or a cat. But by making gradual adjustments to the weights (via the application of a learning rule based on a measurement of the difference between the error and the correct response), the network can come to learn to make the correct classification.

Churchland proposes to identify concepts with attractors in hidden unit activation space. For each unit in the hidden layer, we can represent its level of activation along a dimension. The multiple units thus define a multidimensional state space. The presentation of a photograph to the network will result in a pattern of activation across the units that can be defined as a single point in activation space. The points corresponding to presentations of dogs will cluster closer together in activation space than the points corresponding to presentations of cats. The network's concept of dogs is a region of activation space, the center of which determines a dog that would be perceived as the prototypical dog.

Churchland's account of concepts seems to supply a case for a kind of concept empiricism relevant to addressing the subjectivity claim. Of course, we need to put aside the very difficult question of how concepts would be concepts of sensations as opposed to concepts of distal stimuli that trigger sensations. We will simply assume that the concepts are concepts of sensations. Additionally, we need to assume that the concepts involved in knowing what it is like to see red are learned. Whatever concepts are acquired, they are acquired only when or after the sensations are had. This is in keeping with K+.

However, these simple networks have serious shortcomings as models. Feedforward networks, lacking lateral and recurrent connections, are poor models of consciousness, for they lack recurrent connections and for similar reasons are poor models of concepts, for they cannot account for inferences (insofar as inferences are spread out over time, because only recurrent networks can sustain dynamic patterns of neural activation). Of course, this suggests that we should consider slightly more complicated neural models of concepts, ones that have lateral and feedback connections in addition to feedforward connections.

One such model is the one that figures centrally in what Damasio and Damasio (1994) call "convergence zones." According to Damasio and Damasio, a convergence zone is a neuronal grouping in which multiple feedback and feedforward connections from separate cortical regions converge. A convergence zone generates patterns of activity across widely separated neuronal groupings by sending signals back down to multiple cortical regions. Damasio and Damasio also postulate that convergence zones form hierarchical organizations in which higher level convergence zones are connected to other, lower convergence zones. The lowest levels of the hierarchy would be pools of neurons that are not themselves convergence zones but supply information that would get bound in convergence zones. Convergence zones account for inference insofar as the lateral and top-down connections allow for the endogenous triggering of conceptual representations: One thinks of mammals because one was previously thinking of dogs as opposed to mammals because an actual mammal triggered the perceptual application of the concept.

Convergence zones provide not only models of inference but a more flexible kind of recognition one might associate with genuinely conceptual systems. Cohen and Eichenbaum (1993) hypothesize that the hippocampus is a locus of convergence zones. The flexible kind of recognition is illustrated as follows. Eichenbaum et al. (1989) showed that rats with hippocampal lesions can be trained to prefer certain stimuli, but the preferences will not be exhibited in contexts that differ significantly from the initial training conditions. The rats demonstrate their conditioned preference by moving toward the target odor. A hippocampus-damaged rat, when presented with two odor sources, A and B, can be trained to prefer A to B. This rat will demonstrate this preference even after a sustained delay period. However, if the rat is presented with the preferred odor A, along with some odor N, which differs from the nonpreferred odor B that accompanied A in the learning trials, the rat will demonstrate no preference whatsoever. Healthy rats do not exhibit such a lack of preference—their preference is demonstrated even in novel situations, such as the presentation of A with N.

Given the convergence zone model, we can turn to casting doubt on the phenomenal concepts proposal: Why couldn't top-down or lateral connections suffice for concept acquisition? Whatever set of changes in connections in a network suffice for the acquisition of a concept, in particular, the concept involved in knowing what it is like to see red things, why couldn't those changes be brought about by means other than the perceptual presentation of red things or even activations of the neural areas constitutive of having an experiences as if one were seeing a red thing?

Whatever knowing what is like consists in, it is the downstream effects of having certain experiences. Why couldn't the resulting structures be installed without having such causes? Such a situation is at least possible in theory. Dennett illustrates the possibility in terms of the fanciful thought experiment of "Swamp Mary":

> Just as standard Mary is about to be released from prison, still virginal with regard to colors...a bolt of lighting rearranges her brain, putting it by Cosmic Coincidence into exactly the brain state she was just about to go into *after* first seeing a red rose. (She is left otherwise unharmed of course; this is a thought experiment.) So when, a few seconds later, she is released, and sees for the first time, a colored thing (that red rose), she says just what she would say on seeing her *second* or *nth* red rose. "Oh yeah, right, a red rose. Been there, done that." (2005, p. 120)

What I am suggesting here is less fanciful than Swamp Mary. What I am suggesting is the possibility that concepts in low-level convergence zones can be instilled by having the requisite connection weights modified via lateral influence from other low-level convergence zones and top-down influence from high-level convergence zones. If there were a technique whereby the nonfeedforward installation of a concept can be achieved, then physically omniscient Mary would *know* that technique. Of course, it is open whether she would thereby be able to employ the technique. The phenomenal concepts proposal constitutes a claim to the effect that such a thing would be impossible.

That such a thing would not be possible is a bold *empirical* conjecture about the way humans are wired, at least insofar as we are looking to the structure of concepts to supply a possible explanation of the alleged subjectivity of phenomenal character. But perhaps a different kind of case can be made, namely, if we look to the conditions that determine the representational contents of concepts, we will see what makes phenomenal concepts the only concepts capable of representing phenomenal character. In the next section, I examine some content-based considerations regarding whether phenomenal character is subjective.

5. The Content of Concepts Defense of Subjectivity

There are two ways to attempt to spell out how an account of representational content can secure the subjectivity of phenomenal character. The first involves the contents of perception. The second involves the contents of introspection.

In Mandik (2001), I attempted to give a neurophilosophical account of subjectivity whereby the reason certain phenomenal characters are one-way knowable is because they are representational contents of perception such that what is represented can only be represented by those perceptual states. Assuming that perceptual representations have their contents due to certain kinds of causal interactions that allow them to function as detectors of (typically) environmental properties, I suggested that there may be a certain environmental property such that there is only one "detection supporting causal interaction" the property can enter into, and furthermore, the unique detector is the perceptual representation itself.

I discussed how such a view of uniquely representable properties might be based in an understanding of egocentric representations. Egocentric representations include those mentioned previously in connection with the lowest levels of the visual processing hierarchy, such as LGN and V1 neural activations that represent stimuli in retinocentric spatial locations. I argued that the notion of egocentric representation generalizes to nonspatial examples and developed, in particular, an account of the egocentricity of temperature representations in thermoperception (Mandik, 2001, pp. 194–196).

As Akins (2001) has pointed out, the outputs of thermoreceptors do not simply reflect the triggering temperatures but also what part of the body the temperature is being applied to and what temperature was previously at that portion of the body. Whereas Akins argued that such states are not representations, I argued that they are representations, just not representations of subject-independent properties. As such, what is detected is not a given temperature, but instead "whether the given temperature is, for example, too hot, too cold, or just right. The property of being too hot cannot be defined independently of answering the question 'too hot for whom?'" (Mandik, 2001, p. 195).

What it means for all of these representations to be egocentric is that they don't simply represent things; they represent those things in relation to the representing subject. I argued that such representations have contents that are one-way representable. I attempted to illustrate this feature in terms of imagistic or pictorial representations, wherein part of what is represented is what something looks like from some literal point of view.

> Consider a pictorial representation, such as a photograph of a complex object like the Statue of Liberty. Given the point of view from which the photograph was taken, only a fraction of the surface of the statue is explicitly represented in the photograph. Certain regions seen from one angle would be obscured from another angle. Consider the set of regions that are captured by the photograph: the set of all and only the regions explicitly represented in the photograph....
>
> In specifying the set comprised of all and only the spatial regions captured in the image, one does not carve nature at the joints, but instead carves nature into a gerrymandered collection of items that would be of no interest apart from their involvement in a particular representation. That much of neural representation is concerned with such gerrymandered properties should not come as an enormous surprise. For instance, it makes sense that an animal's chemoreceptors would be less interested in carving nature into the periodic table of elements and more

interested in carving nature into the nutrients and the poisons—categories that make no sense apart from the needs of a particular type of organism. (Mandik, 2001, p. 197)

Another way I illustrated the idea of one-way representable properties was by reference to an example of Dennett's concerning the torn halves of a Jell-O box a pair of spies used as unique unforgeable identification. As I described the case, "the only *detection supporting* causal interactions that one piece of the Jell-O box enters into are causal interactions involving the other piece of the box" (Mandik, 2001, p. 198). As Dennett describes the case, "The only readily available way of saying what property M is [the property that makes one piece of the Jell-O box a match for the other] is just to point to our M detector and say that M is the shape property detected by this thing here" (Dennett, 1997, p. 637).

This completes the sketch of the content-based defense of the subjectivity of phenomenal character based on egocentric representations. However, I've grown to have misgivings about whether egocentric representations can serve as a basis for genuine subjectivity. To see this, let us focus on the Jell-O box example and what an introspective analog would be. If I had a torn Jell-O box half, one way I can identify it as such is to match it to its torn partner. But subsequent to that, I can stick it in my pocket and travel far away. Later in my journey, I reach into my pocket, fish around for it, and easily find it. I can do so even if it is not the only thing in my pocket. There may be a coin and a tube of lip balm in there as well. But I am able to identify the torn Jell-O box half without literally retracing my steps and tracking down its partner. It is strictly false, then, that the only way I can identify that torn Jell-O box is by the matching process. There are multiple ways I can represent that half. I can represent it as the thing that matches the thing in my pocket. One might think there is an essentially demonstrative element involved here, that the box half is essentially represented in virtue of there being some point at which I was able to point to it and say it is that thing detected by this thing. But this is not obviously correct. It seems open for someone who never was in a position to demonstratively refer to the Jell-O box half to refer to it by description, like "the largest thing that Mandik had in his pocket last Wednesday."

So even if there were environmental properties that only entered into detection-supporting causal interactions with certain sensory states, it seems dubious that those sensory states constitute the *only* representations of those properties. Suppose Jones has such sensory states, and Smith does not. Even if Jones's sensory states are the unique detectors of those environmental properties, Smith can still represent those properties. Smith can represent them under such a description as "the environmental properties uniquely detected by Jones's sensory states."

The availability of this kind of move does not seem to depend on any kind of story about representational content. E. Schier ("Representation and the Knowledge Intuition," unpublished paper) has criticized the Mandik (2001) account of subjectivity and offered as superior a substitute that differs primarily in relying on an isomorphism-based instead of causal-covariance-based theory of representational content. It's not clear, though, that replacing the account of representational content is going to protect the account from the charge that Smith can represent the content of Jones's sensory states as "the environmental properties uniquely detected by Jones's sensory states."

Is this kind of move cheating? If a picture is indeed worth a thousand words, then isn't it cheating to say that whatever a picture P represents, the same thing can be represented by the description "whatever P represents?" Even if the "whatever P represents" move is somehow disqualified, the following move remains open: Just add words to the description. Why couldn't a sufficiently long description represent all of the same things without itself being a picture? Analogously, why couldn't a conceptual representation of what it is like to have an experience represent all of the things the experience does without itself being the experience or the consequence of having had the experience? I want to continue to address such questions but by shifting focus slightly. I want to turn from the question of whether perception uniquely represents environmental properties to whether introspection uniquely represents certain mental properties.

To see the kind of pressure that can be applied against the proposal that introspection allows us to represent uniquely representable properties, it will be useful to first consider a neurophilosophical proposal from Churchland concerning what qualia are. Beginning with a focus on color qualia, Churchland identifies them with certain properties in a neural network modeled in accordance with Land's theory of color vision.

According to Land, human color vision is reflectance discrimination, which is accomplished via the reception of three kinds of electromagnetic wavelengths by three different kinds of cones in the retina. In terms of a neural network and state-space representations, Churchland identifies color qualia with points of a three-dimensional state-space wherein the dimensions are defined by the three kinds of cells and their preferred ranges of electromagnetic wavelengths. Churchland identifies color sensations with neural representations of colors, that is, with neural representations of spectral reflectance. Sensations are points in three-dimensional color space and perceived similarity between colors is mirrored by proximity in this neural activation space. Churchland generalizes the account to include qualia from other sensory modalities.

Emphasizing how the account allows for a representation of qualia aside from simply having them, Churchland writes:

> The "ineffable" pink of one's current visual sensation may be richly and precisely expressible as a 95 Hz/80 Hz/80 Hz "chord" in the relevant triune cortical system. The "unconveyable" taste sensation produced by the fabled Australian health tonic Vegemite might be quite poignantly conveyed as a 85/80/90/15 "chord" in one's four-channeled gustatory system (a dark corner of taste-space that is best avoided). And the "indescribable" olfactory sensation produced by a newly opened rose might be quite accurately described as a 95/35/10/80/60/55 "chord" in some six dimensional system within one's olfactory bulb.
>
> This more penetrating conceptual framework might even displace the commonsense framework as the vehicle of intersubjective description and spontaneous introspection. Just as a musician can learn to recognize the

constitution of heard musical chords, after internalizing the general theory
of their internal structure, so may we learn to recognize, introspectively, the
n-dimensional constitution of our subjective sensory qualia, after having
internalized the general theory of their internal structure. (1989, p. 106)

In later work, Churchland emphasizes how such an identity theory allows one
to predict falsifiable data about consciousness. The data in question are not just
third-person accessible data. He makes an excellent case for this in his recent (2005)
"Chimerical Colors: Some Novel Predictions from Cognitive Neuroscience," in
which very odd color experiences are predicted by a neural model of chromatic
information processing. In brief, the differential fatiguing and recovery of opponent processing cells gives rise to afterimages with subjective hues and saturations
that would never be seen on the reflective surfaces of objects. Such chimerical colors
include shades of yellow exactly as dark as pitch-black and "hyperbolic orange, an
orange that is more 'ostentatiously orange' than any (non-self-luminous) orange
you have ever seen, or ever will see, as the objective color of a physical object"
(Churchland, 2005, p. 328). Such odd experiences are predicted by the model that
identifies color experiences with states of neural activation in a chromatic processing network. Of course, it's always open to a dualist to make an ad hoc addition
of such experiences to their theory, but no dualistic theory ever predicted them.
Furthermore, the sorts of considerations typically relied on to support dualism—
appeals to intuitive plausibility and a priori possibility—would have, one would
have expected, ruled them out.

Prior to familiarity with the neural theory, who would have predicted experiences of a yellow as dark as black? One person who would not have thought there
was such an experience as pitch-dark yellow is Ludwig Wittgenstein, who once
asked, "Why is there no such thing as blackish yellow?" (1978, p. 106). I think it
is safe to say Wittgenstein would be surprised by Churchland's chimerical colors.
I know I was, and I literally grew up reading Churchland. However, to be certain
that we have an example of someone who is surprised—for I would like to conduct
a thought experiment about them—let us consider someone, call him Larry, who
has seen yellow and black and in general all the typical colors a normally sighted
adult has seen.

Suppose that Larry has never had a chimerically colored afterimage, such as
hyperbolic orange or pitch-dark yellow. Suppose that he is aware of none of the
neuroscience that predicts the existence of such experiences. Now, let us compare
Larry to Hyperbolic Mary. Like Jackson's Mary, Hyperbolic Mary knows all of the
physical facts about how human color vision works, including the predictions of
chimerically colored afterimages. Suppose also that, like Mary toward the end of
Jackson's story, Hyperbolic Mary has been let out of the black and white room and
has seen tomatoes, lemons, grass, cloudless skies, and the like. In short, she has had
the average run of basic color experiences. Let us stipulate that she has had all the
types of color experiences that Larry has had.

The crucial similarity between Mary and Larry is that not only have they seen
all of the same colors, neither has had chimerically colored afterimages. Neither has

experienced hyperbolic orange or pitch-dark yellow. The crucial difference between Larry and Hyperbolic Mary is that only Hyperbolic Mary is in possession of a theory that predicts the existence of hyperbolic orange and pitch-dark yellow. Here is the crucial question: Who will be more surprised on experiencing chimerical colors for the first time, Larry or Hyperbolic Mary?

I think it's obvious that Larry will be more surprised. I also think this has pretty significant implications for what we are to think the knowledge of what it is like consists in. One thing that knowing what it is like consists in is something that will determine whether one is surprised. Fans of Jackson's Mary must grant this, for they are fond of explicating her ignorance of what it is like in terms of her alleged surprise at seeing red for the first time. Well, Hyperbolic Mary is *less* surprised than Larry on seeing chimerical colors for the first time. This shows that she must have more phenomenal knowledge—more knowledge of what it is like to have certain experiences—than he did. Mary was able to represent, in introspection, more properties of her experiences than Larry. Her introspective capacity was augmented by her neuroscientific concepts.

Does this example suffice to show that *all* knowledge of what it is like can be had without the requisite experiences? No, it does not. But it does help show—especially in concert with the other considerations spelled out in this and the previous section concerning the structure and content of concepts—just how beholden to empirical considerations the subjectivity intuition is. For the subjectivity intuition to be true, quite a bit that is actually up in the air concerning the neural bases of concepts would have to be true. No one should believe the subjectivity "intuition" until further arguments are given. We should be skeptical of claims that the subjectivity of phenomenal character is known by *intuition*. If it is to be known at all, it is to be known via neurophilosophy, and the neurophilosophical considerations weigh more heavily against subjectivity than in favor of it. In other words, the resultant neurophilosophical case more strongly supports subjectivity eliminativism than subjectivity reductionism.

Another issue that the tale of Hyperbolic Mary and Larry helps bring out is my concluding point: If it is unreasonable to expect Larry to predict the possibility of hyperbolic orange, pitch-dark yellow, and the like, then it seems unreasonable to predict, on introspection and intuition alone, the *impossibility* of preexperiential knowledge of what it is like to see red. It is unreasonable, then, to think introspection and intuition suffice for establishing the subjectivity of consciousness.

Acknowledgments

For detailed comments on earlier drafts, I am grateful to Torin Alter and John Bickle. I am grateful for feedback from audience members of a presentation of this material in the CUNY Graduate Center Cognitive Science Symposium, especially

David Rosenthal, Jared Blank, Michael Klincewicz, Peter Langland-Hassan, David Pereplyotchik, Dan Shargel, Josh Weisberg, and Ben Young. I am also grateful for discussion of this and related material with readers of my *Brain Hammer* blog, especially David Chalmers, Tanasije Gjorgoski, Eric Schwitzgebel, Nick Treanor, Chase Wrenn, and Tad Zawidzki.

REFERENCES

Akins, K. (2001). Of sensory systems and the "aboutness" of mental states. In W. Bechtel, P. Mandik, J. Mundale, and R. Stufflebeam (Eds.), *Philosophy and the Neurosciences: A Reader*. Oxford: Blackwell.

Beaton, M. J. S. (2005). What RoboDennett still doesn't know. *Journal of Consciousness Studies* 12: 3–25.

Bickle, J., Mandik, P., and Landreth, A. (2006). The philosophy of neuroscience. In E. Zalta (Ed.), *Stanford Encyclopedia of Philosophy* (Spring 2006 edition). Available at: plato. stanford.edu/archives/spr2006/entries/neuroscience.

Churchland, P. M. (1979). *Scientific Realism and the Plasticity of Mind*. Cambridge: Cambridge University Press.

Churchland, P. M. (1989). *A Neurocomputational Perspective*. Cambridge, Mass.: MIT Press.

Churchland, P. M. (2005). Chimerical colors: Some novel predictions from cognitive neuroscience. In A. Brook and K. Akins (Eds.), *Cognition and the Brain: The Philosophy and Neuroscience Movement*. Cambridge: Cambridge University Press.

Cohen, N., and Eichenbaum, H. (1993). *Memory, Amnesia, and the Hippocampal System*. Cambridge, Mass.: MIT Press.

Damasio, A., and Damasio, H. (1994). Cortical systems for retrieval of concrete knowledge: The convergence zone framework. In C. Koch (Ed.), *Large-Scale Neuronal Theories of the Brain*: Cambridge, Mass.: MIT Press.

Dennett, D. (1997). Quining qualia. In N. Block, O. Flanagan, and G. Güzeldere (Eds.), *The Nature of Consciousness*. Cambridge, Mass.: MIT Press.

Dennett, D. (2005). *Sweet Dreams: Philosophical Obstacles to a Science of Consciousness*. Cambridge, Mass.: MIT Press.

Dretske, F. (1995). *Naturalizing the Mind*. Cambridge, Mass.: MIT Press.

Eichenbaum, H., Matthews, P., and Cohen, N. (1989). Further studies of hippocampal representation during odor discrimination learning. *Behavioral Neuroscience* 103: 1207–1216.

Hume, D. (1739). *A Treatise of Human Nature*. Reprint, P. H. Nidditch (Ed.). Oxford: Oxford University Press, 1978.

Jackson, F. (1982). Epiphenomenal qualia. *Philosophical Quarterly* 32: 127–136.

Lamme, V., Super, H., and H. Spekreijse, H. (1998). Feedforward, horizontal, and feedback processing in the visual cortex. *Current Opinion in Neurobiology* 8: 529–535.

Lewis, D. (1983). Postscript to "Mad pain and Martian pain." In D. Lewis (Ed.), *Philosophical Papers*, vol. 1. New York: Oxford University Press, 13–32.

Lewis, D. (1990). What experience teaches. In W. Lycan (Ed.), *Mind and Cognition*. Cambridge: Basil Blackwell, 499–518.

Mandik, P. (2001). Mental representation and the subjectivity of consciousness. *Philosophical Psychology* 14: 179–202.

Mandik, P. (2005). Phenomenal consciousness and the allocentric-egocentric interface. In R. Buccheri, A. C. Elitzer, and M. Saniga (Eds.), *Endophysics, Time, Quantum and the Subjective*. Singapore: World Scientific.

Mandik, P. (2006a). The introspectability of brain states as such. In B. Keeley (Ed.), *Paul M. Churchland: Contemporary Philosophy in Focus*. Cambridge: Cambridge University Press.

Mandik, P. (2006b). The neurophilosophy of consciousness. In M. Velmans and S. Schneider (Eds.), *The Blackwell Companion to Consciousness*. Oxford: Basil Blackwell.

Mandik, P. (2008). An epistemological theory of consciousness? In A. Plebe (Ed.), Philosophy in the Neuroscience Era, special issue of *Journal of the Department of Cognitive Science*.

Nagel, T. (1974). What is it like to be a bat? *Philosophical Review* 83: 435–450.

Nemirow, L. (1980). Review of *Mortal Questions. Philosophical Review* 89: 473–477.

Nemirow, L. (1990). Physicalism and the cognitive role of acquaintance. In W. Lycan (Ed.), *Mind and Cognition*. Oxford: Blackwell, 490–499.

Papineau, D. (1999). Mind the gap. In J. Tomberlin (Ed.), *Philosophical Perspectives*, Vol. 12, *Language, Mind and Ontology*. Oxford: Blackwell, 373–388.

Pascual-Leone, A., and Walsh, V. (2001). Fast backprojections from the motion to the primary visual area necessary for visual awareness. *Science* 292: 510–512.

Tye, M. (1995). *Ten Problems of Consciousness: A Representational Theory of the Phenomenal Mind*. Cambridge, Mass.: MIT Press.

Tye, M. (2000). *Consciousness, Color, and Content*. Cambridge, Mass.: MIT Press.

von der Heydt, R., Peterhans, E., and Baumgartner, G. (1984). Illusory contours and cortical neuron responses. *Science* 224: 1260–1262.

Wittgenstein, L. (1978). *Some Remarks on Color*. G. E. M. Anscombe (Ed.). Oxford: Blackwell.

Zeki, S. (1983). Colour coding in the cerebral cortex: The reaction of cells in monkey visual cortex to wavelengths and colour. *Neuroscience* 9: 741–756.

INDEX

CPSIA information can be obtained
at www.ICGtesting.com
Printed in the USA
BVOW07s0845230417

481712BV00010B/13/P